D1522898

EQUINE ——— LAMENESS

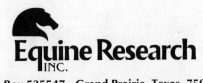

P.O. Box 535547   Grand Prairie, Texas 75053
(U.S. & Canada) 1 (800) 848-0225
(Other Countries) 1 (972) 660-3897

Written by

Christine King, BVSc, MACVSc, MVetClinStud,
research staff of Equine Research, Inc.

and

Richard Mansmann, VMD, PhD

Editor/Publisher

Don Wagoner

Disclaimer

Every effort has been made in the writing of this book to present quality information based on the best available and most reliable sources. Neither the publisher nor the authors assume any responsibility for, nor make any warranty with respect to, results that may be obtained from the procedures described herein. Neither the publisher nor the authors shall be liable to anyone for damages resulting from reliance on any information contained in this book whether with respect to examination procedures, feeding, care, treatments, drug usages, or by reason of any misstatement or inadvertent error contained herein.

Also, it must be remembered that neither the publisher nor the authors manufacture any of the drugs, feeds, veterinary equipment, or other products discussed in this book. Accordingly, neither the publisher nor the authors offer any guarantees of any kind on such items—nor will they be held responsible for the results that may be obtained from the use of any of those items.

The reader is encouraged to read and follow the directions published by the manufacturer of each drug, feed, or product which may be mentioned herein. And, if there is a conflict with any information in this book, the instructions of the manufacturer—or of the reader's veterinarian—should, of course, be followed.

To ensure the reader's understanding of some technical descriptions offered in this book, brand names have been used as examples of particular substances or equipment. However, the use of a particular trademark or brand name is not intended to imply an endorsement of that particular product, nor to suggest that similar products offered by other companies under different names may be inferior. Also, nothing contained in this book is to be construed as a suggestion to violate any trademark laws.

Introduction

Lameness is one of the most common problems in horses, and a primary reason why horses fail to perform to their owners' or trainers' expectations. More training time is lost, more competitions are missed, and more careers are prematurely ended because of lameness than for any other condition.

This book analyzes the causes, diagnosis, and management of the many and varied problems that can cause lameness in horses. By understanding how a condition develops, the owner or trainer is better equipped to prevent it, or at least recognize it early enough for treatment to be successful.

No book can take the place of an experienced veterinarian. But it is hoped that this book will bridge the communication gap that sometimes exists between horse owners or trainers and their veterinarians.

Contents

SECTION I
INVESTIGATING LAMENESS

CHAPTER 3

SECTION II
PRINCIPLES OF THERAPY

CHAPTER 4

CHAPTER 5

CHAPTER 6

SECTION III
DISEASE PROCESSES
&
THEIR MANAGEMENT

CHAPTER 7
HOOF CONFORMATION & SHOEING OPTIONS 187

CHAPTER 8
JOINT PROBLEMS 245

CHAPTER 9

CHAPTER 10

CHAPTER 11

CHAPTER 12

CHAPTER 13

CHAPTER 14

Section IV
Treatment of Specific Conditions

CHAPTER 15
THE FOOT

CHAPTER 16
THE PASTERN & FETLOCK 693

CHAPTER 17

CHAPTER 18

CHAPTER 19
THE UPPER FORELEG 799

CHAPTER 20
THE HOCK 833

CHAPTER 21

CHAPTER 22

APPENDIX

INVESTIGATING LAMENESS

This section introduces and defines many of the concepts and terms that are used throughout the book. It also describes and discusses the tools and techniques veterinarians use to diagnose and treat lameness.

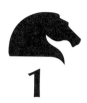

1

DEFINING LAMENESS

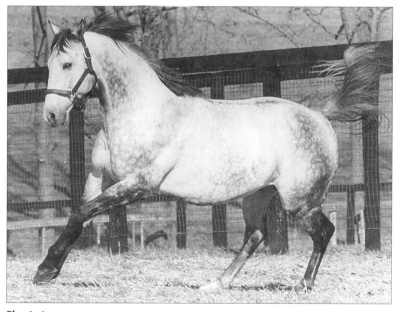

Fig. 1–1.

Lameness can be defined as a gait abnormality that is caused by pain and/or restriction of movement. For example, restriction of movement may occur when fibrous, or scar tissue limits normal joint motion. But with most conditions, pain is the primary cause of lameness. In conditions that involve both pain and restriction of movement, it can be difficult to know how much each factor contributes to the lameness. However, the distinction is important because in many cases pain can be relieved, while mechanical restriction often is due to permanent changes.

ELEMENTS OF LAMENESS
Pain

Pain occurs when sensory nerve endings in the tissues are stimulated. Sensory nerves transmit messages, such as temperature, pressure, and pain, from the tissues to the brain. These nerves can be stimulated by direct trauma, such as a blow, a cut, or a fracture. They can also be stimulated when the tissues they supply (such as skin, tendons, and muscles) are overstretched. When tissues are damaged by direct trauma or overstretching, inflammation develops and can become a persistent source of pain *(see Chapter 5)*. Infection also causes inflammation and pain.

Pain from inflammation may not be noticed by the horse, or show up as lameness until it exceeds the horse's tolerance level, or pain threshold. This threshold is unique to each horse: some horses are very stoic and tolerate a higher level of pain than others. Knowing the horse's attitude toward pain is important in interpreting subtle signs of pain. An owner or trainer who is familiar with the horse's pain threshold is less likely to disregard low-grade pain in a stoic horse, or overreact to minor lameness in a sensitive horse.

Pain tolerance is also an important factor in managing lameness. Progressive, degenerative conditions, such as navicular syndrome,

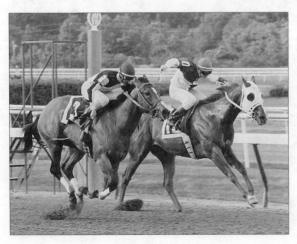

Fig. 1–2. Pain from inflammation may not show up as lameness until it exceeds the horse's tolerance level.

often do not cause consistent lameness until they reach a certain stage and the pain exceeds the horse's tolerance level. Although the degenerative changes cannot be reversed, the lameness often improves or disappears when the pain is reduced with rest, anti-inflammatory therapy, and shoeing and training adjustments.

Mild to moderate inflammation may only cause pain when the horse is moving, or when pressure is applied to the inflamed tissues during examination. However, the horse is aware of a very painful condition, such as a joint infection or a fracture, both during movement and at rest. Some horses with chronic, low-grade lameness "warm out" of the lameness during exercise, probably because activity increases blood flow to the tissues. This warms the tissues and increases their elasticity *(see Chapter 4)*. Warmth also desensitizes (numbs) the nerve endings, which allows normal movement and reduces the pain.

Mechanical Restriction of Movement

Mechanical restriction of movement means that the normal function of a body part (joint, muscle, etc.) is physically prevented by changes in the tissue's structure. Fibrosis, which is thickening or fusing with fibrous (scar) tissue, is the most common cause of mechanical restriction in horses. The body repairs most damaged tissues with fibrous tissue, which is not as elastic as the original tissue. As a result, normal movement of the repaired tissue may be restricted.

When fibrosis involves a joint capsule, tendon, or muscle, it can cause a permanent, non-painful change in the horse's stride.

In some cases it is failure, rather than restriction, that affects normal movement. For example, complete rupture of a muscle, tendon, or ligament can result in profound changes in the stride. Nerve

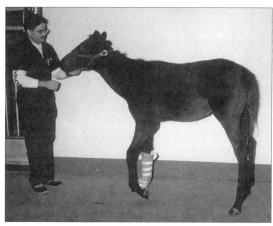

Fig. 1–3. If a motor nerve is damaged, the muscles it supplies cannot contract. (In this case, the radial nerve is damaged.)

damage can also cause an obvious change in the horse's movement. Normally, a muscle contracts when it is stimulated by its motor nerve—the nerve that transmits impulses from the brain and spinal cord to the tissues. If the motor nerve is damaged or cut, the muscle cannot contract (unless it is artificially stimulated). The result is a non-painful gait defect.

Gait Abnormalities Often Confused With Lameness

Not all gait abnormalities constitute lameness. Some are caused by poor conformation, and simply represent the way that particular horse is "genetically programmed" to move. Examples include:

- paddling—swinging the foot out as it is brought forward
- winging—swinging the foot in as it is brought forward
- plaiting—crossing one leg in front of the other as the horse walks or trots (common in pigeon-toed horses)

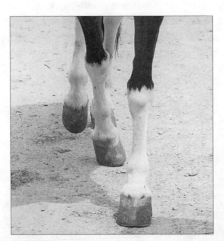

Fig. 1–4. Plaiting is common in pigeon-toed horses.

Incorrect use of some pieces of equipment, such as overchecks, side reins, and martingales, and improper shoeing can cause "mechanical" gait abnormalities. Improper shoeing can also exaggerate the abnormal gaits listed above. In some cases attempts to correct the gait may actually cause lameness in these horses.

People who are unfamiliar with Standardbreds may think that their typical gaits are abnormal. These horses often have a side-to-side "rolling" action when they are pacing. They also have an awkward-looking, shuffling, four-beat gait when trotting or pacing slowly (more of an amble than a trot). However, these are normal variations, and are neither gait abnormalities nor lameness.

Peruvian Paso and Paso Fino horses also have a four-beat gait called the Paso, which is a type of running-walk. These horses have a

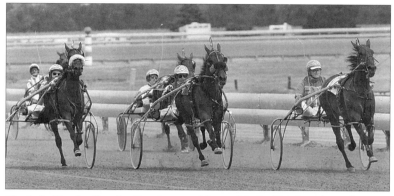

Fig. 1–5. Standardbreds often have a side-to-side "rolling" action when they are pacing.

moderately high-stepping action, in which the lower leg swings out from the knee. This gait is normal for these breeds. Some Arabian horses and Warmbloods have a wide-based hindlimb action at the trot that may also be considered normal for those particular horses.

Bridle Lameness

Bridle lameness is a fairly common false lameness. The gait abnormality is only seen when the horse is ridden; it disappears when the horse is exercised without the rider, or with a different rider. Bridle lameness can be diagnosed by first watching the horse being ridden, and then watching the horse move normally without the rider.

There are several possible causes of bridle lameness. The bridle or saddle may be causing the horse discomfort. However, in most cases the rider is the cause of the lameness. If the rider is tense, the horse may become tense, and its stride becomes short and choppy. If the rider is too far forward, too far back, or off to one side, the horse's balance may be affected, which

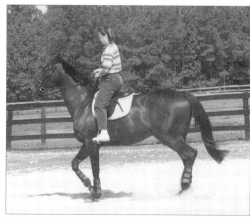

Fig. 1–6. If the rider is tense, the horse becomes tense, and its stride becomes short and choppy.

can alter its stride. These positions can also result in back pain, which may affect the horse's gait *(see Chapter 22)*.

Many riders are stronger or more tense on one side of their body. This can cause a bridle lameness that is worse on one side or in one direction. If the rider sends the horse vague or conflicting signals, this can also cause an intermittent "lameness." The horse may take only a few "lame" strides, and then move normally for several strides. Usually the lameness coincides with something the rider is doing at the time. Many horses with bridle lameness refuse to perform a balanced, rhythmic trot. Instead, they have an uneven, irregular trot, or they try to break into a canter.

With several conditions that genuinely cause lameness, the horse may "warm out" of the lameness. This may appear to happen with bridle lameness, so it is easy to mistakenly conclude that the horse is lame. But actually, the "lameness" disappears as the horse and rider adjust to each other.

Bridle lameness can become a habit for some horses, and it may take some time to retrain the horse to move normally when ridden. The trainer must identify and correct the source of the problem. He or she may need to alter the fit and position of the saddle and bridle, and use a bit that the horse tolerates well. The rider must also examine his or her role in the situation.

IDENTIFYING THE LAME LEG

Most experienced owners and trainers can tell when a horse is lame and which leg is involved, even if the lameness is mild. But in some cases all that the rider or driver can say is that the horse is a little "off," or it is not performing normally. It may have lost a little speed, is refusing jumps or knocking down rails, or is reluctant to perform a particular maneuver. There may be other reasons for these behavioral problems, including temperament, training, and illness. But it is always wise to investigate the possibility that the horse has a musculoskeletal problem—the most common reason for reduced athletic performance in horses.

While generalizations can occasionally be misleading, there are some reliable ways to determine which is the "lame," or affected leg.

Abnormal Stance

In some cases, the way the horse chooses to stand is a sign that there is a problem in a particular limb. The abnormal stance may be

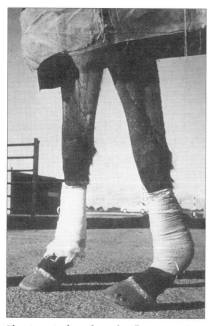
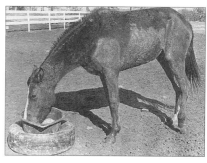
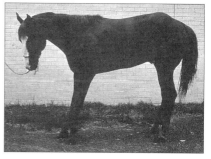

Fig. 1–7. Left: When the flexor tendons are severed, the fetlock drops and the toe tips up. Top Right: This horse is pointing its left hind toe because of a hoof wall abscess. Bottom Right: The typical laminitis stance.

as subtle as the horse resting one hindleg more than the other, or standing with one forefoot slightly forward of the other. More obvious examples include:

- dropping of the fetlock and tipping up of the toe in a horse with severed flexor tendons
- pointing of the toe in a horse with a hoof wall abscess
- the typical laminitis stance

Using Sound

As it is moving, the horse shifts some of its weight off the painful leg. This makes the footfall of the lame leg sound a little quieter, and of a higher pitch than usual. The footfall of the opposite, normal leg is louder and duller than usual because that foot is planted down more heavily. Also, the rhythm of the gait is often changed. These differences are most noticeable in shod horses that are walked or trotted on a firm surface, such as asphalt.

Using sound is not a major part of the lameness evaluation. But the

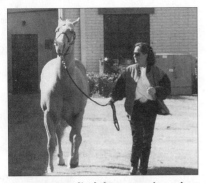

Fig. 1–8. Forelimb lameness is easiest to see from in front of the horse.

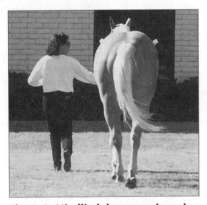

Fig. 1–9. Hindlimb lameness is easiest to see from behind the horse.

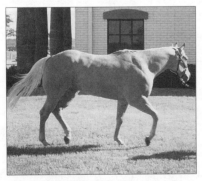

Fig. 1–10. It is important to watch the horse from every angle.

experienced horse owner, trainer, or veterinarian uses sound almost instinctively, without being fully aware of its contribution to the overall picture of lameness.

Observations of Motion

Forelimb lameness is easiest to see by watching the horse from the side or front. Hindlimb lameness is easiest to see from behind the horse. However, in every case, no matter how obvious the lameness, it is important to watch the horse from every angle (front, back, and side). This gives a complete picture, which is particularly important when examining a horse with an obscure lameness that may involve more than one leg.

Mild or moderate lameness is generally not obvious at the walk, so most gait evaluations are performed at the trot. Most lameness problems are made more obvious by increasing the speed from the walk to the trot. But, it is difficult to evaluate lameness at the canter or gallop. Because it is a simple, symmetrical gait, the trot is also better for identifying subtle differences between the left and right legs. *(Veterinarians use a grading system to describe the degree of lameness; see Chapter 2.)*

Head Nod

In many cases of forelimb lameness, the horse's head rises when weight is placed on the lame leg, and drops when the horse's weight shifts to the normal leg *(see Figure 1–12)*. This gives the impression that the horse is "nodding" as it walks or trots. When the horse steps onto the painful leg the head is raised and the body tenses in an effort to keep some of the weight off that leg. As a result, more of the horse's weight is transferred to the normal leg as it is set down. The head nod is easiest to detect when standing in front of the horse, and is usually obvious at the trot. Horses with severe lameness may also have a head nod at the walk. If the horse is lame in both forelegs, the head nod is much less obvious, and may even be absent because the horse's weight is evenly distributed.

In some cases the head nod is due to lameness in the hindleg on the same side as the supposed lame foreleg. For example, the head nod may indicate that the problem is in the right foreleg when it is actually in the right hindleg. This is because the horse takes some of the weight off the painful right hindleg. It throws some of its weight forward by lowering its head and transferring its weight onto the left foreleg—the diagonal weight-bearing partner at the trot. It then appears that the horse's head is lowered as weight is placed on the left foreleg, and raised when weight is placed on the right foreleg. This falsely incriminates the right foreleg as the site of lameness. *(As confusing as this may seem, it usually only occurs in horses with a moderate to severe hindlimb lameness, which is obvious from the side or rear of the horse.)*

Hip Hike

The hip hike or hip lift is the hind end equivalent of the head nod. It is seen in cases of moderate to severe hindlimb lameness. When viewed from behind the horse, the points of both hips normally move up and down slightly as the horse trots. This movement is often

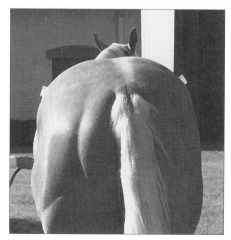

Fig. 1–11. A hip hike is often easier to see if a marker is attached to the point of each hip.

11

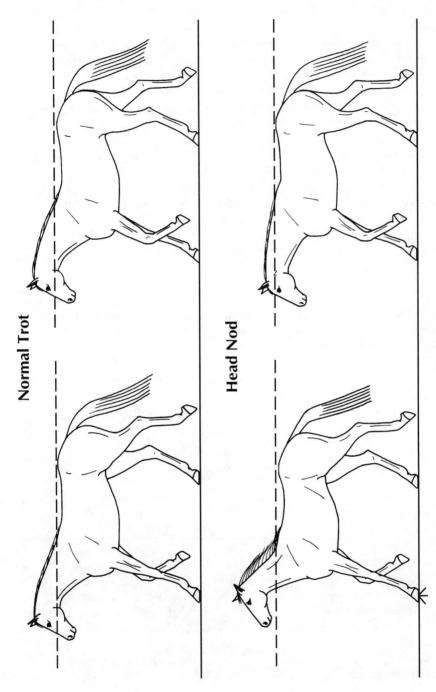

Normal Trot

Head Nod

Fig. 1–12. Top: A normal trot. Bottom: A head nod due to pain in the left forefoot.

easier to see if a marker, such as a piece of light-colored tape, is attached to the point of each hip so that it can be seen from the rear of the horse. If the horse has a hindlimb lameness, the tape on the affected side rises higher than the tape on the normal side. As weight is placed on the lame leg the horse tenses and attempts to lessen the load on that leg. This raises the point of the hip higher than normal during that phase of the stride.

Reduced Arc of Foot Flight

The foot normally makes an arc as it is raised from the ground and brought forward to take another step. The height of the arc may be reduced if the horse is reluctant to flex a joint (or joints) in the affected leg. As a result, the horse does not lift the foot as high as normal. In some cases it drags the toe along the ground. A lowered arc is easiest to see when watching the horse from the side as it walks or trots in a straight line. It is sometimes visible as drag marks on the ground. A scraping or dragging sound may also be heard as the horse is trotted on a solid surface. Wearing or "dubbing" of the toe often occurs in these horses.

When the horse is reluctant to flex a joint in a hindleg, it appears stiff-legged in that limb, and has a reduced arc of foot flight. The hock does not flex as much, and the fetlock does not sink to the same level as in the normal leg. This can be seen from the side and the rear of the horse. It is not as consistent or as obvious in the forelegs.

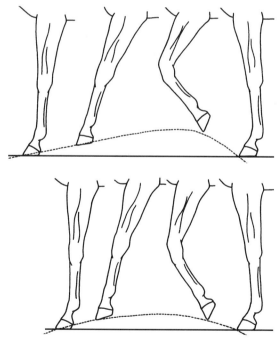

Fig. 1–13. Top: Normal arc of foot flight. Bottom: Reduced arc of foot flight. Note also the slightly reduced stride length.

Reduced Stride Length

The length of the stride may also be reduced. It may be a subtle change, such as the horse not tracking up to cover its forefoot print with its hindfoot. (Although, lazy horses that are not lame also may not track up.) Or, it may be as dramatic as the short stride and abrupt placement of the hindfoot in a horse with fibrotic myopathy *(see Chapter 10)*. A reduced stride length is easiest to see by watching the horse from the side as it is trotted in a straight line. Working the horse on a soft surface, such as sand or dirt, makes it easy to see the forefoot print and the placement of the hindfoot.

Abnormal Foot Placement

A normal horse that is walking or trotting on a level surface places its foot flat as it lands. A variety of conformational problems can cause the horse to land unevenly, although this does not necessarily constitute lameness. But in a horse that normally moves and lands evenly, abnormal foot placement can be an indication of pain. It also provides some clues as to the location of the problem. For example, a horse with a painful condition in the back part of the foot, such as "sheared heels" or navicular syndrome, attempts to spare the heels from concussion by landing toe-first. A horse with a deep hoof wall crack or "gravel" on one side of the foot often places the foot slightly askew, so that little or no weight is placed on the painful side. A more obvious example of abnormal foot placement is seen in horses with laminitis. Pain in the front part of the foot causes these horses to shuffle along, landing heel-first. *(Foot conditions are discussed in Chapter 15.)*

Supporting or Swinging Limb Lameness

Some veterinarians define a lameness as either a *supporting* limb or *swinging* limb lameness, in an effort to better identify its cause. The reasoning is that pain involving the foot, a bone, or a joint surface is worse when weight is placed on the leg. This is when the lame leg is the supporting leg. Pain involving soft tissues, such as tendons and joint capsules, is worse when they are asked to function. This is when the lame leg is "swung" forward. Pain or mechanical restriction involving these soft tissues results in a shorter stride length.

The distinction between these two types of lameness is easiest to make by working the horse in a circle, either led, longed, or free-schooled in a round pen. A supporting limb lameness is worse when the affected leg is to the inside, and so is bearing proportionally more weight. For example, a supporting limb lameness in the left leg is worse when the horse is circled to the left. In contrast, a swinging limb lameness is worse when the affected leg is to the outside. For example, a swinging limb lameness in the right leg is worse when the horse is circled to the left. This is because the horse must swing the outside leg further forward when working in a circle. As a result, the shortened stride length is more obvious when the affected leg is to the outside.

(This observation is not always reliable. It is often impossible to define a lameness as one or the other. Each leg performs both roles during each stride, and some lameness problems involve more than one structure.)

SPECIFIC GAIT ABNORMALITIES

Certain conditions cause a distinctive gait abnormality. In some cases it is so characteristic that a diagnosis can be made just on the abnormality alone. Examples include:

- stringhalt—hock flexion is exaggerated
- fibrotic myopathy—the horse is unable to swing the affected hindleg as far forward as normal, and so plants the foot down early, in an abrupt manner
- upward fixation of the patella—either the stifle is "locked" with the leg extended behind the horse, or the hindlegs "buckle" as the horse walks down a slope
- sweeney—the shoulder joint can "pop" or partially dislocate to the side when weight is placed on the leg
- spinal cord diseases—interruption of nerve impulses can cause ataxia (incoordination), stiff-legged or high-stepping action, and weakness

Shoulder Lameness

"Shoulder lameness" is a common complaint, although the shoulder is an uncommon site of lameness. When most people refer to shoulder lameness, they are describing a gait abnormality that involves a reduced arc of foot flight and stride length. It appears as if the horse is guarding, or protecting the shoulder joint by not allowing the normal range of movement. In reality, this gait abnormality is usually caused by pain in the back half of the foot. The horse is reluctant to put weight on its heel, so it "minces along," taking short steps and landing toe-first. This is often mistaken for shoulder lameness.

Joint pain does not cause a characteristic gait abnormality. Using terms such as "shoulder lameness" or "stifle lameness" can be misleading and can interfere with thorough investigation of the problem.

NON-MUSCULOSKELETAL CAUSES OF LAMENESS

There are a few conditions that do not directly involve the structures of the legs or back, but which can cause lameness.

<table>
<tr><td>**More Information**</td></tr>
<tr><td>The skin is not considered to be part of the musculoskeletal system. But because several skin conditions can cause lameness, they are discussed in Chapter 13.</td></tr>
</table>

Pleuritis

Pleuritis is inflammation of the pleura, which is the membrane that lines the chest cavity and covers the lungs. In most cases pleuritis is caused by bacterial infection. When the lungs are also infected, the condition is called pleuropneumonia. Most cases of pleuritis in horses occur after long-distance transport; hence the common name, "shipping fever."

Pleuritis is a painful condition; horses with pleuritis frequently appear lame because moving the forelegs worsens the chest pain. Often these horses stand with their elbows held out slightly, and are very reluctant to move. Other signs of pleuritis include:

- depression
- fever (above 102°F)
- poor appetite
- a rapid, shallow breathing pattern

Laminitis may occur as a result of the infection, and can be another cause of lameness in these horses *(see Chapter 15).*

Fractured Ribs

Direct trauma to the side of the chest can fracture the horse's ribs, although this is not a common injury. Because the muscles that anchor the shoulder blade to the body attach onto the ribcage, the horse may be mildly or moderately lame when any of the first six to eight ribs are fractured. In some cases the diagnosis can be made by palpation. Although, radiographs may be necessary to confirm the diagnosis and identify fluid (especially blood) within the chest cavity. Unless the horse's condition is worsened by hemorrhage or infection in the chest cavity, rib fractures usually heal uneventfully with 2 – 3 months of rest.

Painful Ovaries

Fillies and mares occasionally develop a vague hindlimb lameness that appears to be the result of pain associated with their ovaries. This lameness can occur at any stage of the estrous ("heat") cycle, not just when the mare has a large follicle on one of her ovaries. Presumably, movement of the hindleg puts pressure on the wall of the abdomen and the abdominal contents, including the tender ovary. In most cases, the mare is only lame for a couple of days, and the lameness disappears without treatment. But it may return when the mare is at the same stage of her next estrous cycle.

This condition should be suspected when any filly or mare repeatedly shows mild to moderate lameness in one hindlimb, with no obvious problems in the leg itself. A behavior change, such as aggression or irritability, is another sign that the mare's ovaries should be examined. When the veterinarian performs a rectal examination, palpation of the ovary on the "lame" side causes the mare discomfort.

Although the lameness usually disappears on its own, it also responds to nonsteroidal anti-inflammatory drugs (NSAIDs; *see Chapter 3*). Oral hormone therapy (such as Regu-mate®) or progesterone implants placed beneath the skin on the side of the neck can prevent this problem.

Mastitis

Mastitis is inflammation of the mammary glands, or udder. In most cases it is caused by bacterial infection. Mastitis is fairly uncommon in horses, and it usually only occurs in lactating (nursing) mares. The signs include a swollen udder and a hungry foal—the udder is so painful that the mare cannot tolerate the foal nursing. When the udder is palpated, it is very firm, hot, and painful. This is what causes the lameness: movement causes the hindlegs to bump against the painful udder. Mares with mastitis often take short steps and swing their hindlegs out when they walk.

Treatment involves antibiotic therapy and stripping the infected milk from the udder. The foal must have an alternative source of nourishment, such as commercial milk replacer. The prognosis for

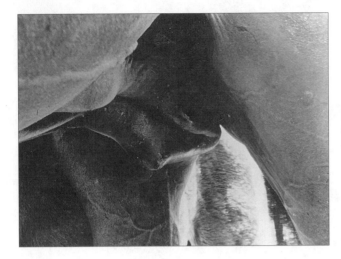

Fig. 1–14. One sign of mastitis is a swollen udder.

complete recovery is very good with appropriate therapy. The lameness disappears once the infection is under control.

Scrotal Problems

Racehorse trainers have long believed that compression or rotation of the testicles by the hindlegs can cause vague hindlimb lameness and reduced performance in colts and stallions. Castration often improves the horse's gait and its willingness to work, which reinforces this belief.

Research into this problem is limited, although some veterinarians have found that lameness caused by scrotal problems is more likely in horses with retained testicles. Instead of dropping all the way into the scrotum, one testicle is caught, usually in the inguinal ring of the body wall (in the groin). Horses with this problem are called cryptorchids or "rigs." Surgery to release the retained testicle often improves the horse's gait. But in some cases castration is necessary.

Whether lameness is ever caused by rotation of the testicles remains to be seen. When the testicle is rotated, the spermatic cord that suspends it could be twisted, causing pain. However, injecting local anesthetic around the spermatic cord in these colts usually does little to improve the gait abnormality. (The nerve supply to the testicles is located in the spermatic cord.) This means that the testicles probably are not a source of pain in these horses. Nevertheless, some trainers have found that using a jock strap on these colts can help.

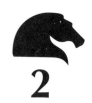

2

LAMENESS EVALUATION

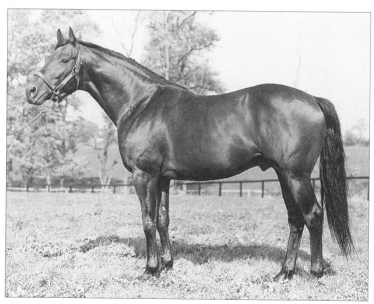

Fig. 2–1.

This chapter describes the methods veterinarians use during a lameness evaluation, or "work-up." It also discusses the uses and limitations of the various diagnostic tools that may be used in making a specific diagnosis.

HISTORY

The more information that is known about the horse and its management, the easier it is to arrive at an accurate diagnosis. Many times the events or management factors of the past few days, weeks, or months can provide clues as to what is causing the lameness. This information is called the history. It is combined with the horse's statistics, such as breed, age, and gender, to narrow down the list of possible problems. Some physical conditions predominate in certain breeds or age groups, or in horses used for a particular purpose. Certain problems are aggravated by exercise, while others may be seen only during a specific maneuver.

Information about shoeing is also important because many conditions are worsened by improper or overdue shoeing, or by sudden changes in the hoof balance *(see Chapter 7)*. Trimming and shoeing can help prevent or manage many conditions, but they can also cause lameness if used improperly.

Sometimes an owner or trainer has already formed an opinion of what the problem is before calling the veterinarian. However, it is important that the history is as complete as possible, no matter how minor or irrelevant a certain piece of information seems. It is very easy to overlook important facts by beginning with a preconceived idea of what the problem is, and concentrating on the obvious. Omissions can mislead the veterinarian and waste time in diagnosing the condition correctly and treating it appropriately.

Record-Keeping

Developing a complete history is made easier, and more accurate if the owner, trainer, or barn manager keeps good records. Also, keeping a record of health problems and other incidents may highlight subtle connections that could otherwise have gone unnoticed. For example, a vague, intermittent hindlimb lameness is sometimes seen in fillies and mares. By recording and reviewing these episodes it may become obvious that the lameness coincides with a certain stage of the estrous cycle *(see Chapter 1)*.

It does not take much time to write down events like visits from the veterinarian or farrier, minor illnesses and injuries, competitions, etc. It is also good to write down any management changes (diet, housing, and training) and treatments in a diary or on a calendar. Recording the date, type, and amount of all medications given also makes it easier to comply with specific competition rules regarding drugs.

Taking a History

The veterinarian might ask the following questions before conducting a physical examination:

- What is the horse's age and breed?

- What is the horse used for?

- Where is the horse housed? (Is it kept in a barn, paddock, pasture, or a combination of these? Is it kept alone, or with company?)

- How long has the horse been lame?

- Was the onset of lameness sudden or gradual?

- Has the horse been lame before? If so, give details.

- Were there any incidents (such as a traumatic injury) that may have caused, or contributed to the lameness? (Note: The injury may not have involved the "lame" leg; all incidents, no matter how minor, should be reported.)

- Has the lameness coincided with a major change in the horse's training schedule, such as an increase in the workload, or a change in activity?

- Since its onset, has the lameness worsened, improved, or remained the same; is it constant or intermittent?

- Is there a pattern to the lameness? (For example, is it worst first thing in the morning, the day after competition, on a particular surface, or during a specific maneuver?)

- Does the lameness worsen or improve with exercise? (That is, does the horse "warm out" of the lameness, or does the lameness get worse during exercise?)

- Since the lameness was first noticed, has the horse been rested? If so, for how long, and with what result?

- Has any treatment been given? If so, what was given, and what was the result?

- Is the horse currently on any medications? If so, what drugs and dose rates?

- Has the horse received any injections (including vaccinations) in the past week? If so, in what part of the body?

- When was the horse last shod? Did the regular farrier trim/shoe the horse? Were there any changes in the trimming or shoeing? What type of shoe does the horse normally wear?

Fig. 2–2.

PHYSICAL EXAMINATION

The aim of the physical examination is to localize the lameness to a specific area, if possible. In cases where the problem is obvious, it is

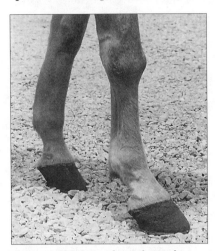

Fig. 2–3. This horse has a bowed tendon on the left foreleg, and a swollen knee on the right foreleg.

equally important that any secondary problems are identified. For example, a horse may have a swollen joint or a hoof wall defect, but also has flexor tendon strain in the opposite leg. It is not unusual for there to be more than one problem in more than one leg, contributing to the lameness.

Every lame horse should be given a complete physical examination, no matter how severe the lameness or obvious the problem. The veterinarian should briefly examine the heart, lungs, and mucous membranes (for example, the gums), and take the horse's rectal temperature. Although this part of the examination may seem unnecessary, some lameness problems are caused by systemic disease that affects the entire body. Examples include:

- joint infection (septic arthritis) in foals
- pleuritis—infection of the chest cavity
- some cases of laminitis

In other instances the musculoskeletal problem may cause systemic illness. Bone infection (osteomyelitis) and a reaction to an intramuscular injection are examples of this type of condition. Fever, depression, and lack of appetite are signs of systemic illness in these horses.

While performing the physical examination, the horse's conformation should be assessed from in front, behind, and both sides. The horse's stance is also an important observation *(see Chapter 1)*. Any obvious asymmetry in the muscles and the position of the bony prominences of the pelvis should also be noted. These characteristics often are easiest to assess by standing back a few feet from the horse.

The order in which the rest of the physical examination is performed

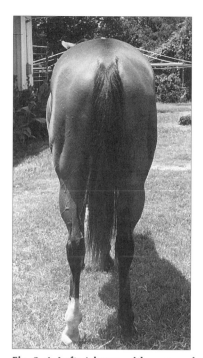 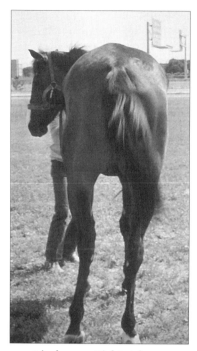

Fig. 2–4. Left: A horse with a normal, symmetrical rump. Right: A horse with an asymmetrical rump due to muscle atrophy on the right side.

varies among veterinarians. Some veterinarians prefer to "zero in" on an obviously abnormal area (such as a swollen joint), and evaluate it carefully before examining the rest of the horse. In this way the relative importance of the obvious problem can be determined early in the examination. A common approach when there are no obvious abnormalities, or when there is more than one problem, is to begin the examination at the feet. The veterinarian then systematically palpates (feels) and manipulates (moves) all four legs, starting at the foot and working up the leg. The neck and back are then thoroughly palpated.

Examining the Feet

The foot is a very common site of lameness, so examination of the feet should be thorough. The feet are evaluated for symmetry of size, shape, wall and heel height, and hoof wall–pastern angle.

Specific abnormalities should also be noted, including:

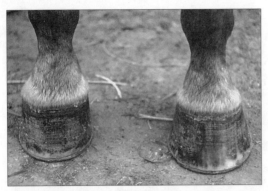

• uneven foot shape and size (mismatched feet)
• horizontal rings in the hoof wall
• contracted heels
• frog atrophy
• hoof wall cracks
• convex or "dropped" sole
(The significance of these findings is discussed in Chapter 7.)

Fig. 2–5. The horse's right forefoot is smaller than the left, which may indicate chronic pain.

While inspecting the foot, the fit and placement of the shoe should be assessed. At the same time, the ground surface of the shoe is assessed for excessive or uneven wear.

Using Hoof Testers

Hoof testers are used to systematically assess the entire hoof (wall, sole, frog, and bars of the heels) for sensitivity or pain. This is an important part of examining the foot. Although using hoof testers is simple, interpreting the results correctly requires considerable experience. The amount of pressure is an important factor. Less pressure should be used in horses with thin soles, and more pressure must be used in horses with thick soles or hard feet.

To be reliable, the results must be repeatable. That is, the horse must consistently respond either when the test is repeated a couple of times in a row, or when the veterinarian comes back to that area after examining the other feet.

Foot Care After the Examination

In some cases, the veterinarian may remove the shoe to exam-

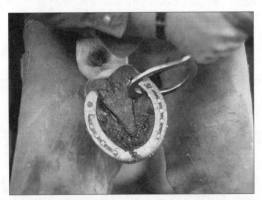

Fig. 2–6. Hoof testers are used to assess the sole, frog, bars, and wall for sensitivity or pain.

ine or treat the foot. The veterinarian may also need to clean and trim the sole. Until the shoe is replaced, it is important to protect the ground surface of the hoof wall from chipping. Wrapping a couple of layers of duct tape around the ground surface of the foot is usually sufficient, unless it will be several days before the farrier can refit the shoe. If so, a more substantial bandage or a protective boot, such as an Easyboot®, should be applied *(see Chapter 4)*. Flat-footed horses also need more protection because the sole touches the ground when the shoe is off.

The other shoes should be left on to protect the feet, and the horse confined to a stall or small paddock and not exercised until the shoe is refitted.

Palpation and Manipulation
Palpation

When palpating the legs and back, the veterinarian is feeling for:
- heat
- pain
- abnormal swellings, described as bony, firm, soft, or fluid-filled
- changes in texture—e.g., abnormal muscle tension (spasm), and replacement of normal tendon with fibrous (scar) tissue

Palpation may involve lightly laying the hand on an area to feel for heat, or it may involve a little more pressure and probing with the fingertips. When assessing the tendons and ligaments at the back of

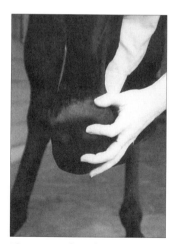 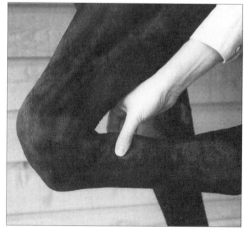

Fig. 2–7. Left: Palpating the knee joints. Right: Palpating the flexor tendons.

the cannon, the tissue can be "kneaded" between the thumb and the first two fingers to check for specific areas of swelling, changes in texture, and pain.

Interpreting the Findings

If the horse flinches or pulls away with only light pressure, the problem is probably in the skin or superficial tissues. For example, bacterial dermatitis or an abscess may cause this reaction. If pain is found only after moderate pressure, a deeper soft tissue (such as tendon, ligament, or muscle) is probably the source of pain. A response to bone pain, such as that associated with ringbone, bone spavin, or an incomplete fracture, usually requires firm, direct pressure. However, not all conditions fit this general guide. For example, a bucked shin can be very painful with only light pressure on the front of the cannon.

It is important to be sure that the response is repeatable: that is, the horse shows signs of discomfort each time the suspect area is palpated. One flinch is not a reliable sign of pain. Some nervous or frightened animals flinch or show other signs of discomfort during palpation even though they do not have a significant problem in that area. So, it is important that the horse's attitude is taken into account when interpreting its reaction. Nervous horses usually stop flinching once they have relaxed and become accustomed to being palpated. In contrast, a horse with a genuinely painful area reacts each time the area is palpated. Moreover, the response may increase with each palpation.

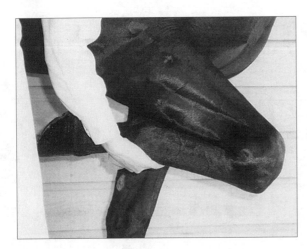

Fig. 2–8. Manipulating the knee joints.

Manipulation

Manipulation involves manually assessing the range of joint mobility while the horse is standing still. It consists of flexing (bending) and extending (straightening) the joint, and where possible, rotating the joint and moving it from side to side. Ideally, each joint in each leg should be manipulated during the physical examination. However, if the horse is in a lot of pain, this part of the examination should be altered or shortened to minimize further damage and pain.

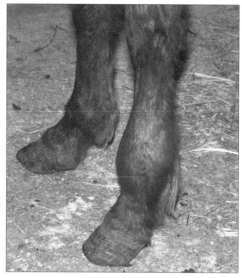

In most cases the range of joint mobility is reduced, usually by fibrosis (thickening with fibrous, or scar tissue). But it may be increased if some of the supporting structures of

Fig. 2–9. The fibrosis surrounding this horse's fetlock dramatically reduces joint mobility.

the joint (in particular, the collateral ligaments; *see Chapter 8*) are damaged. It is important to note that the joints of foals and young horses (less than about 2 years old) usually are more flexible than adult horses.

Abnormal Sounds

Sounds such as pops and clicks are fairly common during joint manipulation, especially in older horses. These sounds, like knuckle cracking or knee clicks in people, usually are not significant.

Crepitus is an abnormal and important finding. Crepitus is a crackling or crunching sensation that may be heard or felt during palpation or manipulation. There are basically two situations that can result in crepitus:

- complete, displaced fractures *(see Chapter 9)*
- gas trapped within the tissues; e.g., in wounds that allow air to be sucked in and trapped beneath the skin, or when gas-producing bacteria invade the tissues

Evaluations With the Leg Down

Each leg should be carefully examined both when the horse is bearing weight on it and when the leg is lifted. Some abnormalities are much easier to see and feel when the horse is bearing weight on the leg. They include:

- joint effusion (excess fluid within a joint)
- soft tissue swellings
- thickening of the flexor tendons or suspensory ligament branches *(see Chapter 11)*
- increased tension in one of the flexor tendons *(see the section on Flexural Limb Deformities in Chapter 14)*

While the horse is standing on the limb, the digital pulses should be evaluated *(see Chapter 4)*. A digital artery runs down each side of the cannon, in the groove between the suspensory ligament and the flexor tendons. The arteries are easiest to palpate as they run across the outer edges of the sesamoid bones at the back of the fetlock joint. Increased pressure in the digital arteries indicates a change in the blood flow to the foot—a very important observation.

Evaluations With the Leg Raised

Conditions that are best assessed with the leg lifted include:

- changes in the texture of the tendons and ligaments
- pain when a joint is manipulated
- changes in the mobility of a joint

When palpating and manipulating the limb, it helps to keep a mental checklist of the structures in the area. In this way the veterinarian ensures that the examination is thorough, and subtle abnormalities are not overlooked.

More Information

Abnormalities of movement may be seen during a gait evaluation. They include head nods, hip hikes, and reduced stride lengths. *See Chapter 1.*

GAIT EVALUATION

The physical examination is usually followed by an evaluation of the horse's gait. This is best performed on a firm, even, level surface. Most veterinarians prefer to conduct a gait evaluation while an assistant walks and trots the horse on a loose lead, so the horse's head is free to move. The gait may also be evaluated by working the horse on a longe line, free in an arena or round pen, or under tack (ridden or driven). The veterinarian watches as the horse is walked and trotted in a straight line, and in a circle to the left and to the right. He or she may also want the horse worked on different surfaces (such as asphalt then sand), and on a slope. If the lameness is only obvious during a specific activity, the veterinarian may ask to see the horse perform that activity.

Lameness Grading System

A grading system has been developed to accurately describe and categorize the severity of the lameness. Using a grading system helps owners, trainers, and veterinarians communicate clearly. What may be "severe" lameness to one person may only be "moderate" lameness to another. The grading system also makes recording the findings of the lameness examination more accurate and reliable for future reference (including repeat examinations).

The severity of the lameness generally is graded on a scale between 1 and 5, as described in Figure 2–10. Veterinarians may also split the grades into halves, such as a grade 2½ lameness. (Some veterinarians

DEGREES OF LAMENESS

Grade	Signs
Grade 1	Subtle lameness; may be inconsistent. Not apparent at the walk, and may not even be consistently seen at the trot.
Grade 2	Consistent, mild lameness at the trot.
Grade 3	Consistent, moderate lameness at the trot, with an obvious head nod (foreleg lameness) or hip hike (hindleg lameness).
Grade 4	Obvious lameness at the walk and trot, with a shortened stride and a pronounced head nod or hip hike. The horse is reluctant to trot.
Grade 5	Severe lameness; extremely reluctant or unable to bear weight on the affected leg during motion and at rest ("three-legged lame").

Fig. 2–10. The lameness grading system.

use a scale between 1 and 4, with 1 being mild and 4 being severe lameness. Because more than one scale is used, it is important to describe the lameness in terms of the grading system: grade "2 out of 5," or grade "1 out of 4.")

The lameness is often a grade worse when the horse is worked in a circle or on a different surface. Thus, it is more accurate to describe the lameness in terms of the different conditions. For example, "The horse is grade 2 of 5 lame in a straight line, and 3 of 5 lame in a circle." A change in lameness grade with the direction of the circle is also an important observation. For example, "The horse is grade 2 of 5 lame in a circle to the left, but 3 of 5 lame in a circle to the right."

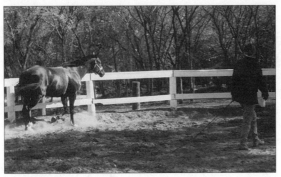

Fig. 2–11. The lameness is often a grade worse when the horse is worked in a circle.

Flexion Tests

A flexion test can be useful for identifying the site of the problem when it is not obvious with a physical examination. The test involves holding a joint fully flexed for 30 – 60 seconds before trotting the horse away. This often aggravates the lameness. In most cases, the horse is more lame for the first six to eight steps after flexion. Sometimes the lameness is worsened for several minutes.

Other indications that the joint is a source of pain include:

- the horse resists joint flexion
- the horse tenses up
- the horse pulls away
- the horse develops quivers in the muscles of the upper leg when the joint is flexed

The principle behind the flexion test is that flexion of a joint places tension on the joint capsule and overlying soft tissues (tendons and ligaments). In some joints, flexion may also place pressure on parts of the joint cartilage and underlying bone, much like a nutcracker.

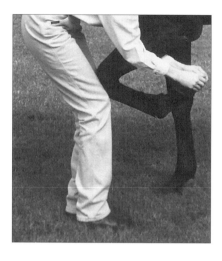 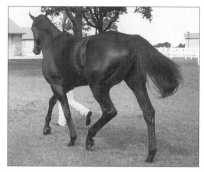

Fig. 2–12. A flexion test. Left: The joints of the lower leg are flexed. Above: The horse is trotted away.

These factors can combine to worsen the pain in an inflamed joint. *(See Chapter 8 for more information on joint structure and problems.)*

Flexion tests can be a source of conflict for owners and trainers when "false positive" results occur during a prepurchase examination *(see Chapter 3)* or pre-competition "vet check." Occasionally, horses that do not have a significant problem in the joint may appear lame for a few steps after a flexion test. This is more likely if excessive pressure was placed on the joint by extreme flexion. Forcing your own wrist into a fully flexed position and holding it like that for a minute has the same result. Stretching the joint capsule and tendons causes pain and a temporary loss of joint mobility when the joint is released.

Flexion tests cannot be relied upon as the sole basis up on which a diagnosis is made. They are simply another means of localizing the lameness to a particular area. In all cases, the opposite leg should be flexed for comparison (assuming it is normal); some veterinarians prefer to flex the normal leg first. If there is any doubt whether the test was positive, it should be repeated after 10 – 15 minutes.

A flexion test may not be as specific as one would think. When using flexion to localize the lameness, it is important to evaluate only one area at a time. However, the fetlock cannot be flexed without also flexing the pastern joint and coffin joint, and the hock cannot be flexed independently of the stifle. So, fetlock flexion can worsen pastern problems (such as ringbone) and can also put pressure on the navicular region. In the hindleg, a positive hock flexion test may be seen even though the stifle is the site of the problem. These facts must be kept in mind when interpreting the results of a flexion test.

DIAGNOSTIC TOOLS & TECHNIQUES

The aim of the physical examination, gait evaluation, and flexion tests is to localize the lameness to a specific area of the leg. However, this is not always possible, as is often the case with multiple site lameness. Other diagnostic techniques often are necessary to locate the problem area(s) and arrive at a specific diagnosis.

Regional (Local) Anesthesia

Regional, or local anesthesia is used to numb, or desensitize an area before a painful procedure, such as suturing a wound. But it can also be used in lameness evaluation to identify the area involved. The principle is a simple one. Local anesthetic is injected into the site, and as the anesthetic is absorbed, sensation (including pain) in the area is temporarily blocked.

Diagnostic Nerve Blocks

Nerve blocks involve injecting local anesthetic under the skin, close to a nerve. As the anesthetic is absorbed into the nerve, the area supplied by that nerve is desensitized. When the painful area is blocked, the lameness should temporarily improve or resolve. By watching the horse during exercise (walking and trotting on a lead or longe line) before and after each block, the problem often can be localized to a particular area of the leg. This method is also a useful way to confirm that a suspect area, which was identified during the physical examination, is the cause of the lameness.

The nerves that supply the lower legs branch like a tree. The "trunk" of the nerve is closest to the body, and the "branches" are closest to the ground. Therefore, the higher up the leg a block is performed, the more nerve branches are blocked and the larger the desensitized area. When using nerve blocks to localize the lameness, it is best to start by blocking the fewest nerves and the smallest area possible. So, the veterinarian begins the nerve blocks at the foot and continues up the leg until the lameness disappears. Other diagnostic procedures, such as radiography and ultrasonography (both discussed later), can then be used to identify the exact cause of lameness.

The nerve blocks commonly used in horses are described below.

They usually are performed in the order in which they are discussed. Each of these blocks involves the Palmar nerve or its branches, which are located in the forelimb.

Palmar Digital Nerve Block

The Palmar Digital (PD) nerves run down the back of the pastern, one on each side of the deep flexor tendon. (The old term for these nerves is the posterior digital nerves.) These nerves provide feeling to the structures in the back third of the horse's foot, including:

- the sensitive tissues (laminae) of the hoof wall, sole, and frog
- the coronet and heel bulbs
- the lower half of the pastern (back part only)
- the deeper structures of the foot: digital cushion, back third of the pedal bone (coffin bone), lateral cartilages, navicular bone and bursa, and deep flexor tendon and its surrounding sheath

(These structures are described and illustrated in Chapters 7 and 15.)

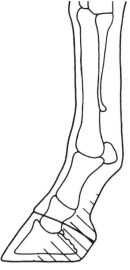

Fig. 2–13. The area desensitized by a Palmar Digital nerve block.

A PD block can be performed with the foot held up and an assistant pulling up on the ergot (the horny structure at the back of the fetlock). Or, it can be performed while the horse is standing on the foot. Because the navicular bone and its associated structures usually are desensitized by this block, it is one of the techniques used to diagnose navicular syndrome. However, just because the lameness improves with a PD block does not mean the horse has navicular pain. Any of the other structures that are desensitized by this block could be causing the lameness.

Low Palmar Nerve Block

The low palmar, or abaxial sesamoidean nerve block, desensitizes the Palmar nerves. These nerves run down each side of the cannon in the groove between the flexor tendons and the suspensory ligament.

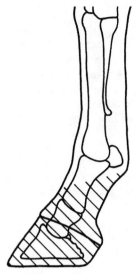

Fig. 2–14. The area desensitized by a low Palmar nerve block.

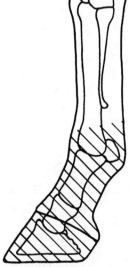

Fig. 2–15. The area desensitized by a 4-point nerve block.

(The old term for this block is the "volar" block.) The nerves divide into the Palmar Digital and Dorsal branches near the base of the sesamoid bones. Blocking both the medial (inside) and lateral (outside) Palmar nerves at or above this point desensitizes the entire foot and at least half of the pastern. If this block is performed at the top of the sesamoids, part of the fetlock and sesamoid bones may also be desensitized, although this is variable.

4-Point Nerve Block

The 4-point nerve block involves the two Palmar nerves and the two Palmar Metacarpal nerves. The Palmar Metacarpal nerves run down the back of the cannon bone, between the splint bones and beneath the suspensory ligament. They supply the front of the fetlock joint after they emerge from under the ends of the splint bones and travel toward the front of the leg. Blocking these four nerves desensitizes the foot, pastern, and entire fetlock joint, including the sesamoid bones.

Other Nerve Blocks

The nerves above the knee or hock may be blocked to desensitize these joints and the entire lower leg. However, because of the large area desensitized, these blocks are not very helpful in localizing the lameness to a particular area. Furthermore, they are more difficult blocks to perform, and they may cause the horse to stumble when so much of the leg is desensitized. Other diagnostic techniques, such as nuclear scintigraphy (discussed later), are better for identifying the site of an obscure lameness involving the upper part of the limb.

Effectiveness of Nerve Blocks

The effectiveness of a nerve block is tested by checking the skin for loss of sensation. This should be done with a pointed but dull object, such as the tip of a ball-point pen. Some veterinarians use a needle, but this can cause bleeding, and unnecessary irritation and pain if the site is not completely blocked. If the block has not worked, repeated testing of the area aggravates the horse, and it may also make the horse "needle-shy." The nerve block must be repeated if skin sensation is not lost.

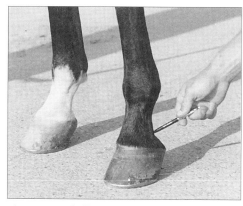

Fig. 2–16. A ball-point pen is used to test the skin for loss of sensation.

The most likely reason for block failure is that not enough anesthetic was absorbed. This may be due to any of the following factors:

- injection too far away from the nerve
- not enough anesthetic injected for the size of the nerve
- testing the skin too soon after injection *(see #2 below)*

Most veterinarians use short, fine needles, and the smallest effective volume of local anesthetic, to avoid blocking nearby nerves. These factors are important when trying to block only one nerve, although it sometimes means that the veterinarian must inject more anesthetic before the block is effective.

Finally, every horse is anatomically unique in some respect. It is not unusual for the nerves of the lower leg to have extra branches or a slightly different path in some horses. This can contribute to block failure, or confusion if the lameness is improved but not completely resolved.

Other Comments About Nerve Blocks

1. The horse must be consistently lame (grade 2 of 5 or greater) for nerve blocks to be useful. If the horse is inconsistently or very slightly lame before the block, it is virtually impossible to see any difference in the gait afterward.

2. Most commonly used local anesthetic drugs take 10 – 15 minutes to desensitize a nerve. The block lasts 1 – 2 hours, depending on the product used and the volume of anesthetic injected.
3. For even more precise identification of the site of lameness, only one side of the leg can be blocked. For example, if a hoof wall defect on the outside (lateral) heel is the cause of the lameness, blocking only the lateral Palmar Digital nerve should resolve or greatly improve the lameness.
4. Joint surfaces and bone lesions (particularly fractures) may not be completely blocked because these structures may receive additional nerve supply from deeper nerves. Other diagnostic procedures, such as a joint block, radiography, and nuclear scintigraphy, may be needed to diagnose these conditions.
5. Although nerve blocks carry very little risk, many veterinarians will not block a leg they suspect may have a fracture. This is a possibility in any horse with sudden lameness after exercise or pasture activity. The fear is that once the pain is lessened by the nerve block, the horse will bear more weight on the leg. This may place enough stress on the bone to turn an incomplete fracture into a complete, displaced fracture—a very serious injury. *(See Chapter 9 for more information.)*
6. Some horses are more lame for several hours after the block has worn off. This may be due to tissue inflammation caused by the drug. Or, it can be caused by an increase in the horse's activity level while the pain was relieved (which aggravated the condition). To minimize swelling and pain, the leg should be bandaged and the horse confined for the next 24 hours. The veterinarian may also recommend anti-inflammatory therapy, such as cold therapy, NSAIDs, etc. *(see Chapter 5)*.
7. All local anesthetic drugs are absorbed into the bloodstream. Because most sports prohibit the use of these drugs in performing horses, the veterinarian should be informed before giving a nerve block if the horse is to be competed within the next week. (Although if the horse is lame, it is unlikely that it will be competing during that time.)

Tissue Blocks

Some areas are best blocked by injecting local anesthetic directly into the tissue. This technique is useful for identifying lameness associated with the origin of the suspensory ligament *(see Chapter 11)*. In fact, this area is difficult to examine or specifically block any other way. Also, injecting local anesthetic around a "splint" *(see Chapter 17)* is a good way to determine whether the bony swelling is causing lameness.

Local anesthetic can also be injected into a tendon sheath or bursa (such as the navicular bursa; *see Chapter 15*).

Intra-articular Anesthesia (Joint Block)

Injecting local anesthetic directly into a joint can temporarily improve or even resolve lameness caused by a variety of lesions, including:

- synovitis—inflammation of the joint capsule lining
- joint capsule damage—e.g. strain and tears
- bone and cartilage fragments—e.g. bone chips and OCD lesions
- damaged or eroded cartilage—degenerative joint disease
- intra-articular ligament damage
  (These structures are described and illustrated in Chapter 8.)

Other conditions may not be completely blocked by this method. This is particularly true of fractures that extend into the joint, and cysts in the bone beneath the joint surface (subchondral bone cysts; *see Chapter 14*).

Performing a joint block also gives the veterinarian an opportunity to evaluate the fluid inside the joint. Joint fluid often dribbles or flows from the needle hub. The veterinarian can collect a sample of this fluid for laboratory analysis before injecting local anesthetic into the joint (see the later section called *Arthrocentesis*).

Minimizing the Risk of Infection

The veterinarian must take care to avoid introducing bacteria into the joint when performing a joint block. For this reason, extra precautions are taken. These aseptic techniques include:

- clipping the hair over the injection site (optional)
- cleansing the skin thoroughly with antiseptic
- using sterile equipment—surgical gloves, syringe, and needle

Bottled drugs are sterile until they are used. Once a needle has pierced the seal and a dose has been removed, the solution may no longer be sterile. So, most veterinarians use a new (unopened) bottle of local anesthetic each time they perform a joint block.

Specific Joint Blocks

Some joints are more difficult to block than others. For example, injections into the coffin joint and shoulder require considerable skill. Some joints are complex: they consist of compartments that may or may not be connected. The knee, hock, and stifle are examples of such joints. To completely block any of these complex joints, at least two separate injections of local anesthetic are needed. It is common to block only one compartment at a time. This approach allows the veterinarian to localize the lameness to a specific part of the joint.

Interpreting the Results

In most joints, the lameness is improved within about 10 minutes of injection. However, in large joints (such as the stifle and hock) it may take up to 30 minutes. If the lameness only begins to improve after this time in any joint, it may be because the local anesthetic has been absorbed from the joint into the surrounding tissues. Unless this possibility is considered, it is easy to mistakenly assume that the problem is within the joint.

Lameness associated with the origin of the suspensory ligament is a good example *(see Chapter 11)*. Sometimes when the knee is blocked, the lameness improves 30 – 45 minutes afterward. The back pouch of the middle knee joint is very close to the suspensory origin. Local anesthetic that was injected into the knee can leak out and desensitize the suspensory origin. If the suspensory origin is the actual site of the problem, the lameness will improve, but it may appear as if the problem is in the knee.

Radiography (X-Rays)

Radiographs are commonly called "x-rays." A radiograph is produced much like a photograph: a split-second exposure is recorded on film. But instead of using light, radiographs are made when the x-ray beam (an invisible ray of electrons) strikes a special film. The film is protected in a specially designed cassette, or plate, which keeps out light, yet allows x-rays to penetrate. Where x-rays reached the film, the surface of the film turns black when it is developed (processed). Where few or no x-rays reached the film, that portion of the image is white or various shades of gray, depending on how many x-rays penetrated the tissues to reach the film.

X-rays travel freely through air, but they are completely prevented from reaching the film by very dense substances, such as lead. Most other substances and tissues are between these two extremes. Soft tissues, such as skin, muscle, tendon, and joint capsule, allow most of the x-ray beam to pass right through them (except where the muscle mass is more than a few inches thick). So, unless there is a distinct difference in tissue densities, such as calcification within a tendon, or an air-filled puncture wound, radiography is not very useful for identifying soft tissue lesions.

Bones allow only a few x-rays to pass through them. So, as long as the beam is intense enough, radiographs can provide detailed information about the surface and interior of bones.

Techniques

Equipment

The basic equipment necessary for taking plain, or routine radiographs includes an x-ray machine and x-ray film in its plate. With high-powered x-ray units, most parts of the

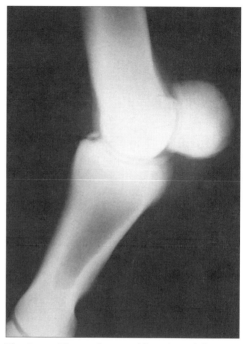

Fig. 2–17. The surface and interior of the bones are clearly visible on this radiograph, but the soft tissues around the fetlock and pastern do not show up well.

horse may be radiographed. University veterinary hospitals and some of the larger private veterinary practices have these machines. In adult horses, good quality radiographs of the pelvis are difficult to get without anesthetizing the horse and laying it on its back. The smaller, portable x-ray units that many equine veterinarians carry in their trucks are good for taking radiographs of the feet and lower legs. Some machines also produce fairly good radiographs of the elbow, shoulder, stifle, and neck.

For ease and safety, the veterinarian may place the x-ray plate in a specially designed holder that has a long, adjustable handle. This allows the assistant who is holding the plate to stand back from the x-ray beam. Plate holders for foot radiographs are often made out of a block of wood with slots cut in it for the plate. Wood does not show up well on the radiograph, so it is a good material for this purpose.

Radiographs become part of the veterinarian's medical records. The name of the horse and its owner, the name of the veterinarian or the practice, and the date on which the radiographs are taken should be recorded on the film. The specific radiographic view and the particular limb being radiographed should also be recorded on the film.

Procedure

Preparation

The ideal area for taking radiographs is a quiet, confined (but not too small) space, with minimal distractions and no human or animal traffic. The area should have a level, even floor, and a reliable electrical supply. It can be very difficult to take good quality radiographs in a less-than-ideal environment. So, it is sometimes best to transport the horse to the veterinarian's clinic.

Before taking radiographs, dirt, mud, bandages, and medications (especially iodine preparations and clay-based poultices) should be removed from the leg. These materials can show up on the radiograph. Likewise, the hoof should be thoroughly cleaned out, and washed if necessary. The grooves (sulci) of the frog, and any hoof wall defects should be packed with Play-Doh™, or a similar material. Play-Doh has about the same density as the hoof wall and soft tissues. Packing the frog sulci and other crevices before taking the radiographs eliminates the air shadows that would otherwise be seen over the pedal (coffin) bone and navicular bone. These shadows can make accurate interpretation of the radiographs difficult.

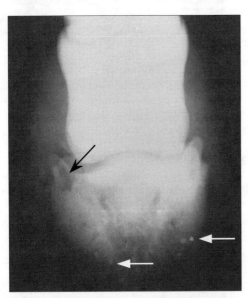

Fig. 2–18. This foot was not cleaned out or packed. Note the shadow [black arrow], gravel [white arrows], and dark v-shaped area (frog sulci) overlying the pedal bone.

The horseshoe and nails can also prevent thorough evaluation of the pedal bone and navicular bone. So, the veterinarian may remove the horse's shoe before taking radiographs of the foot. It is usually best to wait until the films have been developed and the veterinarian is satisfied with the radiographs before replacing the horse's shoe, in case more radiographs are needed.

The horse must be adequately restrained by a competent assistant. To encourage the horse to stand quietly, the handler can lift up a foreleg and hold it while the radiograph is taken. Some horses also require sedation.

Radiographic Views

Radiographs are two-dimensional images of a three-dimensional structure. Therefore, more than one view is necessary for thorough evaluation. This is especially important when radiographing complex structures, such as the

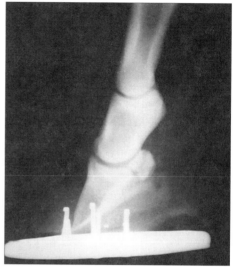

Fig. 2–19. The shoe or nails can obscure the area of interest.

knee or hock. Altering the angle only a few degrees highlights different bones, possibly revealing a hidden lesion.

Routine radiography of the lower limbs should include four standard views:

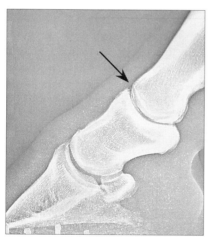
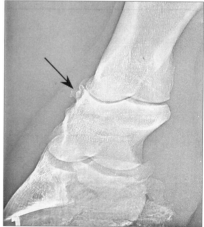

Fig. 2–20. Left: There are only mild changes visible around the pastern joint. Right: But altering the angle a few degrees reveals obvious bony proliferation. (Note: These images are xeroradiographs.)

- **dorso-palmar**—The horizontal x-ray beam passes through the leg from front to back (dorsal surface to palmar surface). Dorso-palmar radiographs of the feet are either taken with the heel raised on a special stand, or by directing the x-ray beam at a 60° angle to the bottom of the foot.
- **latero-medial**—The horizontal x-ray beam passes through the leg from outside (lateral surface) to inside (medial surface).
- **dorso-lateral oblique**—The horizontal x-ray beam passes front-to-back through the leg from a position midway between the front and the outside of the leg.
- **dorso-medial oblique**—The horizontal x-ray beam passes front-to-back through the leg from a position midway between the front and the inside of the leg.

Terminology

Cranio-caudal: the x-ray beam passes from front to back, above the knee or hock.
Plantar: the term used for the back part of the lower hindlimb.
Ventro-dorsal: the x-ray beam is directed upward from below the horse.
Lateral: the x-ray beam passes from the left to right side, or vice-versa.

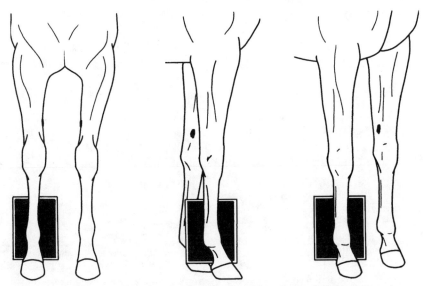

Fig. 2–21. Radiographic views. Left: A dorso-palmar view. Middle: A latero-medial view. Right: A dorso-lateral oblique view.

These views can be reversed when radiographing the hindlimbs. For example, a plantar-dorsal (back-to-front) view is often far easier to take than a dorso-plantar view.

There are a few other views that are sometimes used when radiographing the legs. A flexed latero-medial involves holding the joint flexed while the radiograph is taken. A skyline is where the x-ray beam is directed downward (vertically) along the front or back of the leg.

Where possible, radiography of the upper part of the legs should include a latero-medial and a cranio-caudal view. When radiographing the neck, a lateral view should be taken; a ventro-dorsal view may also be attempted. It is impossible to get useful lateral radiographs of the pelvis in adult horses. But with a powerful x-ray machine, a ventro-dorsal view is usually possible, either under general anesthesia or while the horse is standing.

Taking and Processing the Radiograph

Once the equipment and the horse are prepared, the plate containing the film is placed behind the leg or other body part. The veterinarian can then adjust the position of the machine and the plate as necessary. The beam is "coned down" (narrowed) so that it is more focused and there is less scatter of radiation.

Exposing the film takes a fraction of a second for most parts of the leg. However, it is important that the horse, the plate, and the x-ray machine are perfectly still for that split-second. If there is any movement, the radiograph will be blurry. Once all the radiographs are taken, the films must be developed in a dark room before they can be examined. (This can either be done manually or with an automatic processor.)

Safety Issues

Occasional exposure to x-rays does not present a health risk to the horse or its handler. However, high levels of exposure can cause cancer, bone marrow abnormalities, infertility, arrested growth, and birth defects. Only those people required to restrain the horse and hold the x-ray plate should remain in the immediate area while radiographs are taken. Everyone should stand clear of the x-ray beam at all times. Children and pregnant women should never be permitted to stand nearby while radiographs are being taken.

Everyone who is assisting should wear a lead-lined apron and lead-lined gloves—the x-ray plate should *never* be held with bare hands. Ideally, the plate should be fitted into a holder which has a long handle so that even gloved hands are not exposed to the x-ray beam.

43

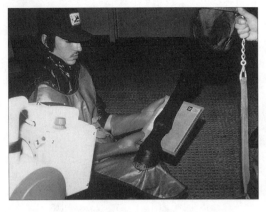
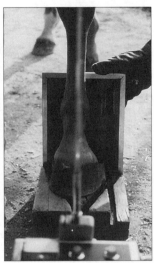

Fig. 2–22. Lead-lined apron and gloves protect the assistants, although a holder with a long handle would be even better.

Sources of Error
Poor Quality Radiographs

Poor quality radiographs are useless at best, and misleading at worst. This is particularly true if an important lesion is missed, or an

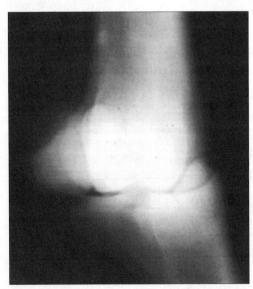

Fig. 2–23. Poor quality radiographs are useless, and should be repeated.

artifact (such as a smudge or scratch on the film) is mistaken for a lesion. So, if any of the radiographs have poor definition or insufficient detail, or if shadows or marks cover the area of interest, they should be repeated.

Errors can occur at any stage in the production and processing of radiographs. For example, improper technique may result in an image that is too dark (overexposed) or too light (underexposed). Also, if the horse, plate, or x-ray machine moved while the radiograph was taken, the image is blurry.

Holding the plate while several radiographs are taken can be a boring and tiring job. To avoid movement, the assistants should pay attention to the task, and hold their breath while the radiograph is taken. It also helps to wait until the veterinarian is ready to take the radiograph before moving the plate into position.

Failing to Find a Lesion

Even with good quality radiographs, the lesion may not be found under certain circumstances.

Early or Mild Lesions

It can take a few weeks for bone lesions to become obvious on radiographs. Early or mild changes may not be apparent at first. For example, early ringbone or bone spavin, both of which involve new bone production, can be difficult to detect. Similarly, mild osteoporosis (loss of bone density) may be missed. A potentially more serious situation involves incomplete fractures, or complete fractures that are not displaced (separated). The fracture line may not be evident for several days after injury, and even then, it may only be seen on one view.

Of Interest
There must be at least a 40% change in the density of the bone before a lesion can be seen on a radiograph.

Lesion Hidden Behind Another Bone

Sometimes structures are superimposed on one another. To avoid missing a lesion because another structure is covering it, more than one view of the area should be taken. In some cases, the veterinarian needs to repeat a view, or take serial views, moving around the leg a few degrees at a time. While this can be time-consuming and costly, it is often essential for identifying subtle, yet important lesions.

Interpretation

As with any specialized technique, it takes training, experi-

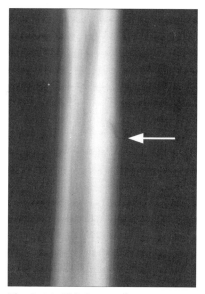

Fig. 2–24. This incomplete cannon bone fracture was visible only after several days.

ence, care, and patience to interpret a radiograph correctly. An experienced veterinarian is not content with just finding an obvious lesion. Instead, he or she thoroughly examines the entire radiograph, looking for other lesions and secondary changes. With all the different factors affecting radiographic quality, the veterinarian may need to repeat some radiographs or take additional views before giving an opinion.

Other Radiographic Procedures
Contrast Radiography

Routine radiography is not very good at showing soft tissue lesions, unless there is a distinct difference between the radiographic characteristics of the lesion and the surrounding tissues. In joints, tendon

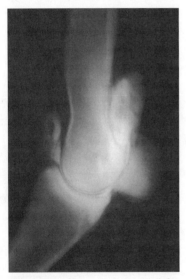

sheaths, and infected tracts, the soft tissues can be highlighted by injecting contrast material into the space or tract. This substance absorbs the x-rays and prevents them from reaching the film. As a result, the space or tract is made more obvious by the white contrast material that fills it. This technique is called contrast radiography. *(Compare Figure 2–25 with Figure 2–17.)*

Severe damage to a joint capsule or tendon sheath can be diagnosed if the contrast material escapes into the surrounding tissues. The depth and path of puncture wounds and draining tracts (formed by a deep abscess or bone infection) can also be identified using contrast radiography.

Fig. 2–25. The contrast material highlights parts of the fetlock that are not visible with plain radiography.

Occasionally, the veterinarian may inject air, which does not block x-ray transmission, into a joint to highlight cartilage defects or irregularities in the joint capsule. These abnormalities may be impossible to see if the joint space is filled with contrast material. But sometimes they can be highlighted when they are surrounded by a black "halo" of air.

Myelography

Myelography is a specific type of contrast radiography that is sometimes used to diagnose cervical vertebral malformation (CVM, or "wobbler" syndrome; *see Chapter 12*). Performing a myelogram involves anesthetizing the horse and injecting a sterile contrast solution into the spinal canal at

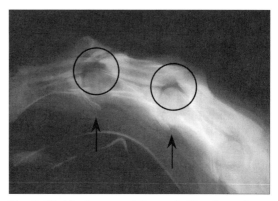

Fig. 2–26. Myelogram of the neck. The dye columns narrow (circles) at the intervertebral joints (arrows).

the base of the skull. The thin columns of contrast material (the dye columns) are narrowed where the spinal cord is being pinched or compressed by the vertebrae.

Myelography is not without risk. It is usually only performed in horses with obvious neurologic problems, including incoordination and weakness. It is often difficult for these horses to get up after anesthesia. Also, the contrast material has caused seizures in a few horses. Myelography is also a costly procedure. For these reasons, it is generally only recommended to confirm the diagnosis for insurance purposes.

Xeroradiography

Xeroradiography uses a conventional x-ray machine, but requires special film, and a specialized x-ray plate and processing technique. The amount of detail is far superior to plain radiography. However, the costs are much greater, the procedure is more difficult, and more radiation is needed to produce xeroradiographs. Because of these factors, xeroradiography is unavailable in many places. Its main advantage is superior image quality when plain radiographs do not provide sufficient detail, or when a lesion is suspected but not found on plain radiographs.

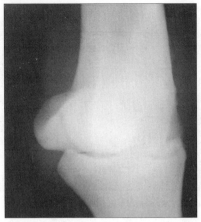 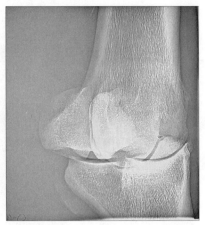

Fig. 2–27. On the left, a plain radiograph of the fetlock. On the right, a xerorad-iograph of the same area. Note the enhanced detail in the image on the right.

Fluoroscopy

Fluoroscopy is a radiographic technique that provides a computer-derived image instantly. The area of interest can be evaluated on a monitor while the horse is being radiographed. Small, portable fluoroscopy units are popular with some veterinarians because an area, such as a joint, can be viewed from several angles just by moving the arm of the fluoroscope. There is no need to process films before the radiographs can be evaluated. Also, the veterinarian does not have to return to take more views if the radiographs did not turn out well.

However, portable fluoroscopy has a few drawbacks:

- the image quality is not as good as plain radiography
- it is sometimes difficult to produce a good quality "hard copy" (a video, paper printout, or film that is a permanent record of the examination)
- only the feet and lower legs can be imaged well; most portable units are not powerful enough to image the upper legs or body
- the unavoidable scatter of x-rays presents a potential health hazard to people nearby

These factors can combine to limit the usefulness of the procedure for diagnosis and for monitoring healing. Nevertheless, fluoroscopy can be a useful screening technique to confirm the presence and exact location of a lesion. Plain radiography can then be used to take good quality images of the specific area for detailed evaluation and future reference.

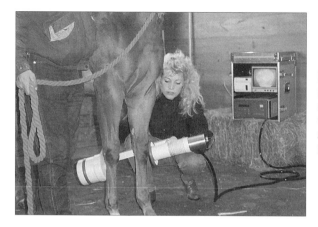

Fig. 2–28. With a portable fluoroscopy unit, an area can be viewed from several angles just by moving the fluoroscope.

Ultrasonography (Ultrasound)

Ultrasonography is commonly used for examining soft tissues. A vibrating crystal in the transducer, or probe, emits ultra-high-frequency sound waves. When these ultrasound waves strike tissue, some waves are transmitted through it. Others are reflected back to the transducer; this is called an "echo."

Ultrasound images, or sonograms, look a little like radiographs, in that the background is black and the tissues are white. Wherever a sound wave is reflected back to the transducer, the resulting image is white. The density of the tissue determines how much of the ultrasound wave is reflected back. Tissues that contain a lot of collagen reflect more of the wave, and therefore produce a bright, white image. In technical terms, these dense tissues are called hyperechoic or echogenic. Structures with a very good blood supply, such as muscle, produce less of an echo than tissues with fewer blood vessels.

Clear fluid, such as normal tendon sheath or joint fluid, reflects virtually none of the sound wave, so the resulting image is black. This is called anechoic. A darker area within a bright, white tissue is described as hypoechoic. For example, an area of disrupted fibers within a flexor tendon is hypoechoic *(see Chapter 11)*.

This ability to identify soft tissues of

Terminology
Collagen: microscopic fibers that provide the strength and resilience in skin, tendons, ligaments, etc.
Hyperechoic/Echogenic: generating an echo.
Anechoic: generating no echo.
Hypoechoic: generating less echo than normal.

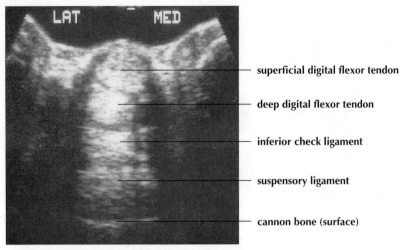

superficial digital flexor tendon

deep digital flexor tendon

inferior check ligament

suspensory ligament

cannon bone (surface)

Fig. 2–29. A sonogram showing the tendons and ligaments at the back of the cannon.

different densities makes ultrasonography very useful for diagnosing a variety of soft tissue lesions.

Quality Control

Many university veterinary hospitals have large, sophisticated ultrasound machines that produce very high quality images. The versatility and image quality of the smaller, portable machines may not be quite as great, but they can still produce good quality images.

Many of the same factors that can affect the quality of a radiograph can also affect the ultrasound image. (See the previous section on *Radiography*.)

Preparation

The procedure is best conducted in a quiet area where there is nothing to distract or startle the horse. The equipment is expensive and easily damaged, and must be placed very close to the horse. So, some veterinarians take the precaution of sedating the horse or restraining it in stocks for the examination. The image is displayed on a monitor, which is easiest to see when the examination is performed in a darkened area. If a suitable area is not available , it is usually best to transport the horse to a veterinary hospital.

Air is not a good conductor of ultrasound waves, and even the small amount of air that is trapped between the horse's hair and the skin is enough to prevent a useful ultrasound image. Therefore, in most cases the hair must be clipped from the area of interest before the examination. In horses with very fine or thin hair, soaking the hair with alcohol and applying a thick layer of contact gel may be sufficient. But if the image quality is not good, the examination must be suspended until the hair is clipped away. It is not necessary to shave the skin; clipping with fine blades is enough. Shaving can cause small, painful nicks, and possibly even skin inflammation (dermatitis) in sensitive-skinned horses. In all horses, the skin should be cleaned of dirt, mud, scabs, and other debris before the examination.

Views

The sound wave is directional, so the view is influenced by the angle of the probe. Rotating the probe even a few degrees alters the image. There are two standard views. One is cross-sectional, which is a horizontal "slice" through the tissue. The other is longitudinal, which is a vertical "slice." Using the flexor tendons as an example, a cross-sectional view gives an image that is like cutting through a rope and looking down onto the cut ends of the fibers *(see Figure 2–29)*. A longitudinal view is like slicing lengthwise along the rope and looking at the fibers as they run down the rope.

Interpretation

Training and experience are very important in making and correctly interpreting ultrasound images. To the unpracticed eye, a sonogram is little more than a mess of white streaks. A detailed knowledge of the anatomy and normal appearance of the tissues in the area is also important for accurate diagnosis.

Artifacts, or false lesions are usually hypoechoic or anechoic. They are very easy to create by slightly altering the probe's angle. To be certain that a lesion is real, it should be found in the same location repeatedly. It should also be visible in both cross-sectional and longitudinal views.

The ultrasound examination is a process of moving the probe up and down the leg. It is often difficult to represent the entire examination in a few still images ("hard copies"). Thus, most veterinarians are reluctant to express an opinion on the still image from an examination with which they were not involved. It is impossible to be certain that the lesion is not an artifact if the veterinarian was not present when the image was taken.

Common Uses

Ultrasonography is often used to examine the tendons and ligaments of the lower leg. Several types of lesions can be identified, and measured for comparison as healing progresses:

- thickening—best seen and measured on the cross-sectional view
- fiber disruption—often seen as a hypoechoic or anechoic area within the tendon or ligament, on either view
- fibrosis—replacement of the normal tissue with echogenic fibrous tissue, as a result of injury
- avulsion—where the tendon or ligament is torn from its attachment to the bone
- fluid accumulation in the tendon sheath—echogenic adhesions (fibrous bands) may also be visible in the normally black fluid

Virtually every other soft tissue that is not covered by bone can also be examined using ultrasound. Bone reflects essentially all of the signal back to the transducer. So, ultrasonography is of no use in evaluating the interior of bones, or structures beneath bone or calcified tissue. However, lesions that damage the bone surface can often be seen with ultrasonography. For example, bone infection (osteomyelitis) may be diagnosed with ultrasonography, particularly if fluid or pus accumulates at the damaged bone surface. Fractures and trauma that results in a fragment of bone being lifted off the surface may also be identified with ultrasonography.

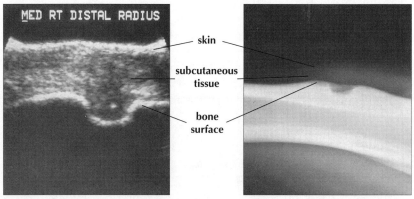

Fig. 2–30. On the left, an ultrasound image of osteomyelitis involving the bone surface. On the right, a radiograph of the same area.

Doppler Ultrasonography

Doppler ultrasonography provides information on the volume, speed, and direction of blood flow in a vessel. It is mostly used to determine the significance of a heart murmur, but it can be used to determine whether blood flow through a particular artery or vein is normal. If, for example, a vessel is crushed or is blocked with a blood clot, doppler ultrasound can identify the problem and measure how much blood is getting through. This technique is occasionally used to assess blood flow in the iliac arteries in the hindquarters *(see Chapter 21)*.

Nuclear Scintigraphy (Bone Scan)

Nuclear scintigraphy involves injecting radioactive particles (radionuclides) intravenously and measuring their uptake in the tissues. Tissue uptake is assessed with a gamma camera, either a large fixed unit, or a small hand-held unit. An area of increased tissue uptake of the radionuclide is called a "hot spot." There are basically two causes of increased tissue uptake:

1. Inflammation—which causes increased blood flow to the damaged tissue.
2. Increased activity of bone-forming cells—e.g. a healing fracture, or an active physis (growth plate).

Not all "hot spots" are abnormal. The physes of young horses normally show increased uptake. The age of the horse and the location of the physes must be kept in mind when interpreting scintigraphs (scans).

Different tissues can be targeted by using specific radionuclides and "carrier" particles, and by timing the examination for maximum tissue uptake. For example, if the lesion is suspected to involve soft tissue, scintig-

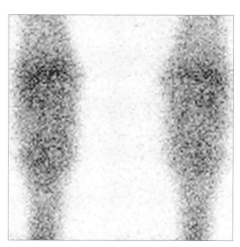

Fig. 2–31. Normal physes in the knees of a young horse.

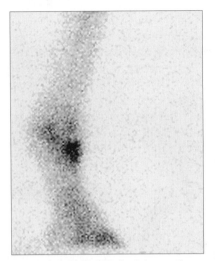 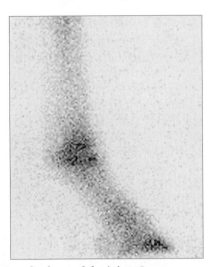

Fig. 2–32. The left fetlock has a "hot spot" at the front of the joint. Compare this area with the normal right leg.

raphy must be performed within about 30 minutes of injection because the radionuclide is quickly cleared from soft tissues. If the lesion is suspected to involve bone, the scan is usually performed about 4 hours after injection. This is because it takes more time for the radionuclide to bind to the minerals in the bone. It is possible to scan soft tissues and bone in the one horse. But this requires scanning the horse immediately after injection, and then rescanning it 3 – 4 hours later.

Typically, both forelegs or both hindlegs are scanned at the same time. It is important for both the normal and the abnormal leg to be imaged. This way, any increased or suspicious uptake of the radionuclide in the lame leg can be compared with the uptake in the other leg. This is particularly important in horses less than 4 years old because their active physes can easily be misdiagnosed as an abnormal site. Bilateral lesions (present in both legs) can be misleading in horses of any age. Thus, correct interpretation of bone and soft tissue scans requires training, experience, and a thorough physical examination.

Uses and Limitations

Nuclear scintigraphy is a very useful technique for identifying the site(s) of obscure or multiple limb lameness, back pain, and incomplete fractures *(see Chapter 9)*. It can sometimes identify bone lesions several days before they are visible on radiographs. It is also a good way to monitor healing of the lesion over time. Once the lesion has healed, the uptake in the area returns to normal.

All four legs and the back can be scanned in one session if necessary, so abnormal areas that were not found during the physical examination or gait evaluation may also be identified. Scintigraphy can also help confirm that there are no significant problems in cases of "bridle lameness" *(see Chapter 1)*. However, nuclear scintigraphy should not be used to replace a thorough work-up.

Scintigraphy does not provide detailed information about the nature of the lesion. All that can be determined is that there is increased blood flow or cell activity in the "hot" area. Other procedures, such as radiography and ultrasonography, are needed to make a definite diagnosis.

Nuclear scintigraphy is a relatively involved, time-consuming, and expensive procedure. The gamma camera and the computer that compiles the images are costly to purchase and maintain. The facility and the staff handling the radionuclides must be registered by the State Health Department. After injection with the radionuclide, the horse must be kept in a specially-prepared stall at the hospital. Its manure and urine must be collected and stored for at least 24 hours, or until they are no longer radioactive. In addition, everyone handling the horse during this time must wear gloves and protective boots. These factors limit the availability of this procedure to university veterinary hospitals and a few well-equipped private practices.

Arthrocentesis (Joint Tap)

Inflammatory or infectious problems within a joint or tendon sheath may be diagnosed by collecting a sample of synovial fluid. Synovial fluid collection should be performed aseptically to minimize the risk of contaminating the joint or tendon sheath with bacteria. (See the earlier section on *Intra-articular Anesthesia* for more information.)

Visible Characteristics

There are several visible characteristics of the fluid that the veterinarian uses to assess the health of the joint (or tendon sheath). This includes the color and

Definitions
Synovial fluid fills a joint space, tendon sheath, or bursa; it nourishes, lubricates, and protects the structures.
Fluid collection from a joint is called arthrocentesis. Fluid collection from a tendon sheath is sometimes called synoviocentesis.

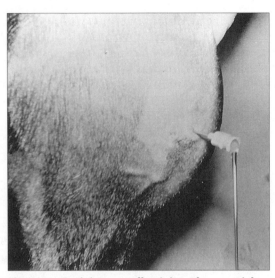

Fig. 2–33. Draining a swollen joint. The synovial fluid appears normal, if excessive.

cloudiness, and the presence of any particles or strands of material. Normal synovial fluid is clear, with a pale yellow tint. There should be no flecks or strands floating in it, and no blood.

Bleeding into the joint may occur during sample collection, especially if the joint is inflamed. Or, it may have occurred during the traumatic incident or condition that damaged the joint. Fresh bleeding during sample collection is usually obvious as streaks of blood in the normal-colored synovial fluid. Bleeding due to joint damage usually results in a fluid sample that is uniformly red or orange.

Normal synovial fluid is viscous, or slippery, like clean motor oil.

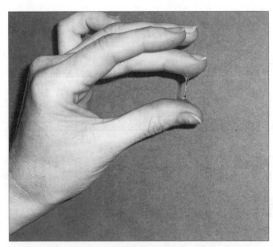

Fig. 2–34. Normal synovial fluid should "string" between the finger and thumb.

This quality can be assessed by placing a drop of fluid on the ball of the thumb and rubbing a finger across it. Normal fluid also strings, which means it forms a thin band when the finger and thumb are separated by an inch or so. Abnormal synovial fluid is more like water: it is not slippery, and it does not string.

Another simple test involves setting the

sample aside to see if it clots. If the protein concentration is abnormally high, a yellow clot forms in about 10 – 15 minutes. To the veterinarian, the formation of a clot is a useful piece of information when laboratory analysis is not immediately available.

Laboratory Analysis

Laboratory analysis of the fluid can provide important information about the condition. A high protein concentration means there is inflammation or infection within the joint or tendon sheath. The white cell count (cells that respond to tissue damage or infection) is another important piece of information. There are very few white cells in normal synovial fluid. A slight increase in the number of white cells in the fluid is sometimes seen in horses with severe joint inflammation. But a moderate or dramatic elevation in the white cell count generally indicates a serious infection. The proportions of the different types of white cells, and the appearance of the cells under a microscope can also provide valuable information about conditions within the joint or tendon sheath.

The presence of bacteria in a sample with a high white cell count is definite proof of infection. However, it is common for no bacteria to be found in a sample from an infected joint. One of the ways the body controls infection within a joint is to produce more synovial fluid. This dilutes the bacteria, the toxins they produce, and any harmful inflammatory substances *(see Chapter 5)*. Thus, it is unlikely that the laboratory staff will find these microscopic organisms in a fluid sample. Culture of the fluid is usually necessary to confirm infection, identify the bacteria that are responsible, and select the appropriate antibiotic(s).

> **More Information**
>
> Managing joint infection (septic arthritis) is discussed in Chapter 8.
>
> Managing tendon sheath infection (septic tenosynovitis) is discussed in Chapter 11.

Bacterial Culture and Antibiotic Sensitivity

Synovial fluid and pus samples can be cultured (incubated) to encourage whatever bacteria are present to multiply. This is usually done by taking a drop of fluid or a swab stick and wiping it over the surface of a culture plate, or adding it to a nutrient solution. The culture plate and nutrient solution contain substances the bacteria need to survive and multiply. After incubating the plate or solution at

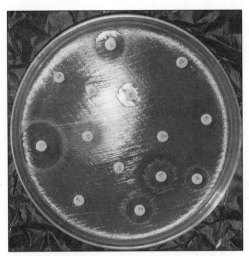

Fig. 2–35. Small paper discs containing specific antibiotics are laid onto the surface, and the culture plate is incubated for 24 hours.

body temperature for 24 – 48 hours, it is examined for bacterial growth. The bacteria can be identified by the colonies they form (or a change in the color or cloudiness of the solution), and by their appearance under a microscope.

The sensitivity, or susceptibility of the bacteria to various antibiotics can be tested by sampling a colony and wiping the sample over a fresh culture plate. Small paper discs that contain specific antibiotics are laid onto the plate surface, and the plate is then incubated for 24 hours. The most suitable antibiotics for treating the infection are those that prevent the bacteria from growing around them. However, this does not necessarily mean that the antibiotic will be 100% effective in resolving the infection in the horse. Many different factors can reduce the effectiveness of an antibiotic *(see Chapter 5)*. Nevertheless, bacterial culture and sensitivity is a good starting point in most cases.

If the horse has already received antibiotics, bacterial culture and sensitivity is often unrewarding or misleading. *Therefore, it is important that antibiotics are only given on veterinary advice.*

Other Tests
Urinary Excretion of Electrolytes and Minerals

The kidney is the main organ that controls the body's electrolyte and mineral balance (although the bowel also controls mineral absorption). If the body is low in a particular element, the kidney conserves it. If there is a dietary excess of an element, the kidney excretes it in the urine. In this way the kidney maintains a fairly constant concentration of that element in the body. These facts can be used to diagnose some metabolic bone and muscle problems. Dietary calcium-phosphorus imbalances *(see Chapter 9)*, and exertional rhabdomyolysis ("tying up"; *see Chapter 10*) are two examples.

The urinary fractional excretion (FE) of an electrolyte or mineral can be determined by collecting some urine from the horse and then taking a blood sample immediately afterward. The concentrations of the electrolyte or mineral in the urine and blood are then compared.

Horse urine normally contains a lot of calcium, much of which settles out as tiny crystals when the urine sample is allowed to sit for a time. So, measuring the concentration of calcium in the urine can be quite inaccurate. However, because the body's calcium balance is intimately tied to the phosphorus balance, measuring the FE of phosphorus can provide information about the horse's calcium and phosphorus status. An FE of phosphorus that is higher than normal occurs when the diet contains too much phosphorus or too little calcium.

Potassium is normally found in high concentrations in horse urine. When the diet does not provide enough potassium, the FE of potassium is low. An FE of potassium that is lower than normal is sometimes seen in horses with exertional rhabdomyolysis. Small changes in the FE of sodium and magnesium have also been reported in some of these horses.

The diet is an important consideration when interpreting FE results. Horses on fresh grass or alfalfa hay have a high FE of potassium. If electrolyte supplements or salt are fed in large amounts, the FE of sodium and chloride may also be greater than normal.

Treadmill Gait Analysis

High-speed treadmills can be useful for evaluating horses with subtle or obscure gait abnormalities. The horse can be observed dur-

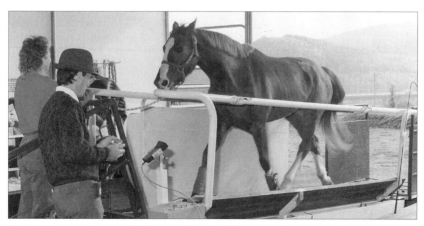

Fig. 2–36. Exercise on a high-speed treadmill is a good way to determine whether lameness is the primary problem in horses that perform poorly.

ing any gait from a walk to a gallop, either on the level or on an incline. It can also be videotaped for later frame-by-frame study. This can help veterinarians and farriers diagnose and manage a variety of conditions. Exercise on a high-speed treadmill can also be a good way to determine whether lameness or another condition (such as lower airway disease) is the primary problem in horses that are performing poorly.

Thermography

One of the hallmarks of inflammation is an increase in blood flow, and therefore heat in the inflamed tissue. The heat is transmitted to the skin, and can be felt with the fingers or palm. Thermography is a more sophisticated and sensitive means of identifying differences in the body's surface temperature. By comparing one leg with another, it is possible to detect small differences in the surface temperature. The temperature is increased in inflammatory conditions, and decreased when blood flow to a particular area is reduced. For example, blood vessel constriction, or obstruction with a blood clot results in a lower surface temperature.

Good quality thermography units can measure small changes in the surface temperature—differences that are not detectable with the hands. This allows much earlier detection of many conditions. If the horse is rested, examined, and treated appropriately, more serious or permanent damage may be prevented.

However, thermography cannot specifically identify which structure is involved, or which disease process is present. It can identify inflammation, but it cannot tell the difference between the minor bumps and strains of training and a more serious condition, such as a bowed tendon. Other diagnostic methods must be used to make a specific diagnosis.

Exercise causes a marked increase in

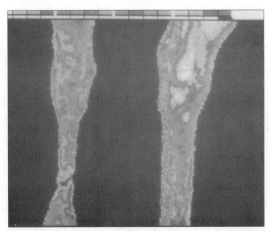

Fig. 2–37. The horse's left hock has areas of increased temperature (light patches).

blood flow to the skin, which lasts for several hours. This fact limits the usefulness of thermography for evaluating inflammation or lameness immediately after exercise.

Electromyography

Electromyography (EMG) is a method of determining whether a muscle and the nerve that supplies it are functioning normally. Fine, needle-like probes are inserted into the muscle. The electrical activity in the muscle is recorded onto a paper strip, much like an electrocardiogram (ECG). The activity at rest and during muscle contraction can be compared with normal values, either in the conscious horse or under general anesthesia.

Conditions that result in an abnormal EMG recording include:

- loss of nerve supply to the muscle—either as a result of nerve damage or spinal cord disease
- severe muscle damage—resulting in the replacement of muscle with fibrous tissue
- abnormally excitable muscle cells—such as occurs in horses with hyperkalemic periodic paralysis, or HPP *(see Chapter 10)*

Muscle Biopsy

Muscle biopsy involves collecting a small piece of muscle with a special biopsy needle or scalpel and examining it microscopically. Muscle biopsy is used to diagnose certain muscle disorders, including polysaccharide storage myopathy in draft horses and chronic ER *(see Chapter 10)*. It is also used to confirm Equine Motor Neuron Disease (EMND; *see Chapter 12*).

CT and MRI

Computerized tomography (CT) and magnetic resonance imaging (MRI) are sophisticated diagnostic techniques that have been used in human medicine for years. Some of the larger veterinary schools now have CT machines, or access to CT or MRI by arrangement with a nearby human hospital. However, because of the location, size, and shape of the equipment, veterinary use is mostly limited to small animals. It is possible to image young foals and small ponies. But in adult horses, only the head, neck, and lower legs can be imaged. The animal must be anesthetized, because it must remain perfectly still for several minutes. Anesthesia adds to the expense and risk of the procedure.

Computerized tomography involves the generation of x-rays by a circular tubehead that rotates around the patient. A computer processes the information gained from multiple angles. It then produces an image that provides either a detailed cross-sectional view through the bones and soft tissues, or a three-dimensional image of the bone's surface.

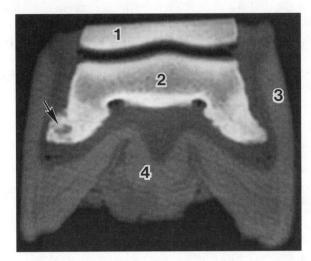

Fig. 2–38. A computerized tomography image of a pedal bone lesion [arrow].

1. Second pastern bone
2. Pedal bone
3. Hoof wall
4. Frog

Magnetic resonance imaging has not yet been adapted for diagnostic use in adult horses. Currently, it is only used in research. Nevertheless, MRI studies of the feet and lower legs of euthanized horses have shown that this could be a very valuable diagnostic tool. The image quality and amount of detail are vastly superior to ultrasonography. As well as identifying soft tissue lesions that can be seen with ultrasonography, MRI can reveal such lesions as:

- cartilage defects in the joints and on the navicular bone
- changes in the sensitive laminae of the hoof wall
- tiny lesions in the tendons and ligaments (including the ligaments of the navicular bone)

Portable MRI units are being developed for diagnostic use in horses, so this technology may soon be available to equine veterinarians.

IMAGING TECHNIQUES & THEIR USES

Imaging Technique	Tissues Imaged
Radiography	**Bones**
Contrast Radiography	Soft Tissue Cavities
Myelography	Spinal Canal
Xeroradiography	Bones
Fluoroscopy	Bones (Feet and Lower Legs Only)
Ultrasonography	**Soft Tissues and Bone Surfaces**
Doppler Ultrasonography	Blood Vessels
Nuclear Scintigraphy	**Bones or Soft Tissues**
Thermography	**Skin and Superficial Tissues**
Computerized Tomography	**Bones and Soft Tissues**
Magnetic Resonance Imaging	**Soft Tissues and Bones**

Fig. 2–39. A summary of the imaging techniques and their primary uses in lameness investigation.

3

PREPURCHASE
EXAMINATIONS

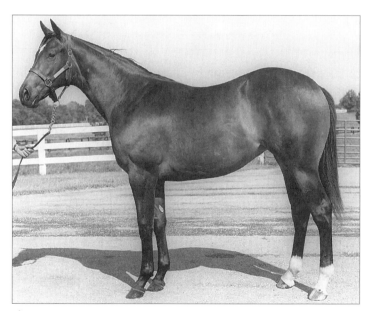

Fig. 3–1.

A prepurchase examination is the examination of a horse by a veterinarian before it is purchased. Some owners and trainers call this procedure a "vet check." Whether buying a racehorse, sport horse, or yearling, the structure and function of the musculoskeletal system are important aspects of the prepurchase examination.

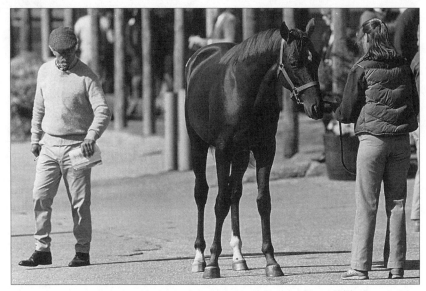

Fig. 3–2. Many factors are important when deciding whether a horse is suitable.

This procedure is important because no horse is perfect. Although an experienced horseperson usually can detect most faults or defects, a veterinary examination can reveal medical facts about the horse that may not be obvious. The veterinarian can give a qualified opinion on the significance of any faults the buyer detected, as well as those found during the examination. Having this information reduces—but does not eliminate—the buyer's risk.

PRELIMINARY COMMENTS

The horse's suitability for its intended function does not depend solely on the outcome of the veterinary examination. Several other factors are important, including:

- age
- gender
- build
- training

- breed
- height
- temperament
- performance history

Unless the buyer is an experienced horseperson, it is a good idea to have someone else evaluate the horse and advise on whether it is suitable. This person may be a friend with horse experience, a trainer, an acquaintance who is actively involved in the particular sport, or a professional bloodstock agent. The veterinarian can give some advice in this area, such as verifying the horse's age, and discussing the breed in general or that horse's conformation in particular. But it is up to the buyer, with input from the advisor, to decide whether the horse will suit his or her needs now and in the future.

Veterinarian's Role

The veterinarian's role is to thoroughly examine the horse and explain to the buyer the significance of any physical abnormalities, in relation to the horse's intended use. There are several things the veterinarian cannot or should not do with regard to the prepurchase examination findings:

- "pass" or "fail" the horse
- guarantee the horse's usefulness for a specific purpose
- predict the length of time the horse will continue to perform its intended function
- make judgements about the horse's value
- dictate whether the horse should be purchased

The decision to purchase the horse is the buyer's responsibility, and it should not be made solely on the outcome of a prepurchase examination.

The buyer should choose a veterinarian who is experienced with prepurchase examinations, and has a good knowledge of the activity the horse will be performing. For example, when buying a reining horse, it is wise to select a veterinarian who has some experience with reining horses. Likewise, a horse intended for racing should be examined by a veterinarian who is familiar with that type of racing.

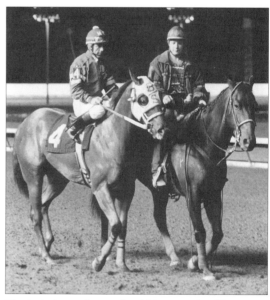

Fig. 3–3. A racehorse should be examined by a veterinarian who is familiar with that type of racing.

Farrier's Role

A farrier will be needed if the veterinarian removes the horse's shoes to examine or radiograph the feet. This gives the buyer's regular farrier an opportunity to evaluate the horse's feet without the shoes. Even if the shoes are not removed, it is worthwhile having the farrier inspect the horse's feet before purchase. The farrier's opinions regarding foot shape, conformation, and current shoeing can alert the buyer to foot problems that may develop over time.

The appointment with the farrier should be made for the day after the prepurchase examination. This gives the veterinarian time to repeat any tests or radiographs before the farrier replaces the shoes. Until then, it is important to bandage or otherwise protect the horse's feet *(see Chapter 4)*.

Before the Examination

To present the horse in its best light, the seller should take care not to make major changes to the horse's management in the week before the prepurchase examination. In particular, the shoeing should not be changed. Also, the horse should not be vaccinated within a week of the examination. Shoeing changes and injection reactions can cause lameness. *(Intramuscular injection reactions are discussed in Chapter 10.)*

When arranging the prepurchase examination, the buyer should tell the veterinarian what the horse will be used for, what is known about the horse's history, and what problems have already been noticed. This information helps the veterinarian decide what

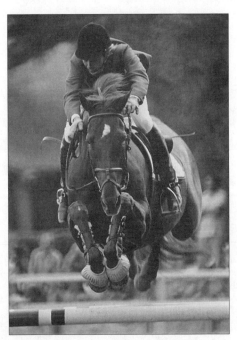

Fig. 3–4. The scope of the examination depends on the purpose for which the horse is bought.

special equipment and tests to include, and on what areas to focus.

If possible, the buyer should be present for the prepurchase examination, and should also try to meet with the veterinarian later to discuss any radiographs taken. The veterinarian can demonstrate and explain the findings far better in person than over the phone.

THE PREPURCHASE EXAMINATION

The prepurchase examination of a performance horse usually consists of three parts: examination of the horse while at rest, while being led or longed, and while being ridden (or driven). This procedure is different from, and more comprehensive than a routine physical examination, an insurance examination, or the investigation of a specific lameness problem.

Examination at Rest

Physical Examination

Every horse, no matter what its intended use or purchase price, should be given a thorough physical examination. This examination should include:

- measuring the horse's heart rate, respiratory rate, and rectal temperature
- evaluating the gum color and capillary refill time
- listening to the heart, lungs, and bowels with a stethoscope
- examining the teeth to verify the horse's age and check for major tooth problems
- examining the eyes, including the retina at the back of the eye

The examination is best performed in a stall or some other area where the horse is settled and relaxed. A darkened area is needed to examine the eyes because darkness causes the pupils to dilate. This allows the veterinarian to examine the back of the eye.

Examining the Horse Outside the Stall

Before examining the feet, legs, and back in detail, they should be observed for symmetry. This evaluation is best made in a well-lit, level area. There should be enough space for the veterinarian to stand back 6 – 12 feet and compare both sides of the horse. This is often difficult to do in a stall.

Symmetry, or the lack of it, is an important observation. The left and right sides of the horse should mirror each other. If not, is it due to swelling on one side or atrophy (loss of bulk) on the other? This question is best answered with palpation: using the fingers and hands to check for pain, heat, abnormal swellings, and changes in texture.

Each foot should be thoroughly examined, and each leg carefully palpated, both while the horse is bearing weight on the leg, and while the leg is raised. With the leg raised, each joint should be manipulated, checking for pain and changes in the range of joint motion. The neck and back should also be carefully palpated. *(Examining the feet, and palpation and manipulation are discussed in Chapter 2.)*

While examining the feet and legs, the veterinarian should test the heel bulbs of both forefeet for sensation. If a Palmar Digital neurectomy has been performed ("nerving"; *see Chapter 15*), the horse may have no skin sensation in its heel bulbs. Prodding the heels with the tip of a ball-point pen is usually all that is necessary to check for sensation. If there is any doubt, the veterinarian may clip the hair from the sides of the pastern to look for surgical scars.

Examination While Led or Longed

The second part of the examination is the gait evaluation. The horse is observed while it is walking and trotting, either led or longed. The veterinarian watches the horse for any sign of lameness, and looks at how the horse places each foot and moves without the rider.

One of the best ways to detect subtle lameness is to trot the horse in a small circle, less than about 30 feet (10 meters) in diameter. The surface should be firm and level or slightly inclined. The horse can

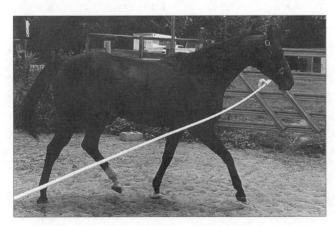

Fig. 3–5. One way to detect subtle lameness is to trot the horse in a small circle.

be trotted either on a lead rope or longe line. The tight circle places tension on the sides of the feet and lower joints. So, it can reveal low-grade lameness that was not obvious when the horse was trotting in a straight line.

Most veterinarians also perform flexion tests on each of the horse's legs during the gait evaluation *(see Chapter 2)*. Some normal horses are a little uneven for the first few steps after joint flexion, but they should quickly recover a normal, even trot after a couple of strides. If there is any question of whether the test was positive, it should be repeated after a few minutes. But in all cases, the results of the flexion tests should be viewed in context with the other examination findings. A questionable flexion test in a horse that is not lame and has no other abnormalities probably should be disregarded.

If the gait evaluation reveals lameness, the veterinarian may re-examine the affected limb to identify the site and possible cause(s). *However, the buyer is not responsible for having the cause of the lameness investigated.* When a horse is found to be lame during a prepurchase examination, the buyer must decide whether to have the veterinarian investigate the cause (at the buyer's expense), or suspend the examination. If it is suspended, the buyer must then decide whether to reject the horse or reschedule the prepurchase examination once the lameness is resolved.

Examination While Ridden or Driven

Observing the horse while it is being ridden or driven is an important part of the prepurchase examination. In this phase the veterinarian can put everything together by watching the horse perform. The veterinarian may have the rider/driver put the horse through certain maneuvers to better determine the importance of any suspicious findings. For example, the veterinarian may ask to see an eventer as it jumps, watch a barrel racer run barrels, or observe a dressage horse as it

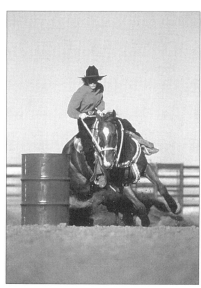

Fig. 3–6. The veterinarian may ask to see a barrel racer run barrels.

performs an extended trot or some collected movements.

Although the buyer and advisor are responsible for deciding on the suitability of the horse, some veterinarians like to observe how well the rider and the horse work together. If for no other reason than rider safety, the veterinarian may comment on the interaction between the horse and the rider. "Bridle lameness" *(see Chapter 1)* may also become apparent during this phase of the examination.

Young or Unbroken Horses

> ### More Information
>
> Developmental orthopedic disorders (DODs) may be present at birth or develop as the foal grows. They include:
>
> • angular limb deformities
> • flexural limb deformities
> • physitis
> • osteochondrosis
>
> (These problems are discussed and illustrated in Chapter 14.)

Although young or unbroken horses cannot be ridden or driven, they can be exercised in a round pen or arena. But in young horses, conformation is as important as how the horse moves. Conformation, particularly of the feet and legs, is one of the major factors that determine whether the horse is likely to develop exercise-related conditions during its working life.

Many conformational defects begin as developmental orthopedic disorders. These problems are much more common than exercise-related injuries or degenerative conditions in young horses. Most of them are obvious at rest, so examining the young horse while it is standing is just as important as observing it during exercise.

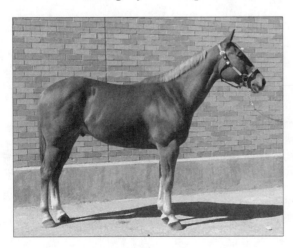

Fig. 3–7. A young horse with less-than-ideal conformation may develop exercise-related problems during its working life.

Racehorses

With racehorses (Thoroughbreds, Quarter Horses, and Standard-breds) it is often useful to watch the horse at the track, during warm-up and speed work. These horses can be difficult to evaluate on a lead and most have not been taught to longe. In many cases the horse is more cooperative after it cools down following track work. This often is a better time to watch the horse walk and trot on the lead, and to perform the flexion tests.

Measuring the heart rate and respiratory rate, and listening to the heart and lungs within 5 – 10 minutes of exercise is a good idea in all horses intended for athletic competition.

ADDITIONAL TESTS

The most important parts of the prepurchase examination are the physical examination and the gait evaluation. When these examinations reveal problems that could affect the horse's usefulness, the veterinarian may recommend additional tests to more fully determine the nature and implications of the condition. In

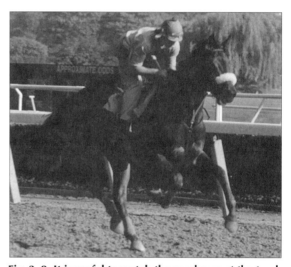

Fig. 3–8. It is useful to watch the racehorse at the track.

other instances the veterinarian may suggest a particular test because the horse's breed or activity makes it more prone to specific problems. *However, these tests are not intended to be the primary basis upon which the decision to buy the horse is made.* The results must be viewed in context with the other findings.

Some of the tests that may be recommended include:

- radiography
- nuclear scintigraphy
- endoscopy ("scoping") of the horse's nasal passages, throat, and windpipe
- ultrasonography
- electrocardiography (ECG)
- blood tests

Depending on the horse's intended use and the findings of the physical examination, the veterinarian may also recommend more specific examination of a particular organ system. For example, a neurologic examination may be warranted in a young, awkward horse *(see Chapter 12)*. If the buyer plans to eventually breed from a mare or stallion, a reproductive examination is worthwhile. If there is any doubt about the significance of an abnormality, the veterinarian may have a veterinary specialist examine the horse or review the examination findings and test results.

Terminology
Radiography: "x-rays" **Ultrasonography:** "ultrasound" **Nuclear Scintigraphy:** "bone scan" (See Chapter 2 for more information on these techniques.)

Radiography

Radiographs may be included in the prepurchase examination for:

- to determine the nature and extent of bone or joint problems that were identified or suspected during the physical examination
- to examine the areas of the horse that are considered high-risk for a particular breed or activity
- to establish baseline radiographs of the high-risk areas for future reference

"High-risk" areas are those parts of the leg that sustain the greatest amount of stress during athletic activity. For example, the hocks are high-risk joints in Standardbred racehorses, dressage and eventing horses, and Western performance horses. In gallopers, the fetlocks and knees are the high-risk joints. The forefeet also are common sites of performance-limiting problems in Thoroughbreds, Quarter Horses, and Warmbloods.

Interpreting the Results

It has been said that "riders don't ride x-rays; they ride horses." This means that *the radiographic findings should be considered in context with the findings of the rest of the examination.* Questionable or inconclusive radiographic findings can be misleading if they are not interpreted in context. For example, minor abnormalities in the navicular bones may not be significant if: 1) the horse has symmetrical, well-shaped feet, 2) did not respond to hoof testers, and 3) was not lame under any circumstances, particularly when circled on a hard surface. *(Navicular bone changes are discussed in Chapter 15.)*

The horse's purpose can influence the significance of some radiographic findings. For example, an older horse being purchased as a schoolmaster for an inexperienced rider will likely have some radiographic changes in its joints and/or feet. As long as the horse can perform to the buyer's satisfaction, these changes may be acceptable. However, if those same changes are found in the joints or feet of a younger horse intended for show jumping, they may be highly significant, particularly if the horse is being bought as an investment.

No horse is perfect; in fact, the more experienced or "seasoned" the horse, the more likely that it has faults. It is up to the buyer, after considering all the information, to decide what faults he or she can accept. Although the schoolmaster may have some foot or leg problems, two questions must be answered: "How is the horse coping with them?" and "Can the buyer tolerate and manage them?" The buyer should bear in mind that a change in the horse's management may worsen some joint and foot problems. Such changes may include a different arena or work surface, a new training program, or a heavier or less experienced rider.

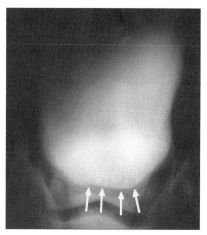

Fig. 3–9. Mild radiographic changes in navicular bone may not be significant.

Other Imaging Procedures

Ultrasonography is often recommended to evaluate a thickened tendon or suspensory ligament. However, ultrasonography cannot always detect early or mild lesions. Torn fibers or fibrosis (scar tissue) indicates a potentially performance-limiting problem, but finding no abnormalities does not necessarily mean the tendons and ligaments are normal.

Some veterinarians recommend nuclear scintigraphy to pinpoint problem areas that may not have been evident during the physical examination or gait evaluation. Scintigraphy may also help establish the significance of certain radiographic findings. For example, if the horse described above (with minor navicular bone changes) is "scanned," and the feet appear normal, this is extra evidence that the navicular bone changes are not currently significant.

Blood Tests

There are several reasons why the veterinarian may take a blood sample during the prepurchase exam. All horses should have a current Coggins' test for Equine Infectious Anemia (EIA), particularly in areas where the disease is common. If the horse has not been tested in 6 – 12 months, it should be retested. A Coggins test is mandatory before shipping a horse interstate or internationally. Other tests may also be required if the horse is leaving the country after purchase.

The veterinarian may recommend a complete blood count and blood chemistry panel to help evaluate certain organ systems, such as the liver and kidneys. These organs cannot be evaluated during a physical examination. Some owners and trainers request a blood test for Equine Protozoal Myeloencephalitis (EPM; *see Chapter 12*). *However, because the results of this blood test can be misleading, it is not recommended during a prepurchase exam.*

Some veterinarians routinely collect a blood and/or urine sample from the horse for drug testing. It is up to the buyer to decide if or when the sample is submitted to the drug testing laboratory. The sample can be frozen and stored for several months if necessary.

THE PREPURCHASE REPORT

Once the examination is complete and the results of any tests are known, the veterinarian makes a report to the buyer. Whether or not the results are reported verbally, they should always be reported in writing. The style and content of the written report varies among veterinarians, although they should all follow the guidelines set out by the American Association of Equine Practitioners. The written report may simply be a letter that summarizes the findings. Or it may be a detailed form that lists the tests performed and the results. Some veterinarians also request that the seller complete and sign a questionnaire of the horse's medical history, including all medications the horse has received in the last 3 weeks. Having this information in writing may help protect the buyer because the seller is legally bound by the information.

In some cases the examination may have a dual purpose: prepurchase and insurance examination, if the sale is successful. In these instances the forms provided by the insurance company must also be completed. 🐴

(Pages 77 – 80 contain the AAEP guidelines, a sample prepurchase report form, and a sample seller's questionnaire.)

Guidelines for Reporting Purchase Examinations

In an effort to better serve its members and their clients, the Board of Directors of the American Association of Equine Practitioners approved guidelines in 1988 to be used in reporting the results of purchase exams. These guidelines were updated and approved by the Board of Directors in 1991. They are as follows:

1. All reports should be made in writing.
2. The report should contain:
   a. A description of the horse with sufficient specificity to fully identify it.
   b. The time, date, and place of the examination.
3. The veterinarian should list all abnormal or undesirable findings discovered during the examination and give his or her qualified opinion as to the functional effect of these findings.
4. The veterinarian should make no determination and express no opinion as to the suitability of the animal for the purpose intended. This issue is a business judgment that is solely the responsibility of the buyer that he or she should make on the basis of a variety of factors, only one of which is the examination and report provided by the veterinarian.
5. Veterinarians should separately record, and retain in their file, a list and description of all the procedures performed in connection with the purchase examination, but the examination procedures need not be listed in detail in the report.
6. The veterinarian should qualify any findings and opinions expressed to the buyer by making specific references to tests that were recommended but not performed on the horse (x-rays, endoscopy, blood, drug, EKG, rectal, nerve blocks, laboratory studies, etc.) at the request of the person for whom the examination was performed.
7. The veterinarian should record, and retain in their file, the name and address of parties involved with the examination (buyer, seller, agent, witness, etc.).
8. A copy of the report and copies of all documents relevant to the examination should be retained by the veterinarian for a period of years not less than the statute of limitations applicable for the state in which the service was rendered. Local legal counsel can provide advice as to the appropriate period of retention.

The spirit of these guidelines is to provide a framework which will aid the veterinarian in reporting a purchase exam and to define that it is the buyer's responsibility to determine if the horse is suitable for him [sic].

Fig. 3–10. The American Association of Equine Practitioners (AAEP) Guidelines for Reporting Purchase Examinations.

Prepurchase Examination Report

Date: _____ Time: _____   Location: _____

Buyer: _____   Seller: _____
Address: _____   Address: _____
City, ST: _____   City, ST: _____
Phone: _____   Phone: _____

Horse: _____   Intended Use: _____
Breed: _____   Sex: _____ Age: _____
Color & Markings: _____
Brands & Tattoo: _____

Physical Examination

From the organ systems that are readily available for examination, the following were noted:

Temp: _____ Pulse: _____ Respiration: _____
Mucous Membranes: _____ Digital Pulses: _____

AUSCULTATION:
  Heart: _____
  Lungs: _____
  Abdomen: _____

ORAL EXAMINATION: _____

SKIN: _____

EXTERNAL UROGENITAL: _____

EYE EXAMINATION:
  Direct Exam: _____
  Ophthalmoscope: _____

SHOEING:
  Date Last Shod: _____
  Remarks: _____
  _____

N = Normal   NR = Not Requested

Fig. 3–11. A prepurchase examination report. This is only one example: different veterinarians use different forms.

Musculoskeletal

LEFT FRONT LEG:
   Palpation: _____
   Hoof Testers: _____
   Flexion Tests: _____

RIGHT FRONT LEG:
   Palpation: _____
   Hoof Testers: _____
   Flexion Tests: _____

LEFT HIND LEG:
   Palpation: _____
   Hoof Testers: _____
   Flexion Tests: _____

RIGHT HIND LEG:
   Palpation: _____
   Hoof Testers: _____
   Flexion Tests: _____

BACK: _____

GAIT:
   Straight Line: _____
   Circle: Left: _____   **Right:** _____
   Under Tack: _____

RADIOGRAPHS: _____

OTHER TESTS: _____

ADDITIONAL REMARKS: _____

Blood/Urine Sample Taken for Drug Test: yes/no
Owner's Release and History Signed: yes/no

   The above information was discussed with the buyer and/or representative during the examination.

Signature: _____

Witnesses: _____

_____

Prepurchase Examination History
(Owner/Agent to fill out)

Date: _____ Time: _____   Location: _____

Owner: _____   Agent: _____
Address: _____   Address: _____
City, ST: _____   City, ST: _____
Phone: _____   Phone: _____

Horse: _____   Present Use: _____
Breed: _____   Sex: _____ Age: _____
Sire: _____   Dam: _____
Brands & Tattoo: _____
Color & Markings: _____

1. How long have you owned the above-named horse? _____
2. Who was the previous owner? _____
Address: _____ Phone: _____
3. As owner: ___ agent: ___ (check one), I declare that the above-named horse has
not had any medication in the past three weeks, except: _____
_____

4. I further declare that the above-named horse has not had any medical or surgical
treatment except: _____
_____
_____

5. If this horse is a mare, is she pregnant? _____
6. Has this horse's tail carriage been altered? _____
7. To my knowledge, there are no defects in this horse's family, except: _____
_____

8. To my knowledge, this horse does not have any bad habits, except: _____
_____

Vaccines and Date Last Given: _____
_____

Deworming Schedule and Date Last Given: _____
_____

_____
Signature   Date

Fig. 3–12. A questionnaire for the seller. This is only one example: different veterinarians use different forms.

PRINCIPLES OF THERAPY

In this section, the therapeutic procedures and drugs mentioned throughout the book are discussed. Some are treatments that the owner or trainer can perform. Others are only performed by a veterinarian. The treatments are discussed in fairly general terms. Specific recommendations are given in later chapters, which deal with particular lameness problems.

4

PHYSICAL THERAPIES

The goal of any therapy should be to help the body heal itself. The body is programmed to repair damaged tissues, including bone, tendons, ligaments, etc., and will attempt to do so if given an opportunity. Often people claim success with a particular therapy, when it was the body's own healing processes that were responsible. Some conditions resolve or substantially improve without treatment if the horse is rested for long enough. However, in most instances the owner or trainer desires a rapid return to training

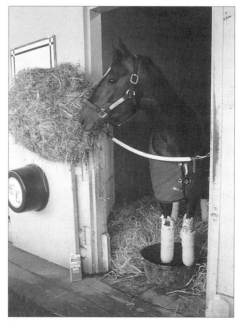

Fig. 4–1.

and competition. *This result can only be achieved with early, accurate diagnosis, and prompt and appropriate treatment.* Early veterinary intervention can often prevent further damage and secondary problems, allowing healing to proceed.

Healing always takes time. However, it may be assisted (and sometimes accelerated) in various ways. The choice of therapy and its success are determined by the diagnosis: which tissues are damaged, and to what extent. There are degrees of tissue damage, ranging from mild inflammation to complete disruption. *(Figure 4–2 illustrates this concept using bone and tendon injuries as examples.)* A single traumatic event may cause complete disruption if the tissue is suddenly and massively overloaded. But in other cases tissue damage may be the result of repeated stress and strain on the tissue. Over a period of days, weeks, or even months, the stress finally leads to breakdown.

DEGREES OF TISSUE DAMAGE

Tendon Injuries	Bone Injuries
bruise (bump or kick)	bruise (bump or kick)
strain (fibrous covering stretched)	periosteal tear (fibrous covering torn)
mild tendonitis (a few fibers damaged)	microfracture
bowed tendon (many fibers damaged)	incomplete fracture
tendon rupture	complete fracture

Fig. 4–2. Different degrees of tissue damage, from mild inflammation to complete breakdown. Tendon and bone injuries are used as examples.

An experienced veterinarian uses the diagnostic tools discussed in Chapter 2 to determine the nature and extent of the tissue damage. Pain—often seen as lameness—is usually the symptom that owners and trainers first notice and about which they are most concerned.

But assessing the degree of pain is not necessarily a good way to gauge the severity of tissue damage. Again using bone and tendon injuries as examples, a superficial bone problem, such as bucked shins, is often more painful than a severe tendon injury, such as a bowed tendon. Furthermore, within a particular tissue, pain does not always increase in proportion to the severity of the injury or the size of the damaged area. For example, a "stone bruise" can be just as painful as a pedal bone fracture. To complicate matters even more, the outward signs of pain can vary among horses. Some horses are very stoic; others appear to be overly sensitive to pain.

Pain relief is one of the main goals of therapy, both for the horse's comfort and the owner's peace of mind. However, pain is "nature's cast"—the body's way of slowing activity or immobilizing an area to protect the injured tissues. *Relieving pain without addressing the cause can be harmful,* especially if the horse is permitted unrestricted activity or continued in training.

REST

Rest from training and competition is the most valuable resource there is. The body can repair most tissue damage once the cause and any aggravating factors are removed. In athletic horses, vigorous exercise often causes or aggravates an injury.

Rest does not necessarily mean stall confinement. Some conditions (for example, chronic joint disease and intramuscular injection reactions) are improved by daily light exercise. Other conditions, in particular exertional rhabdomyolysis ("tying up"), may actually be brought on by stall confinement.

Throughout this book, rest just means a break from the regular training and competition schedule. For minor injuries this may involve decreasing the workload but continuing some type of regular exercise. Or, giving the horse a few days off may be all that is necessary before returning to the normal training schedule.

More Information
See Chapter 8 for information on joint disease.
See Chapter 10 for information on muscle problems, including IM injection reactions and exertional rhabdomyolysis.

For more serious injuries, the rest period may be divided into three phases:

- Restriction phase—confinement in a stall or small paddock. This phase may last for as little as a few days, or as long as a few months, depending on the injury.
- Regeneration phase—paddock or pasture turnout. This phase can last from a few weeks to several months.
- Rehabilitation phase—a program of light, controlled exercise that gradually increases in intensity. This phase prepares the horse for the return to normal activities or another type of regular activity.

Restriction Phase

The ideal environment for the restriction phase of the rest period depends on the condition being treated. For example, fractures and wounds require immobility for best healing in the initial stages, so the veterinarian recommends stall confinement. In contrast, some muscle and tendon problems heal best when the horse is allowed limited activity, such as is provided by a small paddock.

Another point to consider is the horse's temperament. Some horses do not respond well to confinement. They are in more danger of aggravating the injury if they remain stabled than if they are kept in a pen or small paddock. Restless or excitable behavior may also result in a new problem that could prolong the rest period. In some cases the new injury is more serious than the initial condition.

Having an appropriate facility is sometimes another factor that influences where the horse spends the rest period. If the veterinarian advises stall confinement, but a suitable stall is not available, the horse's owner needs to make other arrangements. The horse may have to be moved to another facility for the confinement period.

It is important to note that pasture turnout is not a suitable substitute for stall or paddock confinement. Some horses, particularly young, fit horses, are so excitable or active that they exercise in the pasture almost as much as when they are in training.

Stall Confinement

When a horse is confined to a stall for more than about 24 hours, its grain should be reduced by at least half, or stopped altogether. The horse's energy requirements are much less while it is being rested than when it is exercised regularly. Continuing to feed the horse grain while it is not being exercised can lead to exertional rhabdomyolysis, laminitis, and gastro-intestinal problems. Reducing the grain also helps to keep the horse settled and calm, and helps to control its body weight. These are important considerations when managing musculoskeletal problems.

For healthy digestion and attitude, good quality grass hay should always be available, or fed in small amounts throughout the day. The other basics—clean water, fresh air, light, and good bedding—should not be overlooked, especially if the horse is to be confined for several weeks. The space, feed, and water require-

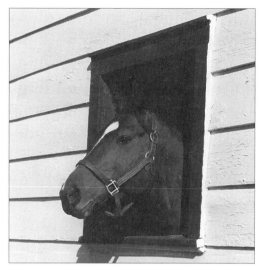

Fig. 4–3. It is important to keep the horse calm in the stall.

ments of a mare and her nursing foal are greater than those of a single horse, no matter how young the foal. These factors must be considered when confining a mare and foal.

It is important to find the best way to keep the horse calm in the stall. Many horses prefer the company of other horses, and are more settled when they can see and hear other horses. Some horses are overexcited by other horses, and should be confined in a quiet area with limited horse activity. Other horses are not choosy about the company of horses, but they may be overexcited by a particular person, other animals (dogs, cattle, donkeys, etc.), or vehicles. Finding what makes the horse overexcited and avoiding these factors is very important. This will ensure that stall confinement is uneventful, and successful in its purpose of promoting healing.

Paddock Confinement

The ideal paddock size for restriction is between 24- and 48-feet square. The square shape makes it easier to catch the horse in a corner. The size provides enough room for the horse to move about, yet not be so active that it injures itself or reinjures the damaged area. (This paddock size is also useful for exercising a mare and foal.)

If such a paddock is not available, a larger paddock can often be modified to fit these specifications. Owners and trainers who plan to rest injured horses on a regular basis should construct at least one

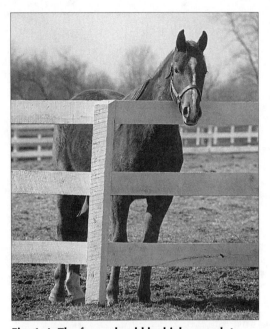

Fig. 4–4. The fence should be high enough to discourage the horse from jumping out.

such paddock. The fence should be at least 4 feet high to discourage spirited horses from jumping out. Good fencing materials for this paddock are steel pipe, or timber posts and solid wire mesh (either V-mesh or 2-by-4 wire).

The best type of footing for this paddock is sand. It drains well in wet weather, does not turn to mud, and is excellent for preventing or managing laminitis. The paddock should be close to the barn. That way the horse does not have to walk very far from its stall to the paddock, and the staff always has the horse in view. The footing between the barn and the paddock should be firm and free of rocks. Shade in the paddock is important in the warmer months. In the winter, having an open aspect allows the paddock to dry out quickly. When planning a rehabilitation paddock, planting trees that lose their leaves in the fall suits the purpose best. When planted just outside the paddock, they provide shade in summer and allow the paddock to dry out in winter.

Regeneration Phase

After stall or small paddock confinement, the veterinarian may recommend turning the horse out into a larger paddock or pasture. The restriction phase allowed the damaged tissue(s) to heal, unhindered by the strain of activity. The regeneration phase is aimed at giving the healed tissues time to regain sufficient strength to withstand the rigors of training. For example, radiographs may show that the fracture has healed in only 6 – 8 weeks. But the bone may take several months to increase its density and strength enough for training and competition. Thus, for serious injuries this second phase of the rest period is just as important as the initial restriction phase.

Pasture turnout has some other benefits. First, even a small amount of activity can limit the restrictive effects of scar tissue in the healed area. Scar (fibrous) tissue is relatively inelastic. When it forms between two tissues that normally move against one another (such as two muscles), it can restrict normal movement. Second, activity helps the horse regain some of the muscle tone it may have lost during stall confinement.

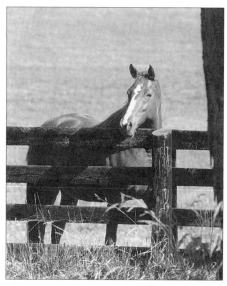

Fig. 4–5. The regeneration phase gives the healed tissues time to regain strength.

If the horse has been confined to a stall or small pen for several weeks, it may be inclined to be too active when first turned out. It is often best to put the horse in a small paddock for a few days. This allows the horse to get used to its freedom before being turned out into the pasture. If this is not possible, the veterinarian can sedate the horse before turning it out. However, some horses take a few days to settle down in the pasture. It is usually not practical, and may not be safe, to keep the horse sedated for that long.

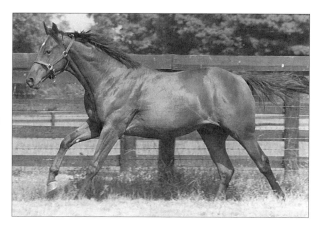

Fig. 4–6. Some horses take a few days to settle down in the pasture.

The length of the pasture turnout phase depends on which tissues were damaged, the extent of the tissue damage, and the rate of healing. It also depends on the horse, the type of work the horse must perform, and the training and competition schedule. So, it is sometimes very difficult to give specific recommendations for a particular problem. (**Note:** Throughout this book, general guidelines for restriction and pasture rest are given for each condition. However, these times are quite broad, and are included to just give an idea of the average time required.)

The veterinarian usually re-evaluates the horse toward the end of the recommended rest period. If the horse is still lame, pasture rest must continue (or the problem must be re-evaluated). If the horse is not lame, and the veterinarian is satisfied that the injury has completely healed, the horse can begin the rehabilitation phase.

Rehabilitation Phase

How quickly the horse can be returned to its normal activity level depends on the nature and severity of the injury, and the length of time the horse has been rested. Unless the horse has been out of work for only 1 – 2 weeks, the return to regular exercise and training should be gradual. No matter how pressing the competition schedule, the horse should not be pushed through this phase more quickly than recommended by the veterinarian. It is not worth the risk of reinjury for the sake of a few weeks or one competition.

In most cases a program of light and gradually increasing (graded) daily exercise is the best approach. The factors that may be gradually increased during rehabilitation are:

- **Speed**—Most graded exercise programs begin with walking, either hand-walking, "ponying," or riding. They gradually increase to trotting or cantering over a period of days or weeks, depending on the injury.
- **Duration**—An exercise session may last for only 5 – 10 minutes at first. It is then gradually lengthened over several days or weeks.
- **Slope**—Exercise should initially be restricted to a level surface. Hill work should not be introduced until the horse's fitness and the particular injury allow. If a treadmill is used, the slope or incline can be gradually increased week by week.

The owner or trainer should merely *exercise* the horse, and not actively train it during the rehabilitation period. The aim is to allow the body time to strengthen the healed tissue(s) in response to the gradually increasing workload. Too vigorous or prolonged activity for the sake of teaching the horse or improving fitness can slow this process, and may cause reinjury.

If training has been suspended for several weeks or longer, the horse must be conditioned after the rehabilitation phase as if it were just beginning a new training program. Although it may have been exercising regularly for several weeks (as rehabilitation), the horse may not be fit enough for regular activities.

Other Options

If appropriate facilities are available, and the horse is cooperative, the horse's activity level may be graded by placing it in a larger enclosure every

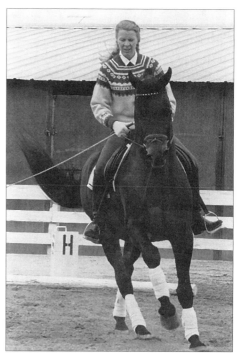

Fig. 4–7. Active training can slow healing, and may cause reinjury.

couple of weeks. For example, the horse may graduate from a 12 x 12 foot stall, to a 24 x 24 foot paddock, to a larger paddock, and then to a pasture. One advantage to this approach is that the horse is less likely to race around the pasture than if it was moved directly from a stall to the pasture. However, the amount of exercise a horse takes in the pasture varies from one horse to the next. Some lazy horses get little or no exercise, while other horses constantly race around the fences. It is often better to longe, ride, or drive the horse each day, rather than relying on how active the horse is in the pasture.

Swimming promotes or maintains cardiovascular fitness without placing any load on the legs. It can be very useful for rehabilitating some joint and tendon injuries. However, swimming and wading are not advisable after most muscle injuries because the horse must work hard against the water. Also, swimming in a pool, pond, or tank is not recommended after surgical procedures or wounds, until the skin has completely healed. The water can contain harmful bacteria that could cause wound infection.

Light Exercise as Therapy

Some conditions benefit from light exercise during the initial healing stages. Exercise can aid the healing process in several ways:

- Activity stimulates blood flow, which is essential for healing.
- Movement prevents or limits adhesion formation (fibrous bands) between tissues that normally move against one another, such as a tendon and its surrounding sheath.
- Gentle exercise puts a little tension on the injured area. This encourages the body to lay down collagen fibers (repair tissue) in the direction of the greatest load.
- Regular activity is important for the horse's morale. It may also reduce the chances of the horse galloping off and injuring itself further when first let out after a long period of stall confinement.

Regular exercise can also help prevent colic, exertional rhabdomyolysis ("tying up"), and respiratory diseases, particularly chronic obstructive pulmonary disease (COPD). These problems are far more common in stabled horses than in horses kept in a paddock or pasture.

If the aim is simply to stimulate circulation and give a stabled horse an outing, the horse can be grazed on a lead for 20 – 30 minutes. Or it can be quietly walked around on a level, even surface for 10 – 15 minutes, two or three times per day. This is usually enough to resolve fluid buildup in the lower legs ("stocking up") and to give the

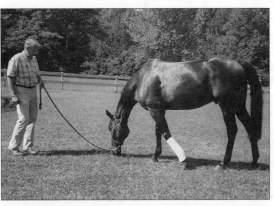

Fig. 4–8. Grazing a horse gives it fresh air and improves its attitude.

horse some fresh air and a new outlook. However, the horse should not be grazed or walked if there is any risk of aggravating the injury.

Most tendon and ligament injuries heal best when a light, graded exercise program is begun within a few days of injury. With these injuries, inactivity can slow or prevent the tissue's return to normal function. It may also lengthen the overall rest period.

Regular Exercise for Chronic Disease

Daily exercise can improve or help manage several chronic or recurrent conditions. Degenerative joint disease, exertional rhabdomyolysis, and sacro-iliac subluxation are three such conditions. The goal is to prevent the problem from returning, or minimize its effects so that the horse can continue to be as useful as the condition allows. Prolonged periods of inactivity in horses with such problems could end the horse's working life.

> **More Information**
>
> Tendon and ligament injuries are common in athletic horses. Managing them with a graded exercise program is covered in Chapter 11.

BANDAGING & SPLINTING

Bandages have many uses, from wound management to support. It is common for the veterinarian to bandage a horse's foot or leg and advise the owner or trainer to monitor and change the bandage regularly. This section deals with the practical details of bandaging the feet and legs, and monitoring the bandage.

Applying a splint to an injured leg is an important first-aid technique with which every owner and trainer should be familiar. This section also discusses the practical aspects of splint placement.

Materials

Standard Bandage

The following materials are needed for a standard bandage: wound dressings, padding, bandages, and adhesive tape.

Wound Dressings

Sterile, non-stick dressings, or antiseptic ointment and gauze pads are best for covering wounds under bandages. These materials make dressing changes less painful for the horse, and less disruptive to the wound surface. They may be purchased at any drug store.

Padding

Padding beneath the bandage is very important for applying a comfortable and effective bandage that does not slip or cause pressure sores (discussed later).

Materials that are suitable for padding underneath the bandage include roll cotton, sheet cotton, "Combine" dressing, large-size disposable baby diapers, and quilted leg wraps. The padding material should be long enough to wrap around the leg at least once, and wide enough to cover the lower leg from the coronet to the knee or hock.

Bandages

The choice of bandage depends on its purpose, and on the veterinarian's preference. The most suitable bandage width for wrapping horses' legs is 4 inches (10 cm). This width is easy to handle, conforms to the leg better than wider bandages, and covers the leg more evenly and economically than narrower bandages. One or a combination of the following bandage types may be used.

Lightweight Gauze Bandages

Lightweight gauze, non-stretch bandages generally are only used under a more substantial bandage. They are good for smoothing out the padding and providing an even, well-contoured base for the outer bandage. They are inexpensive and easy to apply, but they usually cannot be reused.

Stable or Track Bandages

Stable or track bandages are good for support wraps and for protecting the legs during exercise or transport. However, they do not provide as much tension as stretch bandages, which is important when applying pressure wraps (discussed later). Stable or track bandages can be washed and reused, and so are a good choice for bandaging over wounds.

Self-adhesive, Conforming Bandages

Self-adhesive, conforming (or stretch) bandages, such as Vetrap™ or Co-Flex™, are very good general-use bandages. However, they often do not provide as much support or protection as the thicker stable or track bandages. The self-adhesive bandages conform to the leg very well. But it is possible to put them on too tightly if there is not enough padding beneath them. These bandages can be reused once or twice if they are carefully removed.

Adhesive Bandages

Adhesive bandages, such as Elastikon®, provide good support and protection. They conform to the leg well, and can be applied with enough tension to make an effective pressure bandage. However, they are generally more expensive than other disposable bandages.

Adhesive Tape

A roll of 1-inch (2.5 cm) wide adhesive tape, such as masking tape, is often useful for securing the end of the bandage.

Foot Bandage

Some specific materials are needed for bandaging the foot:

- A sterile dressing or piece of roll cotton soaked in iodine solution—used to cover wounds or deep defects in the hoof wall or sole.
- A plastic bag or heavy duty plastic wrap—used to cover the dressing and encase the entire foot, making the bandage waterproof.
- Or, a disposable baby diaper—used as a combined dressing and waterproof padding material. The diaper should be big enough to cover the entire foot and lower pastern. For most adult horses at least a medium size diaper is needed.
- Adhesive bandage or water-resistant adhesive tape (e.g. duct tape)—used to secure the bandage in place.

(The technique for applying a foot bandage is described later.)

Splint

To effectively immobilize the lower leg, extra padding and bandaging materials are needed. With foals and small ponies, two layers of padding-and-bandage may be all that is required. But with larger horses, extra support may be necessary. A common splint material is 4-inch

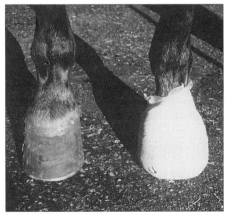

Fig. 4–9. A foot bandage, using plastic and Elastikon.

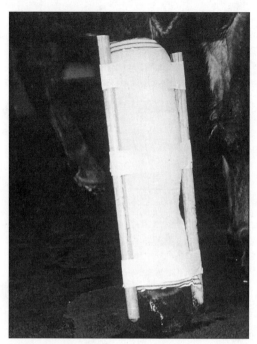

Fig. 4–10. A splint on an adult horse.

(10 cm) diameter PVC pipe, cut lengthwise in half or thirds. Narrow pieces of wood, cut to fit, also make good splints. *(Correct splint length and placement are discussed later.)*

Bandaging Techniques
Standard Bandage

No matter what the purpose of the bandage, some basic principles should be followed. One approach to applying a standard bandage is described below:

1. Adequately restrain the horse before applying the bandage. The safest position for applying a bandage to a horse's leg is squatting down beside the leg—not in front of, or underneath the horse. It is not safe to kneel or sit beside the horse in case it moves suddenly.

2. Remove all dirt, mud, and debris (including shavings) from the leg. If it has been washed, or a wound has been cleansed, thoroughly dry the leg. Otherwise moist dermatitis (skin irritation from constant moisture) may develop under the bandage.

3. If there is a wound on the leg, place a sterile non-stick dressing, or antiseptic ointment and a gauze pad over it before bandaging the leg.

4. Apply at least one layer of thick (minimum ¼ inch, or 6 mm, compressed) padding to the leg. Add a second layer if the first is not thick enough. Wrap the padding around the leg and overlap it. Smooth out the wrinkles so the padding conforms to the leg, and there are no folds of padding to create areas of extra pressure on the skin. The padding (and bandage) must extend to the joints above and below the affected area. For example, rather than only bandaging the middle of the can-

non, extend the bandage from the fetlock to the base of the knee. This minimizes swelling above and below the bandage, and reduces the risk of pressure sores under the bandage.

5. Begin the bandage about ½ inch (1.2 cm) from the top or the bottom of the padding—not in the middle. To prevent the padding from loosening while applying the bandage, have someone hold it in place, or use short pieces of masking tape to anchor it.

6. Unroll the bandage onto the leg with the roll facing outward, not in toward the leg. Overlap the beginning of the bandage once to anchor it in place. Then unroll the bandage, working down (or up) the leg in a spiral, each turn of the bandage covering one-third to one-half of the previous turn. Apply the bandage with even tension all the way down the leg. When the bottom of the padding is reached, spiral the bandage back up (or down) the leg until it is completely unwrapped. **Note:** Leave about ½ inch of padding exposed at the top and bottom of the bandage.

7. If the bandage does not have Velcro® tabs, secure the end of the bandage with a few pieces of masking tape. (Even if the bandage has tabs, masking tape can be used for added security.) *Do not wrap the tape all the way around the leg—this can create a ring of excess pressure.* Instead, cut a couple of 3-inch (7.5 cm) lengths of tape. Fold each strip over at one end, creating a tab for easy removal. Then stick the strips side-by-side over the end of the bandage.

8. Check the tension of the bandage by inserting two fingers, flat against the leg, at the top or bottom. It should be possible to slide the fingers underneath the bandage and have them fit snugly. If the bandage is too tight or too loose, it should be removed and reapplied.

9. Wrap a couple of layers of adhesive bandage (such as Elastikon) around the top and bottom of the bandage, catching both the hair (or hoof wall) and the bandage with each turn. This pre-

Extra Information

The easiest place to begin a bandage is in the middle of the leg, because this prevents the padding from unraveling. However, this makes the bandage tighter in the middle, rather than having even pressure along its length. Uneven tension can cause pressure sores, especially over the tendons.

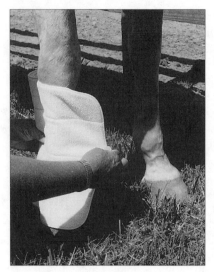

Fig. 4–11. Apply at least one layer of thick padding to the leg.

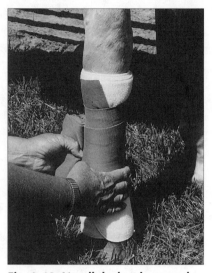

Fig. 4–12. Unroll the bandage, working down (or up) the leg in a spiral.

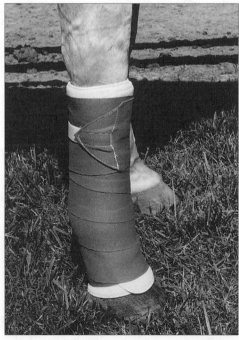

Fig. 4–13. Completed standard bandage.

vents bedding material and dirt from working its way under the bandage. Before applying the adhesive bandage, unroll, then loosely reroll the first 12 inches (30 cm). This makes it less likely that the adhesive bandage will be applied too tightly.

Bandaging the Knee

It is difficult to keep a bandage on the knee because the leg narrows just below the knee. The bandage loosens as the horse flexes its knee when it moves and lies down. Another problem with bandaging the knee is that pressure sores quickly form over the bony points at the back and the inside of the leg. Applying a firm bandage to the knee prevents slipping, but it makes pressure sores more likely.

These problems can be prevented by first applying a standard bandage from the pastern or fetlock to the bottom of the knee. The standard bandage acts as a base for the knee bandage. A light layer of padding is then applied to the knee, and the knee is bandaged in either a spiral or a figure-eight pattern. It often helps if a layer of lightweight gauze bandage is placed over the padding. The gauze smooths it out and makes a snug, well-contoured base for the outer bandage. This outer bandage can be a self-adhesive conforming bandage, or an adhesive bandage. With either method (spiral or figure-eight), the bony point at

> ### Definition
>
> The bony point at the back of the knee is the accessory carpal bone.
>
> The bony point on the inside of the leg is the distal radial eminence.
>
> (See Chapter 18 for illustrations.)

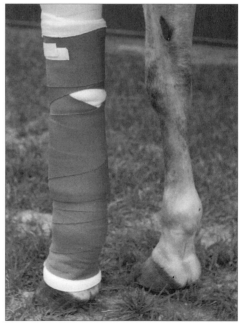

Fig. 4–14. A knee bandage using a standard bandage as a base. The bony point at the back has been left out.

the back should be left out. That is, the bandage should go around, not over it.

Bandages tend to loosen over the front of the knee and tighten at the back of the knee. So these areas should be checked at least twice per day, and the bandage replaced as needed. For added security, a couple of layers of adhesive bandage can be wrapped around the top of the knee bandage. *(See Step 9, in the earlier section on applying a Standard Bandage.)*

Sometimes the bandage is only needed for a day or so. In these cases the veterinarian may apply a light wrap to the knee using an adhesive bandage over very little padding, and no standard bandage below. This method is often used to protect the incisions after ar-throscopic surgery. The adhesive bandage can be stuck to the hair above and below the knee for added security. Some veterinarians prefer to bandage over the bony projections and then cut a slit in the bandage over the accessory carpal bone. However, care is needed to avoid cutting the skin.

Bandaging the Hock

The hock can also be a difficult area to bandage effectively. Hock bandages often slip or loosen, and pressure sores tend to develop over the point of the hock, and along the back of the Achilles ten-dons. As described for the knee, a standard bandage can be applied to the lower leg, up to the base of the hock. A light layer of padding and a bandage is then applied in a spiral pattern, starting at the base of the hock and working upward.

The bandage stays in place better, and pressure sores are less likely if it is a little firmer on the lower part of the hock (up to, but not in-cluding the point of the hock). It should be a little looser on the up-per part of the hock. An extra strip of padding along the Achilles tendons and over the point of the hock may also help prevent pressure sores. It is not necessary to leave the point of the hock exposed—this can create excess pressure over the Achilles tendons. The figure-eight pattern does not work well on the hock. The bandage often slips into two sections and creates pressure over the Achilles tendons *(see Figure 4–16).*

A layer of lightweight gauze bandage over the padding, and a couple of layers of adhesive bandage at the top can help

Definition

The Achilles tendons are the large pair of tendons at the back of the thigh, which attach onto the point of the hock.

(See Chapter 20 for an illustration.)

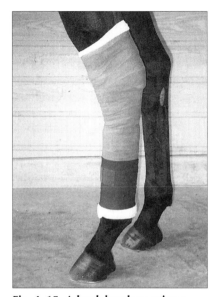

Fig. 4–15. A hock bandage using a standard bandage as a base, and including the point of the hock.

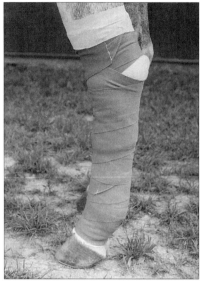

Fig. 4–16. This hock bandage places too much pressure on the Achilles tendons.

secure the bandage. Some veterinarians apply an adhesive bandage directly to the hock, as described for bandaging the knee.

Bandaging the Foot

There are several ways to bandage a foot. Any method that keeps the bandage in place and dry, and that does not create pressure sores is suitable. One method that is quick, easy, and economical uses disposable baby diapers and duct tape. The diaper should be large enough to encase the entire hoof and the lower part of the pastern.

With the leg raised, any necessary medication, poultice, or dressing is applied to the foot. The diaper is placed over the bottom of the foot, plastic side out, and wrapped up over the hoof wall and heels. The foot is then wrapped in duct tape so that the whole hoof is encased. To prevent slipping, the bandage should extend to the middle of the pastern. When wrapping the hoof wall, quite a bit of tension can be used, but the bandage should not be tight around the coronary band or pastern. The "two finger" method of checking the tension also applies to this bandage. *(See Step 8, in the earlier section on applying a Standard Bandage.)* To prevent bedding material or dirt from getting into the bandage, the duct tape should be continued up

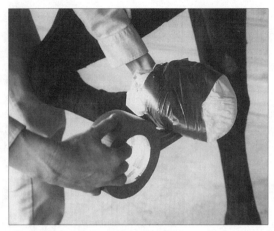

Fig. 4–17. Applying a foot bandage.

over the top of the bandage, loosely sticking it to the hair *(as described in Step 9)*.

If other padding material is used instead of a diaper, a sheet of plastic should be placed over the dressing or padding before the foot is bandaged. It is important that the bottom of the foot is not packed with so much dressing material that it puts pressure on the sole when the horse is standing. This causes pain, and may even cause sole bruising.

Active horses quickly wear through the bottom of the foot bandage, especially at the toe. To prevent this, an extra layer or two of tape can be wrapped around the ground surface of the hoof wall at the toe. Alternatively, a strip of rubber tire inner tube can be taped to the bottom of the foot at the toe. In all cases the horse should be confined to a clean stall or a small paddock that has a soft, dry surface.

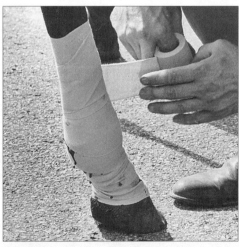

Fig. 4–18. Applying a pressure bandage over a bleeding wound.

Pressure Bandage

A pressure bandage is often necessary to stop hemorrhage from a wound. It is a modification of the standard bandage described earlier. Ideally, a sterile dressing should be placed over the wound, and a thin layer of padding material applied around the leg. Although any kind of bandage will do in an emergency, the self-adhesive conforming bandages (such as Vetrap and

Co-flex) are best. They are easy to put on with speed and tension, and they need no extra fasteners.

A pressure bandage should be applied firmly enough to stop, or at least slow the bleeding. If the bleeding continues, a second bandage should be applied over the first. However, such a tight bandage should not be left on the leg for more than 15 – 20 minutes. This is usually enough time for most wounds to stop bleeding. *(Managing bleeding wounds is discussed in Chapter 13.)*

Another type of pressure bandage may be used to reduce swelling and edema in a leg. The same amount of padding recommended for a standard bandage should be used for this pressure wrap. The bandage should begin at or below the coronet, and extend up the leg as far as the swelling goes (or as far as is practical). It is important to start wrapping the bandage at the coronet. In this way the tissue fluid is forced up and out of the leg as the bandage is applied. The bandage should be firm, but not as tight as the pressure bandage used to control hemor-

> ## Definition
>
> **Edema:** accumulation of tissue fluid, causing swelling.
>
> **(Limb edema can be mild or severe, involving one leg or all four legs. Causes and management are discussed in Chapter 13.)**

rhage. As the swelling goes down, the bandage becomes a little looser, so it is not necessary to remove it any sooner than a normal bandage.

Exercise Bandages

Exercise bandages are used to protect the lower legs from trauma, such as interference. They also give the fetlock joint, flexor tendons, and suspensory ligament a little support during strenuous activities. Overextension of the fetlock occurs during exercise. In extreme cases the back of the fetlock hits the ground. This amount of joint extension places extra strain on the flexor tendons, suspensory ligament, and sesamoid bones.

The standard bandage described earlier does not provide much resistance to fetlock overextension during strenuous exercise. But there are exercise bandages that "sling" the back of the fetlock. They can reduce fetlock overextension, without restricting normal joint motion or significantly affecting the horse's gait. The bandages are applied directly to the legs without padding. They should be put on just before exercise, and removed immediately afterward.

"Rundown" bandages and "speed patches" usually consist of adhesive bandages that are applied without padding around the fetlocks.

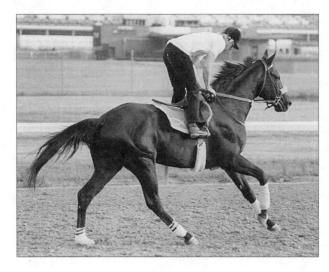

Fig. 4–19. Exercise
bandages protect
the lower legs
from trauma.

They are used to protect the skin over the backs of the fetlocks from injury during strenuous exercise, such as galloping. They should be applied just before exercise, and removed immediately afterward.

Monitoring and Changing the Bandage

Whenever a bandage is left on for more than a few hours, it must be checked at least twice per day for the following signs:

- looseness, slipping, or twisting
- swelling above or below the bandage
- wetness
- odor
- lameness or discomfort (rubbing or chewing, and stamping)

If any of these signs is noticed, the bandage should be removed and the leg inspected closely before another bandage is applied.

How frequently a bandage needs to be changed depends on its purpose. For example, a support bandage can be left in place for a few days, provided it was correctly applied and the horse remains comfortable. In contrast, bandages that cover wounds need to be changed more frequently, particularly if the wound is oozing. A bandage over an open (unsutured) wound may need to be changed every day at first, so that the wound can be inspected and the soiled padding replaced. Frequently changing the bandage in these cases can help prevent moist dermatitis under the bandage, and may also prevent wound infection. However, in wounds with extensive skin loss, changing the dressing too often can upset the granulation bed and slow wound healing *(see Chapter 13)*.

Wounds that involve open joints or tendon sheaths leak much more fluid than other types of wounds. In these cases the bandage may need to be changed two or three times per day, or as often as necessary to keep the wound clean and the padding dry. This also prevents bacterial growth in the bandage.

Except for when wearing exercise bandages, the horse should be confined to a stall or small paddock while the leg is bandaged. This helps prevent the bandage from being soiled or loosened. It also reduces movement in the injured area. Under no circumstances should a horse be put in a large paddock or pasture and left unattended while wearing a bandage. If the end of the bandage comes undone and the bandage unravels, the horse may become frightened or trip on the end of the bandage. Either way, the horse may be seriously injured.

Bandage Chewing

The most common reason why horses chew on their bandages is *discomfort:*

• the bandage may be too tight
• a pressure sore may have developed under the bandage
• the bandage may be loose and irritating the wound
• shavings or dirt may be trapped beneath the bandage
• the bandage may be wet, and moist dermatitis has developed
• the wound may be infected and causing discomfort (independent of the bandage)

Some horses chew at their bandages just to amuse themselves, especially if they are bored. In this situation, there are several things that can be tried:

1. A diversion, such as hay or a stall toy.
2. Commercial products that taste terrible and so discourage bandage chewing.
3. Restraint devices, such as a neck cradle or cross-ties.

But it is more important to find out why the horse is chewing at the bandage than to find a way to prevent it from doing so. The bandage should be removed and the leg carefully inspected for a source of irritation before it is assumed that the horse is just bored or misbehaving.

Pressure Sores

Bandages that are too tight can cut off the blood supply to the skin and underlying tissues. This can cause a pressure sore if the bandage is left on for more than a few hours. Pressure sores occur most often over the back of the flexor tendons and the front of the cannon. They can also develop around the fetlock (particularly the front and back), around the coronet and heel bulbs, and over the bony prominences of the knee and hock. The thickening that develops before a pressure sore over the flexor tendons is commonly called a "bandage bow" *(see Chapter 11).*

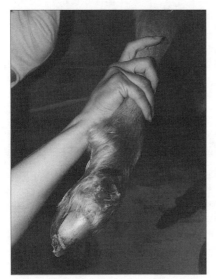 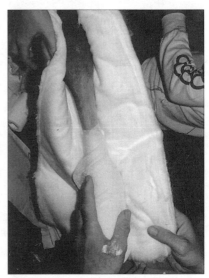

Fig. 4–20. Left: A pressure sore on the pastern of a young foal. Right: The veterinarian places extra padding over this area before reapplying the splint.

Pressure sores can become worse before they improve. Some skin may be lost with the bandage, but it often takes several days for all of the dead skin to slough (lift away). Once they have healed, pressure sores may leave a permanent scar or white hairs at the site. *(Treating pressure sores is discussed in Chapter 13.)*

To prevent pressure sores, plenty of padding should be used, and the bandage applied with even tension over its entire length. It must be checked at least twice per day and the horse monitored for signs of discomfort (bandage chewing or rubbing, stamping, and lameness). Tight pressure bandages should not be left on for more than 15 – 20 minutes.

Splinting Techniques

Veterinarians use splints for a variety of treatment purposes, including stabilizing a joint after dislocation and correcting angular or flexural limb deformities in young foals. But there are also situations in which the owner or trainer must apply a splint as a first-aid procedure. For example, a lacerated flexor tendon or a fracture below the knee or hock needs immediate splinting to avoid further damage. It is important to support and protect the injured area while waiting for the veterinarian to arrive, or before transporting the horse to a veterinary hospital.

Using Bandage Materials

A thick bandage can act like a splint if enough padding material is used and the overlying bandage is applied firmly. To be effective, the bandage must extend from the hoof to the joint above the injured area. At least two layers of thick padding should be used and the bandage applied with as much tension as possible. (As long as plenty of padding is used, pressure sores will not result from such a firm bandage.) It is often necessary to add another layer or two of thick padding and a firm bandage over the first one to immobilize the leg.

This type of bandage is called a modified Robert Jones bandage. It is most useful for immobilizing the joints of the lower leg, although it can stabilize the knee or hock if it is extended to just below the elbow or stifle. It is a very comfortable bandage, but it uses quite a lot of bandage material. A suitable alternative can be constructed with pillows or blankets, and stable bandages. *The key is to*

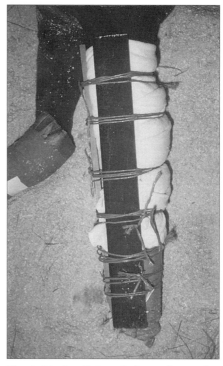

Fig. 4–21. A splint made from pieces of wood and baling twine. The foot is included in the bandage and splint.

use plenty of padding and apply the overlying bandage with as much tension as possible so that the horse cannot flex its leg.

Using PVC or Wood Splints

Struts of PVC pipe (cut lengthwise in half or thirds) or wood can add stability to a bandage for injuries of the lower leg. A standard bandage with plenty of padding should be applied from the hoof to the joint above the injured area. The splints can then be firmly taped to the outside of the bandage with duct tape. In an emergency, rope or baling twine will do, as long as it is tied firmly over plenty of padding.

The exact placement of the splints depends on the injury. In most cases it is best to use two splints: one at the side and one at the front or back of the leg. When in doubt, use more splints, rather than less. The goal is to immobilize the leg until the veterinarian can assess the injury.

No matter where the splints are placed, they should extend from the ground to the top of the bandage. When splinting a fracture or severed flexor tendon, a splint should be applied to the front or back

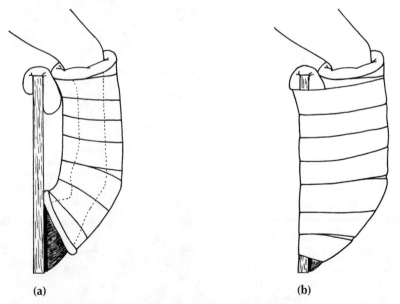

(a)   (b)

Fig. 4–22. Applying a splint for a severe lower leg injury:

(a) Apply a standard bandage to the leg. Flex the horse's fetlock slightly and place the foot flat against the splint. (Add padding at the top if necessary.)

(b) Firmly tape or bandage the leg to the splint.

of the leg so that the horse cannot place the foot flat and bear weight on the leg. This can be achieved by applying the splint while the toe is pointed. It is often easiest to apply this splint to the front of the leg. But if the horse is trying to place the foot flat or put weight on the leg, the splint provides more stability if it is placed at the back of the leg. The fetlock is slightly flexed and the foot is flat against the splint.

Upper Leg Injuries

To effectively support an injured area, the bandage and splints should immobilize the joints above and below. However, it is not possible to immobilize the elbow or stifle this way. Nevertheless, for fractures of the upper leg, bandaging and splinting as far up the leg as possible prevents movement at the knee or hock, and stops the leg from swinging below the fracture. This can make the horse more comfortable, and it makes moving a little easier.

A modified Robert Jones bandage or standard bandage with extra padding should be extended to just below the elbow or stifle. A long board or pole (such as a broom handle) should then be firmly taped to the outside of the bandage. It should extend from the ground to the withers for a foreleg injury, or level with the point of the hip for a hindleg injury.

Splinting Foals

Some foals are born with, or develop deviations of the limbs *(see Chapter 14)*. Sometimes veterinarians correct these deviations with splints. Serious problems can result from improper splinting in foals, so this is a procedure that only a veterinarian should perform.

Pressure sores are more likely in a foal than in an adult horse. This is because the foal's skin is thinner, and it has less soft tissue to protect its bony prominences. So, plenty of padding material must be used beneath the splints. The guidelines given earlier for monitoring bandages also apply to foals with splints. Signs of discomfort may not be as obvious in young foals; they should be monitored even more closely than adult horses.

Wherever possible, the foot should not be included in the splint so that the foal is encouraged to place the foot normally and bear weight on the leg. The bottom of the splint can rub on the coronet or pastern and create a wound if the splint extends lower than the bandage. This problem can be prevented by careful bandaging and frequent monitoring.

The splints should not be left on for more than about 8 hours at a time. (Although, if they are applied correctly, the bandages need not

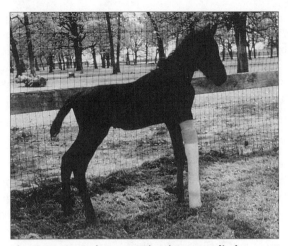

Fig. 4–23. Sometimes veterinarians treat limb deviations in foals by splinting the leg.

be changed this often.) Forcing the legs to straighten can be a painful process for the foal, and pressure sores can develop quickly.

If both legs are splinted (which is often necessary), the foal may have difficulty getting up to nurse with its splints on. Frequently removing the splints, and helping the foal up in between times, ensures that the foal gets enough milk.

Regularly replacing the splints also allows the veterinarian to evaluate the degree of correction, and the need for further treatment. Foals' legs respond very quickly—for better and for worse—so frequent re-evaluation is important. In many cases physical therapy (passive flexion and extension, gentle exercise) and a little time are of more benefit, and cause fewer problems than splints. *(See the later section on Passive Motion Exercises.)*

SPECIFIC PHYSICAL THERAPIES

Rest and controlled exercise are commonly used and effective physical therapies that were discussed earlier. Cold therapy is another common and useful procedure. It is discussed in the *Anti-Inflammatory Therapy* section of Chapter 5. Following are brief discussions about some other physical therapies.

Heat Therapy

Heat causes blood vessel dilation (vasodilation) in the skin and superficial tissues. This improves the blood flow to the injured area, and so can speed healing. However, in the first 2 – 3 days following injury, increasing the blood flow can worsen the swelling and restart bleeding from damaged blood vessels. So, heat therapy should not begin until at least 2 days after injury, particularly if bruising or hemorrhage has occurred. It can be useful at any later time during the healing process, but it has little effect on old, fibrous swellings.

Other benefits of heat therapy include:

- reduced pain by desensitizing (numbing) nerve endings
- relief of muscle spasms
- increased joint mobility by relaxing or softening the surrounding tissues (joint capsule, supporting ligaments, etc.)

Moist heat refers to the use of warm water. Warm hosing, standing the horse in a tub of warm water, or placing a warm, wet cloth over the area are examples of moist heat. "Sweats" and poultices can also provide moist heat. (The primary function of a poultice is to draw fluid from the tissues. But it can also retain, and possibly generate heat if it is applied warm and covered by a bandage.) Liniments and "braces" also generate heat by causing inflammation in the skin. However, their benefit in increasing blood flow to structures beneath the skin is questionable. *(These treatments are discussed in Chapter 5, in the section on Anti-Inflammatory Therapy.)*

Dry heat refers to the use of heating pads and heat lamps, usually visible red or infrared light. No matter which method is used (moist or dry heat), it is important to make sure that the skin is not burned, and the horse does not become overheated. Alternating hot and cold therapy (to cause vasodilation then vasoconstriction) can be useful for reducing soft tissue swellings.

Hydrotherapy

Water can be a useful tool in relieving inflammation and discomfort, and treating wounds. Hosing an inflamed area provides cold or heat therapy, depending on the water temperature. It also stimulates blood flow and lymphatic drainage in the skin and superficial tissues by massaging the area. (The lymphatic system consists of a network of small lymphatic

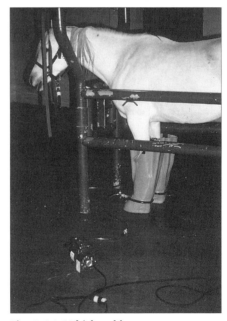

Fig. 4–24. Whirlpool boots.

vessels that drain excess fluid from the tissues and return it to the bloodstream. *See Chapter 13 for more information.*)

The massaging effect is also the main benefit of the whirlpool boot, a device that fits over the horse's leg and is filled with water. Turbulence is created by a small pump that blows air through the water. Walking the horse in small waves at the beach can have the same effect. Sea water is also very good for cleansing wounds. However, pool, pond, and river water may contain harmful bacteria, so these water sources should not be used in horses with surgical or traumatic wounds.

Swimming

Swimming as a form of hydrotherapy or rehabilitation can be very good for restoring and maintaining fitness in horses with foot and leg injuries. There is minimal strain on the lower leg structures while the horse is supported by the water. However, it should not be used for horses with major muscle problems. Swimming is very hard work for the horse, and it can worsen exercise-related conditions such as exertional rhabdomyolysis ("tying up").

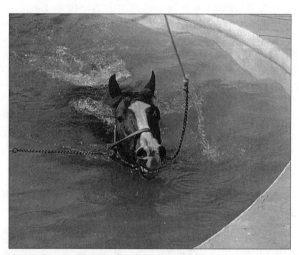

Fig. 4–25. Swimming is good therapy for certain lameness problems.

With any therapy that uses water or moisture, the skin should be thoroughly dried after each treatment. This prevents moist dermatitis (skin irritation from excess moisture).

Massage

Massage is most useful for identifying and relieving muscle spasms, and improving circulation in the skin and superficial tissues. It involves pressing, rubbing, or kneading an area with the fingers and hands. Some therapists also use their elbows or a massage device, such as a tennis ball or wooden roller, for large or deep muscle groups. There are massage machines that do all the work, but there is no substitute for the sensitivity of skilled hands in detecting and treating abnormal areas.

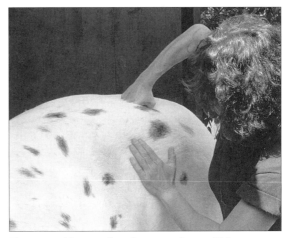

Fig. 4-26. Massage involves pressing, rubbing, or kneading an area with the fingers and hands.

There are several books that include the locations and fiber directions of the major muscle groups of the horse, and descriptions of the various massage techniques. *(Call Equine Research, Inc. at 1-800-848-0225 for the latest publications.)* The main points to remember are 1) do no harm, and 2) use techniques that are comfortable for the therapist and the horse. Relieving a muscle spasm may initially cause the horse some discomfort. However, the pain should not be severe, and should only be temporary if massage is performed correctly.

Areas that are very painful and swollen should not be massaged—this can do more harm than good if the horse has a serious problem. Instead, it is important to have a veterinarian examine the horse to determine why the area is so painful. Infected areas or areas with recent bruising or hemorrhage should not be massaged.

Massage is a procedure that an owner, trainer, or groom can learn and routinely perform. But it is generally worth having an experienced equine therapist evaluate the horse and advise specific massage techniques for the problem area. Either the therapist or the owner or trainer can then continue daily massage until the injury is resolved.

Making a short massage part of the horse's daily routine is an excellent way to detect and treat injuries early; in effect, it is a preventive procedure. Massage prior to exercise can reduce the potential for injury by relaxing the muscles, relieving any muscle spasms, and identifying possible problem areas. It can also calm the horse and improve its attitude.

Passive Motion Exercises

Passive motion is a physical therapy in which the therapist moves a specific part of the horse's body. The horse is only passively involved in the motion.

Movement—flexion, extension, and stretching—can stimulate blood flow to healing tissues. It can also prevent adhesions (restrictive fibrous bands). This therapy is most useful in managing severe joint disease and muscle problems. It can also help foals with flexor contracture, or "contracted tendons."

Flexion/Extension

Gentle, repeated flexion and extension of a joint has several benefits:

• it moves joint fluid around the joint space
• it improves blood flow to the soft tissues of the joint
• it prevents or breaks down fibrin bands within an infected joint—these bands can develop into adhesions
• it prevents fibrosis (fibrous tissue production) in the joint capsule—this helps to maintain joint mobility
• it helps remove pus from the joint in horses with septic arthritis
• it helps prevent or resolve flexor contracture

Flexion/extension involves lifting the horse's leg (if it is standing) and slowly flexing, then extending the joint. The procedure can be repeated 20 – 30 times, at least twice per day. The range of flexion and extension depends on the condition being treated, and on the state of the joint. For example, in horses with severe joint disease, it is best to flex or extend the joint just until resistance is felt or the horse indicates it is uncomfortable. In foals with flexor contracture, it is necessary to extend the joint as far as possible, and hold it in that position for 5 – 10 seconds. But in all cases, flexion/extension should be gradual and never forced.

Some joint conditions, such as septic arthritis, are extremely painful, and it may be necessary to perform these passive motion exercises despite the horse's pain. The benefits outweigh the temporary discomfort. *However, this procedure should never be used without veterinary approval.* It is very important not to be extreme when manipulating these joints. In the early stages of treatment the joint

> ## More Information
>
> Passive motion exercises can mean the difference between a useful joint and a chronically painful joint. Joint structure and joint problems, including septic arthritis, are discussed in Chapter 8.

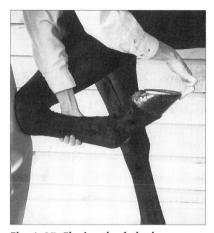 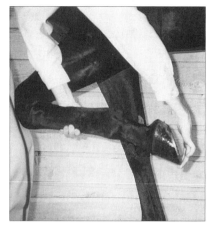

Fig. 4–27. Flexing the fetlock.   Fig. 4–28. Extending the fetlock.

should be flexed and extended only slightly, with just 10 – 12 repetitions per session. As the condition improves, the range of flexion and extension, and the number of repetitions can be increased.

Using heat therapy before flexion/extension can improve the elasticity of the soft tissues (joint capsule, tendons, and ligaments). This can make the procedure less painful and more effective. NSAIDs *(see Chapter 5)* can also help relieve the discomfort in horses with very painful joint conditions.

Stretching

Muscle problems are very common in athletic horses. No matter what the cause, muscle tension and spasms can limit performance, and possibly lead to more serious muscle injury *(see Chapter 10)*. Gently stretching and relaxing a muscle can:

- relieve muscle spasms
- improve muscle blood flow
- prevent or minimize adhesions between muscles

The horse's muscles can be passively stretched by using the horse's legs as levers. For example, lifting the hindleg and drawing it forward (toward the horse's belly) stretches the muscles at the back of the thigh. Muscles must be stretched lengthwise, so it is useful to know the locations and fiber directions of the major muscle groups when devising stretching exercises. This information can be found in several books on physical therapies. *(Call Equine Research, Inc. at 1-800-848-0225 for the latest publications.)*

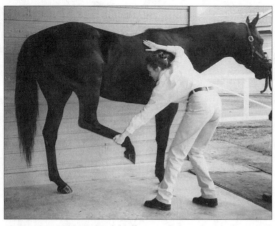

When stretching a muscle, it is important that the muscle is lengthened gradually, and not to its greatest extreme. Muscles should never be jerked suddenly or forced to stretch. After the muscle is stretched to the point of resistance and held in that position for about 5 seconds, it should

Fig. 4–29. Lifting the hindleg and drawing it forward stretches the thigh muscles.

be slowly released and allowed to relax. This procedure can be repeated 10 – 20 times, once or twice per day. As in human athletes, using a stretching routine on the horse before exercise can help prevent muscle injuries during athletic activity.

Chiropractic Manipulation

Chiropractic manipulation, or adjustment, is aimed at restoring the normal alignment of the vertebrae. Malalignment of the small intervertebral joints causes spasms in the muscles that support and move the spine. It can also compress the nerves as they leave the spinal cord at that location. As anyone who has suffered from them can attest, a muscle spasm or a "pinched nerve" causes pain and loss of mobility, which can be debilitating.

Chiropractic manipulation uses controlled force on the affected part of the spine in a direction that will realign the intervertebral joints. (The sacro-iliac joints can also be manipulated; *see Chapter 22*). Some people claim that because of the size of the horse's spinal column and the large muscle mass surrounding it, repositioning the vertebrae along the back is not possible. They suggest that the benefits of chiropractic manipulation are solely due to the relief of muscle spasms. Whether or not this is the case, manipulation by a skilled equine chiropractor can help many horses with neck or back pain.

As with all other forms of therapy, an accurate diagnosis is essential for a successful outcome. Also, the principle of "do no harm" should be foremost in the mind of the horse owner and the chiropractor.

Serious damage to the spine or spinal cord can result from improper manipulation of the neck or back. Only reputable chiropractors with extensive equine experience and an excellent reputation should be allowed to work on a horse. (In some places it is against the law for a chiropractor to work on a horse without a veterinarian's recommendation.)

Repeat adjustment is often necessary if the horse is permitted to reinjure the area with vigorous exercise. Regular massage therapy and stretching exercises may help prevent further problems in some horses.

> **More Information**
>
> **The spinal column is a very complex structure. It consists of over 30 bones (vertebrae) and over 100 joints.**
>
> **(See Chapter 22 for illustrations and detailed explanations.)**

Acupuncture

Acupuncture is an ancient Chinese art of healing. In theory, it restores the balance between the body's positive and negative forces (Yin and Yang), thus allowing the body to heal itself. The underlying principle is one of meridians—energy pathways that interconnect the body's organs with each other and with the body surface. Stimulating an acupuncture point on the body surface affects the energy flow to the organ associated with that point, and to other connected organs.

While the actual physiology may never be completely understood, there is no disputing the beneficial effects of acupuncture for many conditions. Acupuncture is often used to temporarily relieve pain and promote healing. However, as with any form of therapy, an accurate diagnosis is essential for a satisfactory outcome. A properly trained veterinary acupuncturist is skilled in diagnostic procedures, as well as in the art of locating the acupuncture points on the horse. (Using human charts for horses leads to poor results.) Electronic point-finders are available, but they are not always as accurate as the fingers of a skilled acupuncturist.

Traditionally, acupuncturists use fine needles to stimulate the points. More recently, low-level lasers have been used in place of needles. Some veterinary acupuncturists also inject sterile saline solution into the area to provide more long-lasting stimulation of that acupuncture point.

With any method, several treatments are often required before a response is seen. But some horses substantially improve after the first treatment.

Acupressure

Acupressure uses localized pressure instead of needles or lasers to stimulate acupuncture points. The fingertips or a small wooden or metal ball may be used to apply direct, focal pressure over the points. As with acupuncture, a thorough knowledge of the acupuncture points on the horse is necessary for success.

Homeopathy

Homeopathic remedies are made from natural sources, such as plants, animal products, and minerals. They are used to restore the body's natural balance and promote healing. There are hundreds of homeopathic remedies, each with a specific mode of action. The appropriate remedy is chosen for the particular symptoms the patient shows. But because the symptoms may vary among patients, there is no standard remedy for a specific condition.

Success with homeopathy requires extensive knowledge of the homeopathic remedies and their effects in horses. Although these remedies are from natural sources, some are potentially toxic. Thus, the principle of "do no harm" should be followed, and an experienced veterinary homeopath should be consulted before treating a horse with a homeopathic remedy.

Therapeutic Ultrasound

Ultrasound involves ultra-high frequency sound waves. When used as a therapeutic tool, it has two basic effects: thermal (warming) and non-thermal. The thermal effects are similar to those of heat therapy: increased blood flow, relief of muscle spasms, and increased elasticity of soft tissues (including fibrous tissue) in the treated area. The primary non-thermal effect is the stimulation of cell activity in the treated area.

There is some scientific evidence that therapeutic ultrasound improves the rate and quality of tendon repair. It also speeds bone metabolism in fracture sites within the first 2 weeks after injury. However, it has been shown to delay repair in fractures older than about 2 weeks. When used on healthy bones, prolonged use of ultrasound (over about 1 month) can result in loss of mineral from the bones (osteoporosis).

Therapeutic ultrasound should not be used immediately after a soft tissue injury or on an infected area. This is because it stimulates blood flow and can, therefore, worsen the swelling and pain. However, when begun about 3 days after injury, it can be useful in promoting healing of tendon, ligament, and muscle injuries.

The depth of tissue penetration depends on the frequency of the ultrasound waves (measured in megahertz, or MHz). In general, the lower the frequency, the deeper the penetration. Most of the units used for soft tissue therapy have an effective penetration depth of 1 – 3 inches (2.5 – 7.5 cm), depending on the frequency used.

Because ultrasound is poorly transmitted through air, the hair over the treatment area may need to be clipped. If the hair is short and fine, it can just be soaked with alcohol. A coupling gel should be applied to the skin and transducer (probe) to ensure that no air is trapped between the hair and the skin. Alternatively, for lower leg injuries, the horse can be stood in a tub of water. The therapist treats the leg by holding the transducer under the water an inch (2.5 cm) away from the leg. (Water is a good transmitter of ultrasound waves.) With either method, the transducer should be kept at a 90° angle to the skin, directly facing the skin surface. It should be kept moving through-

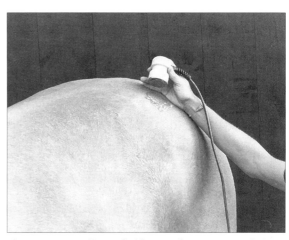

Fig. 4–30. Coupling gel aids sound wave transmission.

out the treatment. Each treatment should last 15 – 30 minutes, repeated once per day for at least 2 weeks.

Laser Therapy

Low-level lasers stimulate healing by increasing cell activity. The therapeutic effects also include increased blood flow, pain relief, and improved nerve regeneration in treated areas.

Terminology
LASER: Light Amplification by Stimulated Emission of Radiation. **Surgeons use "hot" lasers to make incisions and stop bleeding. Physical therapists use "cold" lasers of low intensity to promote tissue repair.**

Laser therapy can be used to promote healing in traumatic and surgical wounds, and in tendon and ligament injuries. It is of most benefit in acute (recent) conditions. But because it increases blood flow, it should not be used for 2 – 3 days after injury, especially in areas where bruising or hemorrhage has occurred.

The depth of tissue penetration depends on the wavelength. Most therapeutic lasers have an effective penetration depth of only ⅜ – ⅝ inch (1 – 1.5 cm). But some physical therapists are using lasers with a penetration depth of over 2 inches (5 cm).

The laser should be held against the skin, and kept moving slowly throughout the treatment. The injury should be treated for 20 – 30 minutes each day, or every other day for at least 2 weeks. *The laser beam is potentially harmful to the eye, so the beam should never be pointed at an eye.*

Magnetic Field Therapy

Magnetic field therapy stimulates blood flow and cell activity in the treated area, thereby promoting healing. It also reduces pain, apparently by direct action on the nerve endings. Its uses include:

- stimulating wound healing
- reducing soft tissue swelling
- improving joint mobility
- enhancing muscle and tendon repair
- reducing back pain

Because it stimulates blood flow, magnetic field therapy should not be used on infected areas, or areas where recent bruising or hemorrhage has occurred.

Magnetic blankets, leg boots, and wire coils are available for use in horses. They use either solid magnets or electromagnetic energy (mains or battery operated). Treatment should last for at least 30 minutes per day, for a minimum of 2 weeks.

Electrical Tissue Stimulation

Electrical tissue stimulation uses low voltage electrical current to stimulate cell activity. Electrodes are placed against the horse's skin and a very low voltage electrical current is passed between the electrodes. The current sometimes causes a skin sensation or muscle contraction, which may make the horse stamp or shift its weight

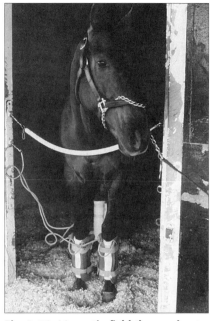

Fig. 4–31. Magnetic field therapy boots.

when first applied. But that is the only adverse effect of this therapy.

Electrical stimulation can be used on any soft tissue, including swellings such as hematomas and edema (accumulation of tissue fluid). But its most common uses are for muscle and nerve injuries, and pain relief.

Electrical Muscle Stimulators

Electrical stimulation is valuable for preventing or reversing the muscle weakness and atrophy that often follows muscle or nerve damage *(see Chapter 10)*. It replaces the normal nerve stimulation of the muscle group. Electrical muscle stimulation can also improve circulation in the area and help prevent or break down adhesions (fibrous bands between the tissues).

Effective treatment causes the muscles to contract. This can initially be uncomfortable for the horse, so the lowest possible setting should be used that still causes muscle activity. Treatment can be started within 1 – 2 days of injury. It is continued daily for up to 30 minutes at a time, until normal muscle and nerve function are restored.

Faradic Stimulators

The earlier devices, called Faradic stimulators, used a fairly crude stimulus that often caused uncomfortable muscle contractions. They have been replaced by units that allow more refined and specific treatment of a particular muscle, rather than a whole group of muscles.

Trophic Stimulators

Trophic stimulators produce a stimulus that causes little or no uncomfortable sensation. The muscle activity they produce is much more controlled than the Faradic stimulators. An electrode is placed at each end of the muscle to be treated, and the power is gradually increased until the muscle contracts. Most units allow two areas to be treated at once, with separate controls for each. In this way, the corresponding muscle on the opposite side of the body can also be treated.

Transcutaneous Electrical Nerve Stimulation (TENS)

TENS units are used to relieve pain. The pulsed electrical stimulus blocks the pain signals from the affected area. These units may also be used to stimulate muscle contraction and increase blood flow to an injured area. However, as with any physical therapy, the source of the pain should be located and treated before using this device.

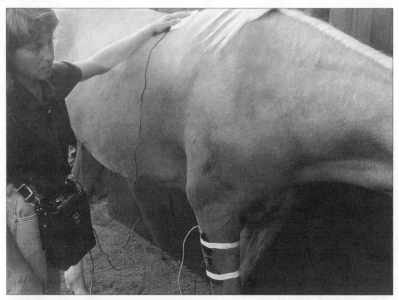

Fig. 4–32. Electrical tissue stimulation uses low voltage electrical current to stimulate cell activity.

ROUTINE FOOT CARE

Foot care is important in all horses, both healthy and lame. The foot is the "pedestal" that supports the horse, the base on which it stands and moves—in other words, "no foot, no horse." It is devastating when a severe injury responds to therapy, yet the horse must be euthanized because it develops severe, unresponsive laminitis ("founder"). By closely observing the feet each day, foot problems may be prevented, or at least detected early enough to be successfully treated.

> **More Information**
>
> Foot conditions are discussed in Chapter 15, including:
>
> Laminitis
> Foot abscesses
> Sole bruises
> Thrush
> Quarter cracks
> White line disease

Assessing the Digital Pulses

Blood supply to the sensitive tissues of the hoof wall is a critical factor in the development of laminitis. Often the earliest sign of laminitis is a strong pulse in the arteries that supply the foot—the digital arteries. For this reason, the digital pulses in all four feet should be assessed regularly. In horses that are prone to laminitis, or that are ill or very lame, the digital pulses should be felt at least twice every day.

The digital arteries run down each side of the leg, in the groove between the suspensory ligament and the flexor tendons (toward the back of the leg). They are easiest to feel as they run beside the sesamoid bones, toward the back of the fetlock. (It is very difficult to feel a pulse unless the artery can be pressed against a bony surface.)

To locate the arteries, cup the back of the fetlock, placing the thumb on one side and the first two fingers on the other. Slowly move the fingers and thumb toward the back of the fetlock, pressing lightly until the pulses are felt. These arteries are quite small in diameter (about ⅛ inch, or 3 mm), and too much pressure blocks them, making it impossible to feel a pulse. However, too little pressure makes it difficult to find the arteries, so the pressure should begin lightly, and gradually increase until the pulse is felt. As a guide, it takes about the same amount of finger pressure as that needed to feel a pulse at a person's wrist.

The strength of the pulse in the digital arteries normally is fairly light, and is about the same as that felt at a person's wrist. In horses with laminitis or an inflammatory condition in the foot, such as an abscess or bruise, the digital pulses in that leg are very strong, or

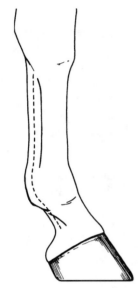

Fig. 4–33. The location of the digital artery.

"bounding." Sometimes the foot problem is very localized, and only involves one side of the foot. In these cases the pulse may be strong on the affected side of the leg, and normal on the other. Thus, it is best to feel the artery on both sides of the leg at the same time. It is worthwhile practicing several times either on the same horse or on different horses to become proficient at finding and assessing the digital pulses.

Environment

Good stable and pasture management are essential for preventing and treating many foot problems. Bad footing, such as a paddock that contains a lot of rocks, should be avoided, particularly in horses that already have a painful foot problem. Horses that must stand all day in a dirty stall or a muddy paddock are prone to developing infectious foot conditions, including thrush and foot abscesses. They are also vulnerable to pastern dermatitis *(see Chapter 13)*. At the other extreme, horses that live in dry, sandy lots are at risk of developing hoof wall problems, such as cracks and white line disease. Fresh, dry shavings can sometimes overdry the hooves and cause hoof wall problems. Excessive drying also makes the hooves hard and inelastic, which adds to the concussion on the feet and lower joints of the leg during exercise.

The worst situation is one that causes the feet to alternate between being very dry and very wet (waterlogged). For example, the horse is kept in a

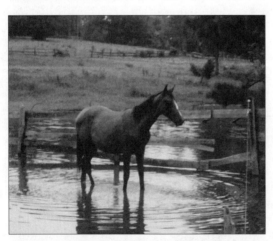

Fig. 4–34. The environment should help the horse maintain a normal balance of hoof moisture.

dirt paddock that is very hard and dry, until a week of rain turns it into a muddy lake. This can make it impossible for the hoof to maintain a normal moisture balance. The aim should always be to provide an environment that allows or helps the foot to maintain a normal balance of hoof moisture. In this case, it would be best to move the horse into a stall or sand pen until the paddock dries out.

Daily Hoof Care
Cleaning the Feet
Every horse, whether healthy or lame, should have its feet cleaned out each day, regardless of the type of horse, housing, or shoeing. Firm strokes with a hoof pick, starting at the heels and paying particular attention to the grooves (sulci) of the frog, are needed to do a thorough job. The hoof pick does not hurt a normal foot. So, enough pressure should be used to remove all mud, bedding, and manure that is packed into the bottom of the foot. Leaving material in the frog sulci can lead to thrush, a superficial infection that can progress to frog deterioration and lameness. One sign of thrush is sensitivity when the frog is picked out.

Finally, a stiff-bristled brush should be used to thoroughly clean any remaining material from the bottom of the foot. The frog and sole can then be inspected for defects or imbedded objects, such as nails, wire, and stones.

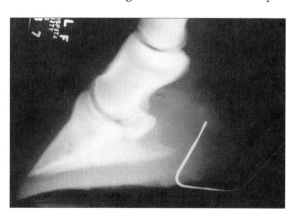

Fig. 4–35. Embedded wire can be missed if the foot is not thoroughly cleaned.

Care of Pads
Horses that have full sole pads need extra attention. The pad keeps the sole moist and provides an ideal environment for bacteria and fungi to multiply. The back of the pad can be sealed with latex bathroom sealer to prevent bedding material, gravel, and mud from being sucked in and trapped under the pad. However, sealing the back of the pad does not prevent moisture from leaking in around the edges.

If the horse is kept in a well-managed stall, and exercised in a clean, dry area, it is often best to leave the back of the pad unsealed. Each day a hoof pick should be used to remove any dirt and manure covering the pad, and any debris from the back of the pad. Every 1 – 2 days a dilute antiseptic solution should be injected under the pad using a syringe (without the needle). Dilute Betadine®, Nolvasan®, and white vinegar are suitable products.

Hoof Moisture and Hoof Dressings

Hoof moisture refers to the water content of the hoof wall and sole. It is essential for maintaining the hoof's resilience and elasticity. The hoof wall and sole are somewhat porous, in that moisture can enter and exit. Too much water makes the hoof soft and easily "deformed," and too little water makes it hard and brittle. The factor that most influences hoof moisture is the foot's environment. Maintaining the moisture balance of the horse's feet should be a daily duty for the owner or groom. If adjusting the horse's environment is not possible, hoof dressings can help.

Oil-based hoof dressings can improve the moisture retention in dry hooves, and help prevent waterlogging in hooves that spend all day in wet conditions. Most commercial hoof dressings contain either animal or vegetable-based oils. Some also contain mineral oil. But it is important to note that some mineral-based oils (such as motor oil) are harmful.

The hoof dressing should not be allowed to accumulate. The hoof wall and sole should be cleaned with a stiff brush to remove the oil and dirt from the previous day, before a fresh coat of dressing is applied.

Astringent substances, such as formalin (formaldehyde) and concentrated copper sulfate solution ("bluestone"), should be used with caution—and only as a specific treatment. These solutions can overdry the hoof when used too often. Extensive rasping of the hoof wall can also reduce the foot's ability to retain moisture because it removes the outer waterproof layer. Alcohol-based hoof paints should be removed after each show because they, too, can overdry the hooves.

Dietary Supplements

A balanced ration containing good quality feeds is the most important dietary aid to healthy hooves. Horses with thin, flaky hoof walls that crack and split may also benefit from having biotin added to their feed. Biotin is a vitamin that is essential for healthy hair, skin, and hoof growth. It does not speed up the *rate* of hoof growth. But it can improve the *quality* and resilience of the hoof wall as new horn is produced. Other dietary supplements, such as methionine, lysine, and gelatin can also improve hoof quality in some horses.

Some veterinarians and farriers have found that feeding vegetable oil for several months can make the hooves too soft. So, this additive probably should not be given to horses that tend to lose their shoes.

Hoof "First-Aid"
Removing a Shoe

If a horse's shoe is loose and twisted out of position, it must be removed right away. Otherwise, the hoof wall may be damaged and the horse's opposite leg injured. Unless the farrier is nearby, the owner or trainer must remove the shoe. In every other situation, the horse's shoes should be left on until the farrier or veterinarian makes a recommendation. If just one nail is loose and sticking out, it should be removed; however, the shoe itself should be left on.

The tools required to remove a shoe without damaging the hoof wall include:

- clench cutter (a chisel-like tool) and hammer; or, the clenches can be filed off with a hoof rasp, or cut off with pincers, although this can blunt the pincers
- shoe pullers or pincers

It is much easier to remove a shoe with the proper equipment. However, in an emergency, the clenches can be straightened with a flat-headed screwdriver and a hammer, and the shoe can be pulled off with pliers.

The shoe should never be pulled without first straightening or cutting all of the clenches. Pulling the shoe without attending to the clenches takes a lot of effort. More important, it damages the hoof wall, making it difficult to put on another shoe for several weeks.

Once the clenches are straightened or cut off, the heel of the shoe is grasped with shoe pullers or pincers. The shoe is then levered up by pushing the handle of the pincers toward the toe. The shoe is loosened a little at a time by alternating between each side of the foot, working from the heel toward the toe. Once at the toe, the shoe should be removed by levering the pincers back toward the heels. This avoids tearing away the hoof wall at the toe.

After the shoe is removed, the foot should be protected (as described below) until the farrier can replace the shoe. It is not necessary to remove the opposite shoe, unless it is also loose and out of position. While the shoe is off, the horse should not be worked.

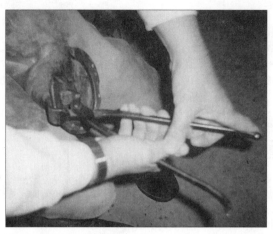

Fig 4–36. It is much easier to remove a shoe with the proper equipment.

Trimming the Hoof Wall

There is no substitute for the knowledge and skill of an experienced farrier, so regular trimming of the hoof wall should be left to the farrier. But sometimes a horse loses a shoe and has a broken piece of hoof wall hanging loose, yet the farrier cannot see the horse for a couple of days. In this case, pincers, a hoof knife, or another suitable tool should be used to cut off the piece of wall. This "first-aid" procedure can help prevent further tearing of the hoof wall. Protecting the bare foot until the shoe can be replaced is also important in preventing further hoof wall damage.

Protecting the Bare Foot

It is very important to protect the foot while the shoe is off. Duct tape makes a useful "first-aid" treatment when the shoe cannot be immediately replaced. A couple of layers are wrapped around the ground surface of the hoof. A more substantial foot bandage (discussed earlier) should be used if more protection or a waterproof covering is needed.

Protective boots, such as Easyboots, can help prevent further injury and infection in many hoof conditions. These boots are more resilient and waterproof than bandages, although this can work against them if the foot is wet when they are put on, or if water leaks in the top. The boot creates a warm, dark, humid, protected environment around the foot, which encourages bacteria and fungi to multiply. Therefore, the boot should be removed and cleaned out at least once

> **Note**
>
> It can be very difficult to reshoe a horse with a painful foot problem, such as laminitis or a subsolar abscess. Moreover, the horse usually needs the shoe for protection. In these cases, unless the shoe is hanging off, it is best to leave it on.

per day. While the boot is off, the leg should be closely inspected for signs of rubbing on the coronet and pastern. If the boot is rubbing the leg, it should be left off or padded.

No matter how the bare foot is protected, it is best to confine the horse to a clean, dry stall or small paddock until the shoe is replaced.

Hoof Treatments

Poultices and Soaks

Several foot conditions, including bruises, abscesses, and "gravel," are improved or resolved with poultices or "soaks." The aim is to improve blood supply with warmth, and draw infected material from the foot. A poultice provides more concentrated therapy than soaking, and works for several hours. Soaking is only effective while the horse is standing in the solution. Furthermore, a poultice only takes a few minutes to apply, whereas soaking is time-consuming.

The most common poultice used in horses is based on absorbent clay powder or paste. Some veterinarians prefer to use ichthammol as a hoof poultice. This black paste has some antibacterial properties, and stimulates blood flow to the damaged area. Poultice-dressings, such as Animalintex®, are also useful for treating hoof conditions. Some hoof wall abscesses eventually break out at the coronary band, which is the point of least resistance for the pus that builds up under the hoof wall. Thus, the poultice and bandage should cover the coronet for the best results. *(See Chapter 5 for more information on poultices.)*

There are commercial products available for soaking the feet, but a concentrated solution of Epsom salts (magnesium sulfate) is very effective. A concentrated solution is made by adding a handful of Epsom salts to a bucket of warm water, stirring the solution and adding more salts until they no longer dissolve. The horse's foot is then placed into the solution for at least 15 minutes.

Wet poultices and "soaks" can saturate and soften the hoof, so the foot needs extra attention and protection after these treatments. The foot and leg should be rinsed off and dried with a towel, and the horse should be made to stand in a clean, dry area until the hoof wall is completely dry. A bandage or protective boot can then be applied to the foot.

Reducine® Rub

Some veterinarians and farriers recommend rubbing the coronet with a mildly irritant ointment, such as Reducine®. This can improve blood flow to the coronary band and increase the rate of hoof wall growth. Unlike other counter-irritant treatments (such as "blisters"), this one is effective in stimulating blood flow to the "target" tissue because the coronary band—which generates the hoof wall—is an extension of the skin. *(Counter-irritants are discussed in the Anti-Inflammatory Therapy section of Chapter 5.)*

Before treatment the hair is clipped from the coronet, around the entire hoof. A small brush (such as a toothbrush) is then used to rub the ointment into the skin around the coronet each day for 7 days. Treatment is stopped for one week, then the process is repeated.

Reducine usually causes mild scurfing of the skin. However, if the area becomes very painful and irritated, treatment should be stopped. This treatment should never be used in horses with any condition that already affects the coronet. Such conditions include wounds, "gravel," quarter cracks, and acute laminitis.

DISEASE CONTROL

Some lameness problems are caused by infectious agents, such as bacteria or viruses, that can be spread to other horses. For example, the neurologic disease Equine Herpesvirus type 1 (EHV-1) myeloencephalitis generally begins as a mild respiratory infection that readily spreads from horse to horse *(see Chapter 12)*.

Other infectious conditions may pose a health risk to the horse's handlers. Certain bacteria that cause wound or joint infections in horses are very pathogenic (disease-causing). They can infect any superficial wound on a person's hands or arms, unless some basic precautions are taken when handling the horse's wound and soiled bandages. On the other side of the coin, unsanitary conditions and poor hygiene can cause wound infection in the horse. Following are some standard disease control measures that can limit the spread of harmful organisms in horses and the people treating them.

Managing Infected Wounds

Any wound that is draining pus should be treated as though it is infective. Whether it is a superficial wound, an infected joint or tendon sheath, or an abscess, the material that is draining from the wound can spread bacteria into the horse's environment. This contaminates the bedding, stall, and equipment. It can also spread bacteria onto the hands of the person treating the wound.

Following are some recommendations for dealing with potentially infective discharges:

1. Remove the horse from its stall before treating the wound. It is difficult to prevent contamination of the bedding when bathing the wound. Also, it is easier to clean a concrete wash-stall or paved aisleway after treatment.
2. Wear rubber or latex gloves when handling the wound and soiled cleaning materials and bandages.
3. Place a plastic trash can liner under the horse's foot. That way, most of the drainage from the wound lands on the bag, rather than on the floor. Discard the bag after each treatment.
4. Dispose of all soiled cleaning materials and bandages immediately in a fly-proof trash can.
5. Wipe up all pus and blood, and disinfect the treatment area (discussed later) after each treatment. Also, clean and disinfect all cleaning utensils, such as buckets and bowls. This step is important in preventing the spread of infection to other horses. (Lining the bucket or bowl with a plastic bag or trash can liner can help keep it clean.)
6. Control the fly population around the barn. Use baits, and remove or cover preferred breeding areas, including manure, soiled bedding, and discarded feed.

Isolation

Isolating infected or exposed horses is an important part of controlling the spread of viral infections. The principles of effective isolation are as follows:

- restrict the movement of people, animals, and inanimate objects through the isolation area
- restrict airflow between the isolated animal and the rest of the group

All animal traffic should be controlled, including horses, dogs, cats, poultry, other livestock, rodents, and wildlife. The inanimate objects most likely to transmit infection include feed and water containers, grooming tools, bedding, manure, surface water, tack, stall cleaning tools, and the shoes or boots of the people entering the stall.

Ideally, an isolated horse should be kept at a different location from the rest of the herd. However, this is often impossible, so compromises are usually necessary. Where possible, the affected horse should be placed in a separate barn. A less effective alternative is to put the horse in a stall at the end of the barn and rope off the area directly in front of the stall. There should be at least one empty stall between the infected horse and the other horses. That end of the barn should be closed off to reduce airflow through the remainder of the barn.

There are several other procedures that can limit the spread of infection:

1. Attend to the healthy horses before the isolated horse.
2. Restrict the number of people handling the isolated horse. The more people that come in contact with the horse, the greater the risk of spreading the infection.
3. Handle the horse as infrequently as its medical condition and basic needs allow. Every exposure is an opportunity for infection to be spread.
4. Keep a separate set of stall cleaning tools, buckets, halters, and grooming equipment for the isolation area, and thoroughly clean and disinfect all of these items after the horse has left the isolation area. Assume all in-contact items are infected. Dispose of the bedding, uneaten feed, and unused water carefully.
5. Wash up thoroughly after each contact with the horse, and clean or change boots if necessary.
6. Control the fly population in and around the isolation area.
7. Limit the isolated horse's exercise. This avoids exposure to other horses and contamination of the environment (feed and water containers, fences and gates, pasture, etc.).

The length of time the horse must remain isolated depends on the infection. For example, when EHV-1 is involved, the affected or exposed horses should be isolated for at least 3 weeks. The veterinarian who regularly attends the facility is the best person to give more specific recommendations for this and other diseases.

More Information

Viral infections that may cause lameness include:

- **Equine Herpesvirus type 1 (EHV-1)**
- **rabies**
  (See Chapter 12)
- **Equine Viral Arteritis (EVA; see Chapter 13)**

Hygiene and Disinfection

Many species of pathogenic bacteria can survive in the horse's environment for several weeks or more. This is especially true if they are protected by organic material such as manure, discharges (mucus, pus, etc.), bedding, or soil. Once a horse has recovered from a potentially contagious condition, or has been moved out of the stall, the bedding should be removed and composted or burned. The feed and water containers should also be removed and cleaned. Discharges, saliva, blood, and diarrhea should be cleaned off all surfaces and equipment, ideally with a high pressure hose or hot water. Steam cleaning is very effective for thoroughly cleaning stalls and equipment. This is an important step because some disinfectants are inactivated (made ineffective) by organic material *(see Figure 4–37)*.

The stall floor, walls, and door; stall cleaning tools; feed and water containers; and all in-contact equipment, such as halters, twitch, and brushes, should then be treated with disinfectant. Clorox™ is the most widely effective common disinfectant. Its other advantages are its availability and low cost.

With any disinfectant, the dilution instructions on the container should be followed exactly. Using too little disinfectant is ineffective, and using too much may be harmful. All exposed surfaces should be completely saturated with disinfectant, and the disinfectant should be left on the surface for the recommended time (which varies among products). The disinfectant should be rinsed off only if so advised on the product label. But feed and water containers should always be thoroughly rinsed before they are reused.

The stall and equipment should be left until completely dry before being used for another horse. Most bacteria cannot stand drying—they need either water or moist organic material to survive outside the horse.

(Figure 4–37 at the end of the chapter is a table of common disinfectants and their effectiveness.)

Rabies

A dramatic (but fortunately uncommon) example of a transmissible disease is rabies. The virus that causes this deadly disease is readily spread in the saliva from an infected animal. If the people handling the infected horse are not extremely careful, they are at risk of spreading or developing the disease. Saliva from a horse that is suspected of having rabies should be treated like pus: all contact with this potentially infective fluid should be avoided. Any horse suspected of having rabies should be isolated, and the procedures discussed for isolating horses strictly followed. In particular, the number of people handling the horse must be kept to a minimum. *(See Chapter 12 for more information on rabies.)*

ACTIVITY OF COMMON DISINFECTANTS

	Bacteria	Bacterial Spores*	Fungi	Viruses	In the Presence of Organic Matter‡	In Hard Water
Quaternary Ammonium	+	–	+	+	±	+
Phenols	+	–	+	+	+	+
Hypochlorite	+	+	+	+	±	+
Iodophors	+	±	+	+	–	±
Chlorhexidine	+	–	–	–	±	±

Fig. 4–37. The activities of some common groups of disinfectants.

Quaternary Ammonium—compounds with "ammonium" in the chemical name
Phenols—compounds with "phenol" in their chemical name
Hypochlorite—the active ingredient in bleach products, such as Clorox™
Iodophors—iodine-based compounds, for example povidone-iodine (Betadine®)
Chlorhexidine—the active ingredient in Nolvasan®

+ = effective
± = somewhat effective
– = ineffective

* spores are the dormant, resilient stage of the bacterial lifecycle
‡ organic matter includes manure, blood, pus, mucus, other secretions, bedding material, and dirt

5

MEDICATIONS

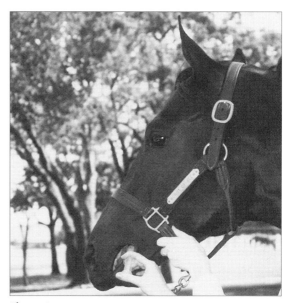

M edica- tions are often an important part of treating lameness. Many are drugs the veterinarian in- structs the owner or trainer to give the horse. Common examples include NSAIDs, such as phenylbutazone, and certain antibi- otics. Other drugs, such as joint medi- cations, are given only by the veteri- narian.

Fig. 5–1.

ANTI-INFLAMMATORY THERAPY
The Process of Inflammation

Most conditions that cause lameness involve inflammation. So, a basic knowledge of the inflammatory process is important for understanding the benefits, limitations, and harmful effects of anti-inflammatory treatments.

Cells can be damaged by various insults, including trauma, toxins produced by bacteria, and interruption of the blood supply. When cell damage occurs, a chain reaction in the cell's outer membrane causes inflammatory substances to be released into the surrounding tissue fluid and nearby capillaries. These inflammatory substances have the following effects in the damaged tissue:

1. Vasodilation (blood vessel dilation) in the area surrounding the damage.
2. Vasoconstriction (blood vessel constriction) in the damaged blood vessels.
3. Clumping of platelets—the small particles in the bloodstream that assist blood clotting.
4. Leakage of fluid (plasma) from the capillaries.
5. Pain.
6. Migration of white blood cells from the bloodstream into the damaged tissue.

These effects are responsible for the outward signs of inflammation:

- pain
- swelling
- heat
- redness

The pain is due to 1) direct stimulation of the nerve endings in the damaged tissues, 2) increased sensitivity of the nerve endings caused by some inflammatory substances, and 3) tension on the tissues and skin as a result of the swelling. Heat, swelling, and redness are caused by vasodilation and fluid leakage from the capillaries.

Loss of function is another result of inflammation. It is a loose term that probably has as much to do with the pain and swelling as with any functional changes in the damaged tissue.

Effects of Inflammation

Some of the inflammatory substances stimulate tissue repair by attracting and activating fibroblasts. These cells produce collagen, the microscopic fiber that gives tissues their strength. New cells are then laid down on the collagen framework. Thus, inflammation is an important part of the body's response to injury—a vital first step in the healing process. However, each component of the inflammatory process can be harmful when it is allowed to escalate, or is unopposed. In essence, each of the actions listed earlier have both positive and negative effects.

To prevent or at least minimize further tissue damage from the negative effects, some of the inflammatory substances have opposing actions. For example, inflammation results in both vasodilation and vasoconstriction. These two effects counteract or balance each other, so that neither is permitted to go to extremes. This system ensures that the inflammatory process is kept under control and the positive effects are greater than the negative effects.

The effects of each component of the inflammatory process are discussed below and summarized in Figure 5–2.

Vasodilation

Vasodilation increases blood flow, bringing more oxygen and nutrients to the injured tissues. It also delivers white blood cells and antibodies (immune system proteins) to the damaged area. This is essential for controlling infection at the site of injury. An increase in blood flow also helps remove waste products and cell debris from the area. Vasodilation also causes heat, which increases cell activity. So, it speeds up the activity of the white blood cells (see below), and the healing process.

However, the increase in blood flow also causes an increase in fluid leakage from the capillaries, which increases the swelling and pain.

Vasoconstriction

Vasoconstriction in the damaged blood vessels helps to limit blood loss. It also limits the spread of inflammatory substances to nearby tissues. However, it reduces blood flow to the injured area. As a result, less oxygen, nutrients, white blood cells, and antibodies reach the tissue, and the cells' waste products are not efficiently removed.

Severe or prolonged interruption of the blood supply can result in cell damage, which leads to further inflammation. When the blood supply is inadequate, the cells release harmful substances called "free radicals," which are unstable oxygen molecules. They can damage other cell membranes and cause those cells to release inflammatory substances, thus continuing the inflammatory process. Severe damage to the cell membrane may cause the cell to rupture and release its contents (including enzymes) into the surrounding area. This can also damage other cells.

THE BALANCING EFFECTS OF INFLAMMATION

	Positive	Negative
Vasodilation (in surrounding area)	• increased blood flow brings oxygen, white cells, and antibodies to the damaged tissues • also removes waste products and cell debris • heat increases cell activity	• increases fluid leakage, which worsens the swelling
Vasocontriction (in damaged vessels)	• reduces blood flow, limits hemorrhage • limits spread of inflammatory substances	• decreases oxygen supply and waste removal • can result in cell damage if severe
Platelet Clumping	• clots reduce blood flow & limit hemorrhage • limits spread of inflammatory substances	• decreases oxygen supply and waste removal • can result in cell damage if severe
Capillary Leakage	• allows white blood cells and antibodies to leave the bloodstream and enter the tissues • swelling reduces mobility in the injured area	• swelling causes pain and can reduce blood flow (with the same results as above)
Pain	• makes the horse protect the injured area	• discomfort
White Blood Cell Response	• some produce antibodies • others destroy and remove bacteria, and remove damaged cells	• enzymes released by activated white blood cells can damage other cells, causing release of more inflammatory substances

Fig. 5–2. The components of inflammation and their positive and negative effects.

Platelet Clumping

Some of the inflammatory substances that cause vasoconstriction also cause the platelets to clump together and form tiny clots within the vessels. This response is important for controlling bleeding and limiting the spread of inflammatory substances. However, it can also reduce blood flow in the injured tissue, with the same results as vasoconstriction.

Capillary Leakage

An increase in the permeability (leakiness) of the capillaries has the positive effect of allowing white blood cells and antibodies, which are large molecules, to easily move into the damaged tissues. However, the negative effect is that it allows plasma (the liquid portion of the blood) to escape from the capillaries. The result is swelling and reduced blood flow in the injured area.

On a larger scale, swelling has the positive effect of reducing mobility in the injured area. However, if the swelling is severe, the increased pressure within the tissues can compress the smaller blood vessels and reduce blood flow to the injured area. Swelling also causes pain by putting tension on the skin.

Pain

Pain also has both positive and negative effects. It makes the horse protect the injured area from excessive movement and further injury. However, the cost is discomfort.

White Blood Cell Response

White blood cells are very important because some produce antibodies and others destroy and remove any bacteria that have invaded the injured tissue. They also remove damaged cells and other debris from the site of injury.

The white blood cells are attracted to the damaged area by specific inflammatory substances called leukotrienes. These substances also activate the white blood cells to perform their functions. One of the ways activated white blood cells kill bacteria is by releasing potent enzymes. However, these enzymes can damage the surrounding tissue. The newly damaged cells release more inflammatory substances, and the process of inflammation continues.

Definition

Enzymes are complex molecules that aid cell reactions. They can damage other cell membranes when released.

Inflammatory Cycle

Although inflammation is essential for the healing process, some of the effects can cause further cell damage if they are left unchecked. This can create a vicious cycle of damage and inflammation. But, unless there is extensive tissue damage, repeated injury, or infection, the inflammatory process is self-limiting. It winds down and resolves on its own in time, usually a minimum of 3 days.

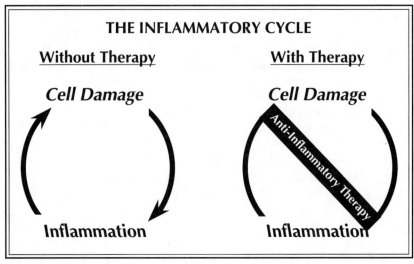

Fig. 5–3.

However, in many cases the amount of tissue damage requires anti-inflammatory therapy to reduce the harmful effects of inflammation, and make the horse more comfortable. The anti-inflammatory therapies commonly used in horses are discussed in the following sections.

Physical Anti-Inflammatory Therapies

Although this chapter is about medications, certain physical therapies have anti-inflammatory actions. They include cold therapy and combination therapies, such as "sweats" and poultices.

Cold Therapy

Cold is a very effective method of temporarily relieving inflammation. Cold causes the blood vessels in the skin and superficial tissues to constrict. It also desensitizes (numbs) nerve endings, providing temporary pain relief. Cold therapy can be performed several ways.

Specific Methods

Hosing

Hosing the affected area with cold water for 10 – 15 minutes, several times per day helps to reduce the signs of inflammation.

Standing in Cold Water

Standing the horse in a stream or pond, or in a tub of cold water can also help reduce inflammation in the feet and lower legs. However, standing the horse in muddy water is not advisable for injuries that also involve a wound.

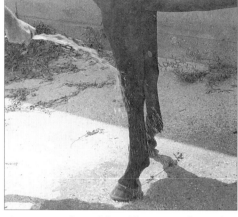

Fig. 5–4. Hosing with cold water reduces the signs of inflammation.

Ice Pack

Commercial ice packs are available for cooling a specific area, although a plastic bag of crushed ice is just as effective. A bag of frozen peas conforms to the leg very well, and it can be refrozen and used several times if necessary. (**Note:** The peas should not be eaten if they have been thawed more than once.) The ice pack can be held over the affected area, or it can be bandaged in place, if possible.

Wet Bandage

A stable or track bandage and a quilted leg wrap are good materials to use for a wet bandage. *Elastic bandages or any other material that may shrink when wet should never be used for this*

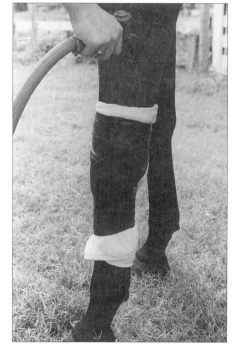

Fig. 5–5. The bandage should be repeatedly soaked to keep it cold and wet.

Extra Information
Epsom salts are crystals of magnesium sulfate.
Rubbing alcohol is also called isopropyl alcohol.
Note: Alcohol should not be added if there is an open wound or skin irritation on the leg.

purpose. The padding and bandage are saturated with cold water before being applied to the leg. For a colder, more "bracing" treatment crushed ice, rubbing alcohol, and Epsom salts can be added to the water. The wet padding and bandage should be applied to the leg with just enough tension to keep them in place. The bandage should either be removed once it becomes warm or repeatedly soaked to keep it cold and wet.

Ice Boot

Commercial ice boots are available for cooling the lower leg. But an effective ice boot can be made out of a plastic trash can liner (kitchen size or larger) and duct tape. A stocking is made by wrapping the bag loosely around the leg and securing the bottom of the bag at the pastern or hoof with duct tape. The boot is then filled with crushed or cubed ice so that the injured area is completely covered. If necessary, the top of the bag can be loosely taped to the leg to help keep it up.

Length of Treatment

After about 10 minutes, cooling the skin causes reflex vasodilation in the area. This warms the tissues, so cold therapy is of little benefit after this time. Therefore, it should only be applied for 10 – 15 minutes at a time. It should be repeated as often as possible during the first 2 – 3 days after injury. By about the third day, the benefits of cold therapy are minimal, unless inflammation persists. If this is the case, the reason for the persistent inflammation should be investigated.

With the exception of the ice pack, these cold therapies involve wetting the skin. The area should be thoroughly dried after each treatment to avoid moist dermatitis (irritation and inflammation of the skin), particularly on the lower legs.

Bandaging

Applying a firm, well-padded bandage over the injured area can help reduce the signs of inflammation. It restricts swelling and minimizes movement and further injury of the damaged tissues. However, the bandage should not be so firm that it restricts blood flow. *(Bandaging techniques are discussed in Chapter 4.)*

Anti-Inflammatory Drugs
Nonsteroidal Anti-Inflammatory Drugs (NSaids)

Nonsteroidal anti-inflammatory drugs, or NSAIDs are among the most common anti-inflammatory therapies used in horses. They relieve inflammation by blocking some of the same inflammatory reactions that corticosteroids block, yet they are not steroids. Hence, their rather involved name. (Corticosteroids are discussed later.)

The NSAIDs that are used in horses include:

- phenylbutazone (PBZ or "bute"; formerly butazolidin, or Btz)
- flunixin (Banamine®)
- ketoprofen (Ketofen®)
- meclofenamic acid (Arquel®)
- dipyrone
- aspirin
- ibuprofen
- indomethacin
- naproxen

Actions

NSAIDs work by preventing the production of some of the inflammatory substances released by damaged cells. Some inflammatory substances cause pain, so *NSAIDs relieve pain by resolving inflammation,* not by just blocking pain. By reducing the negative effects of inflammation these drugs can also promote healing. So, they are not merely masking the horse's pain—they are a valuable therapy when used correctly.

The results of effective NSAID therapy include pain relief (analgesia) and reduction in the other signs of inflammation: heat, swelling, and redness. These drugs can also reduce a fever. When some of the inflammatory substances enter the circulation, they act on the heat regulation center in the brain. In effect, these substances turn up the body's "internal thermostat." NSAIDs can reduce or resolve a fever by preventing the production of these inflammatory substances. However, fever is an important sign of infection. It may also help the body resolve the infection by inactivating the bacteria or viruses, and enhancing the immune response. Suppressing the fever eliminates a very useful signal that the disease is worsening or the treatment is ineffective. So, these drugs should not be used without veterinary advice in a horse with a fever.

Most NSAIDs do not block leukotriene production. Leukotrienes are the inflammatory substances that cause white blood cells to migrate into the injured area and become activated to fight infection and remove damaged cells. Thus, NSAIDs do not prevent the white cells from performing these important functions. This is one of the important differences between NSAIDs and corticosteroids, which do block leukotriene production. Although, some of the newer NSAIDs, in particular, ketoprofen, may inhibit leukotriene production.

Side Effects of NSAIDs

High doses of NSAIDs given for several days can have some harmful effects. They include ulceration in the stomach (and occasionally the colon) and kidney damage. These effects primarily relate to the fact that NSAIDs effectively block production of prostaglandins, some of the inflammatory substances produced by damaged cells. At high doses, a few of these drugs—in particular, aspirin—can also slow blood clotting.

Gastric Ulcers

The stomach lining normally produces hydrochloric acid and digestive enzymes. These substances are important for digestion. However, they can also "digest" the stomach lining, resulting in ulcers. There are several ways the stomach protects itself from damage. Specialized cells in its lining produce mucus and bicarbonate. The mucus coats the inside of the stomach, and the bicarbonate helps neutralize the acid. Production of these protective substances is stimulated by certain prostaglandins: PGE_2 and PGI_2. These prostaglandins also increase blood flow to the cells lining the stomach, and

NSAIDs

Positive Effects	Negative Effects

• relieve inflammation
  - pain relief
  - reduce swelling, heat, and redness
• most do not inhibit the white blood cell response to tissue damage and infection
	• suppression of fever can mask signs of infection
	• suppression of prostaglandin production can cause gastric ulcers and kidney damage
	• pain relief without diagnosis can lead to further damage if exercise continues

Fig. 5–6. The effects of NSAIDs.

they reduce acid production, which further protects the stomach. NSAIDs reduce the normal production of these protective prostaglandins in the stomach. As a result, the acid and enzymes can ulcerate the stomach lining.

There are several anti-ulcer drugs that can help prevent NSAID-induced gastric ulcers in horses.

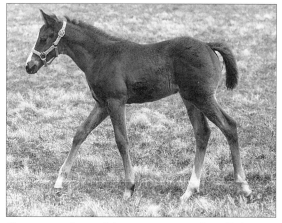

Fig. 5–7. Foals receiving NSAIDs may benefit from anti-ulcer drugs.

It is more important to use these drugs when treating foals with NSAIDs because foals are more prone to gastric ulcers than adult horses. Sucralfate and histamine blockers (like Tagamet™ and Zantac™) are the more commonly used drugs. The newer drugs that are being tried in horses include a synthetic PGE (misoprostil) and an acid-inhibitor (omeprazole).

The harmful effects of NSAIDs on the stomach may also be reduced by feeding corn oil (approximately ½ cup twice per day for an adult horse) for the duration of NSAID treatment. Corn oil contains linoleic acid, which the body can make into PGE2. The oil may also help by coating the stomach and physically protecting it from acid and enzyme damage.

Kidney Damage

The "protective" prostaglandins are also normally produced in the kidneys, where they maintain good blood flow through the kidneys. This action is vital for effective filtering of the body's waste products. NSAIDs suppress these prostaglandins, reducing blood flow in the kidneys, which can lead to kidney damage. This is most likely if the horse is dehydrated, because dehydration further reduces blood flow to the kidneys.

Kidney damage can be prevented or minimized by reducing the daily dose of the drug to the lowest effective level as soon as possible, and keeping the course of treatment short. Ensuring that the horse has plenty of fresh drinking water is also important.

Administration Issues for NSAIDs

There are several other important points about NSAID use.

1. Effective treatment begins with an accurate diagnosis. It is inadvisable to give a lame horse an NSAID and continue to work it, without identifying the cause of the lameness. If lameness is due to early tendonitis or an incomplete fracture, for example, serious damage is likely if the horse continues in training. *The cause of the lameness should be identified before treatment begins.*

2. The inflammatory products released by damaged cells are not the only substances that cause pain. Although NSAIDs can relieve the discomfort of many conditions, they cannot completely resolve the pain of a serious injury such as a fracture or an infected joint. Increasing the dose of an NSAID to increase the analgesic effect is ineffective, and can be harmful.

3. Gastric ulcers and kidney damage generally develop only after high doses of NSAIDs have been given for several days. Therefore, with most NSAIDs, the veterinarian prescribes an initial dose rate, then tapers it down over the next few days. If the horse needs NSAIDs for several days, the dose should be reduced to the lowest effective level within 3 – 4 days.

4. In chronically lame horses, such as those with osteoarthritis, the horse may need to remain on a low dose for months or years. If, for any reason, treatment is stopped or the horse's condition worsens (such that the low dose is no longer effective), the veterinarian usually begins the course again. That is, rather than simply restoring or continuing the low dose, the higher dose is given and tapered back down over the next few days. Whenever an event (such as shoeing or transport) is likely to increase the horse's discomfort, the veterinarian may recommend giving the higher dose that day, and for the next 2 – 3 days.

5. The effectiveness against musculoskeletal pain varies among NSAIDs. For example, aspirin and dipyrone are relatively poor pain-relievers in lame horses. The effectiveness can also vary with the type of problem. For example, phenylbutazone often is better than ibuprofen for tendon and ligament injuries. But ibuprofen can sometimes be more effective for joint pain, such as osteoarthritis in old horses. Furthermore, the effectiveness of a particular NSAID may vary among horses with the same type of problem. Thus, the veterinarian may recommend different drugs in different situations.

6. Giving more than one NSAID at a time greatly increases the potential for gastric ulcers and kidney damage. Also, it does not relieve pain any better than one well-chosen NSAID given at an appropriate dose rate.

In view of these considerations, it is best to leave the decision to use NSAIDs, together with the choice of drug and dose rate to the veterinarian.

> ## Note
>
> The choice of drug and dose rates are not given in this book. *They are decisions that only the veterinarian who is examining and treating the horse should make.* The reader is encouraged to discuss these issues with his or her veterinarian whenever a question arises.

Corticosteroids (Cortisone)

Corticosteroids are commonly called "cortisone." They mimic the effects of cortisol, a hormone that is produced by the adrenal glands. Cortisol is released by these glands in response to stress, and its effects on the body are complex and wide-ranging. Because the actions of corticosteroids mimic those of cortisol, they have similar effects on the body.

The more frequently used corticosteroids in horses are prednisolone (Depo-Medrol®), dexamethasone (Azium®), and triamcinolone (Vetalog®). These drugs are given orally, intramuscularly, intravenously, or intra-articularly, depending on the formulation and the condition being treated.

Actions and Harmful Effects

Corticosteroids are very potent anti-inflammatory drugs. They effectively block the production of the inflammatory substances discussed earlier. They can also stabilize or protect cell membranes from breakdown. This prevents the release of harmful cell contents (especially enzymes) into the surrounding area, and further tissue damage.

However, corticosteroids also inhibit the production of leukotrienes, which are the inflammatory substances that attract and activate white blood cells. This action has both positive and negative effects. By blocking the activation of white blood cells, corticosteroids also block their harmful effects, in particular, the release of destructive enzymes. Thus, corticosteroids can prevent tissue damage by these "aggressive" cells.

However, the negative effect is that corticosteroids decrease the number of white blood cells that are attracted to the site, and reduce their bacterial killing power. As a result, the body may not be able to effectively control bacterial infection when these drugs are given. Corticosteroids also reduce the production and activity of fibroblasts, which are the cells that produce collagen—the fiber responsible for tissue repair. This effect can result in slower healing, and a weaker repair site.

Corticosteroids suppress the white blood cell response to tissue damage and infection both at the site of injury (locally), and throughout the body (systemically). This effect is known as immuno-suppression—suppression of the immune response. It is potentially very serious because it reduces the body's ability to fight off infection. Furthermore, the potent anti-inflammatory effects suppress the signs of infection: pain, heat, swelling, etc. at the site of injury, and fever. As a result, the infection can escalate, with little opposition from the immune system and few outward signs to alert the owner, trainer, or veterinarian.

The margin of safety between the therapeutic (positive) effects and the potentially harmful effects is very narrow with these drugs. In fact, there is an overlap between the positive and negative effects with the white blood cell function. Immunosuppression—a harmful effect—can occur at the same dose rates that must be used to control inflammation. Thus, *these drugs should always be used with caution,* and never without (or against) veterinary advice.

CORTICOSTEROIDS

Positive Effects	Negative Effects

• relieve inflammation
    - pain relief
    - reduce swelling, heat,
      and redness
 	
• stabilize cell membranes to
  prevent further cell damage
	• suppress white blood cell
	  response to tissue damage
	  and infection
	• slow tissue repair
	• mask signs of further tissue
	  damage and infection
	• cause immuno-suppression
	• alter adrenal-pituitary hormonal
	  balance
	• can cause abortion
	• can cause gastric ulcers
	• can cause laminitis

Fig. 5–8. The effects of corticosteroids.

Other Effects of Corticosteroids

Corticosteroids can have other, more general effects on the body, including:

- upset in the normal hormonal balance between the adrenal gland and the pituitary gland in the brain
- abortion, if given in the last few months of pregnancy
- gastric ulcers, as with NSAIDs
- laminitis ("founder")

Corticosteroids can cause laminitis by making the blood vessels in the feet more sensitive to catecholamines. Catecholamines, such as adrenaline, are hormones that are produced in response to stress. They are potent substances that cause blood vessel constriction, especially in the extremities. The result is reduced blood flow to the sensitive tissues of the hoof wall—the event thought to begin the destructive process of laminitis.

Laminitis is more likely in large, heavy horses, particularly show horses. These horses are already under stress, which stimulates cortisol and catecholamine release. Also, they typically are overfed in relation to the amount of work they are required to perform. Thus, these horses are prime candidates for laminitis, whether due to illness, too much

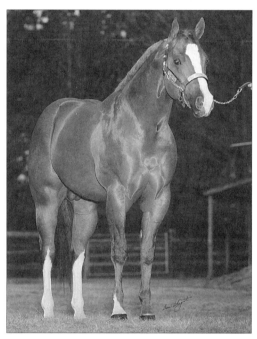

Fig. 5–9. Laminitis is more likely in large, heavy horses, particularly show horses.

grain, corticosteroid administration, or any other cause. *(See Chapter 15 for more information on laminitis.)*

Corticosteroids have legitimate uses in show horses. However, other anti-inflammatory options should always be considered before corticosteroids are used. If, after corticosteroids are given, the horse becomes short-strided, or if the digital pulses become stronger, the veterinarian should be called immediately. *(Finding and assessing the digital pulses is discussed in Chapter 4, in the section on Routine Foot Care.)*

Administration Issues for Corticosteroids

Some corticosteroids last only a few hours, while others last for several weeks. Harmful effects are more likely with the longer-acting products, and when high doses of any corticosteroid are given repeatedly.

Even though the drug may be injected into a joint, some of it is absorbed into the general circulation, and could cause harmful effects. It can also be detected in a pre- or post-competition blood or urine sample. (Using corticosteroids for treating joint disease is discussed in the later section on *Joint Medications.*)

Dimethyl Sulfoxide (DMSO)

Dimethyl sulfoxide, or DMSO is a potent anti-inflammatory drug that is often applied to the skin (topically) in horses. Occasionally, the veterinarian may give it orally, or inject it intravenously or intra-articularly for specific conditions. When given intravenously, DMSO can reduce inflammation and edema (accumulation of tissue fluid) within the brain and spinal cord. For this reason, veterinarians commonly give DMSO to horses with neurologic disease.

The anti-inflammatory effects of DMSO primarily relate to its ability to scavenge and inactivate "free radicals": harmful chemicals that are released from damaged cells. DMSO can also stabilize cell membranes, which prevents them from releasing enzymes into the surrounding area. These anti-inflammatory actions relieve pain. They may also improve blood flow to damaged tissues, promoting tissue repair. In addition, DMSO has some antibacterial properties.

Definition
The blood-brain barrier prevents cells and large molecules from leaving the bloodstream and entering the tissues of the brain and spinal cord.
(The nervous system and neurologic diseases are covered in Chapter 12.)

Precautions

DMSO is rapidly and completely absorbed through the skin and other tissue barriers, including joint capsules and the blood-brain barrier. It carries with it any other compound that is added to it. Thus, DMSO is often used as a "vehicle" to aid topical absorption of a variety of drugs, including NSAIDs, corticosteroids, and antibiotics. But for this reason, products that contain mercury, strong

DMSO

Positive Effects	Negative Effects

• relieves inflammation
  - pain relief
  - reduces swelling, heat, and redness
• does not inhibit the white blood cell response
• reduces edema (accumulation of tissue fluid); especially useful in the brain and spinal cord
• stabilizes cell membranes to prevent further cell damage
• anti-bacterial
• penetrates tissue barriers
• acts as a "vehicle" for other drugs
	• carries harmful compounds through the skin
	• can blister the skin when used topically
	• possible human health risk

Fig. 5–10. The effects of DMSO.

iodine, or other potentially toxic substances should never be added to DMSO.

Because it is such a concentrated solution, topical DMSO can irritate, and possibly even blister the skin if it is overused. So it should only be used once per day, or once every other day in sensitive horses. Treatment should be stopped for a couple of days if irritation develops. Unless the aim is to "sweat" the leg, the skin should not be covered after DMSO is applied.

DMSO is rapidly absorbed through human skin, and there have been some concerns about the possible risks of cancer and birth defects in humans. If for no other reason than to avoid the unpleasant taste within a few seconds of skin contact, DMSO should be applied to the horse's leg with a small, soft brush, such as a paint brush.

MSM

Methyl sulfonylmethane (MSM) is a substance that is related to DMSO, and it appears to have some of the same anti-inflammatory actions. MSM is available as a powdered feed additive. It can help some horses with chronic, low-grade lameness, such as degenerative joint disease.

Herbal Products

Natural, plant-based analgesic (pain-relieving) or anti-inflammatory products have become popular with some horse owners. These "herbal" products have few, if any, harmful side effects, and are therefore safe in virtually all horses. Their other main advantage is that, because they are not considered drugs, their use is not prohibited in performing horses. However, these products are not as potent as the anti-inflammatory drugs. Their use should be reserved for minor injuries.

Combination Therapies

Sweats

A "sweat" is a combination of medication and a plastic wrap. In most cases the medication includes DMSO and another anti-inflam-

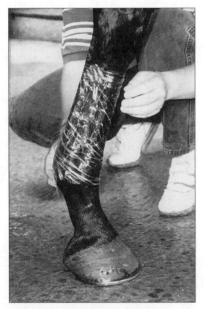

matory product, such as an NSAID or corticosteroid. Some veterinarians also add an antibiotic to the mixture. The medication is painted on the leg, and the area is covered with plastic (such as Saran™ wrap). A stable or exercise bandage is then applied over the plastic wrap.

This combination of therapies uses warmth beneath the plastic wrap to increase blood flow in the injured area. Although increasing blood flow to an inflamed area can increase the swelling, the bandage prevents further swelling. At the same time, the increased blood flow increases absorption of the anti-inflammatory medication.

Fig. 5–11. Applying a "sweat."

"Sweats" are often used on soft tissue swellings, such as bruises and sprains. But they can also be useful in reducing inflammation in a more serious injury, such as a bowed tendon. Superficial wounds that appear to be infected can be "sweated" with just an antibiotic ointment, such as nitrofurazone, under the plastic wrap and bandage. For back pain the horse's back can be "sweated" by applying the medication and covering it with plastic wrap and a blanket.

In most cases the veterinarian leaves the "sweat" in place for 8 – 12 hours (or overnight). It can be reapplied the next day if necessary. Some "sweat" preparations—particularly those that contain a high proportion of DMSO or a liniment—can irritate and blister the skin. So, they should not be over-used in sensitive horses.

Poultices

Poultices are products that can reduce the signs of inflammation by drawing fluid, either excess tissue fluid or pus, from an area. They work in the same way that salt or sugar absorbs water from its environment. Poultices are most effective when there is a break in the skin, such as a puncture wound or a defect in the hoof wall. Normally, intact skin and healthy hoof wall allow very little moisture to escape. When applied cold, the poultice also has the effect of cold therapy. When applied warm, the poultice stimulates blood flow to the injured area.

Most of the poultice products that are used in horses are based on a very absorbent, powdered clay, such as bentonite, kaolin, or aluminum silicate (Fuller's Earth). These products are available either as a powder to which water must be added, or as a premixed paste. Glycerin is another compound that draws fluid to itself, and is used in some poultice preparations. Sugar and Epsom salts (magnesium sulfate) also absorb, or draw fluid, and they make inex-

> **Note**
>
> An accurate diagnosis is essential for a successful outcome. Resolving the inflammation without identifying its cause can lead to more serious injury.
>
> For example, if there is pain, heat, or swelling in a flexor tendon, it is inadvisable to "sweat" the leg and then return the horse to training, without having the veterinarian examine the leg. If the inflammation was due to mild tendonitis (early bowed tendon), exercise can cause serious tendon injury.

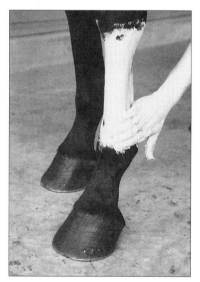

Fig. 5–12. Applying a poultice.

pensive and effective poultices. At high concentrations, sugar is also antibacterial because bacteria require moisture to survive. A paste of sugar and iodine ("sugardine") is a common and effective treatment for hoof infections.

Other "therapeutic" ingredients, such as menthol, camphor, and eucalyptus oil, are often added to poultice preparations. But in most cases they do little more than give the product a medicinal scent. Antibacterial agents such as zinc oxide and boric acid, and anti-inflammatory compounds such as methyl salicylate are also commonly added to poultice preparations. However, these products are unlikely to have any real benefit because they merely stay on the skin/hoof surface. The most effective ingredients are the "drawing" agents.

Ichthammol, a coal-tar derivative, is often used as a foot poultice. Its drawing effects are limited, although it does stimulate blood flow to the injured area. It also has some antibacterial properties. Another advantage of ichthammol is that it does not make the foot too moist or soft as many "wet" poultices do. *(The importance of hoof moisture is discussed in Chapter 4, in the section on Routine Foot Care.)*

There is at least one poultice product (Animalintex®) that consists of a dressing which is impregnated with dry poultice material. The dressing-poultice combination can be applied either dry or moist to wounds. It is bandaged in place.

With most other products the poultice is applied as a paste. It is covered with plastic or damp paper and a bandage to keep it moist, and to prevent it from being wiped off. The poultice is usually left in place for 12 – 24 hours, and replaced as many times as necessary.

Counter-Irritants

Liniments, "braces," "leg paints," and "blisters" are all examples of *inflammatory* products, or counter-irritants. When these products are applied to the skin they cause a chemical burn, which can be anywhere from mild to severe. The aim is to cause skin inflammation for the purpose of increasing blood flow to the injured tissues beneath. By creating inflammation, these products are meant to speed healing, which ultimately relieves inflammation.

However, the blood vessels that supply the skin are not the same vessels that supply the deeper tissues. So, causing inflammation in the skin does not necessarily increase blood flow to the structures beneath. In other words, applying a counter-irritant to the skin does little to promote healing of a damaged tendon or joint capsule.

"Firing" (applying a hot iron to the skin) also causes severe skin damage—either second- or third-degree burns. "Blistering" and "firing" are seldom used now because they have been replaced by more effective and humane therapies. When they were commonly used, their purpose was to create skin damage that would take about as long to heal as the underlying injury. The trainer was forced to rest the horse from regular training for several weeks. No matter what their personal views of these treatments, veterinarians agree that it is the period of enforced rest that is of most benefit to the horse.

Following this reasoning, rest alone should be as effective as any of these counter-irritants, *without causing the horse more pain and suffering.*

TETANUS VACCINATION

Tetanus, or "lockjaw," is a highly fatal disease in horses. Tetanus bacteria *(Clostridium tetani)* enter the body through wounds, particularly puncture wounds. They release a toxin that affects the nervous system, resulting in agonizing muscle spasms and eventually, death from respiratory failure. *(Tetanus is discussed in more detail in Chapter 12).*

The tetanus organisms are commonly found in the horse's bowel and, therefore, in manure. So, every wound and deep defect in the hoof wall or sole poses a tetanus risk. Tetanus is very difficult to successfully treat, but it can easily be prevented by regular vaccination.

Tetanus Toxoid and Antitoxin

The tetanus vaccine, or *toxoid,* consists of inactivated tetanus toxin. When the vaccine is injected into the body, the immune system produces antibodies (protective immune proteins) against the toxin. The toxoid takes at least 2 weeks—probably longer—to produce enough antibodies to protect the horse against tetanus. But the immunity lasts up to 12 months after the initial course or annual booster.

Tetanus *antitoxin* is a preparation of purified horse antibodies to the tetanus toxin. In effect, it is an "antidote." The antitoxin provides immediate, but short-lived protection: only 7 – 10 days. Occasional cases of acute liver failure (Theiler's disease) have been reported in horses a few weeks after tetanus antitoxin was administered. The actual cause

Definitions
Tetanus *toxoid* is the vaccine.
Tetanus *antitoxin* is the short-acting "antidote."

is unknown, but it is possible that a virus in the antitoxin is involved. Because of this small but real risk, many veterinarians avoid using tetanus antitoxin in any circumstance. Instead, they urge their clients to keep all horses currently vaccinated with tetanus toxoid.

Administration Issues

Tetanus toxoid generally is given intramuscularly. It can cause mild muscle soreness at the injection site for 1 – 3 days. The pain is due to an immune-related inflammatory reaction in the muscle. Most horses do not show any signs of this reaction. But depending on where the injection was given, and how severe the inflammatory reaction is, the horse may be short-strided or mildly lame for a couple of days. This is more likely when the vaccine is injected into the muscles at the front of the chest or back of the thigh.

More Information
Treating vaccine-related muscle pain, and the preferred sites for intra-muscular injection are discussed in Chapter 10.

Tetanus antitoxin is usually given subcutaneously: by injection beneath the skin. It often causes a small lump at the injection site for 12 – 24 hours after injection. The lump appears immediately because it is a depot of injected fluid just under the skin. It is seldom hot or painful, and it disappears without treatment as the fluid is absorbed.

Vaccination Schedule

Unvaccinated Horses

The initial vaccination schedule for an unvaccinated horse or foal involves two intramuscular injections with tetanus toxoid, given 2 – 4 weeks apart. After that, the horse should receive a single "booster" toxoid injection every year for the rest of its life. Any horse that has a vague or unknown vaccination history, or has not been vaccinated in the last 18 months or so should be treated as if it is unvaccinated. It should receive the initial course of two injections, followed by annual boosters.

Before all surgical procedures, and upon discovery of any wound (no matter how minor), some veterinarians recommend that unvaccinated horses receive both the *toxoid and the antitoxin*. This provides the horse with immediate protection. (The risk of developing Theiler's disease from the antitoxin is weighed against the poten-

ROUTINE VACCINATION SCHEDULE

	Initial	Maintenance
Unvaccinated Adult	Two injections, 2 – 4 weeks apart	single "booster" every year
Foal (from 2 – 3 months old)	Two injections, 2 – 4 weeks apart (plus third injection at 6 months?)	single "booster" every year

Fig. 5–13. The tetanus vaccination schedule (using tetanus toxoid).

tial for the horse to develop tetanus before the toxoid has produced a protective level of antibodies.) To ensure continued protection, the horse must be given a second injection of toxoid 2 – 4 weeks later: the routine initial vaccination schedule.

When giving both the toxoid and the antitoxin at the same time, it is best to give the toxoid intramuscularly and the antitoxin subcutaneously in a different part of the body. This is so the antitoxin will not bind up the toxoid and reduce its effectiveness.

Vaccinated Horses

If a vaccinated horse receives a wound or requires surgery more than about 8 months after vaccination, it is worth giving the horse a booster *toxoid* at that time. This will not harm the horse, and is a small price to pay for peace of mind.

Foals

The best way to ensure that newborn foals are protected against tetanus is to give all pregnant mares a booster toxoid about 1 month before foaling. (If the mare is unvaccinated, she should receive the initial course of two injections, 2 – 4 weeks apart.) This approach ensures that the colostrum has a high level of tetanus antibodies. Foals born to unvaccinated

> **Definition**
>
> **Colostrum:** the antibody-rich milk that the mare produces around the time of foaling.

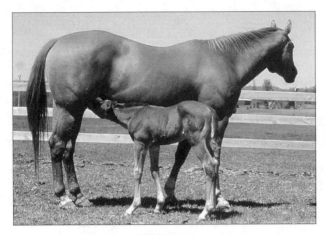

Fig. 5–14. The best way to protect newborn foals from tetanus is to vaccinate their dams during pregnancy.

mares, and foals that may not have received adequate colostrum should be given tetanus antitoxin within 24 hours of birth.

Routine vaccination against tetanus should begin when the foal is 2 – 3 months old. Before this time the antibodies received in the colostrum may prevent the foal's system from responding to the vaccine and producing its own antibodies. Some veterinarians take the precaution of revaccinating foals at 6 months of age, just in case persistent maternal antibodies interfered with the earlier vaccination.

ANTIBIOTICS

Antibiotics are an important part of therapy for many infectious conditions that cause or contribute to lameness. They are also routinely prescribed by veterinarians as a precaution following surgery. However, antibiotics are seldom effective on their own—the cause of the infection must also be addressed. For example, antibiotics are ineffective in resolving the infection while there is a piece of wood buried in a wound.

Choice of Antibiotic

The choice of antibiotic is not a simple matter—not all antibiotics are equally effective. What may work in one instance may be totally ineffective in another. For antibiotic therapy to be successful, the drug must be effective against the bacteria causing the infection. Some antibiotics are active against only a few types of bacteria.

Others are "broad-spectrum," meaning that they have some activity against many types of bacteria.

No single antibiotic is effective against all types of bacteria. Bacterial culture and antibiotic sensitivity testing are often necessary to identify the bacteria that are causing the infection, and to decide which antibiotic is most appropriate *(see Chapter 2).* In some cases the veterinarian prescribes a broad-spectrum antibiotic at the start of treatment. Once the culture and sensitivity results are known (which usually takes 24 – 48 hours), broad-spectrum antibiotics can be discontinued and the most appropriate antibiotic started.

Terminology
In this book "antibiotic" refers to a drug that specifically acts against bacteria. ("Antimicrobial" is another term that some veterinarians use.) Here, only the treatment of lameness is discussed. The horse's regular veterinarian should be consulted for more information.

In some conditions the type of bacteria causing the infection is fairly predictable. So, the veterinarian may decide not to do a culture and sensitivity test, and just use an antibiotic that is usually effective for treating that condition. However, this is a professional judgment; such decisions should never be made by an owner or trainer.

Administration Issues

Many factors can reduce the effectiveness of an antibiotic. But if the owner or trainer ensures that the horse receives all of the prescribed dose at the interval, and for the length of time recommended, some of these factors can be controlled.

Frequency

To be effective, the drug must be given at the prescribed dose rate, and at the specified interval. For example, "twice per day" means every 12 hours, not at 8:00 AM and 4:00 PM. "Three times per day" means every 8 hours, for example, at 6:00 AM, 2:00 PM, and 10:00 PM. If it is impossible to comply with the veterinarian's instructions, other arrangements should be made. For example, another boarder or a staff member can give one of the treatments. Or, the horse can be transported to a lay-up farm or veterinary clinic, where the staff can guarantee that the horse will receive its medication at the prescribed interval.

Duration

In most cases antibiotic therapy is given for at least 5 days, although this varies with the condition being treated. If antibiotics are given before and after surgery simply as a precaution, the veterinarian may discontinue them after 3 days. In cases of septic arthritis or osteomyelitis (joint or bone infections), antibiotic therapy may need to be continued for a couple of weeks. Horses treated for Equine Protozoal Myeloencephalitis (EPM) may need antibiotics for 2 – 3 months at a time.

But no matter what duration is recommended by the veterinarian, it is important to give the entire course of antibiotics. Discontinuing the drugs too soon can allow the infection to return or worsen, even though the condition may appear to have resolved.

Misuse

Antibiotics are among the most misused drugs (along with NSAIDs and corticosteroids). Some owners and trainers, and even a few veterinarians tend to overuse antibiotics, or use them in inappropriate circumstances. Such misuse can lead to poor results, and bacterial resistance to the commonly used antibiotics—a situation that makes control of some infections very difficult.

The following circumstances constitute misuse of antibiotics:

- when they are used without an accurate diagnosis—e.g. fever of unknown origin
- when they are relied upon without removing or treating the cause of the infection—e.g. an infected wound that contains a sequestrum (piece of dead bone)
- when the dose, interval, or duration is different from that recommended by the veterinarian
- when they are used without any knowledge of the type of bacteria causing the infection

To avoid the problems that can result from improper use, **antibiotics should never be given without (or against) veterinary advice.**

Potentially Harmful Effects

As with any other drug, antibiotics are distributed to every cell in the body, so their effects, both beneficial and harmful, can be wide-ranging. This section is limited to a brief discussion of the harmful effects that are more likely with the antibiotics used to treat lameness problems.

Diarrhea

The normal population of bacteria in the horse's bowel is large and very diverse. The horse relies on these bacteria for normal digestion, and protection from potentially harmful organisms in the bowel. Some antibiotics, especially those that are given orally, can upset the balance of bacteria in the bowel by destroying the beneficial bacteria, and allowing harmful bacteria to multiply. The result may be as mild as soft, loose ("cow pattie") manure. Or, it may be as severe as profuse, watery diarrhea, accompanied by fever, toxemia, shock, and death. The veterinarian should be informed if the manure changes consistency while the horse is receiving antibiotics.

Drug Reactions and Allergies

Adverse drug reactions and allergies to antibiotics are extremely uncommon in horses, with one notable exception. Procaine penicillin occasionally causes an adverse drug reaction in horses. This is not an allergic response because it can occur the first time the horse is given procaine penicillin, and it is usually safe to continue to treat the horse with the drug after such a reaction. Allergic reactions need prior exposure to the drug and time to develop antibodies against it. They also tend to become more severe with each exposure to the drug.

The signs of a procaine penicillin reaction include muscle tremors, restlessness, agitation, and hyperexcitability. In some cases the horse appears terrified, and seems to be fleeing from an invisible assailant (sometimes called the "dog biting at the heels" syndrome). Procaine penicillin reactions can be fatal, and those that are not may be alarming and potentially dangerous, both for the horse and the handler. In most cases the reaction subsides without treatment after about 10 minutes. However, during the excitable period the horse can do serious damage to itself and anyone in its way.

In contrast, allergic reactions usually cause large, flat lumps beneath the skin (urticaria), swelling of the face and muzzle, and constriction of the airways,

> **Note**
>
> Procaine penicillin reactions occur when the drug enters the bloodstream too quickly.
>
> To avoid accidentally injecting it into a blood vessel, draw back on the plunger before injecting. If blood is drawn into the syringe, relocate the needle in another part of the muscle. Check for blood again, then *slowly* inject the penicillin.

leading to difficulty breathing. As in humans, an allergic reaction can be rapidly fatal. In some cases the horse may die before showing any signs whatsoever. But again, allergic drug reactions are very uncommon in horses.

Other Effects

Oxytetracycline is an antibiotic, but it is sometimes used to treat flexor contracture ("contracted tendons") in young foals. This drug can damage red blood cells when it is given intravenously. For this reason it should be diluted in sterile saline solution before being given to foals.

Trimethoprim-sulfonamide antibiotics work by blocking folic acid use within the bacterial cell. However, they also block folic acid use in the horse's cells. Folic acid is essential for normal red blood cell production. Long-term use (longer than about 3 weeks) of this antibiotic combination can cause mild anemia.

Several antibiotics can cause kidney damage when given at high dose rates, particularly gentamicin and related drugs. The risk of kidney damage is increased if the horse is also receiving NSAIDs.

The procaine that is added to penicillin to prolong its effect is in the same class of drugs as lidocaine and other local anesthetics. These drugs are prohibited in performing horses, so giving the horse procaine penicillin may produce a positive result in a pre- or post-competition drug screen.

JOINT MEDICATIONS

Medications that specifically target the joints are often used to manage inflammatory and degenerative joint conditions, in particular, degenerative joint disease. Joint medications may also be prescribed after arthroscopic removal of bone or cartilage fragments *(see Chapter 6),* and after recovery from joint infection (septic arthritis).

The joint conditions mentioned here have very different causes. But the common result in each case, and the main reason for treatment with a joint medication, is cartilage damage.

Cartilage Damage

Joint cartilage is composed of cartilage cells in a matrix, or framework of collagen fibers and proteoglycans (large, complex molecules of amino acids and sugars). These substances give the cartilage its

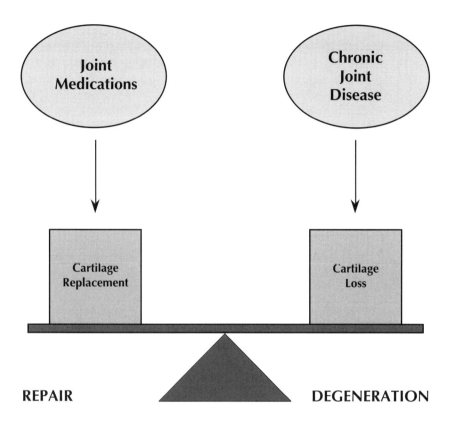

Fig. 5–15. The balance between cartilage repair and cartilage degeneration.

ability to absorb concussion and resist compression. The cartilage components, like any other tissue, are constantly "turned over." This is a process that replaces old or damaged cells with new ones, and replenishes the matrix as needed. In healthy joints there is a balance between loss and replacement of these cartilage components so that the normal thickness of healthy, resilient cartilage is constantly maintained.

The destructive processes within a diseased joint result in part from inflammatory substances and cartilage-degrading enzymes. These products can upset the balance of cartilage loss and replacement, tipping the scale toward depletion of the components that give the cartilage its strength and resilience. This weakens the cartilage, making it more prone to physical damage during exercise.

These destructive substances can also degrade hyaluronic acid, the

Degenerative Joint Disease (DJD) is a chronic, progressive condition that consists of:
- joint capsule fibrosis
- cartilage degeneration

These changes are caused by:
1. Chronic strain and inflammation of the joint capsule and synovium.
2. Repeated, excessive cartilage compression during exercise.

(See Chapter 8 for more information on DJD and other joint problems.)

molecules in the joint fluid that give the fluid its lubricating properties. Hyaluronic acid has a crucial role in maintaining a healthy environment within the joint space and protecting the joint surfaces.

Medical Options

Cartilage has slow and limited repair capabilities. Once significant cartilage damage has occurred, it is unlikely that any medication can do much more than slow the degenerative process. No drug can prevent cartilage damage from physical insult, but several drugs can protect the cartilage by inhibiting the joint's own destructive responses. Slowing the degenerative process may aid cartilage repair by restoring the balance between loss and replacement of the cartilage components.

NSAIDs and DMSO suppress inflammation within the joint. In doing so, they block one of the prime movers of cartilage degeneration: inflammation of the joint capsule lining (the synovium). NSAIDs generally are given orally or intravenously, whereas DMSO is usually applied topically for this purpose.

NSAIDs and DMSO

Positive Effects	Negative Effects
• reduce soft tissue inflammation	• see Figures 5–6 and 5–10 • limited or prohibited in performing horses

Fig. 5–16. Effects of NSAIDs and DMSO on horses with joint disease.

There are three separate groups of drugs that are considered to be specific joint medications:

- corticosteroids ("cortisone")
- hyaluronic acid (HA)
- glycosaminoglycans (GAGs)

Traditionally, these drugs are given by injection directly into the joint (intra-articularly, or IA). However, recent research has found that these products can also be effective when given by other routes, for example, intravenous HA, and intramuscular corticosteroids or GAGs. This approach avoids the possible complications of IA injection: joint infection, cartilage damage by the needle, and chemical irritation of the joint lining (chemical synovitis).

Corticosteroids

The use of corticosteroids to treat joint disease is a controversial issue among veterinarians. This is because when high doses are given repeatedly, corticosteroids can slow cartilage repair and may even accelerate cartilage degeneration. High doses can also inhibit the production of hyaluronic acid in the joint. As a result, the molecules of HA that were degraded by inflammation are not immediately replaced. But there is evidence that low doses can increase HA production in a diseased joint.

> **Reminder**
>
> The actions and harmful effects of NSAIDs and corticosteroids were discussed in the earlier section on Anti-Inflammatory Therapy.

Despite these potentially harmful effects, corticosteroids are potent anti-inflammatory drugs, and so can quickly stop the destructive cycle of inflammation and cartilage degeneration if used with care. A single, low-dose injection of a corticosteroid can very effectively relieve inflammation in the joint, without adversely affecting cartilage repair.

Administration Issues

Corticosteroids can produce a rapid and remarkable response in inflamed joints. But, while a response is usually seen within 24 hours of injection, it is only temporary. It may last from a few days to several weeks, depending on the product, the severity of the joint damage, and how strenuously the horse is exercised after treatment. Repeated IA injection of corticosteroids should be avoided because of the possible harmful effects on the cartilage. Other treatments should be considered for the long-term management of chronic joint disease.

There are two other cautions about the IA use of corticosteroids.

CORTICOSTEROIDS

Positive Effects	Negative Effects
• effectively reduce soft tissue inflammation • may increase HA production (at low doses)	• reduced production of cartilage components, leading to cartilage degeneration (at high doses) • reduced HA production and joint fluid quality (at high doses) • suppression of inflammation and immune response mask signs of joint infection when given IA • prohibited in performing horses

Fig. 5–17. Effects of corticosteroids on horses with joint disease.

First, these drugs suppress inflammation and the immune response within the joint. So, they can mask the signs of joint infection for several days after IA injection—a potentially devastating effect. Second, even though the drug was injected directly into the joint, some of it is absorbed into the bloodstream. Thus, corticosteroids can be detected in pre- or post-competition drug screens, possibly for several weeks after injection with the long-acting steroids. Giving the drug

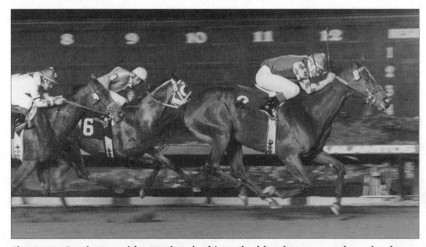

Fig. 5–18. Corticosteroids are absorbed into the bloodstream, and can be detected in pre- or post-competition drug screens.

intramuscularly prevents the first of these problems, and it has the added advantage of treating several joints at once. This can be of benefit in older horses that have DJD in several joints.

Hyaluronic Acid (HA)

Commercial preparations of hyaluronic acid (HA; also just called "acid") can:

- reduce joint inflammation, though not as effectively as anti-inflammatory drugs
- aid in joint lubrication
- help protect the cartilage surfaces from further destruction by harmful inflammatory substances

Injected HA is rapidly cleared from the joint fluid, but some stays in the synovium where it reduces inflammation and stimulates HA production. This explains how signs of joint inflammation are reduced for several weeks in some horses.

HA may aid cartilage repair by reducing the rate of cartilage degeneration, and by restoring a more normal environment within the joint. In other words, HA can help tip the scales toward cartilage repair.

Administration Issues

These products are injected into the affected joint(s), although there is at least one product that can be given intravenously (IV). Giving the medication IV avoids the risks of IA injection, and it also allows several joints to be treated at the same time. However, for this latter reason, a higher IV dose is needed to achieve the same benefits

HYALURONIC ACID (HA)

Positive Effects	Negative Effects
• reduces soft tissue inflammation • improves joint fluid quality by stimulating HA production • aids cartilage repair by protecting cartilage surfaces from inflammatory substances	None Known

Fig. 5–19. Effects of hyaluronic acid on horses with joint disease.

as IA injection. With either route, a single injection of HA is usually all that is necessary. The veterinarian may repeat the treatment every 1 – 2 weeks in horses with chronic joint disease.

Commercial HA products vary in the size, or molecular weight of the hyaluronate molecules. Some veterinarians believe that the higher molecular weight products are more effective and longer-lasting than the lower molecular weight products. The duration of effect can also be increased by using a larger dose of HA.

Incidentally, HA has also been used to treat tendonitis and tenosynovitis (inflammation of a tendon sheath; *see Chapter 11*). The drug is injected into the area of tendon fiber damage, or directly into the tendon sheath. Its anti-inflammatory and lubricating effects apparently reduce inflammation and adhesions (fibrous bands between tissues) at the site of injury. Some veterinarians believe that HA may also speed up tendon fiber repair, although this has yet to be proven.

Glycosaminoglycans (GAGs)

Glycosaminoglycans, or GAGs (such as Adequan®) are large, complex molecules that are similar in structure to the proteoglycans found in normal cartilage. After injection, the body quickly incorporates the GAGs into the cartilage. *Experimentally*, these drugs have some very positive effects:

- they protect the cartilage from further destruction by enzymes
- they increase the production of collagen and proteoglycans
- they stimulate the production of new cartilage cells

They may also increase HA production. The claims that GAGs can prevent further cartilage damage and enhance cartilage repair have earned these compounds the title of "chondro-protective" (cartilage-

GLYCOSAMINOGLYCANS (GAGs)

Positive Effects	Negative Effects
• reduce soft tissue inflammation • experimentally, they reduce cartilage damage by enzymes, and increase production of cartilage components and HA	• can cause chemical synovitis after IA injection • can make joint infection more likely after IA injection

Fig. 5–20. Effects of GAGs on horses with joint disease.

protectors). However, as good as this sounds, no clinical studies have yet proven that these products—when given at the recommended dose rate—protect the cartilage from further damage. Nor has it been proven that GAGs speed up the repair of cartilage defects or improve the quality of cartilage that fills the defects (called "repair cartilage"). Realistically, these products probably are a little more effective than other medications in tipping the scales away from cartilage destruction, in favor of cartilage repair. In practical terms, GAGs can visibly improve some horses with chronic joint disease. But they fail to have any apparent short- or long-term effects in other horses.

Administration Issues

Adequan can be given intra-articularly (IA) or intramuscularly (IM). IA injection with Adequan occasionally causes a severe inflammatory reaction in the joint (chemical synovitis) within about 24 hours of injection. Treatment involves anti-inflammatory therapy: in particular, cold therapy, NSAIDs, and DMSO. In severe cases the veterinarian may also lavage the joint with sterile saline solution *(see Chapter 6)*.

> **Of Interest**
>
> Adequan® is a polysulfated GAG, or PSGAG. Several sulfur molecules are attached to the core GAG.

Adequan also increases the potential for joint infection after IA injection. For this reason, some veterinarians add an antibiotic to the solution before injecting Adequan IA. This precaution is unnecessary when giving the drug IM.

IM injection of Adequan avoids the risk of joint inflammation and infection. In addition, the drug is distributed to every joint in the body. This means that more than one damaged joint can be treated with a single injection. However, a higher dose (at least twice the IA dose) may be needed IM to get the same benefits.

Whether giving Adequan IA or IM, it is usually given as a course of injections, twice per week for 3 – 4 weeks. This drug may be given at up to five times the recommended dose without any harmful effects.

There are several oral GAG products available, although they do not appear to be as effective as IA or IM Adequan. These compounds are well absorbed from the intestine. But there is some question of whether they enter the joints in an active form or at a high enough concentration to be very effective. Despite these concerns, oral GAGs do appear to help some horses with chronic joint disease. 🐴

6

VETERINARY PROCEDURES

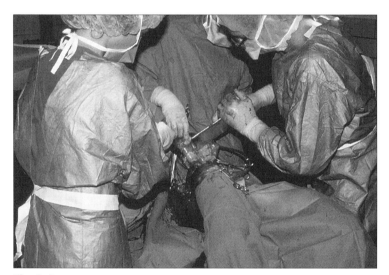

Fig. 6–1.

The procedures described in this chapter are performed by the veterinarian. Typical recommendations for the horse's care after the procedure are discussed. In many cases the veterinarian relies on the owner or trainer to carry out these instructions. Each case is a little different, so the veterinarian will provide specific instructions for managing the horse.

JOINT LAVAGE

Joint lavage is a very important part of managing joint infection (septic arthritis; *see Chapter 8*). Inflammatory substances released by the joint capsule lining, toxins produced by the bacteria, and enzymes released by white blood cells can cause severe damage to the cartilage surfaces. Also, fibrin (a blood-clotting protein) can leak into the joint from the inflamed joint capsule lining, and form adhesions. These fibrous bands can restrict normal joint mobility.

More Information
Inflammatory substances and white blood cells are discussed in Chapter 5, in the section on Anti-Inflammatory Therapy.

Lavage involves flushing the joint with large volumes of sterile saline solution to remove these harmful substances and debris from the joint. In most cases the veterinarian samples the joint fluid for bacterial culture and antibiotic sensitivity testing *(see Chapter 2)* before flushing the joint. Lavage is most effective when performed as soon as joint infection is suspected. The sooner the joint is lavaged, the sooner the infection is controlled and the joint can begin to recover—and the better the chances of a satisfactory outcome. Also, secondary problems, such as cartilage erosions, adhesions, and joint capsule fibrosis, are prevented or minimized if the joint is lavaged early in the course of the disease.

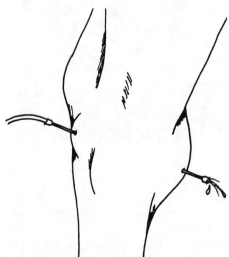

Fig. 6–2. Joint lavage in the hock.

Technique

The veterinarian may lavage the joint using a catheter (about the size of a large needle). This involves placing a sterile catheter in each side of the joint, flushing sterile saline solution through one catheter and allowing the fluid to leave through the other.

If there is a wound that involves the joint capsule, or if the material in the joint is very thick, the veterinarian may instead lavage the joint through a small incision. With this procedure the saline is flushed in and allowed to drain back out through the same hole. Dissolving and removing the pus, fibrin, and other debris can be aided by repeatedly flexing and extending the joint gently during lavage.

The joint is lavaged until the fluid leaving it is clear. This can take as little as 50 – 100 ml in foals, or up to 5 liters in the larger joints (hock and stifle) of adult horses. The procedure may need to be repeated every 1 – 2 days until the signs and joint fluid analysis *(see Chapter 2)* indicate that the infection is controlled and the inflammation is resolving.

Joint lavage can be very painful, so a nerve block or general anesthesia may be necessary. General anesthesia has the advantage of ensuring that the horse remains completely still during the procedure. This minimizes the risks of damaging the cartilage or breaking off the catheter within the joint. Even though the joint may already be infected, it is important that the veterinarian uses strictly sterile techniques to prevent contamination of the joint with other bacteria. Depending on the condition being treated, the veterinarian may inject antibiotics or DMSO into the joint after lavage. If a small incision is used, the joint must be protected from further contamination with a sterile dressing and clean bandage.

Note
Sterile techniques, also called "aseptic" techniques, include:
• clipping the hair
• scrubbing the skin
• using sterile gloves
• using sterile equipment and materials
(See Chapter 2 for more information.)

SURGERY

There is a wide variety of musculoskeletal conditions that may require surgical treatment. Most equine veterinarians have the equipment and skills to perform straightforward surgical procedures, such as suturing deep wounds, periosteal "stripping" in foals with angular limb deformities, and removal of a fractured splint bone. But other, more complicated surgical procedures may need to be performed by an equine surgeon who has the specialized equipment and advanced training necessary to perform these procedures.

Arthroscopic surgery and surgical repair of a fracture are examples of procedures that may require referral to a specialist equine sur-

Definitions

Collateral ligaments: short, strong ligaments at the sides of a joint.
Joint capsule: fibrous, outer covering of a joint.
Synovium: membrane that lines the joint capsule and produces synovial fluid.

(Joint structure and diseases are discussed in Chapter 8.)

geon. Because the two procedures are mentioned in several places throughout the book, their uses, techniques, and post-operative care are discussed below.

Arthroscopic Surgery

Arthroscopy uses a rigid endoscope with a fiberoptic cable and light source to examine the interior of joints. Specially designed instruments are used to remove bone and cartilage fragments from the joint. Soft tissues within the joint, such as the fibrous pad at the front of the fetlock, can also be trimmed or removed from the joint with the arthroscopic instruments.

Arthroscopy has several advantages over the older technique, called arthrotomy, which involved making a relatively large incision in the skin and joint capsule. Although arthroscopy may be more expensive, its advantages over arthrotomy include:

- less trauma to the soft tissues of the joint: collateral ligaments, joint capsule, and synovium
- better view of the joint's interior, allowing the surgeon to determine the extent of cartilage and soft tissue damage
- easier to locate and remove bone and cartilage fragments, and identify smaller secondary lesions
- faster post-operative recovery and return to athletic activity
- better prognosis for athletic usefulness in some cases
- better cosmetic result

Technique

The procedure is performed under general anesthesia, with the horse either on its back or on its side. The standard surgical principles of sterility are very important with this procedure. All items that touch the surgical site after it has been prepared for surgery (clipped and scrubbed with antiseptic) must be sterile.

At the start of the procedure the surgeon uses a needle to inflate the joint with sterile saline solution. A small incision (less than ½ inch, or 12 mm long) is then made in the skin, subcutaneous tissue, and joint capsule. The arthroscope is inserted into the joint, and the joint surfaces are examined. Once the bone/cartilage fragment (or soft tissue lesion) is found, a second small incision is made in a position that allows an instrument to be inserted into the joint for retrieval of the fragment. This second incision is usually made on the other side of the joint. So, the surgeon looks down the scope through one hole and guides the instrument to pick up the fragment through the other hole.

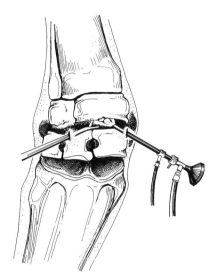

Throughout the procedure, sterile saline solution is pumped through the joint. This keeps the joint capsule inflated and flushes away any blood or debris that may reduce visibility. Once the surgeon has retrieved all the fragments, and inspected and removed any damaged cartilage, the joint is lavaged to remove any remaining debris. In most cases the skin is then sutured, and a light bandage is placed over the joint (in suitable locations).

Fig. 6–3. Arthroscopic surgery allows the joint surfaces to be examined. (The horse is lying on its back for this procedure.)

Post-Operative Care Following Arthroscopy
Initial Care

The horse is confined to a stall or small pen at least until the sutures are removed, which generally takes place about 7 days after surgery. The joint is usually kept bandaged (and the bandage changed as needed) for at least 3 days, preferably until the sutures are removed.

Many surgeons do not prescribe antibiotics after arthroscopic surgery. When antibiotics are given, they are usually given for only 2 – 3 days. Although the risk of tetanus is slight with this procedure, every horse undergoing surgery should be currently vaccinated against tetanus. Most horses seem to be quite comfortable after arthroscopic surgery,

> **More Information**
>
> Medications, including antibiotics, tetanus toxoid and antitoxin, and NSAIDs are covered in Chapter 5.

but surgeons routinely give an NSAID (such as phenylbutazone) for a couple of days. This helps to reduce the inevitable soft tissue inflammation within and around the joint. Hand-walking for 15 – 20 minutes twice per day is also beneficial after surgery, although it is important to check with the surgeon first.

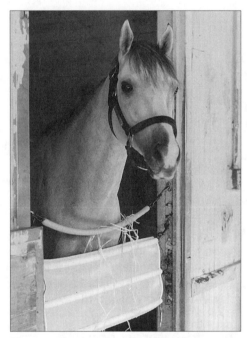

Fig. 6–4. The duration of stall confinement depends on the degree of inflammation and cartilage damage within the joint.

Duration of Turnout

The duration of stall confinement depends on the degree of inflammation and cartilage damage within the joint. It may be as short as a week, or as long as a month following surgery. Likewise, the duration of pasture turnout and rehabilitation may vary from 6 weeks to 6 months *(see the Rest section of Chapter 4).* Full-thickness cartilage defects—those that expose the underlying bone—take at least 3 months to fill in. Even then, the cartilage that fills the defect is not as strong or resilient as normal, healthy cartilage. So, if large bone and cartilage fragments were removed or deep cartilage erosions were found, most surgeons advise at least 3 months of rest before returning the horse to regular exercise. Joint medications, either hyaluronic acid or Adequan, may also be advised, shortly after surgery or just before the horse resumes regular exercise *(see Chapter 5).*

Surgical Repair of Fractures

For fracture healing to proceed as quickly as possible, the fracture site must be stabilized. That is, movement between the pieces of bone must be minimized. In some cases, a thick bandage (with or without splints; *see Chapter 4*) or a fiberglass cast may provide enough stability. However, some fractures require surgical stabilization with metal implants, either bone screws, plates, or pins.

Techniques

Bone Screws and Plates

Fracture stability can sometimes be achieved by attaching the bone fragment to the main part of the bone, or attaching two equally sized pieces to each other with bone screws. The metal screws keep the fracture pieces closely aligned while fibrous tissue, and then bone, bridge the gap and permanently stabilize the bone *(see Chapter 9)*.

The procedure is performed under general anesthesia, usually with the horse lying on its side. A common method, called "lag screw" fixation is performed as follows:

A. A hole is drilled in one side of the bone with a drill bit that is the same width as the outer diameter of the screw thread.

B. The drill hole is then extended across the fracture line and into the other part of the bone with a drill bit the same width as the core of the screw.

C. A thread is then made ("tapped") in this deeper part of the drill hole so that the screw's thread will anchor into the bone.

D. As the screw is tightened, the fracture pieces are pulled toward each other and the fracture line is compressed.

As many screws as necessary are placed across the fracture line to achieve stability. These screws can remain in place for the horse's lifetime. However, the surgeon may decide to remove them once the fracture has completely healed (usually at least 2 months after fracture repair). Bone screws can restrict the normal amount of "give" a bone has, and this sometimes causes chronic, low-grade lameness.

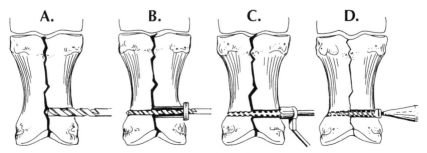

Fig. 6–5. Lag screw fixation of a pastern bone fracture.

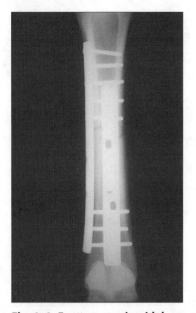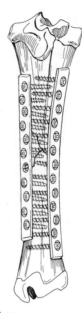

Fig. 6–6. Fracture repair with bone plates.

The screws do not need to be removed in every case. The risk of a second surgical procedure should be weighed against the horse's performance. If the horse is performing satisfactorily, the screws can be left in.

Bone Plates
Some fractures require the extra support of one or two bone plates. The stainless steel plates, and the bone screws that anchor them to the bone, keep the fracture pieces together. The plates also help protect the fractured bone from weight-bearing forces, as well as distracting forces from the tendons and ligaments that attach to the fracture pieces.

Definition

Longbones: long, thick, roughly cylindrical bones such as the cannon bone and radius.

(See Chapter 9 for more information on bones.)

With longbone fractures, two plates are anchored in place with bone screws: for example, one plate on the side and one on the front of the bone. Once the fracture has healed, the plates can be removed, either one at a time or both at once.

Bone screws or plates may also be used to surgically fuse a badly damaged joint. This technique is called arthrodesis.

Bone Pins and Orthopedic Wire
Some longbone fractures can be repaired with an intramedullary bone pin. This pin is a solid metal rod that is inserted into the medullary, or "bone marrow" cavity in the bone's center. Some of these pins can be anchored with bone screws for added fracture stability. The bone screws help prevent the bone pieces from rotating around the pin.

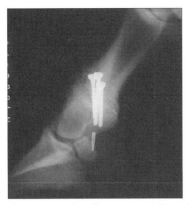 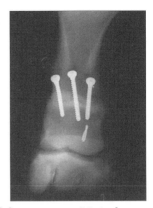

Fig. 6–7. Fusing the pastern joint with bone screws. (Note the drill bit that has broken off in the bone!)

Smaller bone pins are sometimes used for fracture repair of other bones. Examples include the olecranon (point of the elbow) and the calcaneus (point of the hock). The pin runs through the bone fragment, anchoring it onto the main part of the bone. Orthopedic wire is usually combined with these small pins for extra compression of the fracture line. A bone screw is inserted just below the fracture, and the wire is placed in a figure-eight pattern around the base of the pin and the head of the screw. This holds the fracture fragment in place

Fig. 6–8. Left: A bone pin stabilized with bone screws. Right: Bone screws, a bone plate, and orthopedic wire fuse the fetlock joint following a complete sesamoid bone fracture.

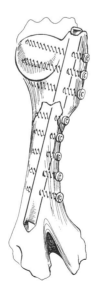 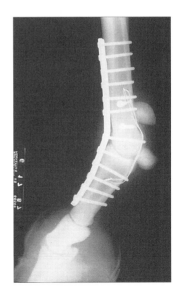

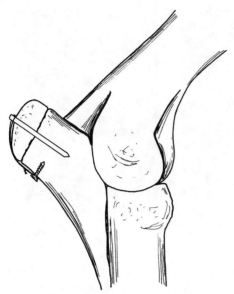

and resists the distracting forces of the muscles that attach onto the fragment.

Orthopedic wire is also used in foals with angular limb deformities. The wire can be wrapped in a figure-eight pattern around bone screws placed on either side of the physis (growth plate). This temporarily prevents growth on that side of the physis. Stainless steel staples are also used for this purpose. *(Managing angular limb deformities and other developmental problems is discussed in Chapter 14.)*

Fig. 6–9. A small bone pin and orthopedic wire used to repair an olecranon fracture.

Bone Graft

Sometimes a fracture is so severe that part of the bone shatters into fragments that are too small to be repaired. These fragments cannot be stabilized, and they commonly lose their blood supply. In these cases the surgeon may remove the fragments and fill the defect with a bone graft, before stabilizing the fracture. Incomplete fractures are sometimes treated by drilling along the fracture line and filling the hole with a bone graft.

Definitions

Cortex: dense, outer layer of a bone.
Cancellous bone: relatively soft, lattice-like bone beneath the cortex.
Osteoblasts: bone-forming cells.

(See Chapter 9 for more information on bones.)

Cancellous bone is a good source of osteoblasts. Filling the fracture site with cancellous bone does not provide any strength or stability to the fracture. But it does provide a matrix, or framework for new bone cells and mineral deposits. Thus, it speeds up the rate and quality of bone production at the fracture site.

Cancellous bone usually is harvested from the point of the horse's hip during surgery. After cutting or chiseling through the cortex at the harvest site, the cancellous bone is scooped out and deposited into the fracture site. The skin over the harvest site is sutured closed, and the wound is managed like any other surgical wound. This procedure does not leave an obvious defect at the harvest site once the area has healed.

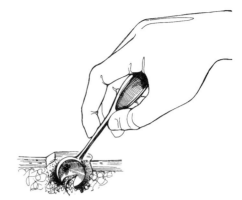

Fig. 6–10. Harvesting cancellous bone for a bone graft.

Post-Operative Care Following Surgical Fracture Repair

Initial Care

Even though the fracture has been stabilized with metal implants, most surgeons take the precaution of applying a fiberglass cast (discussed later) to the horse's leg. The cast helps protect the repaired fracture from the extreme stresses it must withstand when the horse gets up after anesthesia. This is the time when implants are more likely to loosen, bend, or break, or the bone fractures above or below the repair site. In most cases the cast is removed 1 – 2 days after surgery, and replaced with either a thick support bandage or a standard bandage *(see Chapter 4)*.

Damaged bone and the surrounding bruised or traumatized soft tissue are excellent environments for bacterial growth. Therefore, broad-spectrum antibiotics are given before surgery, and continued for at least 5 days. The horse's tetanus status must also be addressed before surgery. NSAIDs are given for several days after surgery, to reduce swelling and relieve discomfort. The precautions necessary with long-term use of these drugs are discussed in Chapter 9. *(Antibiotic therapy, tetanus prevention, and NSAIDs are discussed in Chapter 5.)*

If pus begins to drain from the surgical wound, or if radiographs show that bone infection (osteomyelitis) has developed, the affected screws may need to be removed. Diseased bone may also need to be removed. Depending on the stage of fracture healing and the number of screws that are removed, the fracture may need to be restabilized with extra bone screws or a cast. Osteomyelitis is a very serious complication of surgical fracture repair *(see Chapter 9)*.

Duration of Turnout

Following surgical fracture repair, the horse must be confined in a stall or small pen for at least 6 weeks, or until radiographs indicate that the fracture has healed. As healing progresses, the fracture line is eventually replaced with bone. At the bone surface this may be seen as a bony callus. Once the fracture has healed, the horse can be permitted a limited amount of paddock activity. But it is important that the horse is not suddenly turned out into a pasture after being confined to a stall *(see Chapter 4)*. The healed bone must be gradually loaded so that it can increase its strength and resilience without being damaged by overactivity. *(Rehabilitation following fracture repair is discussed in Chapter 9.)*

CASTS

Fiberglass casts can be used to provide extra stability for a variety of lower leg conditions, including:

- fractures
- wounds (especially on the heel bulbs and pastern)
- hoof wall defects
- tendon lacerations or rupture
- dislocated (luxated) joints
- surgical fusion of a joint (arthrodesis)

A cast can be the primary means of stabilizing a fracture. Or, it can be used after surgical repair of the fracture to protect the metal implants from the extreme forces on the fracture site when the horse gets up after anesthesia.

The support a cast provides can substantially improve the rate and quality of bone and soft tissue healing. However, the cast can create problems of its own, from mild dermatitis (skin irritation) to severe pressure sores and flexor laxity *(see Chapter 14)*. Full limb casts are occasionally used in horses and foals. But these casts are associated with far more problems than a cast that just extends to the knee or hock. In all cases the cast should only be applied by an experienced equine veterinarian who can check on the horse frequently.

Cast Maintenance

Unlike a bandage, a cast cannot easily be removed and replaced just to inspect the leg. Therefore, it is very important that the cast is checked at least twice per day for the following signs:

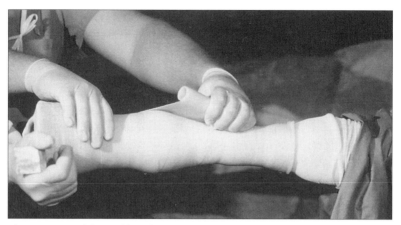

Fig. 6–11. Applying a fiberglass cast.

- soft or wet areas—due to drainage from an underlying wound, or wetting with water or urine
- specific areas of heat—this may indicate a pressure sore
- odor or flies—good indicators of problems under the cast
- cracks or splits in the cast
- abrasions around the top, or swelling above the cast

The horse should also be observed closely for signs of discomfort, such as pawing, rubbing or biting at the cast, and increased lameness. A cracked cast does not provide stability, and it can allow sufficient movement to create pressure sores. So, if the cast is cracked it may need to be replaced. When any of these signs is noticed, the veterinarian should be informed.

Even if all is well, the cast usually needs to be changed at least once during treatment. In young foals the cast must be removed or replaced after 10 – 14 days so that growth is not restricted. Adult horses can usually tolerate a cast for longer. But if the injury requires a cast for several weeks, it should be replaced every 3 – 4 weeks. While the cast is off, the hoof wall should be trimmed. Because the normal forces on the foot are substantially altered while the cast is on, the wall grows rapidly, particularly at the heels, and the heels tend to become contracted *(see Chapter 7)*.

The length of time the leg must remain in the cast depends on the injury. If the cast was only applied to protect the metal implants and fracture repair site as the horse gets up from anesthesia, it usually is removed 24 – 48 hours after surgery. For wounds below the fetlock, the cast usually is left on for 2 – 3 weeks. For a fracture, dislocation, or surgical joint fusion, a cast must be used for 6 weeks to 3 months, depending on the site and severity of the condition.

Cast Removal

Most veterinarians remove fiberglass casts with an oscillating saw. This tool cuts through the cast by rapidly vibrating forward and back, but it only cuts when pressure is applied. However, it is still possible to cut the skin and hoof wall with this saw, so care must be taken. Recently, a polyurethane resin-impregnated padding material has become available for use under casts. As well as reducing the potential for pressure sores beneath the cast, it helps prevent injury to the skin and hoof during cast removal.

When applying the cast, some veterinarians place a piece of braided wire lengthwise beneath the cast (between the padding material and the fiberglass) on each side of the leg. This makes cast removal safe and simple. The veterinarian locates the ends of the wire, and cuts through the fiberglass from the inside out by pulling the wire back and forth in a sawing motion.

When the cast is removed, a thick support bandage may need to be applied for a few days until the joints regain their normal mobility and the flexor tendons their normal tension. The leg can then be "weaned off" the extra support by replacing the thick bandage with a standard bandage, and then leaving the leg unbandaged. A support bandage usually is unnecessary if the cast has been on for 2 weeks or less. *(See Chapter 4 for more information on bandaging.)*

SECTION
III

DISEASE PROCESSES & THEIR MANAGEMENT

This section divides the musculoskeletal system into five parts: the foot, joints, bones, muscles, and tendons and ligaments. Each chapter details the disease processes that affect that part of the musculoskeletal system.

This section also covers problems of the nervous system and skin that can either directly or indirectly lead to lameness. The final chapter in this section discusses developmental problems in foals and young horses.

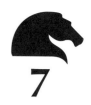

HOOF CONFORMATION
&
SHOEING OPTIONS

The horse's body is supported on four columns—its legs—which, compared with its size and weight, are long and narrow. The foot is the base of the column. The weight of the horse (and rider) is concentrated in the feet, and this pressure is intensified by ground impact forces during motion. Therefore, the foot is under constant pressure, both while the horse

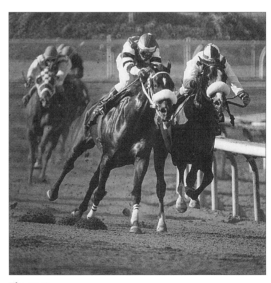

Fig. 7–1.

is standing still and when it is moving. The foot absorbs some of these forces and transmits the rest up the column.

So, it is not surprising that most causes of lameness involve the foot, either primarily or secondarily. This chapter deals with the more common abnormalities of foot shape that can either cause lameness themselves, or cause joint, bone, or soft tissue problems that lead to lameness.

More Information
The internal structures of the foot are described and illustrated in Chapter 15. That chapter is devoted to specific foot conditions, including: • navicular bone problems • laminitis • pedal bone problems • bruises and abscesses • white line disease • quarter cracks

NORMAL FOOT STRUCTURE

The bones and soft tissues of the foot are encased in a capsule of firm, insensitive tissue: the horn of the hoof wall, sole, and frog. This chapter deals mainly with these external structures.

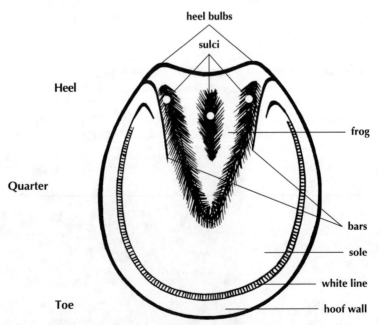

Fig. 7–2. External structures of the foot.

Hoof Wall

At the junction between the skin of the pastern and the hoof wall is a rim of specialized tissue called the coronary band. It consists of blood vessels and the coronary corium, which is the layer of cells that produce the horn tubules of the hoof wall. These tubules are about as thick as hair, and are "glued" together to form the solid hoof wall. The horn tubules grow down the wall, like fingernails grow from the nailbed at the base of the nail. There is a very thin, whitish,

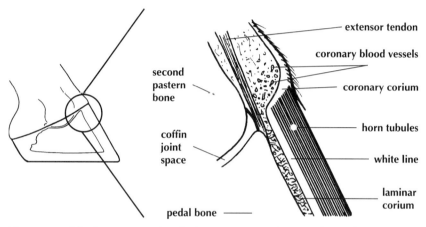

Fig. 7–3. Inside the coronary band, the coronary corium produces the horn tubules that make up the hoof wall.

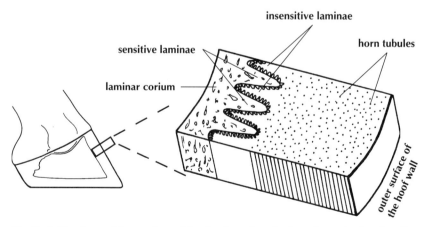

Fig. 7–4. The insensitive and sensitive laminae interlock to form the hoof wall–pedal bone bond.

cuticle-like layer of horn (called the periople) that covers an inch of wall just below the hairline. The periople protects the new wall from excessive moisture or dryness.

The hoof wall consists of a thick, outer layer of horn (which in many horses is pigmented, or dark) and a thinner, white, inner layer. At the ground surface this inner layer forms the "white line." Neither of these layers are supplied with nerves, so they are "insensitive."

Between the inner layer of wall and the pedal (or coffin) bone is another thin layer called the laminar corium. This tissue connects the hoof wall to the surface of the pedal bone. The inner surface of the hoof wall (the white line) has thousands of tiny, finger-like projections called laminae. These projections interlock with similar, tiny corrugations (also called laminae) in the laminar corium overlying the pedal bone. It is this tight bond between the hoof wall and the pedal bone that holds the hoof together. To replace the wall that would normally be worn away at the ground surface (in an unshod horse), the wall must continue to grow. To accomplish this while still maintaining the hoof wall–pedal bone bond, the projections on the inner surface of the wall slowly slide down the corrugations in the laminar corium.

The laminar corium is richly supplied with blood vessels and nerves, which is why the tiny grooves in this part of the wall are often called the "sensitive laminae." Disruption of the blood supply to the sensitive laminae can cause the laminar cells to die. When this occurs the hoof wall–pedal bone bond breaks down, which can allow the pedal bone to rotate or sink *(see the section on Laminitis in Chapter 15).*

On a less devastating scale, pressure from ground impact forces may cause the sensitive and insensitive laminae to separate at various places along the ground surface. With either situation (interruption of blood supply or ground impact forces) these areas of separation are permanent. The laminae do not reattach once they have been torn apart. But, over time the separated area eventually grows out at the ground surface. As the new horn moves down the wall from the coronary band, it can attach to the laminar corium at the previous site of separation (provided the corium is not permanently damaged).

Sole, Frog, and Deeper Structures

The sole consists of an outer layer that grows down from the solar corium overlying the bottom of the pedal bone. The solar corium is

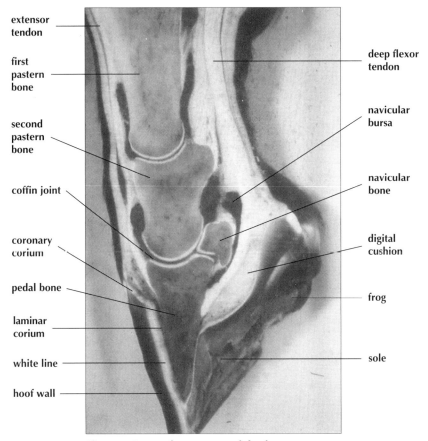

extensor tendon

first pastern bone

second pastern bone

coffin joint

coronary corium

pedal bone

laminar corium

white line

hoof wall

deep flexor tendon

navicular bursa

navicular bone

digital cushion

frog

sole

Fig. 7–5. Internal structures of the foot.

well supplied with blood vessels and nerves, so it is "sensitive" tissue; the outer layer of the sole is "insensitive."

The frog also consists of a thick, insensitive, outer layer and a thinner, sensitive, inner layer. But the outer layer of the frog is much softer and more pliable than the horn of the sole or wall. Directly above the frog is an area of fibrous connective tissue and blood vessels called the digital cushion. This tissue absorbs some of the ground impact forces, protecting the deeper structures of the foot from excessive concussion. It also helps move blood through the foot and back up the leg.

As Figure 7–5 illustrates, the internal structures of the horse's foot are:

- **pedal bone**—also called the coffin bone because it is completely encased in the box-like hoof capsule; this bone is also referred to as the third phalanx (P3)
- **second pastern bone**—also called the short or middle pastern bone, and the second phalanx (P2)
- **coffin joint**—between the pedal bone and second pastern bone
- **navicular bone**—also called the distal sesamoid bone; it forms the back of the coffin joint
- **deep flexor tendon**—begins at the top of the leg and attaches onto the bottom of the pedal bone
- **navicular bursa**—a protective sac between the navicular bone and the deep flexor tendon
- **extensor tendon**—begins at the top of the leg and attaches onto the extensor process at the front of the pedal bone

INFLUENCE OF CONFORMATION

Conformation of the foot and the rest of the limb has an important bearing on the horse's movement and its ability to withstand strenuous exercise. If one or more parts of the limb deviate from normal alignment, the forces on the column are no longer distributed evenly. It is then likely that excessive stresses will damage one or several structures in the limb. In some cases the opposite limb is also affected by this abnormal distribution of weight. Thus, conformation is primarily about function, not the horse's appearance.

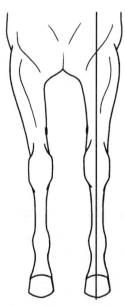

Fig. 7–6. Front View: A line through the center of the limb should perfectly bisect it.

Assessing Limb Conformation

When looking at the horse from the front, it should be possible to draw an imaginary vertical line from the point of the shoulder, through the center of the forearm, knee, cannon bone, fetlock, pastern, and foot. From the rear of the horse, an imaginary vertical line should also perfectly bisect the hindlimb. In other words, all parts of the column should be aligned, with the foot placed squarely under the column.

From the side, a vertical line through the center of the cannon should reach the ground just behind the heel bulbs. (Specific conformation of the foot is discussed later.)

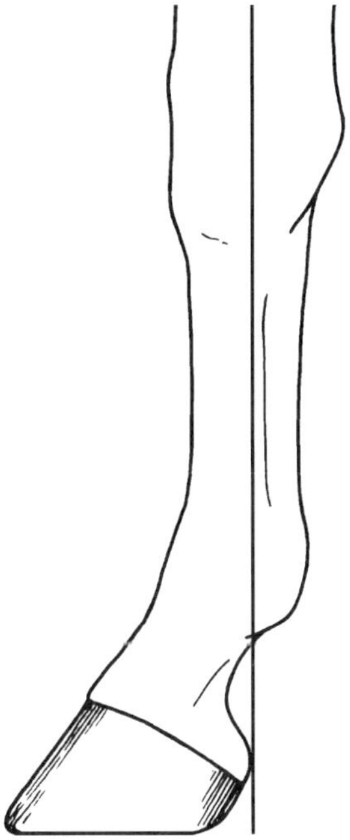

Altering Limb Conformation

In many cases conformational abnormalities begin with a developmental orthopedic disorder, such as an angular or flexural limb deformity. Unless the condition is completely corrected in the young foal, permanent conformational abnormalities commonly result. These defects cannot be corrected once the horse is mature; they can simply be managed, more or less successfully.

Abnormal limb conformation can affect foot shape. For example, an angular limb deformity (ALD) causes uneven loading on the foot and abnormal hoof wall growth. But on the other hand, abnormal foot conformation can adversely affect the rest of the limb. For example, the long toe–low heel foot shape can over-stress the lower joints and flexor tendons, even though the horse has good leg conformation.

The effect the foot has on the rest of the column can sometimes be used to advantage. Using a foal with an ALD as an example, trimming one side of the hoof or using plastic glue-on shoes with "wings" can straighten a mild ALD.

Using the same techniques on older foals or mature horses to correct a conformational defect is ineffective. It can even overstress the joints if the hoof balance is suddenly and dramatically altered.

Fig. 7–7. Side View: A line through the cannon should reach the ground just behind the heel bulbs.

Definitions

Angular Limb Deformity: the limb deviates either to the inside or the outside; "crooked" legs.

Flexural Limb Deformity: abnormal limb angle when seen from the side; "contracted" or lax tendons.

(See Chapter 14 for more information.)

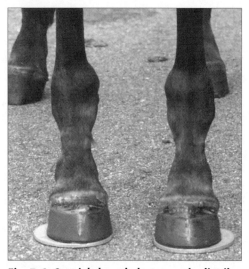

Fig. 7–8. Special shoes help to evenly distribute the forces up the leg.

A horse that is just used for pleasure riding needs only moderately good conformation and coordination to perform its required function. In contrast, a horse that must perform precise or demanding maneuvers, such as reining, jumping, or racing, needs good conformation and excellent coordination, particularly when speed is involved. It can tolerate very little that may interfere with its movement. Conformation problems that may be tolerated in a pleasure horse can limit performance or even lead to orthopedic problems in an athletic horse.

Hoof Balance

Hoof balance is a very important aspect of foot shape. A balanced foot is one in which the horse's weight and the ground impact forces are evenly distributed across the foot and up the center of the column. That sounds simple, but hoof balance is really a complex concept that is very difficult to define. The foot is a three-dimensional structure, so it can be analyzed in three different planes: front-to-back, side-to-side, and top-to-bottom. An important component of hoof balance is side-to-side, or latero-medial balance. When looking at the foot from the front, the height and angle of the wall should

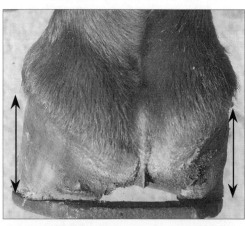

Fig. 7–9. These heels are not the same height.

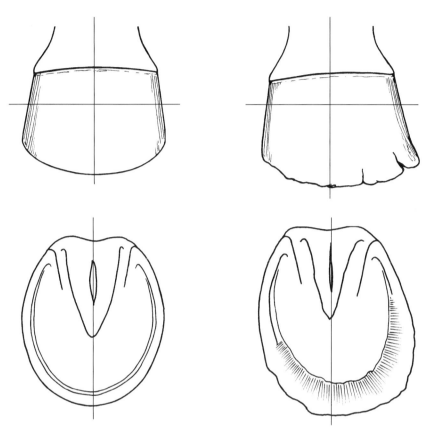

Fig. 7–10. Left: Good latero-medial balance—the two halves are identical, and the ooronary band is level. Right: Poor latero-medial balance—the two halves are uneven and the coronary band is not level.

be identical on both sides of the hoof, and the coronary band should be parallel with the ground. This symmetry should also be obvious when looking at the ground surface of the foot. An imaginary line, drawn from the cleft of the frog (between the heels) to the center of the toe, should bisect the foot into two perfectly matched halves.

Of particular importance is the symmetry of the hoof wall at the heels. In each foot, both heels should be the same height. Heel height can be assessed either with the horse standing (and the heels viewed from behind), or with the foot raised.

Improper trimming and shoeing can affect hoof balance. However, in many cases imbalance results from abnormal conformation of the foot, the leg, or both.

Movement

No matter how hoof balance is defined and measured, it is important to realize that what is found in the standing horse is not always the same as what occurs when the horse is moving. For a variety of reasons (conformation being the main one), the weight-bearing and ground impact forces may not be evenly distributed across the foot when the horse is in motion. In other words, the well-balanced foot may no longer be well balanced once the horse moves.

Foot Placement

When a horse walks on a firm, level surface, it should place the foot squarely on the ground at each step. The outside and inside of the foot, and the toe and heel should all land at the same time. However, many horses do not land normally. The most common abnormality is landing on the outside of the foot. That is, the outside of the foot is placed slightly before the inside, and the horse rolls the foot flat from outside to inside. This abnormality, which is generally due to poor conformation, is most commonly seen in the forefeet. Horses rarely land this way with the hindfeet. Nor do they land on the inside of the foot first when walking in a straight line.

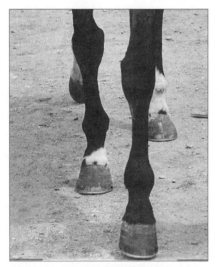

Fig. 7–11. Horses with poor conformation may land on the outside of the foot first.

Painful foot conditions and problems with either the extensor tendon or deep flexor tendon can also cause abnormal foot placement. These horses land with the heel or toe first, or land and remain on one side of the foot to spare the painful side from weight-bearing.

The higher the level of performance demanded of the horse, the more important it is that the horse lands evenly. The forces on the foot and column must be as evenly distributed as possible. Many people assume that an imbalance observed at the walk also occurs at the trot and faster gaits. However, it is impossible to be certain without using high-speed cinematography—filming the horse's feet as it trots, canters, or gallops, and reviewing the video in slow motion. It is often best to video the horse when it is working on a high-speed treadmill. If a treadmill is not available, an alternative is to set the video camera on a

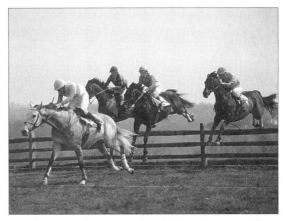

Fig. 7–12. The higher the level of performance, the more important it is that the horse lands evenly.

stand and film the horse moving toward it on a firm, flat surface.

Trimming and shoeing can influence hoof balance and placement for better or for worse. However, in many cases, unbalanced feet and uneven foot placement are due to conformational faults, not the farrier. In most horses trimming and shoeing can only partially compensate for faulty conformation. Sometimes, trimming an abnormal foot to make the horse land evenly can be harmful because it suddenly alters the forces on the foot and the rest of the column. Nevertheless, the farrier should aim to at least improve hoof balance to help equalize the forces on the foot and to ensure that movement is as unrestricted and efficient as possible.

Breakover

Breakover is the term used to describe the moment just before the horse's foot leaves the ground. As the horse begins to take a step forward, the heel is lifted first, and the foot "rolls over" the toe as the horse pushes off. In a perfectly-conformed horse with a balanced foot, breakover occurs at the

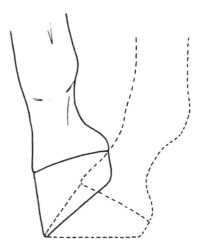

Fig. 7–13. Breakover is the moment just before the horse's foot leaves the ground.

center of the toe. However, in many horses the foot breaks over slightly to the inside or outside of the center. When breakover occurs off-center, abnormal stresses may be placed on the foot (in particular, the hoof wall), and also the joints and soft tissues of the lower leg.

Shoes can be modified to alter breakover. These alterations help the horse by making it easier to break over at the center of the toe. They do not necessarily change the speed of breakover, just its point and direction. Examples include the rolled toe, square toe, and rocker shoe (described at the end of the chapter).

Foot Flight

The term "foot flight" refers to the path the foot travels during a step, from the time it is lifted to when it lands *(see Figure 1–13 in Chapter 1)*. The foot should move in the direction the horse is moving, swinging neither inward nor outward as it is brought forward. The hoof prints should all point in the direction the horse is traveling (even when working in a circle), and the prints made by the left feet should parallel those made by the right feet. Furthermore, the feet and legs should never contact one another during motion.

Abnormalities of Flight

In many cases abnormalities of foot flight are caused by faulty conformation. A horse that "toes out" may "wing," or swing the feet inward during foot flight. Sometimes the foot hits the inside of the opposite leg, causing a minor abrasion, called an interference mark, at the fetlock. If the foot causes an abrasion higher up the leg, the wound is often called a "speedy cut." In most cases this problem is bilateral (occurs in both legs), although it is common for one leg to be worse than the other. To correct this problem, the farrier makes the foot as symmetrical as possible. He or she may also add a heel extension (described later) on the outside branch of each shoe.

> **Definitions**
>
> **Toed Out:** the feet point out slightly, instead of straight ahead; also called "splay-footed."
> **Toed In:** the feet point in slightly, instead of straight ahead; also called "pigeon-toed."

A horse that "toes in" may "paddle," or swing the feet outward during foot flight. Although the horse usually does not interfere when it paddles, paddling places strain on the sides of the joints. So, it is important for the farrier to improve the horse's gait as much as possible.

There are a few other types of inter-ference. "Scalping" occurs when the toe of a forefoot strikes the front of a hindfoot (usually at the coro-net) as the forefoot is lifted to take another step. This only tends to occur at speed. "Forg-ing" occurs when the toe of a hindfoot con-tacts or catches on the shoe of a forefoot. Occasionally sparks fly from this metal-to-metal contact.

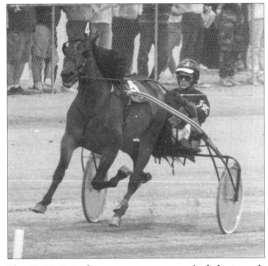

Fig. 7–14. Interference can cause gait defects and abrasions.

"Over-reaching" occurs when a hindfoot contacts the heels of a forefoot. In some cases this may loosen the branches of the front shoe, but in other cases it can cause a wound on the heel bulb or coronet. An over-reaching wound (also called a "grab") can be as mild as a superficial scrape, or it can be as severe as a skin laceration or torn hoof wall at the heel. When an over-reaching wound occurs at the coronet, it can sometimes be difficult to distinguish from the wound left by a hoof wall abscess that has broken out at the heel *(see Chapter 15)*.

Patterns of Interference

There are several patterns of interference, and many situations in which it may occur:

1. A "one-time" event caused by bad footing, such as mud, ice, or sand.
2. A recurring, specific type of interference caused by abnormal conformation (e.g. toeing out).
3. Variable and inconsistent interference problems in a normal horse, caused by fatigue, improperly fitted harness or equip-ment, poor riding or driving skills, or shoeing problems. Sud-den stops and turns may occasionally result in interference, even though none of these factors are present.
4. Variable and inconsistent interference problems in horses with early or mild neurologic disease *(see Chapter 12)*.

Managing an interference problem depends on the cause of the abnormality. If there is any question about the significance of the interference marks, or if the horse is lame, the owner or trainer should consult a veterinarian.

Altering Foot Flight With Weight

Increasing the weight of the hoof and/or shoe increases the height of the foot's arc because the horse must work a little harder to lift its foot. Increasing the weight of the feet in a normal horse results in more exaggerated, or "showy" knee or hock flexion, a trait referred to as the horse's "action." Some horses, for example, Saddlebreds and other gaited breeds, are selectively bred for their exaggerated action. Within virtually every breed there is an innate or ideal action; this characteristic is important when competing in certain show classes. For instance, Quarter Horses have a low action, which is encouraged for showing in Western Pleasure classes. In contrast, Hackneys have a very showy, high action, which is desirable in driving classes.

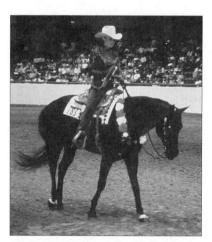

Fig. 7–15. Western Pleasure horses have a low action.

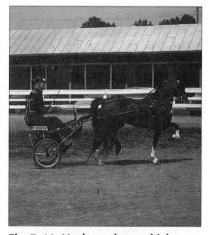

Fig. 7–16. Hackneys have a high, showy action.

Although the action is mostly determined by heredity, it can be altered by:

- the weight of the hoof—leaving more wall at each trimming, or extending the interval between shoeings can increase the action
- the weight and size of the shoe, which may be steel, titanium, aluminum, or plastic—the heavier the shoe, the greater the action
- padding materials—using pads and heavy nails may add to the

weight of the shoe, increasing the horse's action
• any other materials—using materials such as heavy boots and bandages that weigh down the feet or lower legs can increase the action

The way the horse moves can be important for successful performance, especially in competitions in which the judging is based on subjective criteria, such as the horse's action. When aiming to alter the horse's natural action, care should be taken to comply with the shoeing and padding (dimension and weight) rules of the particular competition. It is best to employ a farrier with knowledge and experience of the type of activity the horse is asked to perform.

The long-term effects of altering the horse's action must also be considered. For example, using small, aluminum racing plates on a show hunter to decrease its action and lengthen its stride may be good for the under-saddle classes. However, these shoes do not provide enough support for a jumper. At some point the horse's feet will likely become sore, and as a consequence its action will be affected and its stride shortened. The pain may worsen and cause lameness, which prevents the horse from performing at all. When a lightweight shoe is used for this type of competition, support of the foot is compromised. A heavier, more supportive shoe should be used once the competition season is ended.

Altering the horse's action can also be used as a therapeutic measure. For example, a horse with Equine Protozoal Myeloencephalitis (EPM; *see Chapter 12*) may have muscle atrophy in the hindquarters. Increasing the weight of the hind shoes may encourage an increase in muscle bulk, tone, and strength, and therefore coordination. As a result, the horse's gait may improve, and it may become usable in some capacity.

SHOEING FOR SUPPORT

Not all horses need shoes. However, the horse should be shod when:
• its use causes excessive hoof wear or potential damage to the sole (e.g. rough terrain or hard ground)
• it needs extra traction
• abnormal foot shape results in uneven forces across the foot and up the column

The foot is the base of the column that supports the horse, so a discussion of shoeing should center around the principle of support. *When the base is adequately supported, the column, and therefore the entire horse, is better supported.* By ensuring that the foot has adequate support, it is often possible to prevent, correct, or at least limit the effects of many foot and leg problems.

The three parts of the foot in need of support are:

- the heels
- the wall
- the sole

Heel Support

The heels take a good deal of the weight-bearing and ground impact forces that the foot sustains, particularly when the horse is moving at speed. Heel support is an essential part of column support, so it should be a primary consideration when trimming or shoeing any foot, whether normal or abnormal.

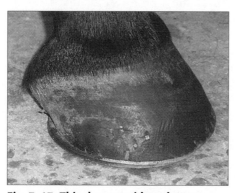

Fig. 7–17. This shoe provides adequate heel support.

Providing adequate heel support can be as simple as ensuring that the shoe is large enough for the horse's foot. An important farriery adage is: "the hoof grows to steel." This means that the foot tends to expand or grow to fit the shoe. However, the opposite is also true: the foot contracts if the shoe is too small. This latter situation is one of the most common shoeing faults. It can set up a vicious cycle in which a shoe that is too small results in a smaller foot. A smaller shoe is then fitted, and the cycle continues. The result is a narrower base, and less effective column support.

Another way to provide heel support is by setting the shoes a little wider at the heels, called "setting the shoe full." Not only does this give the column a slightly wider base while the shoe is on, it can also encourage the heels to widen if the horse is repeatedly shod full. Setting the shoes full can help horses with normal-sized feet, but it is particularly useful in horses with feet that are small for their body size.

In horses that must gallop in muddy conditions, many riders or trainers have their farriers fit shoes to the forefeet that are slightly shorter than normal at the heels. The rationale behind this is that it will help prevent the horse from over-reaching and tearing off the front shoes with the hindfeet. However, this strategy reduces heel, and therefore, column support, so any reduction in the shoe length at the heels should be a slight as possible. In these horses it is worthwhile lengthening the branches of the shoes at the end of the competition season to restore adequate heel support.

Evaluating Heel Support

In the normal foot, the front of the hoof wall and the pastern should be at the same angle to the ground, when viewed from the side. Also, the hoof wall at the heel should have the same angle as the front of the hoof wall and the pastern. If the hoof wall is steeper than the pastern, the foot is "broken forward"; this usually occurs when the heels are too high. If the pastern is steeper than the hoof wall, the foot is "broken back"; a situation commonly seen with the long toe–low heel foot shape (discussed later).

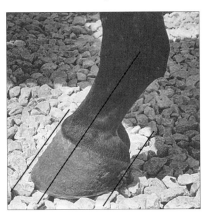 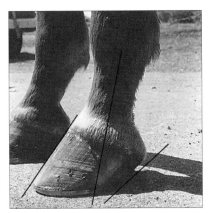

Fig. 7–18. Left: A normal hoof wall–pastern–heel angle. Right: A "broken back" foot—the pastern is much steeper than the hoof wall; the hoof wall angle at the heel is lower than the angle at the front of the foot.

There is another imaginary line that is useful for evaluating heel support. When looking at the leg from the side, with the horse standing squarely, a vertical line drawn through the center of the cannon and continued down to the ground should run just behind the heel bulbs *(see Figure 7–7)*. The back of the shoe should finish just in front of this line if the shoe is providing adequate heel support.

These visual evaluations are only subjective; it is very difficult to grade the severity of abnormalities just with imaginary lines. Nevertheless, they are a good starting point. In horses with obviously abnormal foot shape or angles, more objective measurements are needed. There are three simple, repeatable, recordable assessments that can be used to evaluate heel support:

• measurement of the hoof wall angle
• evaluation of a lateral radiograph of the foot (with the shoe on)
• measurement of the width of the foot, taken at the widest part

These assessments allow the farrier, veterinarian, and owner or trainer to pool their findings and monitor changes in the horse's feet over time.

Hoof Wall Angle

The angle between the front of the hoof wall and the ground surface of the foot (the hoof wall angle) is measured with a protractor that is specifically designed for use on the horse's foot. There are a couple of different protractors available. But no matter which one is used, the person using the protractor must practice with it to ensure that the measurements are repeatable. That is, the same measurement should be obtained when the angle is measured several times in a row.

Each horse, and in fact each foot, has its own natural angles that are determined by the horse's conformation. As a general guide, the forefeet normally have an angle between 48° and 55°, and the hindfeet are typically a few degrees steeper than the forefeet. (Some people do not rely on the actual number. Rather, they visually compare the angle of the hoof wall with that of the pastern and the hoof

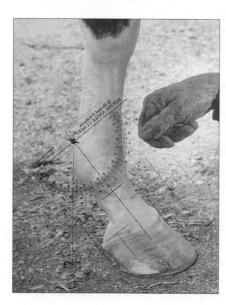

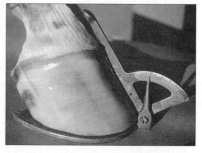

Fig. 7–19. Two types of protractor.

wall at the heels.) The left and right feet should have the same angle, whether evaluating the forefeet or the hindfeet.

The significance of this measurement is in the distribution of forces across the foot. When the hoof wall angle is normal, the weight-bearing and ground impact forces are evenly distributed between the heels, frog, and hoof wall. When the angle is increased, more weight is borne by the wall at the toe, and the long heels sustain more concussion. When the angle is decreased, the heels take more of the weight-bearing and ground impact forces.

Some farriers and trainers, particularly those working with Standardbreds, are very concerned with hoof wall angles, and they record and refer to these measurements at each shoeing. In most cases experienced farriers measure the hoof wall angles simply to double-check what they detected with their eyes. A mistake that owners, trainers, and even veterinarians sometimes make is directing the farrier to alter the horse's hoof angles to a set figure without discussing with the farrier the reasons for the change. The farrier should always be actively involved in any discussion of the horse's feet.

Lateral Radiographs

A lateral radiograph is taken from the side of the horse, with the x-ray beam directed across the foot, from outside (lateral) to inside (medial). This radiograph allows the veterinarian and farrier to see the shoe position in relation to the deeper structures of the foot. It can also reveal bony abnormalities within the foot. In many cases only a single radiograph of each foot is needed, although repeat radiographs may be necessary to monitor a problem over time.

To ensure that the radiograph provides as much information as possible, the veterinarian places the horse's foot on a wooden block. This is so that the x-ray beam is centered on the lower part of the hoof wall, not on the pastern (which is what happens if the foot is placed on the ground).

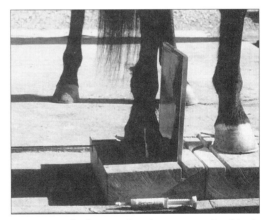

Fig. 7–20. The horse's foot is on a wooden block so that the x-ray beam is centered properly.

In this instance it is best to take the radiograph with the horse's shoe on. If both branches of the shoe are not seen as a single, solid line on the radiograph (because one branch is higher), the radiograph is not a true lateral image and may need to be repeated.

The lateral radiograph can help answer the following questions about shoeing and bony abnormalities within the foot:

1. *Is the shoe properly positioned?* A vertical line drawn through the center of the coffin joint should bisect the shoe; that is, there should be 50% of the shoe in front of this line and 50% behind it. As long as no more than about 55% of the shoe is in front of the line, heel support is probably adequate.

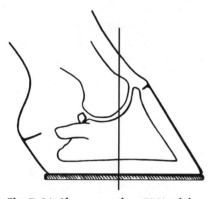

Fig. 7–21. If no more than 55% of the shoe is in front of the line, heel support is probably adequate.

2. *How thick is the front of the hoof wall?* The hoof wall may be thicker than normal if there has been previous separation of the hoof wall–pedal bone bond (discussed earlier).

3. *How thick is the sole?* Thin soles bruise easily.

4. *Is the front of the pedal bone parallel with the front of the hoof wall?* Downward rotation of the tip of the pedal bone may indicate a previous episode of laminitis.

5. *Is the bottom of the pedal bone normally aligned?* The bottom of the pedal bone should be about 5° off horizontal, being slightly higher at the heel than at the toe.

6. *Are the visible surfaces of the pedal bone and navicular bone normal?*

Foot Width

The width of the foot is easily measured by placing a ruler across the widest part of the foot. A wide, normally-shaped foot provides the most column support, whereas a narrow foot provides a smaller and less stable base. In horses with abnormal feet, the foot width should be measured and recorded at each shoeing.

Common Problems Affecting Heel Support

The three assessments discussed above can be used to manage the most common foot problems: long toe–low heel foot shape, mismatched feet, and contracted heels.

Long Toe–Low Heel

The most common abnormal foot shape—a long toe and low heel—affects one or both forefeet. It occurs when the hoof wall grows longer at the toe than at the heel, and it results in a reduced hoof wall angle, both within a shoeing period (6 – 8 weeks) and over time. This abnormality does not necessarily cause lameness. But horses with this foot shape are more prone to exercise-related acute and chronic joint problems and tendon injuries. The long toe–low heel conformation also results

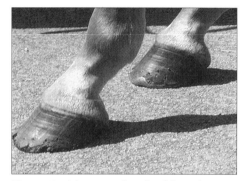

Fig. 7–22. A long toe–low heel foot shape.

in greater concussive forces at the heel. These forces are transmitted to the internal structures directly above the heels (such as the navicular bone and its supporting structures), so this foot shape can also contribute to navicular syndrome *(see Chapter 15)*.

Causes and Effects

The prevalence of the long toe–low heel foot shape is probably due to the Thoroughbred's genetic influence in many modern breeds. Decades of indirect selection for this foot shape (which is falsely thought to be ideal for producing speed) has likely played a major role. This foot shape is an important contributing factor to the common injuries in racehorses: fetlock and knee problems, and bowed tendons.

The harmful effects of chronic heel concussion (in particular, navicular syndrome) may not necessarily show up in a racehorse because most horses are retired from racing before these problems become apparent. However, repeated stress on the heels can be a

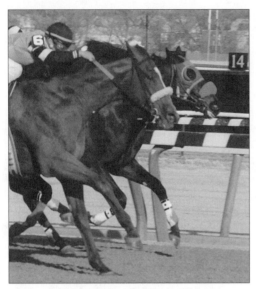

Fig. 7–23. The long toe–low heel foot shape is common in Thoroughbreds.

contributing factor in the development of quarter cracks, which commonly plague race-horses.

A farrier may indirectly encourage this foot shape in a horse that is prone to it. This is done by leaving the toe a little long at each shoeing, for fear of cutting the horse too short and causing lameness. After several shoeings the longer toe alters the foot's balance by setting the horse back on its heels. This puts added pressure on the heels, restricting their growth and creating a vicious cycle of excessive wall growth at the toe and restricted growth at the heel.

Another situation that can contribute to this problem is inconsistent or prolonged shoeing intervals. Increasing the interval between shoeings can result in the heels overgrowing the sides and back of the shoe as the shoe is drawn forward by the lengthening wall at the toe. This can lead to separation, cracking, or chipping of the wall at the heels, and corns. Any condition that compromises the integrity and strength of the wall at the heels can encourage or aggravate the long toe–low heel problem.

Managing the Problem

The long toe–low heel foot shape often cannot be completely corrected, but it can be improved by:

- regular shoeing every 4 – 6 weeks (or as directed by the farrier)
- adequately supporting the heels
- daily exercise

A regular shoeing interval cannot be emphasized too strongly. In horses with chronic foot problems, regular reshoeing is **essential** for continued athletic function. In horses with normal feet, it is an important preventive measure. For horses with the long toe–low heel foot shape, a standing appointment should be made with the farrier for every 4 weeks, or whatever time period the farrier recommends for that particular horse.

Simply ensuring that the shoe is big enough for the foot may be all that is needed to adequately support the heels. Other options include lengthening the branches of the shoes a little, or using an egg bar shoe (described later).

The generating layer of the coronary band (the coronary corium) responds to the forces placed on it through the hoof wall. As with other tissues in the body, the coronary band responds to regular exercise, which both improves blood flow to the coronary corium and encourages new horn production. Therefore, provided heel support by the shoe is adequate, regular exercise can stimulate more normal hoof wall growth at the heels.

If the problem is severe and unaffected by these measures, some farriers use a "four-point" trim to encourage more normal hoof wall growth. This trimming method involves:

1. Removing the excess wall at the toe.
2. Trimming the wall at the heels to move the weight-bearing surface back to the widest part of the frog.
3. "Unloading" the wall at the quarters.

As a result, the even distribution of weight-bearing and ground impact forces in the foot is restored to the four "pillars" of the foot: the two heels, and the hoof wall on each side of the toe (just in front of the frog). A shoe that follows this principle can also be used. However, this procedure must only be performed by an experienced farrier. Sometimes the horse is lame for a few days after a four-point trim. It may need to be kept from hard training for 2 – 4 months afterward, or until more normal wall growth at the heels is underway.

Under-run Heels

When the heels are at a lower angle than the front of the hoof wall, the heels are said to be "under-run" or "under-slung." As a result, the horn tubules grow down the wall at a very oblique angle, and are crushed by the weight-bearing and ground impact forces. This further reduces the height of the heels. Under-run heels are

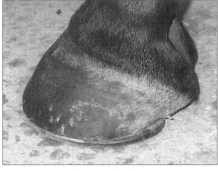

Fig. 7–24. Under-run heels.

the end result of the long toe–low heel foot shape that is left unmanaged.

On its own, this conformation does not necessarily cause lameness, but it does increase the risk of the horse developing painful foot and leg problems. The hoof wall often separates at the quarter in these horses, making hoof wall abscesses, "white line disease," and quarter cracks more likely. The longer the under-run heels are left without proper management, the greater the damage done to the heels.

In horses with mild to moderate under-running, improving heel support by lengthening the branches of the shoe or using an egg bar shoe may be all that is necessary to correct this problem. Shoes that use the frog for support can also be effective in more severe cases. Examples include the heart bar or tongue bar shoe (described later).

When chronic pressure on the abnormal heels, or the resulting separation of the hoof wall at the quarter causes pain and lameness, the veterinarian or farrier may remove the defective hoof wall at the heels. This encourages the growth of healthy hoof wall at a more normal angle. Resection (removal) of the abnormal wall at the heels disconcerts some owners and trainers, sometimes to the extent that they refuse to allow this procedure. However, normal, healthy heels cannot be achieved any other way in these horses. Once the abnormal wall has been resected, the farrier may use one or more of the following techniques:

- trim the toe to help "normalize" the hoof wall angle
- apply a plastic or rubber wedge pad (discussed later) between the wall and the shoe to raise the heels and re-establish a more normal hoof wall angle
- apply a shoe that uses the frog for support for 1 – 3 shoeings; this is usually reserved for horses with very painful heels
- rebuild the hoof wall at the heels with acrylic resin

Mismatched Feet

Mismatched feet is the second most common abnormality of foot shape. With this problem the forefeet are different from one another in size, shape, and hoof wall angle. This problem in itself may not cause lameness, although there is a greater risk of horses with this foot shape becoming lame. Looking at this from another angle, chronic pain in the foot or elsewhere in the limb is a common cause of mismatched feet.

Often one of the feet has a long toe–low heel conformation. In most cases the "good" foot is the lower, wider foot, and the "bad" foot is the narrow, upright one. This is because the horse places less weight on one leg, and as a result, that foot grows more heel and becomes steeper and narrower. The other foot bears more weight, so it spreads and becomes flatter. However, over time this flatter foot may become the problem foot if the long toe–low heel situation continues.

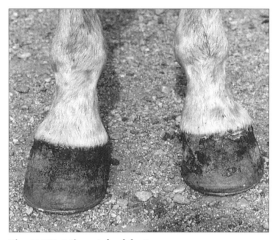

Fig. 7–25. Mismatched feet.

In some horses with mismatched feet, slight muscle atrophy (wasting) in front of the withers may develop after a couple of months, on the side with the narrow, upright foot. This "mismatching" of the muscle mass is easiest to see by standing on a box just behind the horse, and comparing the size and shape of the muscles over the shoulders, just below the withers. The loss of muscle bulk results from uneven loading of the forelegs. The "good" side takes more of the weight, so it does more of the work.

The degree of uneven loading need only be slight to cause mismatched feet. Examples of conditions that can lead to mismatching include:

- any painful condition, whether obvious or subtle, in one leg
- excessive tension on the deep digital flexor tendon ("club foot") in one leg
- any shoe that restricts hoof wall expansion (described later) and causes narrowing of the heels in one foot
- uneven trimming and shoeing

Managing Mismatched Feet

The best way to evaluate and monitor mismatched feet is to compare hoof wall angles and widths over several shoeings. Lateral radiographs are not as important in monitoring this condition. However, an initial set of routine radiographs *(see Chapter 2)* can provide useful information about the possible role of various bony problems, such as a rotated pedal bone or navicular syndrome.

The following case studies demonstrate how monitoring the hoof wall angles and foot width can help determine the cause and significance of mismatched feet.

Case 1:

	Left Forefoot		Right Forefoot	
	Angle	Width	Angle	Width
Before trimming	51°	14.4 cm	54°	13.8 cm
After trimming	53.5°	14.1 cm	54°	13.9 cm
4 weeks later	54°	14.1 cm	54°	13.9 cm

In this case the left and right forefeet previously had not been trimmed or shod evenly; the left foot was lower and wider than the right foot before this shoeing. However, the farrier then trimmed the feet as evenly as possible, and 4 weeks after shoeing, the feet are still similar in angle and width. The minor difference in foot size and shape that was present before this shoeing was easily corrected and was, therefore, of no great significance. Ideally, after three more shoeings the angles would be approximately:

Before trimming	54°	14.3 cm	54°	14.2 cm

Case 2:

	Left Forefoot		Right Forefoot	
	Angle	Width	Angle	Width
Before trimming	54°	12.7 cm	59°	11.5 cm
After trimming	53°	12.5 cm	55°	11.5 cm
4 weeks later	53°	12.5 cm	57°	11.5 cm
6 weeks later	54°	12.5 cm	59°	11.5 cm

In this horse the right forefoot has become steeper and narrower than the left forefoot. At this shoeing the farrier attempted to equalize the angles by trimming extra wall at the heels on the right foot. But the problem is with the horse's foot conformation, not with the farrier. The difference in angles returned within 6 weeks. Shoeing this horse at an interval of no greater than 4 – 5 weeks would hopefully limit the difference in angles between the left and right feet to only about 4° (53° vs. 57°).

Ideally, after a few shoeings at an interval of 4 – 5 weeks, the horse's angles and widths would be approximately:

Before trimming	54°	12.4cm	55°	12.0cm

These results would mean a definite improvement, and successful management of the problem.

However, if after regular trimming every 4 – 5 weeks the measurements are:

Before trimming   54°   12.4cm   59°   11.2cm

it can be assumed that the problem is still active, and is not being managed simply by regular trimming and routine shoeing. It is likely that the horse has heel pain, or pain elsewhere in the right foot or leg, which is causing the mismatching to persist and worsen. The veterinarian should be consulted to determine the site and cause of the problem in this horse.

Contracted Heels

Contracted heels is the term used to describe narrowing of the foot across the heels. Typically, horses with contracted heels grow more wall at the heels than normal. This results in a foot with tall, narrow heels, and a steeper than normal hoof wall angle. This condition is a potential problem because when the heels are narrowed, there is less support at the base of the column. Also, it often leads to shrinkage of the frog (discussed later). Usually both forefeet are affected, although it can occur in only one foot if the forefeet are mismatched. Occasionally, only one heel may be contracted (for example, in horses with "sheared heels"; *see Chapter 15*).

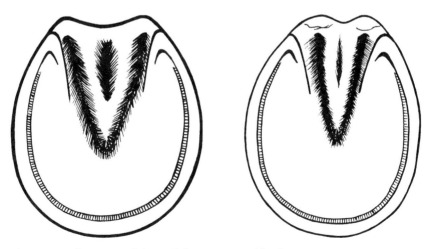

Fig. 7–26. Left: A normal foot. Right: Contracted heels.

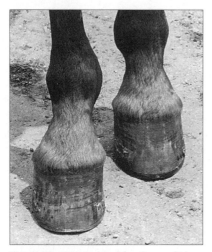

Fig. 7–27. Contracted heels result in narrow, "boxy" feet.

Contracted heels are less common than the long toe–low heel foot shape or mismatching, but horses with contracted heels are more likely to be lame. Concussion on the wall at the heel and on the deeper structures at the back of the foot (notably, the navicular bone) is increased in horses with contracted heels. The heels cannot expand properly, and the frog is prevented from doing its job. As a result, the concussive forces that are normally absorbed and dispersed by these structures are transmitted to the deeper structures of the foot and further up the column.

There are several factors that can contribute to the development of contracted heels, including:

- hereditary predisposition for taller, narrower feet, e.g. Saddlebreds, Morgans, and Standardbreds
- trimming—some breeds are trimmed this way to increase their action for training and showing
- chronic heel pain, which causes the horse to take some of the weight off the heel (common in horses with navicular syndrome)
- flexor contracture of the coffin joint ("club foot")
- chronic laminitis *(see Chapter 15)*
- a shoe with clips or a raised rim that prevents normal hoof wall expansion (discussed later)

Managing a horse with contracted heels involves: 1) identifying and managing the cause, and 2) lowering the heels as much as the horse's conformation and training demands allow. The higher the heels, the narrower the foot becomes, and the greater the concussive forces on the heels.

Wall Support

To support the column, the hoof wall must be strong and resilient. Yet it also needs to be a little pliable (elastic), to withstand and absorb the concussive forces placed on it. When the bottom of the bare foot is examined, the wall at the ground, or bearing surface (from the white line to the outer edge) should be at least ¼ inch (6 mm) thick. It should be roughly even in width all the way around, although it is normal for the wall to be a little wider at the toe than at the quarters or heels. The wall should be firmly attached at the white line all the way around the foot.

Common Hoof Wall Abnormalities

The common problems with the wall are discussed below. Some of these abnormalities disfigure the wall, but more important, they can weaken the wall—an essential component of column support.

Stretched Wall

The toe is a very common site for the wall to widen or be stretched by the ground impact forces, especially in horses with the long toe–low heel foot shape. This is because the wall at the toe is the breakover point—the last part of the foot in contact with the ground as the horse moves forward. When the toe is longer than normal there is more leverage on the wall during breakover. Widening of the wall may be very slight, or it can be quite extensive, particularly in horses with chronic laminitis. In any horse, when the wall at the toe is stretched,

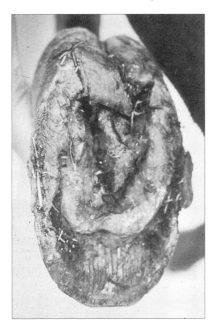

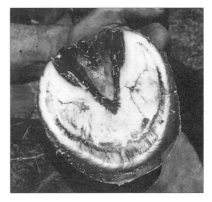

Fig. 7–28. Left: Extensive widening of the wall in a horse with chronic laminitis. Above: Red streaks in the wall between the white line and the sole indicate recent tearing of the blood vessels.

Fig. 7–29.

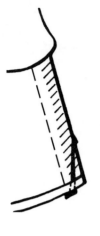

Normal hoof wall—the nail does not touch the sensitive tissues.

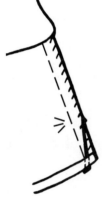

Thin wall—the clench may put pressure on the sensitive tissues.

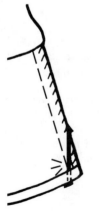

Thin wall—the nail may penetrate the sensitive tissues.

separation at the white line and hoof wall cracks (both discussed later) are more likely.

Stretching of the wall is easiest to see immediately after the foot has been trimmed (before the shoe is set). A common finding is a few red streaks in the wall between the white line and the sole. This indicates recent tearing of the blood vessels in the sensitive tissues of the wall. Bleeding that occurred weeks or months ago is seen as brown staining. Finding evidence of bleeding can be a clue to a prior, mild episode of laminitis.

The farrier or veterinarian looks for the cause of this problem before deciding how to manage it.

Thin Wall

The hoof wall may be thinner than normal if the coronary band produces poor quality horn, or if the wall is excessively rasped to alter its shape or smooth its surface. A thin hoof wall provides less column support, which may increase the load on the other structures of the foot. A thin wall is also at more risk of being stretched or separated. Furthermore, horses with thin hoof walls are more likely to be "pricked" or "nailed too close" when being shod. Usually, the thin wall is the reason for these problems, not an incompetent farrier. Thin walls make it more likely that the nail will put pressure on, or penetrate the sensitive tissues of the hoof wall. When the farrier tightens the clenches, the bent-over end of the clench can also put pressure on the sensitive tissues in a horse with thin walls.

Thin walls are more likely to chip and break, especially if the shoeing interval is too long or a shoe is lost. Horses with thin walls tend to lose their shoes more easily, regardless of the activities they perform. For a nail to be anchored firmly in the wall, the wall must be thick enough to support it. The thinner the wall, the less grasp the nail has, and the more likely the wall will break or the nail will loosen. Either situation makes it more likely that the shoe will be lost.

> **Note**
>
> The farrier should reset the opposite shoe when a lost shoe is replaced, unless the horse was shod less than a week before. Otherwise, the feet are uneven in height. This can encourage mismatching, and can also result in unequal loading of the limbs.

It is often difficult to manage feet with thin walls. In some horses, supplements, such as biotin and methionine, can improve the quality, and hence the thickness of the hoof wall *(see Chapter 4).*

Plastic Glue-On Shoes

Plastic glue-on shoes are sometimes used to protect the ground surface of the foot in foals and in horses with hoof walls that cannot tolerate shoe nails. Plastic shoes come in a variety of sizes, and they have tabs or rims

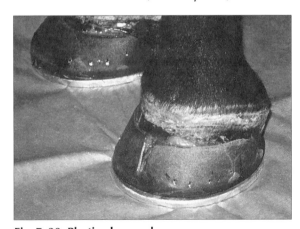

Fig. 7–30. Plastic glue-on shoes.

that are glued to the hoof wall. The more recently developed plastic shoes appear to be very well tolerated and resilient. However, over time, the glue may begin to weaken the wall.

Hoof Wall Rings

Horizontal rings in the hoof wall develop after a period of altered hoof wall growth at the coronary band. The more common causes of

hoof wall rings are:
- inflammation at the coronet
- reduced blood flow to the coronary band
- serious illness, particularly if it involves a fever
- severe stress
- dietary or environmental changes

The rings run around the hoof wall, parallel with the coronary band, and they move down as the hoof grows. In most cases there are just a couple of closely spaced rings. Multiple, separated rings that extend down most or all of the hoof wall indicate ongoing or repeated episodes of illness or stress. Rings that are not parallel with the coronary band, but are wider apart at the heel represent severe changes in hoof wall growth, most commonly as a result of chronic laminitis. The rings are not parallel with the coronet because hoof wall growth at the front of the foot is slower than at the heels in these horses. This results in a slipper-shaped foot—the hallmark of chronic laminitis.

When rings are found in only one foot it usually indicates inflammation at the coronet in just that foot. It could be caused, for example, by a hoof wall abscess or trauma. Rings in both forefeet indicate a condition that involved both feet, such as a mild episode

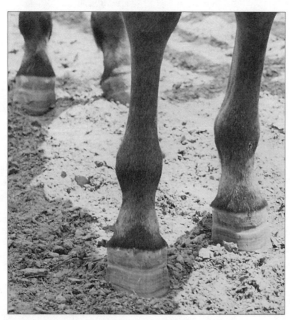

of laminitis. Rings in all four feet represent a situation that affected the entire body, such as illness, severe stress, or laminitis from a systemic problem. These rings are sometimes called "fever rings" because they often develop in horses that have had a fever. Changes in the horse's environment or diet can also cause rings in all four feet. Examples of such

Fig. 7–31. Fever rings in all four feet.

changes include turning out a horse onto pasture immediately after race training, moving the horse a long distance, and suddenly changing the horse's diet.

It is possible to estimate how long ago the problem occurred by looking at how far down the hoof wall the rings have grown. It takes about 12 months for a ring to grow down from the coronary band to the ground surface at the front of the foot, and about 6 months to grow down at the heel. (The hoof wall normally grows at about the same rate at the front of the foot and the heels, but the wall is shorter at the heel, so it takes less time for the ring to grow out there.) A ring that is halfway down the wall at the front of the foot, and very close to the ground at the heels, represents a change that occurred in that foot about 6 months ago.

Rings do not cause lameness, but they do indicate that the hoof wall was stressed in the past.

Flared Wall

The hoof wall may flare out at the toe or on either side of the foot. In most cases the wall grows down normally to about half or two thirds of the way down, and then flares out. Flaring is common in horses with naturally wide, flat ("pie plate") feet, particularly if the shoeing interval is prolonged. Horses with chronic laminitis are especially prone to flaring of the wall at the toe. A horse that had an angular limb deformity (ALD; *see Chapter 14*) as a foal which was not completely corrected may have a slight deviation of the foot and lower leg. This can cause uneven loading of the foot, and flaring on one side of the hoof wall.

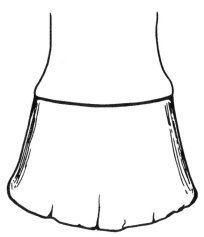

Fig. 7–32. Flared hoof wall.

Separation at the White Line

It would seem that a flared or stretched wall benefits the foot by widening the bearing surface (the base of the column). However, this is an illusion. The stretched or flared wall is actually weaker than a normal wall, and the increased leverage it provides often results in separation of the wall at the white line. This separated area creates a space at the ground surface, between the wall and the sole. The space easily becomes packed with dirt, which can cause further separation as more dirt is pressed into the defect. It can also lead to infection beneath the wall, commonly called "gravel." If the separated area extends along the white line, it is often called "white line disease." *(Managing these problems is discussed in Chapter 15.)*

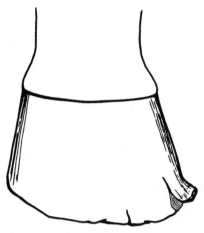

Fig. 7–33. Chipped hoof wall.

Chipping and Breaking

Another common problem in feet that flare is chipping and breaking of the hoof wall if the horse is left unshod. It is often seen in weanlings and yearlings, and mature horses that are exercised or turned out without shoes. The broken hoof wall can act like a hangnail, bending back and putting pressure on the sensitive tissues of the hoof wall at the point of attachment every time the horse bears weight on the foot. This may cause lameness. Infection can develop beneath the damaged wall, and this too can cause lameness.

The broken hoof wall must be cut off cleanly at the point where it is attached. If the piece of wall is not trimmed far enough up and a crevice is left beneath part of the wall, infection can result. It can also allow further separation of the wall above this point as the defect grows down to the ground surface.

Raised Areas

A raised or irregular area on the hoof wall usually does not cause pain or lameness, unless it becomes infected. Nevertheless, it should be monitored closely because its cause and importance may not be immediately obvious.

These abnormalities may represent previous trauma to the coronary band. The inflammation subsides and, as with horizontal rings, the resulting defect in the wall grows down slowly as the hoof grows. Sometimes the raised area is caused by internal separation of the wall. A direct blow to the wall (caused, for example, by knocking a jump or pawing at the bottom of a gate) can cause bleeding in the sensitive tissues beneath the wall. The small hematoma that develops, like a blood blister beneath a fingernail, can cause separation in that area of the wall.

The raised area may also be caused by separation that began at the ground surface and progressed up the inside of the wall (discussed earlier). The top of the defect may cause the hoof wall to bulge slightly. A very uncommon cause of a raised area in the hoof wall is a benign tumor called a keratoma *(see Chapter 15)*.

Cracks

Hoof wall cracks usually are easy to see, although they may sometimes be hidden under hoof dressing, hoof paint, or mud. There are several types, and varying degrees of hoof wall cracks. Most do not cause lameness, although deeper cracks should always be suspected if the horse is lame.

The depth of the crack is the most important evaluation to make. It is the factor that determines whether the crack will cause lameness, and to what extent wall support is compromised. A partial thickness crack begins at the outer surface, but does not extend to the sensitive

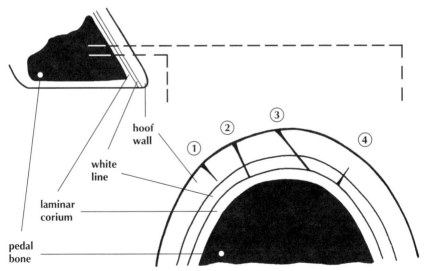

1. Partial thickness crack.
2. Full thickness crack going directly into the sensitive tissues.
3. Full thickness crack angling into the sensitive tissues.
4. Partial thickness crack extending from the inside out.

Fig. 7–34. Various types and depths of hoof wall cracks.

tissues on the inside of the wall. A full thickness crack extends the entire thickness of the wall, down to the sensitive tissues. It is often difficult to distinguish between a partial thickness crack that extends nearly to the sensitive tissues, and a full thickness crack. This is an evaluation for the farrier or veterinarian to make.

Full thickness cracks may have one of three forms:

- the crack goes straight into the sensitive tissues
- the crack angles through the hoof wall, such that the affected sensitive tissues are ¼ inch (6 mm) or so in front of, or behind where the crack starts on the surface
- the crack begins on the inside of the hoof wall and extends to the outer surface

Presumably, in the third instance the ground forces travel up the inner (softer) layer of the hoof wall, along the path of least resistance, and damage the wall from inside out.

Full thickness cracks do not necessarily cause lameness unless they are disrupted by trauma or become infected. Some full thickness cracks can be present for years without causing the horse pain. This is a common situation in horses that are not very active, such as brood-mares. However, when these chronic cracks do cause problems they can be very difficult, if not impossible to resolve. This is because there is often a permanent defect in the sensitive laminae or coronary band (if the crack originated in, or extended to the coronary band).

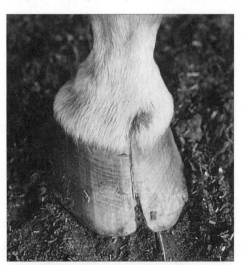

Fig. 7–35. A chronic crack caused by a permanent defect in the coronary band.

Hoof wall cracks should be evaluated and treated as soon as they are first noticed. Many owners are concerned by the slight and temporary disfigurement of the wall that is sometimes the result of treatment. But this area of the wall represents only a very small part of the bearing surface. So, provided the rest of the wall is stable, the horse's training program usually is not disrupted to any great degree. The alternatives, if the crack is not treated appropriately, are infection and further hoof wall damage. These complications may require more extensive and invasive hoof wall resection that could suspend or even end the horse's athletic career.

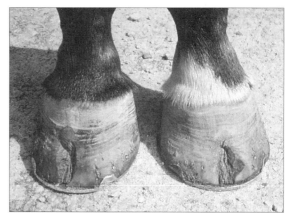

Fig. 7–36. Treatment of full thickness cracks: the cracks have been pared out and shoes with side clips applied.

Horizontal Cracks

Horizontal cracks in the hoof wall usually are caused by trauma to the coronary band, or a hoof wall abscess that broke out at the coronet. These cracks usually do not cause lameness, although the horse probably was lame before the abscess broke out. In most cases the farrier cuts away all of the damaged horn overlying and surrounding the crack so that there are no crevices in which dirt can collect, and cause infection and further separation. This procedure, which is not painful for the horse,

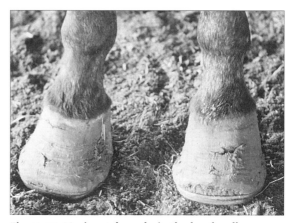

Fig. 7–37. Horizontal cracks in the hoof wall.

leaves a small defect in the wall that eventually grows out completely.

Vertical Cracks

Vertical cracks that begin at the ground surface and are only partial thickness cause few problems. However, they often indicate a decrease in the quality of hoof wall. The owner or trainer should re-evaluate

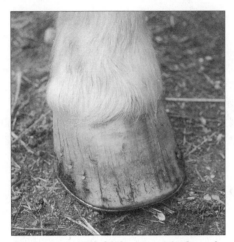

Fig. 7–38. Partial thickness vertical cracks indicate decreased hoof wall quality.

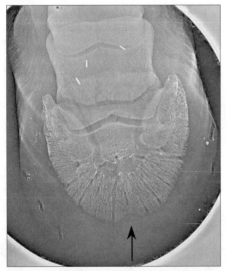

Fig. 7–39. The crena [arrow] at the tip of the pedal bone.

the horse's diet and its environment (as it affects hoof moisture; *see Chapter 4*).

Toe Cracks: Vertical cracks commonly develop at the center of the toe. They are usually full thickness cracks that are accompanied by minor separation and stretching of the wall. The crack may have caused the separation. But just as likely, the stretching and separation could have led to the crack.

Some veterinarians believe that the notch (the crena) that is commonly found in the tip of the pedal bone causes toe cracks. Most veterinarians consider this notch to be normal. However, it could make stretching or disruption of the sensitive laminae (which attach to the pedal bone) more likely at this site. This could cause separation of the wall at the toe, and subsequent cracking.

Cracks at the toe that involve separation of the wall should be treated promptly if "white line disease" is to be avoided. Specific ways a farrier might treat such a crack include:

1. Cutting an inverted V-shaped notch at the ground surface (opening up the crack and the separated area), and packing the defect with cotton soaked in disinfectant.
2. Rasping a horizontal groove in the hoof wall just above the top of the crack, to keep it from progressing up the wall.

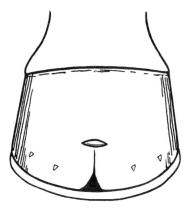
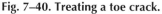

Fig. 7–40. Treating a toe crack.

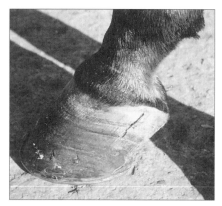

Fig. 7–41. A crack beginning at the coronary band.

Coronary Band Cracks: Vertical cracks can also begin at the coronary band and extend down the wall; these cracks often are not full thickness. They usually are the result of coronary band injury, such as a wound or a direct blow. The crack should be treated by paring away all damaged horn, as described earlier for horizontal cracks.

Complete Cracks: Vertical cracks that extend the length of the wall (either starting at, or extending up to the coronary band) are more common at the quarter. But they can occur in any part of the hoof. These cracks, which usually are full thickness, can occur suddenly or develop slowly. They often cause persistent or intermittent lameness. Factors that can cause these cracks include:

- abnormal foot conformation
- heredity—e.g. long toe–low heels in Thoroughbreds, or narrow, upright feet in Saddlebreds
- inadequate heel support—e.g. the shoe is too small or too short
- abnormal hoof moisture—alternating wet and dry conditions
- trauma, whether a single blow or repeated stress on the hoof wall from a hard or irregular surface—common in racehorses
- any combination of the above

If the cause(s) is not identified and corrected, or at least managed, the crack may persist or return despite treatment. The farrier or veterinarian must do three things when treating complete, full thickness cracks:

1. Cut away the damaged horn—this is most important.
2. Reduce the weight-bearing and ground impact forces on the damaged wall.
3. Consider stabilizing or patching the area.

The damaged horn must be removed from along the crack. Otherwise the sides of the crack can move and pinch the sensitive tissues beneath. Also, the crack must be opened up to prevent or treat the infection that is inevitable if the damaged wall is not removed.

It may take a few treatments to remove all the abnormal horn, while minimizing damage to the unaffected tissue. Over-aggressive resection can damage the normal tissue, so it is usually best to resect the damaged wall in stages, leaving 5 – 10 days between treatments for the exposed tissues to harden.

The forces on the damaged wall can be reduced by cutting an inverted V-shaped notch in the wall at the ground surface, directly over the crack. This defect must be kept cleaned out; a hacksaw blade or flat-headed screwdriver is ideal for this purpose. It is also important to minimize movement and disruption at the coronary band directly above the crack. This can be done by removing a V-shaped piece of wall immediately below the coronary band.

Whether to patch the defect is a matter for consideration. The acrylic patch keeps dirt, manure, mud, and other debris out of the defect while it grows out. However, the most common problem with acrylic patches is that reinfection can occur beneath the patch if the defect is patched too soon after resection. When infection develops beneath the patch, it can be more severe than the infection that was present in the crack before treatment. For this reason, many farriers and veterinarians prefer not to use patches if possible.

Depending on the acrylic used and the farrier's skill, acrylic patches can substantially improve wall support, so they can speed up the horse's return to active training. When correctly applied, they can also encourage normal hoof wall growth by transmitting some of the ground forces to the new horn tubules as they grow down from the coronary band.

> **More Information**
>
> Hoof wall cracks do not always cause lameness. But quarter cracks are an exception—they typically cause chronic, intermittent or persistent lameness. Therefore, quarter cracks are covered in Section IV: Treatment of Specific Conditions, Chapter 15.

Sole Support

The sole is the one part of the hoof that is not designed to bear weight directly. The normal sole is concave, curving away from the

Fig. 7–42. Repair of a hoof wall defect with acrylic and wire. The farrier has resected the damaged hoof wall, which had become separated and infected.

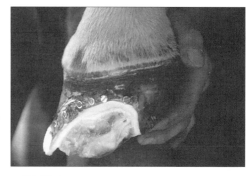

Fig. 7–43. The wires attach the shoe to the wall for extra stability.

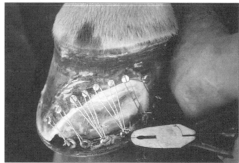

Fig. 7–44. The acrylic is packed firmly into the entire defect.

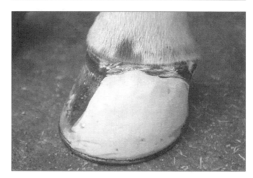

Fig. 7–45. The farrier shapes the acrylic to match the intact hoof wall.

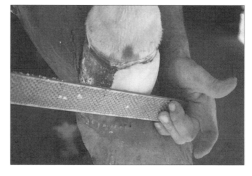

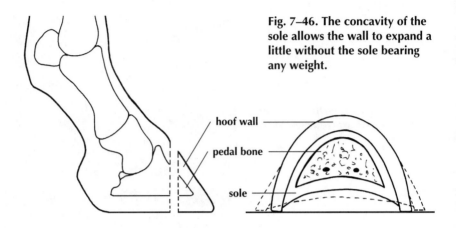

Fig. 7–46. The concavity of the sole allows the wall to expand a little without the sole bearing any weight.

hoof wall

pedal bone

sole

ground surface, with the deepest part being just in front of the point of the frog. This allows the wall to expand a little without the sole bearing any weight.

Conditions that damage or put pressure on the sole are among the most painful foot problems. Horses with flat soles often are intermittently lame, especially when left unshod or trimmed too short. In these horses the flattened sole touches the ground, and pressure on the sole from the horse's weight and the ground forces causes pain.

There are several factors that may cause flat soles, or otherwise allow pressure on the sole:

- heredity—some Thoroughbreds and many draft breeds naturally have large, flat ("pie plate") feet
- poor environmental conditions in unshod horses—e.g. very wet conditions can waterlog the foot, allowing it to spread and flatten; and rough terrain can cause excessive wearing of the wall, which can allow the sole to touch the ground
- over-trimming of the hoof wall—as above for rough terrain
- over-trimming of the sole—thinner soles are more prone to bruising *(see Chapter 15)*
- dried mud, snow, or thick wound dressings packed into the bottom of the foot
- faulty trimming or shoeing, allowing the shoe to touch the sole
- laminitis—rotation or sinking of the pedal bone puts pressure on the sole from above (within the foot), and may cause the sole to drop

Negative factors can add up, making the problem worse. For example, the potential for a flat-footed horse to be trimmed too short is greater than for a normal horse. Also, laminitis in a flat-soled horse can have more serious consequences than laminitis in a horse with normally-shaped feet.

Providing Sole Support

The best preventive measure for horses with flat soles is regular shoeing at an interval of no more than 6 weeks. There are several other ways to provide temporary relief or more substantial sole support:

1. Prevent the shoe from contributing to the problem. One of the most common sources of lameness in flat-footed horses is pressure on the sole from the shoe—the shoe should never put pressure on the sole. Leaving a little extra wall when trimming the foot, and beveling the shoe away from the sole (described later) may be all that is required to prevent lameness in these horses.

2. Raise the sole a few extra millimeters off the ground with a pad. A rim pad is the width and shape of the shoe, and is nailed on with the shoe, between the wall and the shoe. A full sole pad covers the entire underside of the foot. In either case the pad should not touch the sole.

3. Build up the wall with acrylic resin in horses with convex (dropped) soles. A shoe can be nailed onto the resin, raising the sole further off the ground. This procedure requires considerable experience, but it can be very useful in managing complex foot cases, such as horses with chronic laminitis.

Pads

The most obvious benefit of a pad which covers the underside of the foot is that it protects the sole from direct trauma. If the pad is made of a rigid material it can also direct the ground forces away from the sole to the wall. Pads may be made of leather, synthetic materials (plastic, rubber, etc.), or metal. The firmer the pad material, the better the sole is protected, and the more the ground forces are directed away from the sole. Pads (whether full sole or rim) can also help reduce concussion. The more "give" the material has, the more concussion is absorbed and dispersed by the pad.

Pads can be used in many situations, both preventive and therapeutic. For example, the farrier may recommend pads during the drier months to protect a horse with thin soles while the ground is very hard. Or, pads may be used during the winter to prevent snow and mud from packing into the feet and causing sole bruising. Heavy duty plastic or aluminum pads are sometimes used in competitive trail and endurance horses to protect their soles from rocks and

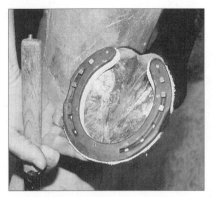
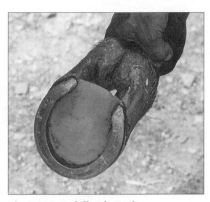

Fig. 7–47. A rim pad.   Fig. 7–48. A full sole pad.

other potential causes of sole trauma. The most obvious therapeutic use is to protect a bruised or otherwise damaged sole.

However, pads can create problems if they are used continually, and if care is not taken. Pads do not prevent the sole from getting wet; water can leak in under the pad at the back of the shoe, and also around the edges of the wall. The pad prevents the sole from drying out, so it creates a moist, dark, protected environment that is ideal for bacteria and fungi to multiply. Also, mud, sand, manure, and other materials can be sucked under the pad as the horse walks if it is not kept in a very clean, dry area. Further, the constant wetness under the pad keeps the sole moist and soft. When the pad is removed, the sole is more easily damaged.

The moist conditions under the pad can also slow healing and encourage infection of a wound that involves the sole or frog. The wound itself can be another source of moisture under the pad if it is draining. The veterinarian must consider these possibilities when requesting that a farrier place a pad over such a wound. It is usually best to wait until the defect in

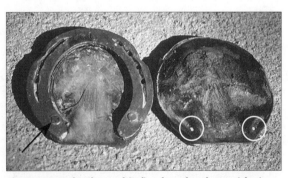

Fig. 7–49. Left: The pad is fixed to the shoe with rivets [arrow]. Right: The underside of the pad (the sole side). Note where the rivets show through the pad.

the sole has dried up and is beginning to fill in with horn (cornify) before placing a pad on the foot. In the meantime, the foot should be covered with a waterproof bandage *(see Chapter 4)*. More severe sole or frog wounds can be covered with a hospital plate.

Rather than using temporary nails or other measures to keep the pad in place while the shoe and pad are nailed on, some farriers use a pad that is fixed to the shoe branches with rivets. However, the rivets may put pressure on the sole at the heels and cause corns, so extra care must be taken when using this pad-and-shoe combination.

Hospital Plate

A hospital plate is a steel plate that is bolted to the bottom of the shoe. Four bolts are used: one on each side of the toe and one at each

Fig. 7–50. A hospital plate.

(a) An egg bar shoe with bolt holes is fitted.

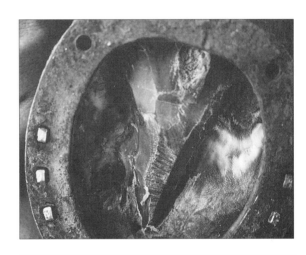

(b) A steel plate is then bolted to the shoe.

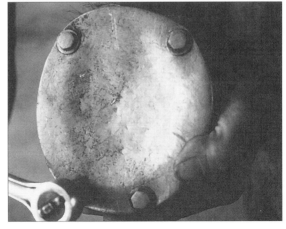

heel, stabilizing the foot and ensuring that the horse breaks over at the center of the toe. The bolts can be undone and the plate removed so that the bottom of the foot can be inspected or treated as often as necessary. After treating the foot, the plate is bolted back in place.

As with rigid pads, the hospital plate both protects the sole from trauma, and directs the ground forces away from the sole to the wall. Hospital plates are used for a variety of conditions that affect the bottom of the foot, from mild bruising to extensive surgical procedures *(see Chapter 15)*. Although there is the initial expense of having the farrier make and fit the shoe and plate, using a hospital plate is more economical in the long run. It is also better for the sole (and the entire hoof) than keeping the foot bandaged. Also, the steel plate may allow the horse to begin activity much sooner than with any other method of sole protection. Gentle exercise can promote wound drainage and improve blood flow to the area, so it can aid healing.

Using the Frog for Support

The frog is a roughly triangular, rubbery structure that lies in between the heels, and covers approximately 25% of the ground surface of the foot. The frog's primary function is to absorb and disperse some of the ground impact forces. The frog must be thick, wide, and healthy to be effective. In a horse with long or contracted heels, the heels do not spread and the frog is not "engaged" when the horse bears weight on the foot. The frog shrinks and becomes less elastic with disuse. As a result, the concussive forces that are normally absorbed by the frog are redistributed to the other structures of the foot and directed up the leg.

The grooves (sulci) deepen in the shrunken frog, and they are ideal places for mud, manure, and other debris to collect. Bacteria that thrive in a low-oxygen environment make good use of this situation. They quickly spread to invade the frog tissue, and cause thrush.

A healthy frog can be a real asset when heel, wall, or sole problems require additional support. The frog can be used to take more of the weight-bearing and ground impact forces, sparing the damaged area. Shoes that use the frog to support the foot include the heart bar, tongue bar, and mushroom shoe (described later).

> **Definition**
>
> **Thrush:** foul-smelling, superficial infection of the frog, which when severe can cause frog deterioration and mild lameness.
>
> **(See Chapter 15 for more information on thrush.)**

Applying pressure to the frog can also support the structures directly above it, notably the navicular bone, deep flexor tendon, and pedal bone. This support may help counteract the pull of the deep flexor tendon on the pedal bone, which is especially useful in horses with laminitis *(see Chapter 15)*. It may also help prevent laminitis in the opposite, weight-bearing foot in a horse with a severe, nonweight-bearing lameness.

A rubber or vinyl frog-shaped pad (such as a Lily Pad™) can be taped to the bottom of the foot, directly over the frog. In an emergency, a roll of gauze bandage can serve the same purpose. No matter which item is used, it is important that the frog support does not extend any further forward than the tip of the frog. Pressure on the sole can cause pain and bruising. If necessary, the pad should be cut to the shape and size of the frog. It is also important that the position of the frog support is checked at least twice per day. Lily

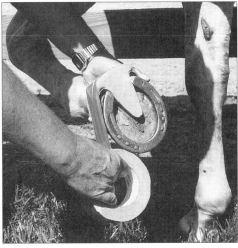

Fig. 7–51. A frog-shaped pad (such as this Lily Pad™) taped to the foot applies frog pressure.

Pads cup the back of the heels, which helps prevent them from shifting. But they can still move and either cause pain or fail to provide adequate support.

SHOEING OPTIONS

Horseshoes were designed to protect the ground surface of the foot from damage and excessive wear, allowing the horse to exercise more freely and for longer on many different surfaces. There are many types of shoes. The ideal shoe depends in part on the horse's use: the weight and style of the shoe should adequately support the foot and help the horse perform its required function safely.

Because shoes are an extension of the foot, they have either a positive or negative effect on foot and column support. An inappropriate or incorrectly fitted shoe can cause or predispose the horse to a variety of problems. For example, shoes with toe grabs can be very un-safe in horses that must make quick turns, such as polo ponies. Also, light aluminum racing plates wear out too quickly and do not provide enough support for a trail or endurance horse.

A few years ago any special shoe or shoeing method was called "corrective" or "therapeutic." However, many farriers and veterinarians now use the word "correct" to describe any shoe that supports the foot, improves hoof balance, and caters to the individual needs of the particular foot. One of the most important aspects of successful shoeing in the prevention or management of foot and leg problems is a good working relationship among the farrier, veterinarian, and owner or trainer. It is up to the farrier and veterinarian, with input and feedback from the owner or trainer, to decide which shoe is best for an individual horse with a specific problem.

There is a wide variety of shoes that may be used to improve foot or gait abnormalities, and to manage leg problems. Some of the shoes were developed with one specific condition in mind, although most have several possible effects and uses. It is beyond the scope of this book to detail the art and science of horseshoeing. Rather, this section briefly describes the more common shoes and devices, which are mentioned in this chapter or elsewhere in the book.

Keg Shoes

A correctly fitted "keg" or regular steel shoe supports the foot well, and it is all that most horses require. There was a time when it was thought that "cold shoeing" with a pre-made (keg) shoe was inferior to "hot shoeing." With hot shoeing, the farrier makes the shoe from a steel bar (using a forge to heat and shape it), and applies the hot shoe to the foot. However, when an experienced farrier shapes the keg shoe to the foot (using an anvil and hammer), rather than trimming the foot to match the shoe, keg shoes can be just as good as hot shoes.

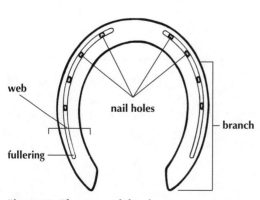

Fig. 7–52. The parts of the shoe.

The parts of the shoe are illustrated in Figure 7–52. Although the fullering (the groove in which the nails are set) may extend back to the heels, the nail holes begin just to the side of the toe, and do not extend any further back than the widest part of the foot. This ensures that the shoe is securely attached to the foot, while still allowing the heels to expand a little as weight is placed on the foot. Occasionally the farrier may need to place one or two nails at the quarter or heel. For example, if a large area of hoof wall has been resected at the front or side of the foot, it may not be possible to place enough nails further forward than the quarter. However, the trade-off is that nails at the quarter or heel prevent the hoof wall from expanding normally. Over time the heels may begin to contract if the farrier must continue to shoe the horse this way.

Of Interest

The keg shoe is so named because it is mass-produced. As the shoes come down the production line, they are collected in a large bin, or keg with others of identical size and shape.

The reverse shoe has also been called the "bank robber's shoe." Horses wearing reverse shoes make hoof prints that head in the opposite direction, "faking out the posse." Another name for this shoe is the open-toe egg bar.

Reverse Shoes

A reverse shoe is a regular shoe that is nailed onto the foot backward (the toe of the shoe is at the horse's heel). This shoe relieves

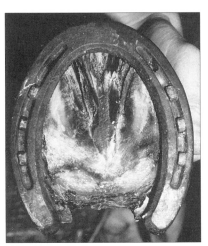

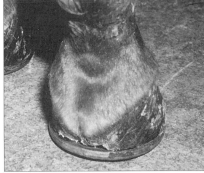

Fig. 7–53. A reverse shoe is a regular shoe that is nailed on backward.

pressure on the wall at the toe, and provides extra support at the heels. It is commonly used in horses with laminitis. Extra nail holes may need to be made in the branches of the shoe so that the nails are not placed any further back than the quarters.

Bar Shoes

Bar shoes are commonly used when extra support of the foot, particularly the heel area, is needed. However, bar shoes do not provide extra heel support unless the branches (and hence the bar) extend further back than the heels. The back of the shoe should protrude at least ¼ inch (6 mm) behind the heels to provide enough heel support. The ideal length depends on the particular problem and the type of activities the horse must perform.

A full bar shoe is a regular-shaped shoe that has a straight bar connecting both branches across the heels. There are several variations on this theme, the four most common being:

Egg bar shoe—This is a regular shoe that has a curved bar connecting the ends of the branches, creating an oval- (or egg-) shaped shoe.

Diagonal bar shoe—Also called a "¾ bar" shoe, this is a shoe with a shortened branch and a straight bar connecting that branch with the end of the normal branch, diagonally completing the circuit. This shoe is often used to manage quarter cracks *(see Chapter 15);* the bar takes weight off the damaged heel while new wall grows down.

Heart bar shoe—The bar that connects the branches on this regular shoe is in the shape of a "V" that overlies the frog. The "V" can either be level with the shoe, or slightly tilted so that it puts a controlled amount of pressure on the frog. This shoe, which uses the frog for additional support of the foot, is sometimes used in horses with laminitis.

Tongue bar shoe—This shoe has features of both the egg bar and the heart bar shoe. A flat "tongue" of metal is welded to the egg bar so that it sits directly over the frog.

Another type of shoe that uses the frog for support is a mushroom shoe, also called a "T" bar shoe. With this shoe, both heels are relieved of all weight-bearing.

Provided the nails are not placed any further back than the quarters, contracted heels are unlikely to develop with bar shoes because the hoof wall can still expand as the horse bears weight on the foot.

Fig. 7–54. Types of Bar Shoes.

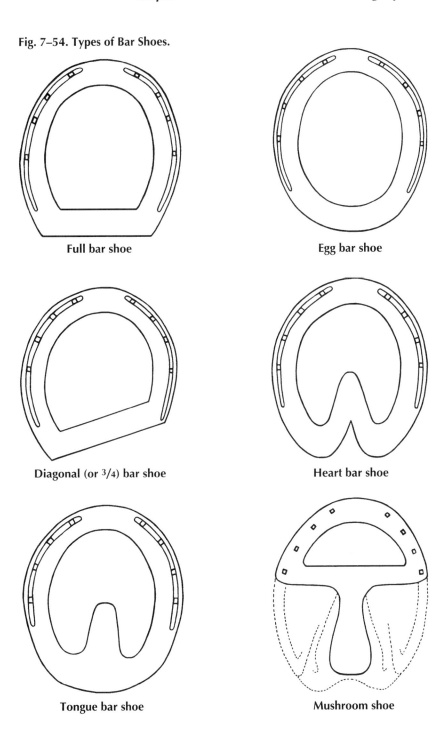

Full bar shoe

Egg bar shoe

Diagonal (or 3/4) bar shoe

Heart bar shoe

Tongue bar shoe

Mushroom shoe

Other Modifications

There are several modifications that can be made to any type of shoe. The more common ones are discussed below.

Fig. 7–55. Types of Clips and Rims.

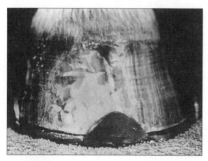

A. Toe clip.

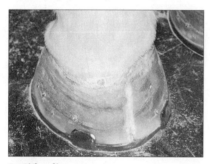

B. Side clips.

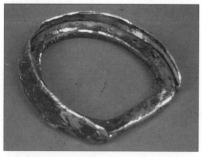

C. Raised rim shoe.

Clips

Toe, side, or quarter clips can be made on any metal shoe by heating the shoe and raising a narrow flange at the outer edge. The farrier can also work them into a "hot" shoe while making it. Toe clips help prevent the shoe from sliding back and creating pressure on the sole behind the toe. Side or quarter clips can help stabilize a hoof wall crack if they are placed on each side of the crack. In horses with a pedal bone or navicular bone fracture, several clips or a low rim can be raised around the outer edge of the shoe to prevent movement and expansion of the hoof wall.

Note: When the clips or raised rim involve both sides of the foot and extend further back than the quarters, they prevent normal expansion of the hoof wall at the heels. This could lead to contracted heels.

Beveled or Slippered Shoe

The shoe can be beveled away from the sole to prevent it from putting pressure on the sole. To do this the farrier grinds down the inner arc of the shoe on the surface that faces the foot. This makes the area of contact between the shoe and the hoof narrower than normal, and concentrates it at the outer part of the wall.

Beveling the branches of the shoe on the outer arc can encourage the heels to spread. As the horse puts weight on the foot, the heel wall slides down the angled shoe. This type of shoe, which is sometimes called a "slipper heel" shoe, can help horses with contracted heels.

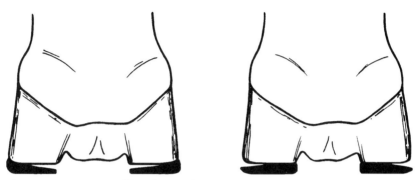

Fig. 7–56. Two types of beveling. Left: Beveling the shoe away from the sole. Right: Beveling the branches of the shoe to the outside.

Rolled Toe Shoe

The farrier grinds down the ground surface of this shoe at the center of the toe so that the front of the shoe is curved when viewed from the side. The actual bearing surface is set back a few millimeters from the tip of the toe. This shoe makes it easier for the horse to break over at the center of the toe.

Square Toe Shoe

The toe of this shoe is flat, rather than round or oval-shaped, giving the shoe a roughly square shape. The foot usually is trimmed to match. The front of this shoe can also be "rolled" for easier breakover.

Rocker Shoe

The front of the shoe is tipped up slightly from the ground surface. Before this shoe is applied, the hoof must be trimmed to match.

Half-Round Shoe

Using a half-round instead of a flat piece of steel to make the shoe can help horses with degenerative joint disease or osteoarthritis *(see Chapter 8)* in the lower leg joints. Because the entire ground surface is rounded, this shoe allows the horse to break over at the most comfortable part of the foot, which may be in a slightly different place each stride. Not only can this shoe relieve the horse's discomfort, it may also prevent further stress on the arthritic joints by allowing the horse to move as efficiently as possible.

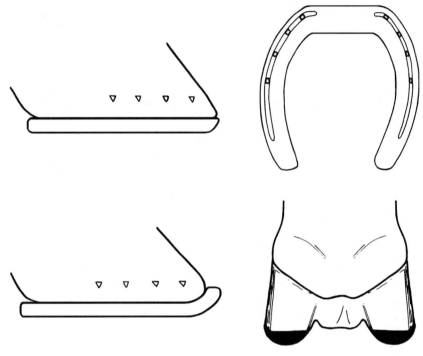

Fig. 7–57. Top left: Rolled toe shoe. Top right: Square toe shoe. Bottom left: Rocker shoe. Bottom right: Half-round shoe.

Raised Heels

The horse's heels can be raised with a wedge pad, which is a plastic or rubber pad that is thickest at the heels and narrows toward the front of the foot. Most wedge pads are only a little wider than the shoe web (that is, they are rim pads). Alternatively, the ends of the shoe branches can be "swelled" or built up to elevate the heels a few degrees.

Raising the heels is commonly used to normalize the hoof–pastern angle in horses with low heels. However, unless the wall at the heels is trimmed properly, the wedge pad or raised-heel shoe can crush the horn tubules at the heels. This is because raising the heels shortens the effective bearing surface of the foot, and therefore alters the direction of forces on the wall at the heels. It is most likely in horses

with under-run heels—
horses that cannot afford
further heel damage, yet
are commonly fitted with
wedges. To prevent
crushed heels, the shoe's
branches should be ex-
tended by ¾ inch (18 mm)
for every 3° the heels are
raised. This ensures ad-
equate heel support.

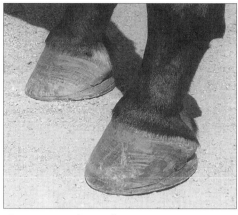

Raising the heels by at
least 7° can reduce ten-
sion in the deep flexor
tendon. It apparently has

Fig. 7–58. Wedge pads.

little effect on tension in the superficial flexor tendon, but it actually
increases tension in the suspensory ligament. So, although raising

the heels can reduce
the pull of the deep
flexor tendon on the
pedal bone (which
can help some
horses with lamini-
tis), the cost is in-
creased strain on
some of the other
support structures in
the limb.

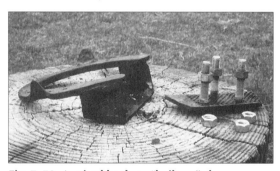

Fig. 7–59. A raised heel, or "built up" shoe.

Extensions

Metal extensions (or "trailers") can be welded onto, or worked into
the toe, back, or side of the shoe to alter foot placement. This modification can be used for a variety of problems. Toe extensions are
sometimes used in foals with flexor contracture of the coffin joint
("club foot"). Plastic glue-on shoes with side extensions ("wings") are
used in foals with angular limb deformities. *(Both conditions are discussed in Chapter 14.)*

Slightly lengthening the branches of the shoe can increase heel
support. Extending one or both branches can also be used to alter
foot flight (discussed earlier). In a horse with severed flexor tendons,
a long heel extension can help prevent the toe from tipping up and
the fetlock from dropping further *(see Chapter 11).*

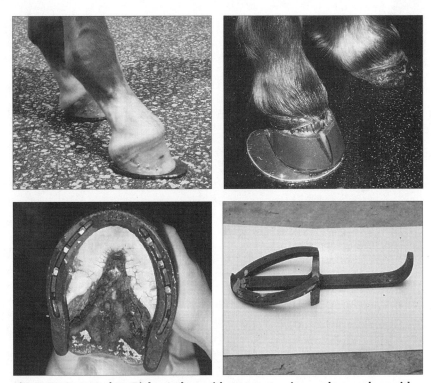

Fig. 7–60. From Left to Right: A shoe with a toe extension; a glue-on shoe with a side extension ("wing"); a shoe with heel extensions; a long heel extension for a horse with severed flexor tendons.

Traction Devices

Slipping and sliding can cause joint, tendon, ligament, and muscle injuries, although in certain sports (notably reining), sliding stops are required. In reining horses, using long hind shoes with wide, smooth webs (without fullering) can help the horse slide better. However, in other sports, a little traction is an advantage to the horse, and may actually prevent injury.

The simplest and most common traction devices to help prevent slipping in difficult terrain are the nail heads and fullering. Horses that must work on bad footing (mud, snow, steep hills, etc.) may need the extra traction provided by heel caulks. Turning over the ends of the shoe branches is another way to increase the horse's traction.

The farrier can also weld small patches of borium onto the bottom of the shoe in several spots, depending on the rider's preference and the horse's need for traction. Studs are useful traction devices in horses that do not need extra traction all the time. They can be screwed into the bottom of the shoe as needed (although the shoe must already have holes drilled for the studs). For example, eventers do not need extra traction dur-

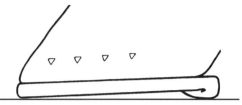

Fig. 7–61. Turning over the ends of the shoe branches is a simple way to increase the horse's traction.

ing the dressage phase of the competition, so the studs can be screwed in before the cross-country or stadium jumping phases and removed right afterward.

Traction and Racing Injuries

Racehorses are often fitted with shoes that have toe grabs and/or traction rims. A toe grab is a narrow metal bar that protrudes from the bottom of the shoe at the toe. It is usually only a couple of millimeters high, and is located just in front of the fullering. With traction rims the outer (or sometimes the inner) edge of the fullering is raised all the way around the bottom of the shoe.

These traction devices reduce slipping, but they also slow breakover, so the feet are not picked up as quickly. This can cause excessive strain on the joints, tendons, and ligaments of the lower leg.

> **More Information**
>
> "Breakdown" injuries occur when the supporting structures of the fetlock are severely damaged. They are discussed in Chapter 16.
>
> Flexor tendon strain is commonly called a "bowed tendon." See Chapter 11 for treatment and prevention.

Recent studies into racetrack injuries in gallopers have found that there is a definite relationship between the use of toe grabs and "breakdown" injuries. Flexor tendon strain also appears to be more common in horses that wear these shoes.

On a firm surface, toe grabs have the same effect as the long toe–low heel foot shape because the metal strip raises the toe slightly. This alters the angle of the hoof wall and tips the foot back onto the heels a little. In horses that already have long toes and low heels, toe grabs can exaggerate this defect. As discussed in the earlier section on *Heel Support*, this foot shape makes the horse more prone to a variety of lower leg injuries during exercise.

Traction rims that run all the way around the bottom of the shoe

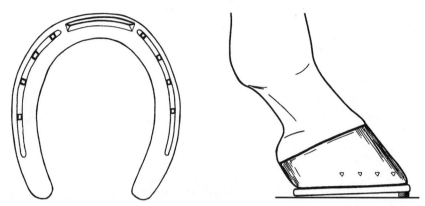

Fig. 7–62. Toe grabs have the same effect as the long toe–low heel foot shape because the metal strip raises the toe slightly.

do not alter the hoof wall angle. The rim keeps the angle the same as it would be with a regular shoe, and simply raises the foot off the ground a few millimeters. So, traction rims may be safer than toe grabs, especially in horses with the long toe–low heel foot shape.

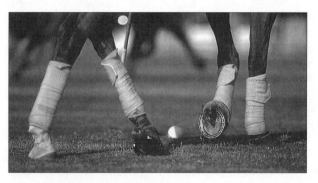

Fig. 7–63. Traction devices, such as these heel caulks, can cause excessive strain on the joints and soft tissues of the lower leg.

Other Drawbacks

Traction devices also prevent the foot from rotating while weight-bearing. Although this can give the horse extra security on loose or slippery surfaces, it can also cause excessive strain on the joints and soft tissues of the lower leg. In some cases it can contribute to fractures.

Having the foot fixed in place while the body and upper leg rotate above it concentrates the twisting forces at the fetlock and pastern. This can cause joint damage or pastern fractures *(see Chapter 16)* in horses that must make sharp turns at speed.

8

JOINT PROBLEMS

Inflammatory and degenerative conditions involving the joints are very common problems in athletic horses. These conditions are discussed in this chapter, as are infectious joint problems and joint dislocation. *(Osteo-chondrosis and the joint problems it can cause are discussed in Chapter 14.)*

JOINT STRUCTURE

A joint is a point of contact between two bones. Most of the joints in the limbs and back are designed to allow some degree of motion (flexion and extension, rotation, or side-to-side mobility), which is essential for locomotion. Some joints are more complex than others, but

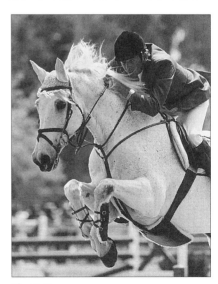

Fig. 8–1.

245

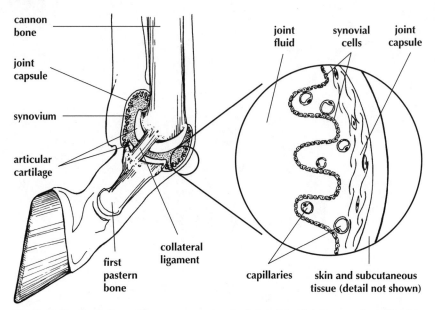

Fig. 8–2. On the left are the components of a joint. (The joint space is stylized for clarity; in reality, the cartilage surfaces meet.) On the right is a detailed view of the joint capsule.

most joints have the same basic components: articular cartilage, joint fluid, and supporting structures.

Cartilage

The contact surfaces of the bones are covered by cartilage, which reduces friction and concussion between the bones, and helps the joint move smoothly and efficiently. Articular cartilage is composed of a framework of collagen fibers and proteo-glycans. Together, these components give the cartilage its unique properties: a "buffer" that absorbs concussion, yet resists compression. Collagen and proteoglycan molecules are produced by specialized cartilage cells. These cells are located toward the base of the cartilage, near the junction with the underlying bone. Like any other tissue, these components are continually being replaced,

Definitions

Articular: involving a joint.
Collagen: microscopic fibers that give tissues their strength and resilience.
Proteoglycans: large molecules that trap water within the cartilage.

or "turned over" to maintain healthy, resilient cartilage.

Joint Fluid

Cartilage does not have a blood supply, so the cartilage cells rely on the fluid that fills the joint space to supply them with nutrients and remove their waste products. Articular cartilage is only a few millimeters thick, so the nutrients and waste products filter

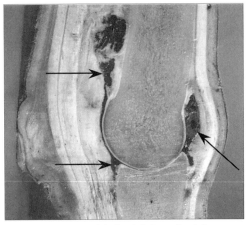

Fig. 8–3. A normal fetlock joint. The joint space [arrows] has been filled with a dark dye.

through it in both directions. This process is aided by exercise, which moves the fluid around the joint space and pumps the nutrients and wastes through the cartilage.

The joint fluid also helps protect the joint surfaces. It contains large molecules of hyaluronic acid that make the fluid viscous, like motor oil in an engine. These molecules reduce friction between the joint surfaces, and also inactivate some of the harmful inflammatory substances that can accumulate in the joint space and damage the cartilage surface. However, in the process, the hyaluronic acid molecules may be degraded.

Supporting Structures

There are several soft tissue structures that stabilize the joint. The joint capsule completely surrounds and encloses the joint. It consists of a fibrous, outer layer (which provides strength) and a thin, inner membrane, called the synovium. The synovium is well supplied with capillaries and produces the joint fluid (or synovial fluid).

Most joints have collateral ligaments on each side to prevent the joint from dislocating to the sides. These ligaments are short, broad, and strong. The tendons and ligaments (and in the upper limb, the muscles) that overlie the joint add to its structural support. Some

---

Definitions

Viscous: slippery.
Capillaries: microscopic blood vessels that supply the cells.

---

joints, such as the knee, stifle, and hip, also have ligaments inside that add support.

SYNOVITIS & DJD

The two most common joint conditions in adult horses are synovitis and degenerative joint disease (DJD). Osteoarthritis, a severe form of DJD, is also discussed in this section.

Definitions and Causes

Synovitis, DJD, and osteoarthritis represent different stages of the same process—different steps along a path of progressive joint disease. Synovitis is the first sign of a stressed joint, whereas the other two conditions represent later stages of joint deterioration. Although the difference between severe synovitis and early DJD may not be very clear in every case, it is important to realize that synovitis is essentially a reversible process. But the changes that occur with DJD and osteoarthritis are largely irreversible. In other words, synovitis is treatable, but degenerative joint disease and osteoarthritis are merely manageable.

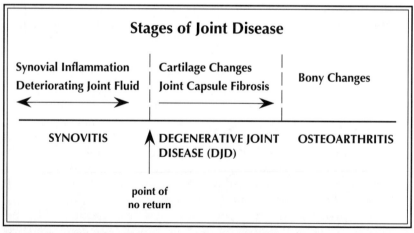

Fig. 8–4. Synovitis, degenerative joint disease, and osteoarthritis are different stages of the same process.

Synovitis

Synovitis is inflammation of the synovium that lines the joint capsule and produces joint fluid. *Capsulitis* is inflammation of the joint capsule, the fibrous outer covering of the joint. Because these two structures are intimately associated, distinguishing between synovitis and capsulitis is often impossible, and is not very useful. In many cases both conditions exist together, because it is difficult to stress the joint capsule without affecting the synovium. The effects of synovial inflammation on the joint are the most important, so, unless otherwise stated, the combined conditions of synovitis and capsulitis are called "synovitis" throughout this chapter.

In most cases synovitis is caused by overstretching of the joint capsule and synovium during strenuous exercise. A single wrong step can also wrench the joint and overstretch the soft tissues. The result in either case is inflammation of the joint capsule and synovium. Inflammatory substances released by the cells in the damaged tissue cause pain, heat,

Note

Arthritis is a general term that just means inflammation of a joint. In scientific terms, synovitis is a mild, reversible form of arthritis. However, most people think of arthritis as chronic joint pain, reduced joint mobility, and permanent disability. Therefore, in this book the word "arthritis" is limited to mean either the severe changes associated with advanced DJD (osteoarthritis), or severe joint infection (septic arthritis).

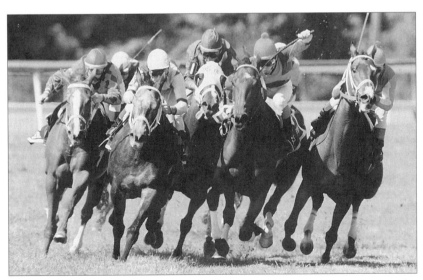

Fig. 8–5. In most cases synovitis is caused by overstretching of the joint capsule and synovium during strenuous exercise.

and swelling. When the synovium is the inflamed tissue, these substances leak into the joint fluid, where they can inflame other parts of the joint and degrade the protective hyaluronic acid molecules. Synovial inflammation also results in an increase in joint fluid production, or joint effusion. The body does this to dilute the inflammatory substances and limit their harmful effects on the joint.

Changes within the joint that are not directly related to the synovium, such as a bone chip or an osteochondrosis lesion, can also cause synovitis. In these cases, only the synovium is inflamed and stimulated to produce more joint fluid. The joint capsule is not affected, unless the joint becomes very distended with fluid.

Chemical synovitis (inflammation of the synovium caused by a medication, such as Adequan) occasionally develops after injection into a joint. Unless it is severe, chemical synovitis may not involve the joint capsule either.

Synovitis is usually self-limiting. That is, it reaches a certain point then resolves on its own, provided the cause does not persist or return. When synovial inflammation persists, the inflammatory substances can begin degrading the cartilage surface, which leads to DJD.

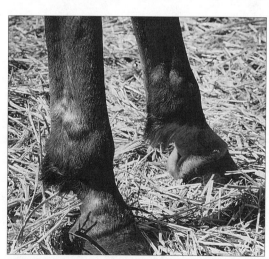

Fig. 8–6. "Windpuffs" are caused by chronic joint distention.

Chronic Synovitis

Chronic synovitis is defined as persistent joint distention: swelling that has been present for over a month. "Wind puffs" and "bog spavin" are examples of chronic joint distention (although "wind puffs" may instead involve a tendon sheath; *see*

Chapter 11). There are at least four possible causes of chronic joint distention:

- repeated bouts of synovitis
- DJD
- bone or cartilage defects within the joint, e.g. a bone chip or an osteochondrosis lesion *(see Chapter 14)*
- stretching of the joint capsule

This last possibility is generally the result of prior episodes of synovitis. The joint may no longer be actively inflamed. But once the joint capsule is stretched—whether by strain, persistent effusion, or both—the distention may remain because the joint continues to fill to its new capacity.

Acute (new or sudden) joint swelling is always important; however, the importance of chronic distention depends on the cause and severity of the initial joint damage. In general, chronic joint distension is unlikely to be significant if heat does not develop and the effusion does not worsen with exercise, the horse is not lame, and the original cause is known. In these horses the swelling may be considered to be a blemish. But if the amount of effusion increases and/or lameness develops with exercise, or the original cause is not known, the possibility of some source of persistent inflammation should be seriously considered.

The different causes of chronic joint distention vary in their impact on the horse's athletic future. So, each case of chronic synovitis should be evaluated by a veterinarian.

Chronic Proliferative Synovitis

Chronic proliferative synovitis (also called villo-nodular synovitis) is a specific type of synovitis that involves the front of the fetlock. It is almost exclusively seen in the forelegs of racehorses, both flat runners and hurdlers.

There is a small pad of tissue attached to the synovium in the front of the fetlock joint. Its role is to protect the bone surfaces at the front of the joint when the fetlock overextends. Fetlock overextension occurs during galloping and jumping—in many cases joint overextension is so extreme that the back of the fetlock touches the ground. If this pad of tissue is persistently inflamed by repeated compression during fetlock overextension, it may become thickened (proliferative) and fibrous. In long-standing cases the pad may also begin to calcify, causing a type of "osselet" *(see Chapter 16).*

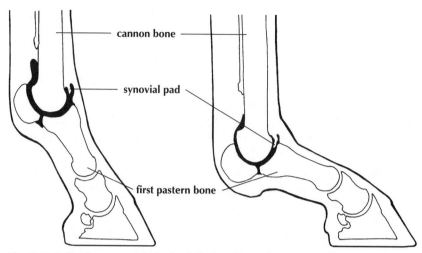

Fig. 8–7. Left: The normal fetlock while standing. Right: Fetlock overextension during strenuous exercise causes the synovial pad to be compressed.

DJD

The hallmark of degenerative joint disease is chronic, progressive degeneration of the joint cartilage. Persistent inflammation of the synovium and joint capsule are also features of this condition. Al-

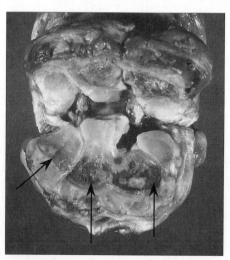

Fig. 8–8. A knee (opened) with severe DJD. The arrows indicate areas of cartilage erosion.

though DJD often affects high-motion joints, such as the fetlock and knee, it is also common in the low-motion joints of the pastern and the lower hock joints.

In most cases, DJD is caused by wear-and-tear of the joint's soft tissues and cartilage surfaces. There are two basic elements of DJD: synovitis and cartilage degeneration.

Repeated, excessive flexion and extension of the joint—such as occurs during many types of strenuous athletic activities—results in synovitis. As mentioned earlier, persistent or repeated synovitis can degrade the joint fluid, making it a thinner and less effective lubricant. It also becomes less effective at protecting the cartilage surfaces from the harmful inflammatory substances released by the synovium.

Meanwhile, the weight of the horse (and rider) compresses the cartilage. Speed, landing after a jump, and sudden turns and stops intensify this effect. Repeated, excessive compression causes the cartilage to become roughened and flattened, and less resistant to compression. The cartilage cells may also be damaged by excessive compression. When these cells are damaged they release enzymes and other substances that degrade the cartilage components (collagen and proteoglycans; discussed earlier), making the cartilage more prone to physical damage. Furthermore, damaged cartilage cells cannot replenish the cartilage components that are destroyed. These cartilage-degrading enzymes can also cause synovitis when they leak into the joint fluid.

This two-pronged attack on the cartilage (from inflammatory substances and compression) creates a vicious cycle of synovial inflammation, deteriorating joint fluid, and further cartilage degeneration. Eventually it results in:

- flattened and eroded cartilage
- increased concussion in the underlying bone
- greater friction within the joint
- chronic pain

Over time, the persistent synovitis that accompanies DJD can lead to fibrous thickening (fibrosis) of the joint capsule, which reduces joint mobility. The fibrosis is more-or-less permanent, as are the cartilage erosions if hard training continues.

Osteoarthritis

Osteoarthritis is the term used to describe advanced DJD, in which bony changes have occurred. These changes may take three forms, which can be present together:

Bone remodeling—the shape of the bone(s) at the joint surface is changed, particularly at the edges of the joint. The most common change seen in osteoarthritic joints is bone spurs on the edges of the bone. This is more frequently seen on the "cuboidal" (block-shaped) bones of the knee and the hock. Bone remodeling is caused by excessive compression from the facing bone(s), and/or uneven forces on the joint. For example, rotation and side-to-side movement in the pastern joint during

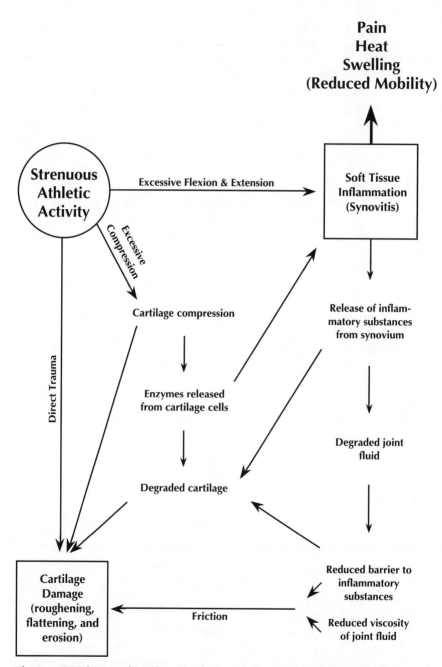

Pain
Heat
Swelling
(Reduced Mobility)

Strenuous Athletic Activity

Excessive Flexion & Extension

Soft Tissue Inflammation (Synovitis)

Excessive Compression

Direct Trauma

Cartilage compression

Release of inflammatory substances from synovium

Enzymes released from cartilage cells

Degraded joint fluid

Degraded cartilage

Cartilage Damage (roughening, flattening, and erosion)

Friction

Reduced barrier to inflammatory substances

Reduced viscosity of joint fluid

Fig. 8–9. DJD is a combination of soft tissue inflammation, deteriorating joint fluid, and cartilage degeneration.

sharp turns and spins is a primary cause of ringbone. Joint instability, caused by damage to the supporting soft tissues, can also result in unusual stresses on the bone, and remodeling.

Exostoses—specific areas of new bone production on the surface of a bone. When they occur around a joint they usually develop where the joint capsule attaches onto the bone. This bony change can occur as a result of overstretching of the joint capsule or collateral ligament. Presumably, it is the body's attempt to strengthen a stress-point. Exostoses can also develop after direct damage, such as a wire cut over or near a joint. When they are large, exostoses may cause a hard swelling around the joint that can be seen or felt.

Narrowing of the joint space—excessive compression and/or extensive cartilage erosion may result in narrowing of the joint space, which can be seen on radiographs. This is most common in the lower hock joints, where the joint space is either narrowed or completely filled in with new bone. Narrowing of the

> ## More Information
>
> Osteoarthritis of the hock is called bone spavin. Hock problems are discussed in Chapter 20.
>
> Osteoarthritis of the pastern and/or coffin joint is called ringbone. Pastern problems are discussed Chapter 16.
>
> Bone problems such as exostoses are discussed in Chapter 9.

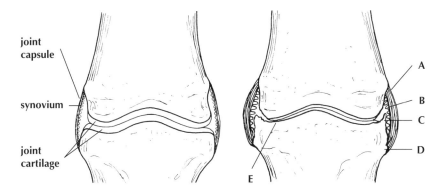

Fig. 8–10. Left: A normal joint. Right: Components of osteoarthritis.

A = joint capsule fibrosis	D = exostosis
B = synovitis	E = eroded cartilage and
C = bone spur	narrowed joint space

joint space can occur in other joints if cartilage erosion is extensive. But it is difficult to confirm unless radiographs of the opposite joint are available for comparison. Septic arthritis can damage enough of the cartilage to cause narrowing of the joint space, as can severe DJD.

An osteoarthritic joint is an "end-stage" condition: the irreversible conclusion to severe joint disease. Certain joints, in particular the pastern joint and the lower hock joints, appear to be more prone to osteoarthritis than other joints. But any joint that is severely damaged can develop these bony changes.

Factors Contributing to Synovitis and DJD

There are several factors that can contribute to the development and progression of these joint conditions.

Training

Overextension of the fetlock and knee during strenuous exercise is a key factor that can lead to synovitis and DJD in these joints, especially in galloping or jumping horses. Overextension becomes more pronounced as the horse begins to tire. This is because the flexor muscles at the back of the forearm become fatigued, and the flexor muscle–tendon unit *(see Chapter 11)* lengthens, allowing the fetlock and knee to overextend further. This can also occur with the flexors of the hindlimb.

Muscle fatigue occurs more quickly in under-conditioned or poorly-trained horses. Regular exercise is important to properly condition all of the parts of the musculoskeletal system—bones, joints, tendons, ligaments, and muscles. So, the "weekend warrior" that stands around all week, and then is made to do a week's work in a day, is more likely to develop joint (and other musculoskeletal) problems than the horse that is exercised more often. Allowing the horse to become or remain overweight can add to the compressive load on the joints.

At the other end of the spectrum, repeated overloading accelerates the degenerative processes in horses that are worked too hard for months on end. One way of looking at this is that the joint, like an engine part, will withstand only so much stress. The limit may be accumulated gradually over the horse's lifetime, or it may be reached in the first few years, depending on how hard the horse is trained and competed. However, unlike an engine part, the joint has some

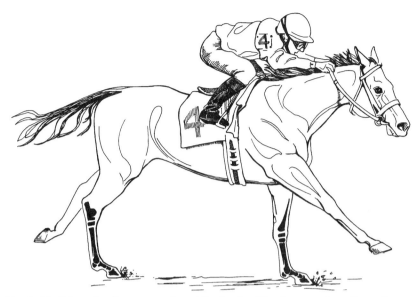

Fig. 8–11. When the flexor muscles at the back of the forearm tire, they allow the fetlock and knee to overextend. The hindlegs can be similarly affected.

capacity to heal. Not allowing the joint enough time to repair accelerates the degenerative process in many athletic horses. As long as the horse continues in training, cartilage damage is greater than cartilage repair. The scales may be tipped toward cartilage repair with proper management (discussed later).

Conformation and Shoeing

Poor conformation and improper shoeing can also play a role in the development of synovitis and DJD, particularly in the lower joints (the knee or hock and below). Toe-in or toe-out foot conformation, base-narrow or base-wide stance, unbalanced feet, or an inappropriate shoe can create abnormal forces on these joints. Long, sloping pasterns and the long toe–low heel foot shape can increase fetlock overextension during exercise. Straight pasterns and upright, "boxy" feet can increase concussion in the lower joints and worsen cartilage compression.

> **More Information**
>
> Foot conformation and shoeing options are covered in Chapter 7.

Fig. 8–12.

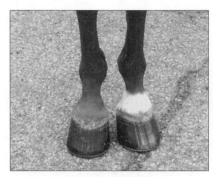

Base-narrow, toed-out stance.

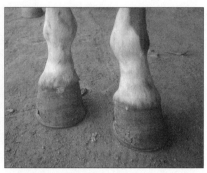

Unbalanced feet and improper shoeing.

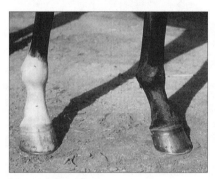

Long pasterns.

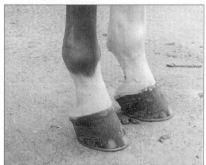

Short, upright pasterns.

Breed and Use

The breed and use of the horse can influence the site and severity of joint problems. For example, Quarter Horse and Thoroughbred racehorses are more prone to knee and fetlock problems because of the extreme overextension in these joints during galloping. In young racehorses, the entire musculoskeletal system is relatively immature, and this can also play a part.

Horses involved in Western sports (roping, barrel racing, reining, etc.) are more prone to hock and pastern problems. The upright conformation of many Quarter Horses adds to the concussive and compressive load on these joints during strenuous activities. But on the whole, it is the extreme forces these joints must withstand during sharp turns, spins, and sliding stops that contribute most to the joint problems.

Hock problems are also seen in dressage horses (of any breed), Saddlebreds, and Standardbred racehorses. This probably relates to the amount of exaggerated hock motion during training and competition.

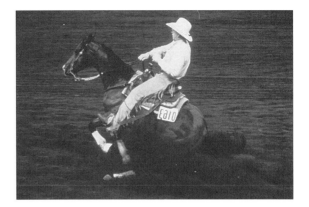

Fig. 8–13. The hocks must withstand extreme forces during sliding stops.

Other Factors

A single traumatic incident, such as stepping in a hole and wrenching the joint, can cause synovitis. It could also lead to DJD and possibly osteoarthritis, especially if permanent changes occur in the joint or its supporting soft tissues. Such changes could include an untreated bone chip, a joint capsule tear, or collateral ligament damage.

Osteochondrosis lesions, such as osteochondritis dissecans (OCD) and subchondral bone cysts, can lead to DJD if they are not treated appropriately. Cartilage erosions, cracks, flaps, or loose fragments are commonly found in joints affected by osteochondrosis, whether or not there are also bony lesions.

Articular fractures that heal leaving a gap or step at the joint surface can cause cartilage damage on the facing joint surface. Severe DJD can rapidly develop in these joints. *(See Chapter 9 for more information on fractures.)*

Definitions

Osteochondrosis: an abnormality of developing bone.

Osteochondritis dissecans: osteochondrosis lesion where a fragment of bone and cartilage has broken off the joint surface.

Subchondral bone cyst: round cavity in a bone near the joint surface.

(Osteochondrosis is covered in Chapter 14.)

Signs of Synovitis and DJD

The typical signs of synovitis and DJD include:
- joint swelling (see below)
- heat felt during palpation of the joint, although this may only be mild, and present only after exercise in horses with low-grade

DJD or chronic proliferative synovitis

• reduced range of joint motion—this is due to pain, joint capsule distention, and, with chronic DJD, joint capsule fibrosis

• pain during flexion of the joint, and a positive flexion test *(see Chapter 2)*

• lameness—the grade depends on the severity of the joint changes, but in most cases synovitis and DJD cause mild to moderate lameness (grade 1 – 3 of 5)

Joint swelling is a consistent feature of synovitis and DJD in the more mobile joints, such as the fetlock, knee, hock, and stifle. These joints must move through a much wider range than other joints, so their joint capsules are looser and more "roomy." In part, the swelling is due to thickening of the joint capsule, but most of it is caused by joint effusion (accumulation of joint fluid). Effusion can be very difficult to detect in other joints because their joint capsules are tighter, which leaves less room for fluid distention.

Because joints have tendons and ligaments that run over them, joint effusion often causes "pouches" of fluid to protrude between the tendons and ligaments. For example, fetlock effusion is mostly seen toward the back of the joint, between the collateral ligament and the suspensory ligament. In the knee, discrete "bubbles" develop over the front of the joint, on either side of the extensor tendons *(see Chapter 18)*. In the hock, effusion may be seen at three or four separate places *(see Chapter 20)*. In each of these joints, pressing the swelling on one side of the joint causes the other side to protrude further.

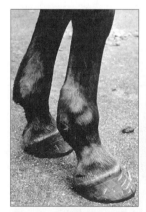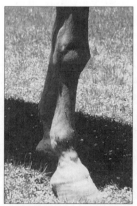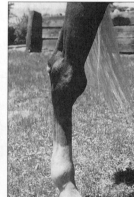

Fig. 8–14. Left: Fetlock effusion. Middle: Knee "bubbles." Right: Hock effusion.

Chronic proliferative synovitis causes a characteristic "doughy" thickening over the front of the fetlock joint, but effusion in the rest of the joint is usually mild. The lameness is also mild; in most cases the primary complaint is that the horse will not stretch out or gallop as fast as it used to.

In horses with mild or early DJD, the presence or degree of effusion and lameness can be inconsistent. The effusion and lameness may improve or resolve with rest, and return or worsen with exercise. This can be very confusing.

Advanced osteoarthritis often causes bony swelling around the joint, and reduced joint mobility (although the lower hock joints are normally immobile). Firm pressure with the fingers may cause a low-grade pain response during palpation of the swelling.

Diagnosis of Synovitis and DJD

History and Signs

Diagnosis is sometimes based just on the history, in particular, the horse's age and use, and the signs. Synovitis is more common in young horses, especially when they begin fast work (racehorses) or hard training (show horses). Because DJD is a chronic, progressive condition which is brought on or worsened by strenuous exercise, it is more often seen in mature athletic horses.

It is sometimes difficult to distinguish between synovitis and DJD based on the signs. Because synovitis is an acute condition, the signs may appear to be more severe than those commonly seen in horses with DJD (which is a chronic condition). However, such generalizations can be misleading.

In basic terms, the feature that distinguishes DJD from synovitis is cartilage degeneration. However, the presence and extent of cartilage damage can be difficult to detect without actually looking at the cartilage, which is impractical. So, if lameness and effusion persist or return, it is usually safe to assume that the changes within the joint may include cartilage degeneration.

Regional Anesthesia

Many veterinarians use nerve blocks to localize the lameness to a particular area of the leg and rule out other potential sites of lameness (such as the foot), even though joint effusion may be obvious. If

More Information
The diagnostic techniques mentioned in this section are detailed in Chapter 2.

there is any doubt that the joint is the sole or primary site of lameness, the veterinarian may perform a joint block. This procedure specifically desensitizes the joint, and in most cases it temporarily resolves lameness caused by synovitis or DJD.

Radiography

Routine radiography cannot reveal soft tissue or cartilage changes, unless there is calcification of the soft tissues or narrowing of the

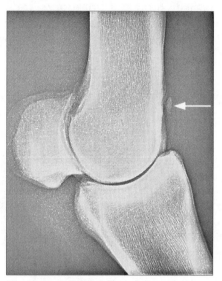

joint space by extensive cartilage erosion. For this reason, it is not much use in diagnosing synovitis and DJD. However, radiography is often performed to determine whether there are any bony changes within or around the joint. It is important to check for bone chips, osteochondrosis lesions, or other bony abnormalities that could complicate matters. It is also worth knowing whether DJD has progressed to osteoarthritis.

Contrast radiography, although not frequently used, is valuable for outlining the enlarged, fibrous pad in horses with chronic proliferative synovitis. Unless there is obvi-

Fig. 8–15. Calcification of the soft tissues at the front of the fetlock.

ous calcification of the pad or loss of bone density at the front of the cannon bone, this condition is difficult to confirm with plain radiography. Contrast radiography may also highlight large cartilage defects and "joint mice" (floating pieces of cartilage; *see Chapter 14*) in other joints. Ultrasonography is another way to identify chronic proliferative synovitis and some large cartilage defects.

Arthrocentesis (Joint Tap)

Arthrocentesis (a joint tap) should be performed if the horse is very lame and the joint is very swollen. Although septic arthritis (discussed later) is not common, it is very important to rule it out in horses showing such severe signs. If the horse is suddenly lame immediately after exercise it is more likely that acute soft tissue damage, such as a joint capsule tear, or a fracture involving the joint is causing the severe joint swelling and lameness. In these two cases it is not unusual for there to be blood in the joint when the fluid is sampled.

In most cases of uncomplicated synovitis or DJD, the joint fluid is thinner and has a slightly higher protein concentration than normal. However, these findings are not very specific, so most veterinarians sample the joint fluid only if they are performing a joint block. The needle is in the joint for the purpose of injecting local anesthetic, so the veterinarian simply examines the joint fluid as it dribbles from the needle.

Other Tests

Occasionally the veterinarian may recommend nuclear scintigraphy to localize the lameness to a joint in the upper part of the leg, such as the shoulder or hip. These joints can be difficult to block with regional anesthesia, and difficult to radiograph well.

Arthroscopy is not a very practical or economical way to diagnose joint disease in most cases. However, if arthroscopic surgery is being performed for another reason (such as bone chip removal), it provides the surgeon with an excellent opportunity to evaluate the cartilage surfaces. At present there is no better way to determine the degree of cartilage damage in horses. *(See Chapter 6 for more information on arthroscopy.)*

Current research is aimed at developing a test to identify some of the cartilage-breakdown products in joint fluid. This test may enable veterinarians to diagnose low-grade DJD much earlier, and start treatment that could halt the destructive progress of the condition.

Treatment of Synovitis and DJD

Synovitis

The first episode of synovitis should be taken seriously, because if appropriate measures are not taken, it could lead to chronic joint problems. Prompt treatment can prevent persistence and recurrence of synovitis, and DJD.

Initial Therapy

The two most important parts of treating synovitis are rest from regular training, and anti-inflammatory therapy (in particular, cold therapy, NSAIDs, and DMSO; *see Chapter 5*). Ideally, the horse should be rested in a stall and/or paddock until the joint has healed. This can take from 10 days to 3 weeks, even though the obvious signs of pain, heat, and swelling may substantially improve in the first few days of treatment. In most cases, anti-inflammatory therapy can be stopped after 4 – 5 days. Cold therapy is usually of limited benefit after this time, and NSAIDs should no longer be necessary.

A support bandage is often useful when treating synovitis of the fetlock. The bandage can aid healing by providing support and warmth, and it may help prevent chronic joint distention. *(See Chapter 4 for information on bandaging.)*

Light exercise, such as hand-walking, for 20 – 30 minutes twice per day during the rest period benefits all horses, but particularly young racehorses. It may actually be harmful to stop all exercise in these horses because the other musculoskeletal components (bones, tendons, ligaments, and muscles) require regular activity to remain in good condition. The aim is to reduce stress on the joints, while still providing a low level of controlled exercise. It is often easiest and safest to walk a young racehorse by "ponying" it (leading it while riding another, quieter horse) or by putting the horse on a slow treadmill or "hot walker." Swimming relieves the joints of their compressive load, so it can also be a useful form of exercise in these horses.

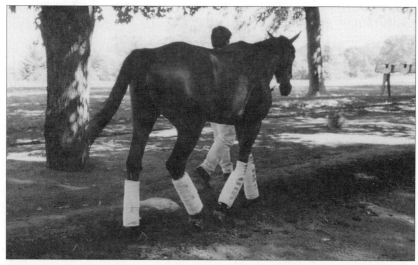

Fig. 8–16. Hand-walking for 20 – 30 minutes twice per day during the rest period benefits all horses, but particularly young racehorses.

Other Medical Options

Joint medications, such as corticosteroids, HA, and Adequan *(see Chapter 5)*, are of most benefit for recurrent synovitis and early DJD. These products are probably overkill in acute synovitis because the joint should respond simply to rest, cold therapy, and NSAIDs. Also, they may mask the signs of joint stress for weeks, which could be harmful if the horse is returned to full training during that time. Still, HA and Adequan may be worthwhile because they help protect the cartilage from damage.

Bone chips and osteochondrosis lesions that appear to be involving and potentially damaging a joint surface should be treated with arthroscopic surgery *(see Chapter 6)* for the best long-term result. As long as bone or cartilage fragments remain in the joint, persistent synovitis and cartilage erosions could develop.

Other Management Recommendations

Synovitis is mostly an activity-related condition, so it can be counter-productive to return the horse to its original intensity of exercise immediately after the rest period. Instead, the intensity and duration of exercise should be gradually increased over a 2 – 3 week period. During this time, the joint should be closely examined before and after each exercise session for return of the signs. *NSAIDs will mask these important signs of joint stress,* so they should not be given once training resumes. If the horse develops heat or swelling in the joint, or if lameness returns, the horse should be rested. The joint should be re-examined by the veterinarian, and the exercise program re-evaluated.

The horse's hoof balance and shoeing should be examined and improved as necessary. Shoes that adequately support the heels are important in every horse, but especially those with the long toe–low heel foot shape *(see Chapter 7)*.

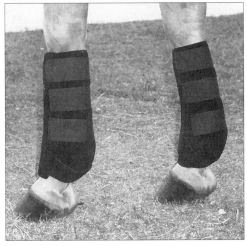

Fig. 8–17. Exercise bandages that "sling" the back of the fetlock can reduce fetlock overextension during strenuous exercise.

Exercise bandages that "sling" the back of the fetlock can reduce the amount of fetlock overextension during strenuous exercise. So they can be useful in horses recovering from fetlock synovitis.

It is important for the horse's long-term athletic future that this acute and treatable condition is not allowed to develop into a chronic problem. An adequate rest period, effective anti-inflammatory therapy, and gradual return to full training reduce the potential for chronic joint disease. These measures also reduce the amount of time the horse is out of training because recurrence is likely if the horse resumes training too soon. They lessen the overall cost of treatment for the same reason.

Chronic Proliferative Synovitis

In early or mild cases of proliferative synovitis, rest and anti-inflammatory therapy may be all that are needed to reduce the inflammation in the pad of tissue. This condition also responds well to corticosteroid injection into the joint. However, if the condition persists or returns, or if the pad has begun to calcify, removing the tissue with arthroscopic surgery is the best long-term option. Not all of the tissue can be removed arthroscopically, and the pad probably regrows to some extent, so the surgery is unlikely to leave the bone surfaces unprotected during strenuous exercise. Provided there are no other problems in the joint, most horses can be gradually returned to training 4 – 6 weeks after surgery.

DJD and Osteoarthritis

Cartilage damage and other permanent changes in the joint often are well advanced by the time the signs of DJD are consistent. Therefore, therapy can only be expected to:

• slow further cartilage degeneration
• promote cartilage repair
• improve the function of the joint
• keep the horse usable in some capacity

Drugs
NSAIDs

NSAIDs are among the most useful drugs for the long-term management of chronic joint disease in horses. These drugs do not merely block the pain, they treat its cause—inflammation. Thus, provided they are used with care, these drugs can keep joint inflammation and pain to a minimum, slowing disease progression and making the horse more comfortable and serviceable.

Depending on the degree of discomfort and the response to treatment, some horses may only need an occasional short course of NSAIDs (less than 2 weeks' duration). Other horses, particularly those with osteoarthritis, may need more prolonged or continuous treatment. If the horse is to remain on the drug long-term, its comfort must be balanced with the potential for side effects when these drugs are overused. The safest approach is to keep the dose at the lowest effective level. The dose may occasionally need to be increased, especially during a sudden cold spell, and for reshoeing and transport, in chronically lame horses.

Most sports prohibit or limit the use of NSAIDs in performing horses. Therefore, the drugs should be withdrawn or the dose reduced in the week leading up to a competition in horses that are "serviceably sound" (not obviously lame).

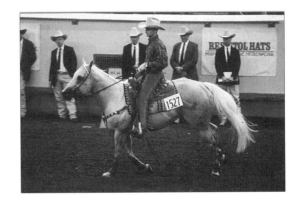

Fig. 8–18. Most sports prohibit or limit the use of NSAIDs in performing horses.

Joint Medications

Corticosteroids are very effective in resolving soft tissue inflammation in horses with DJD. They can rapidly and completely suppress inflammation for days or weeks, depending on the product. However, corticosteroids can slow cartilage repair if they are overused. They also inhibit the immune responses in the joint, making it more prone to infection.

Other joint medications, such as hyaluronic acid (HA) and Adequan, may be of some use in early cases of DJD, but they are generally of limited benefit in advanced DJD and osteoarthritis. Although, having said that, they can help some of these horses. Many horses have DJD in multiple joints, even though the condition may be obvious in only one or two joints. Giving these medications systemically (intravenously for HA and intramuscularly for Adequan) treats multiple joints with one injection. So, while the drug may do little for the obviously diseased joint, it may make the horse more comfortable by improving conditions in other joints.

(These medical options are discussed in detail in Chapter 5.)

Exercise

Strenuous exercise is one of the key factors involved in the development and progression of DJD. Therefore, the intensity of the horse's training program and competition schedule may need to be decreased to reduce joint stress.

The intensity and duration of exercise, and the types of activities the horse can perform, will depend in part on the severity of the signs. For example, if the horse is only slightly lame, and the lameness is resolved with joint medication, the horse may be exercised more-or-less normally. Although, strenuous activities, such as galloping, jumping, sharp turns, and sudden stops, should be kept to a minimum. However, if the horse is moderately lame, and NSAID treatment merely improves the lameness, the intensity and duration of exercise should be lessened accordingly. Provided an accurate diagnosis is made, giving a low dose of an NSAID to make the horse more comfortable during exercise generally will do no harm with DJD. It may even be helpful.

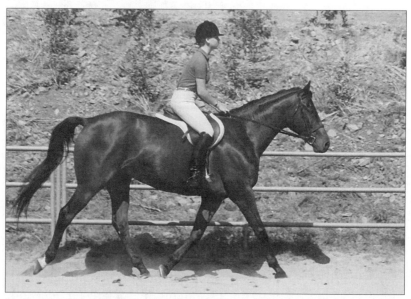

Fig. 8–19. A horse with chronic joint disease should be warmed up for longer.

Another useful sign is whether the horse "warms out" of the lameness (the lameness improves or even disappears during exercise). Horses that "warm out" of the lameness can usually be worked more actively than those that remain the same or worsen with exercise. All horses with chronic joint disease should be warmed up for a longer time before each exercise session, and trained less strenuously than healthy horses. Nevertheless, the horse must be suitably conditioned if it is to perform in an athletic competition. Activities that improve cardiovascular fitness without overstressing the joints, such as swimming and slow work on steep hills, can be substituted for the usual athletic training activities.

Inactivity can be just as limiting to the horse's long-term usefulness and comfort as strenuous exercise. While rest is important in managing synovitis, some activity every day is important in maintaining joint function and mobility once cartilage degeneration, joint capsule fibrosis, or bony changes have developed. Activity improves blood flow to the soft tissues of the joint, and it also increases the elasticity of these tissues. Furthermore, exercise moves the synovial fluid around the joint space (which nourishes the cartilage), and it may also improve the rate and quality of synovial fluid production. Although daily pasture turnout is preferable to stall confinement, many mature horses are not very active in the pasture. These horses should be worked each day, even if this only involves longeing for 10 – 15 minutes.

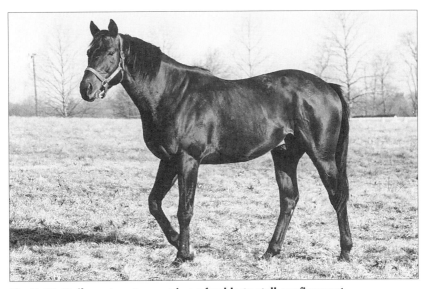

Fig. 8–20. Daily pasture turnout is preferable to stall confinement.

Other Management Recommendations

The type of shoeing required depends on the horse's conformation and particular foot problems, if any. But no matter what shoe the farrier or veterinarian recommends, regular reshoeing is important. It is also important that there is little or no change in the angles of the feet once the farrier restores them to normal *(see Chapter 7)*.

Exercise bandages can help support the fetlocks during strenuous exercise *(see Figure 8–17)*. However, a bandage can do little to reduce the compressive load on the joints.

The ideal footing for horses with chronic joint disease is firm, but not hard. Deep sand or mud stresses the joint's soft tissues, while hard surfaces, such as asphalt or dried clay, add to the concussive forces on the joint cartilage. Irregular surfaces, such as plowed fields, should also be avoided.

The horse's ration should consist of a balanced diet of good quality feeds, with care being taken not to permit the horse to become overweight. Excessive body weight places extra strain on the joints.

Prognosis for Synovitis and DJD

In horses with synovitis, the prognosis for return to full athletic function is very good if the synovitis is an isolated event that is managed properly. Even if a bone chip or osteochondrosis lesion is the cause, as long as prompt surgical treatment is followed by a sufficient rest period, the horse should completely recover in most cases.

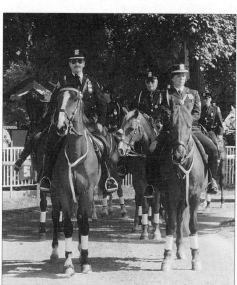

The long-term prognosis for DJD and osteoarthritis is not so good. DJD is one of the most common reasons why an athletic horse cannot continue to compete at its best. Even with appropriate therapy and modifications to the training program and competition schedule, a critical evalu-

Fig. 8–21. A racehorse could become a mounted patrol horse.

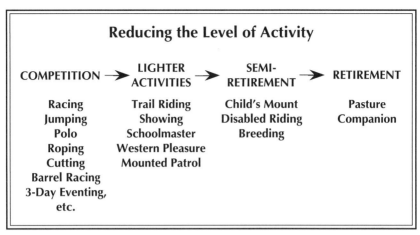

Reducing the Level of Activity

COMPETITION → LIGHTER ACTIVITIES → SEMI-RETIREMENT → RETIREMENT

COMPETITION	LIGHTER ACTIVITIES	SEMI-RETIREMENT	RETIREMENT
Racing	Trail Riding	Child's Mount	Pasture
Jumping	Showing	Disabled Riding	Companion
Polo	Schoolmaster	Breeding	
Roping	Western Pleasure		
Cutting	Mounted Patrol		
Barrel Racing			
3-Day Eventing,			
etc.			

Fig. 8–22. In most horses with chronic joint disease, the level and intensity of exercise must eventually be reduced.

ation of the horse's athletic future is, at some point, inevitable. Some horses continue to perform at their previous level for a time, but in most cases the level and intensity of exercise must eventually be reduced. This may mean, for example, turning a three-day-eventer into a hunter, downgrading a roping horse to a ranch horse, or using a competitive dressage horse as a "schoolmaster" to teach less experienced riders. The horse's athletic ability and attitude are important in determining how much work it will tolerate and what its long-term use will be.

Prevention of Synovitis and DJD

Many people consider synovitis and DJD to be occupational hazards of the athletic horse. However, reviewing the factors involved in the development of these conditions, and preventing them where possible, reduces the incidence or severity in most horses.

SEPTIC ARTHRITIS
Definition

Septic arthritis is a very serious condition that is caused by bacterial infection of the joint space and surrounding tissues. Dramatic changes within the joint can rapidly result in severe disability and permanent joint damage. Septic arthritis can occur in horses of any age; in young foals this condition is commonly called "joint ill."

Causes of Septic Arthritis

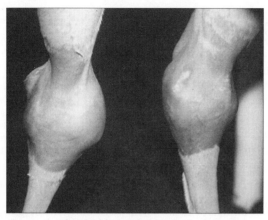

Fig. 8–23. This foal has infection in both hocks.

Foals

In foals in the first week of life, infection can spread to the joints through the bloodstream. In many cases bacteria from the foal's environment enter the body through the umbilical stump. Infection can spread to multiple sites—several joints, the lungs, or other organs—within hours.

Joint ill is most commonly seen in foals that did not receive adequate colostrum in the first 24 hours of life. Because the foal is born without any protective antibodies, it is at the mercy of all kinds of potentially deadly bacteria in its environment if it does not drink enough colostrum soon after birth. The foal's colostrum intake can be determined by measuring the concentration of antibodies in its bloodstream. Foals with a low level of antibodies after 12 – 18 hours of age are at greater risk of developing septic arthritis than foals that received plenty of colostrum within that time.

> **Definition**
>
> **Colostrum:** the antibody-rich milk that the mare produces around the time of foaling.

Adult Horses

In adult horses, spread of infection from the bloodstream to a joint is possible, but it is very uncommon. In most cases the bacteria enter the joint through a wound (either surgical or traumatic) or during arthrocentesis (joint tap). Whether the veterinarian is collecting a sample of joint fluid for analysis or injecting medication into the joint, bacterial infection is a risk every time a needle is inserted into a joint. *(The steps veterinarians take to avoid joint infection are listed in*

Chapter 2 in the section entitled Intra-articular Anesthesia.)

Septic arthritis is more likely after intra-articular injection with corticosteroids or Adequan. Because corticosteroids suppress the immune response within the joint, the infection may go undetected for over a week following intra-articular injection. This delay seriously compromises the chances of successful treatment. If joint pain develops within 24 hours of intra-articular injection with Adequan, it is more likely that chemical synovitis has developed. When joint infection occurs with Adequan, it usually takes at least 3 days to become obvious. *(These drugs are discussed in Chapter 5.)*

Extra Information
The type of bacteria causing the infection may affect the severity of joint disease and the outcome. Streptococcal ("strep") infections do not seem to be as difficult to resolve as Staphylococcal ("staph") infections or infection with bacteria from the bowel, such as *E. coli*.

Effects on the Joint

The bacteria and the toxins they produce cause severe inflammation of the synovial membrane. These toxins, and the inflammatory substances that are released by the synovium and responding white blood cells, also degrade the joint fluid and damage the cartilage *(see Chapter 5)*.

Severe inflammation also causes fibrin to be released into the joint space. Fibrin is a blood clotting protein that can leak from the capillaries in the inflamed synovium. It causes fibrous bands, or adhe-

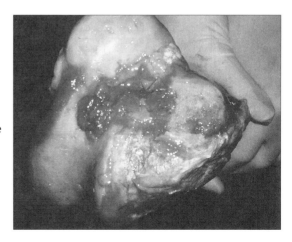

Fig. 8–24. A joint with severe septic arthritis: the cartilage is eroded, and the brown clot in the center is a mass of fibrin and pus.

sions, to form within the joint. These adhesions can make joint lavage (discussed later) difficult, and they can also contribute to the reduced joint mobility that is common after septic arthritis.

Septic arthritis can lead to the most serious type of osteoarthritis a horse can have. Severe changes in the joint can occur within days of infection. If effective therapy is not begun before this time, irreversible changes in the cartilage and soft tissues of the joint can render the joint permanently disabled. Even with early diagnosis and treatment, this may still be the final outcome in some cases.

Signs of Septic Arthritis

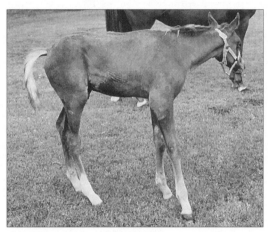

Fig. 8–25. Foals may have more than one affected joint. In this foal, the elbow and stifle are swollen.

Septic arthritis is a very painful condition, so in most cases the affected horse or foal is grade 4 – 5 of 5 lame. The infected joint is hot, and palpation and manipulation cause extreme pain. Although the joint may be very swollen, the swelling may not be confined to the joint space. Bacterial infection of the superficial tissues (cellulitis; *see Chapter 13*) often develops outside the joint capsule, and causes swelling to spread above and below the joint.

Another common sign is a fever. The normal rectal temperature for an adult horse at rest is around 100.4°F, although it can vary. Foals generally have slightly higher rectal temperatures than adult horses, although the temperature should not normally exceed 101.5°F.

It is common for foals to have more than one affected joint, or to have

Note
Normal Body Temperature
Adult Horse
Range: 98.6 – 101.3°F
(37.0 – 38.5°C)
Average: 100.4°F (38°C)
Foal
Range: 98.6 – 101.5°F
(37.0 – 38.6°C)
Average: 101°F (38.4°C)

other joints develop signs of infection over the next few days. In contrast, adult horses generally develop septic arthritis in only one joint.

Diagnosis of Septic Arthritis

Diagnosis can often be based on the history (a wound, surgery, arthrocentesis, or insufficient colostrum in the first 24 hours of life in foals) and the signs. These signs can mimic a fracture involving the joint, so radiographs may be necessary if the history is inconclusive. Radiographs are also useful for determining the prognosis in advanced cases.

In every case, the veterinarian should collect a sample of joint fluid. Visible changes in the fluid that can help the veterinarian confirm the diagnosis include abnormal color, cloudiness, and a change of viscosity. For example, the fluid may be discolored red-brown, or it may be cloudy yellow or white. In some cases it is watery, and in others it is thick and clumpy. This is pus, which is an accumulation of fluid, fibrin, white blood cells, bacteria, and cell debris. A joint does not have to contain pus to be infected, however.

The sample of joint fluid is submitted to a laboratory for analysis, and bacterial culture and antibiotic sensitivity testing. Because bacteria are so small, and effusion (in response to inflammation) dilutes the contents of the joint fluid, the laboratory staff sometimes cannot find any bacteria in the sample. However, if the white cell count and the protein concentration of the joint fluid are greatly increased, septic arthritis should be strongly suspected and treatment should begin. *(See Chapter 2 for more information on joint fluid collection, appearance, and testing.)*

Some veterinarians believe there is a less severe form of joint infection. Others believe that this so-called "low-grade joint infection" is simply severe synovitis. The signs are typical of severe joint inflammation: joint effusion, moderate lameness, and pain during manipulation. However, joint fluid analysis is inconclusive. The protein concentration and white cell count may both be moderately elevated, but no bacteria are cultured from the sample. Treatment varies among veterinarians, with some managing the joint like any case of synovitis (discussed earlier), and others treating the joint as if it were infected. These joints seldom progress to the stage of typical septic arthritis, which adds weight to the conclusion that this is not primarily an infectious condition.

Treatment of Septic Arthritis

Septic arthritis can be very difficult to resolve because the bacteria invade the synovium. It is virtually impossible to remove all of the bacteria from the synovium, so there is the potential for reinfection if treatment is stopped too soon. Furthermore, the joint's inflammatory response to the infection can cause as much, if not more damage than the bacteria. So, for the best outcome, treatment should begin as soon as possible.

These treatments are discussed in Section II: Principles of Therapy.

Lavage

The primary treatment involves lavage: flushing the joint space with large volumes of sterile saline solution, either under nerve block or general anesthesia. In some cases the joint can be lavaged through a catheter. In other cases the veterinarian may lavage the joint through a small surgical incision (an arthrotomy) in the skin and joint capsule. No matter which approach is chosen, lavage is *vital* for removing the destructive bacteria, toxins, inflammatory substances, fibrin clumps, and cell debris.

Lavage may need to be repeated every 1 – 2 days until the infection is under control. Some veterinarians add DMSO to the lavage solution because it is a potent anti-inflammatory agent, and also has some antibacterial properties.

Caution

Antibiotics alone are not enough to successfully treat septic arthritis. When an owner or trainer treats the horse with antibiotics, hoping to resolve the problem, effective treatment is delayed and the chances of a satisfactory outcome are greatly reduced. *This condition must receive immediate veterinary attention.*

Antibiotics

Systemic (intravenous or oral) antibiotics are essential for treating septic arthritis. It may seem to make more sense to inject the antibiotics directly into the joint—the site of infection. However, joint effusion dilutes the antibiotics, and lavage flushes them from the joint. In contrast, systemic antibiotics are delivered to the synovium through the bloodstream, so the infection is attacked at its source (the bacteria in the synovium). Some veterinarians inject antibiotics into the joint after lavage. This may be of some use in "closed" joints, which do not have a wound or arthrotomy incision.

The best approach to antibiotic therapy is to first identify the bacteria causing the infection, and the antibiotic(s) most likely to be effective. However, in most situations, bacterial culture and antibiotic sensitivity results are not available for at least 24 hours, so the veterinarian begins treatment with broad-spectrum antibiotics. Once the results are known, the veterinarian can then switch to the most effective, specific antibiotic(s).

Anti-inflammatory Drugs

NSAIDs are most important in the early stages of joint infection, when reducing the inflammatory response may influence the course or outcome of the disease. Once permanent changes have occurred in the joint, the anti-inflammatory actions of these drugs are of limited benefit. In the later stages of the disease, and as the condition resolves, pain relief is the primary benefit of NSAIDs.

There are a couple of points about NSAIDs that are worth considering. First, high doses of these drugs given over several days can cause gastric ulcers and kidney problems, especially in foals. Second, NSAIDs lower the body temperature of a horse or foal with a fever. Fever is an important sign in these animals, particularly if it persists despite antibiotic therapy. So, NSAIDs can remove one of the important indicators that the disease is worsening and treatment is ineffective. For these reasons, the owner or trainer should closely follow the veterinarian's recommendations regarding the choice of NSAID and the dose rate.

One approach some veterinarians take with NSAID administration in these cases is to give the drug for 3 days, and then withhold it for 2 days (while still continuing with the lavage and antibiotics). This allows the veterinarian to evaluate the joint without the drug's influence. If the pain, heat, swelling, lameness, and fever are reduced on day 5 of treatment (2 days after the NSAID was stopped), this means that conditions within the joint are improving, and the chances of a good outcome are better. However, if the horse is more lame and the joint is more painful on day 5 than it was on day 3 (when it was still receiving the NSAID), or if the fever returns, the treatment program must be re-evaluated. Once the veterinarian has examined the joint without the NSAID, the drug can then be continued as necessary.

Note: Corticosteroids severely compromise the joint's ability to resolve the infection. So, even though they are potent anti-inflammatory drugs, they should not be used to treat an infected joint.

Other Management Recommendations

A sterile bandage should be kept on the infected joint if the joint capsule is open, whether due to the initial wound or an arthrotomy. This bandage must be changed as often as necessary (in some cases at least twice per day). Care must be taken to prevent further contamination of the joint space while the bandage is removed. Thus, the bandage should not be changed in the horse's stall. Instead, the horse should be slowly walked to a clean, dust-free area where there is no draft. Wearing clean latex gloves when changing the bandage helps to reduce the chances of introducing other bacteria into the joint. It also protects the person changing the bandage from infective material that may be draining from the joint.

In adult horses the opposite, weight-bearing limb should be supported with a thick bandage and frog support *(see Chapter 7)* for as long as the horse is severely lame. Laminitis in the weight-bearing limb is a risk in all severely lame horses. So, the digital pulses should be checked at least twice per day for early signs of foot problems in the supporting limb. The horse should be confined to a well-bedded stall until the infection is resolved.

As soon as the horse is able, it should be hand-walked for 10 – 15 minutes twice per day. Alternatively, the owner or trainer can perform passive motion exercises on the limb. These procedures minimize or break down adhesions within the joint, and help limit fibrosis (fibrous thickening) of the joint capsule. They also improve blood flow to the soft tissues. In open joints, passive motion also aids drainage, which is important for removing debris from the joint.

Foals with septic arthritis may also benefit from an intravenous infusion of hyper-immune (antibody-rich) plasma, although this therapy is often too little, too late. It is very important in foals with joint ill or any other infectious condition (such as pneumonia, diarrhea, or an infected umbilicus) that the caretaker carefully examines every joint at least once per day. At the first sign of heat, swelling, or pain in any joint, the veterinarian should be called.

Rehabilitation

Once the infection is resolved, daily light exercise is very important in restoring and maintaining joint mobility. The duration and intensity of each exercise session should gradually increase as the horse's comfort and the condition of the joint allow. With foals, the mare and foal can be hand-walked or turned out into a small paddock for a short time each day. The duration of these activities can be gradually

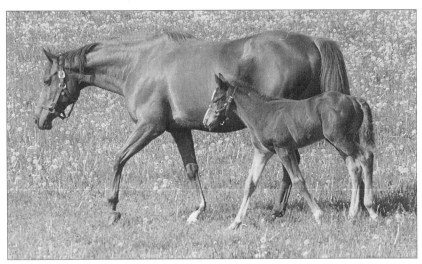

Fig. 8–26. The foal's exercise should be gradually increased until it is ready for unlimited pasture turnout.

increased until the foal is ready for unlimited pasture turnout.

NSAIDs can help make the horse more comfortable during exercise. However, it must be remembered that by this time the horse may have been receiving these drugs for 2 weeks or more. Harmful effects are more likely in this situation, so the veterinarian's instructions regarding the dose rate and interval should be closely followed.

The management recommendations given in the earlier section for horses with DJD and osteoarthritis also apply to horses recovering from septic arthritis. In many cases, the infection causes permanent joint changes, so in essence, these horses do have DJD.

Prognosis for Septic Arthritis

The prognosis for athletic usefulness is guarded in all cases. Permanent, performance-limiting changes in the joint's soft tissues and cartilage surfaces can occur within days of infection. The time frame appears to be an important factor in determining the outcome. Early recognition of the problem, and prompt and aggressive treatment give the horse or foal the best chance of satisfactory recovery. However, even with timely and diligent care, the outcome could still be a chronically lame horse.

Osteoarthritis is a fairly common result of septic arthritis. If radiographs show bony changes within or around the joint, the prognosis for athletic usefulness is poor. If radiographs reveal that the infection has spread to involve the underlying bone (osteomyelitis), the prognosis is very poor. In these cases, euthanasia is often recommended for humane reasons. Osteomyelitis following septic arthritis is more common in foals than in adult horses. Infection of the nearby physis (growth plate) can also occur in these foals; it too has a poor prognosis. The prognosis also is worse if more than one joint is infected. *(See Chapter 9 for more information on these bone problems.)*

WOUNDS AROUND JOINTS

A wound over a joint should be considered a very serious condition until the veterinarian can determine the amount of damage done, if any, to the joint structures. With some wounds it is obvious that the joint capsule has been damaged because the cartilage surface can be seen through the gaping wound. But in other cases it is not easy to be certain that the wound has damaged the joint capsule. Some wounds that damage the joint capsule leak clear, yellow joint fluid when they first occur. However, serum (the liquid portion of the blood, released after the blood has clotted) is also clear yellow, so it can be difficult to know whether the joint space has been opened based on this sign. This is a decision that is best made by the veterinarian. *(See Chapter 13 for first aid care of these wounds.)*

Whenever a wound overlying a joint appears to be deep enough to have damaged the joint capsule, it is best to assume that the joint is infected. If the joint may be safely "tapped" *(see Chapter 2)*, the veterinarian may inject sterile saline solution into the joint to see whether the wound involves the joint capsule. If the saline dribbles out through the wound, the joint capsule has been damaged, and the joint is probably infected. The veterinarian will take extreme care not to introduce infection into the joint while performing this procedure. If the nature or location of the wound means it cannot be done without risking joint infection, the veterinarian will not attempt it.

It is usually of little use to analyze the joint fluid if the wound is fresh because there may be few changes in the fluid for the first 1 – 2 days after injury. Many veterinarians assume the worst, and treat the joint as if it were already infected *(see the section on Septic Arthritis)*. Depending on the appearance and location of the wound, the veterinarian may take a more conservative approach. Conservative treatment may include bandaging the wound, giving intravenous antibiotics, confining the horse, and adopting a "wait and see" approach. The horse's tetanus status should also be reviewed *(see Chapter 5)*.

These wounds often have a better outcome than the typical case of septic arthritis, particularly if the veterinarian examined the horse within a few hours of injury, and promptly began treatment. As with septic arthritis, the length of time between infection and detection has an important influence on the final outcome.

LUXATION (DISLOCATION)

Luxation, or dislocation of a joint can occur whenever the soft tissues that support and stabilize the joint are severely stretched, torn, or lacerated. The joint capsule and the collateral ligaments are the major supporting and stabilizing tissues on the outside of the joint. These and the other support structures are discussed and illustrated at the beginning of the chapter.

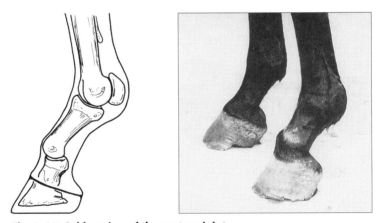

Fig. 8–27. Subluxation of the pastern joint.

The degree of joint instability and bone displacement depends on how much structural support is lost. For example, subluxation (partial luxation) of the shoulder joint in horses with sweeney does not prevent the horse from bearing weight on the leg. Sweeney is a condition that results in loss of the nerve supply to the muscles on the side of the shoulder *(see Chapter 12)*. These muscles help to stabilize the outside of the shoulder joint. When the muscles atrophy (waste) as a result of nerve damage, the shoulder joint is not as stable, and

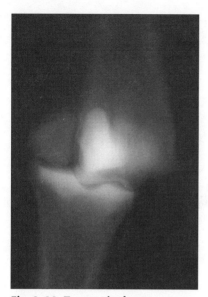

Fig. 8–28. Traumatic damage can result in severe displacement.

the head of the humerus can slip sideways a little when weight is placed on the leg. When weight is taken off the leg, the head of the humerus returns to its normal position within the joint.

In contrast, *traumatic* damage to the joint capsule and/or collateral ligaments can result in severe instability and marked displacement. In some cases, the leg hangs at an abnormal angle below the dislocated joint, and the horse cannot bear weight on the leg. This is a very serious condition that can result in severe osteoarthritis and permanent lameness, despite prompt treatment. If the joint was opened (that is, the skin and joint capsule were damaged) during the injury, infection within the joint further reduces the chance of a satisfactory outcome.

Management of Luxation

Depending on the joint involved and the severity of the displacement, the veterinarian may need to anesthetize the horse to correct the dislocation. This is more likely to be necessary with luxation of a joint in the upper leg. Tension in the muscles that surround or activate these joints can make correction very difficult, even in an anesthetized horse. Relocation is also very painful, which is another reason to anesthetize the horse.

Following correction, the veterinarian may manage traumatic luxation or subluxation of a joint in the lower leg by placing the leg in a cast or thick support bandage (with or without splints; *see Chapter 4*) for several weeks. The collateral ligaments and joint capsule eventually heal, but in many cases the joint is not stable enough to allow normal athletic function, or to prevent osteoarthritis. Some surgeons may try to reconstruct torn collateral ligaments, but the success rate with this surgery usually is fairly low.

In severe cases the joint must be stabilized surgically, using bone screws or a bone plate *(see Chapter 6).* This procedure is called arthrodesis, and it results in permanent fusion (total immobility) of the joint. Arthrodesis of a high-motion joint, such as the fetlock, is merely a salvage procedure. Its main purpose is to allow the horse to bear some weight on the leg with a minimum of discomfort. These horses cannot be used for athletic activities—some are not even comfortable enough to be turned out onto pasture. In contrast, arthrodesis of a low-motion joint (such as the pastern and lower hock joints) may actually result in a rideable horse once the joint has completely fused.

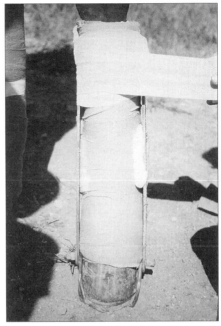

Fig. 8–29. Traumatic luxation of a fetlock treated with a thick support bandage and metal splints (attached to the shoe).

Prognosis for Luxation

In adult horses, traumatic luxation has a poor prognosis for athletic usefulness. Luxation of a joint in the upper leg may require euthanasia because the chance of surgical success is small and the potential for chronic lameness is great. Luxations in foals, small ponies, and Miniature Horses may have a better prognosis because of their smaller size. Foals also have the added advantage of a more rapid rate of healing than adult horses.

Condition	Goals of Treatment	Treatment/ Management	Prognosis for Athletic Function
Synovitis	Prevent further damage Pain relief Prevent recurrence	Rest NSAIDs, cold therapy Hand-walking Review training	Very Good
Chronic Proliferative Synovitis	Prevent further damage Pain relief (±Remove thickened tissue)	Rest NSAIDs, cold therapy ±Corticosteroids ±Surgery	Good
Degenerative Joint Disease	Slow further damage Pain relief Maintain usefulness	NSAIDs Joint medications Controlled daily exercise Review training & use	Guarded for long-term use
Osteoarthritis	Pain relief Slow further damage Maintain some function	NSAIDs Controlled daily exercise Review training & use	Guarded to Poor
Septic Arthritis	Resolve infection Prevent further damage Pain relief	Lavage Antibiotics NSAIDs Hand-walking	Guarded to Poor (Prognosis for Survival: Fair to Guarded)
Luxation	Stabilize joint	Cast or Thick bandage ±Surgery	Foals/Small ponies: Guarded Adults: Guarded to Very Poor

Fig. 8–30. Major joint problems, their treatments, and prognoses.   (± = may or may not be recommended)

LYME DISEASE

Lyme disease is a tick-transmitted disease that is caused by a microscopic organism called *Borrelia burgdorferi.* This disease can also affect people, but it cannot be directly transmitted from a horse to a person, or vice versa. The organism, which enters the horse's bloodstream when an infected tick feeds on the horse, appears to have a preference for joints, as well as the nervous system, eyes, and heart. Thus, the symptoms can involve several body systems. Affected horses may have polyarthritis, neurologic abnormalities, uveitis, or cardiac abnormalities. The arthritis may be simply a mild synovitis, or it can be so severe that the cartilage is eroded by the inflammatory products; this can result in DJD. *(Synovitis and DJD are discussed earlier in the chapter.)*

> **Terminology**
>
> **Polyarthritis:** arthritis involving several joints.
> **Neurologic:** involving the brain and/or spinal cord; *see Chapter 12.*
> **Uveitis:** inflammation of the eye.
> **Cardiac:** involving the heart.

Definite diagnosis is often difficult because the organisms can be hard to find and culture from a blood sample. Antibodies against the organism can be measured in the blood. However, as is often the case with infectious conditions (for example, Equine Protozoal Myeloencephalitis, or EPM; *see Chapter 12*), a positive antibody response simply indicates prior exposure to the organism. It does not necessarily mean the organism is still present in the body or is causing disease. Furthermore, with lyme disease there are a few related, but harmless organisms that can "cross-react," or produce a positive test result. Finding antibodies against *B. burgdorferi* in the joint fluid of an affected horse is probably a more meaningful piece of information than a positive blood test.

Although no controlled studies have been conducted, there are several antibiotics that have been successfully used to treat lyme disease in horses. Anti-inflammatory therapy, in particular, cold therapy, NSAIDs, and DMSO *(see Chapter 5),* is also important in managing this disease. 🐎

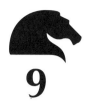

9

BONE PROBLEMS

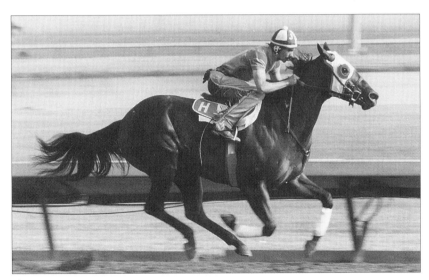

Fig. 9–1.

The bones have several important roles. Apart from enabling locomotion, they support the body and protect the internal organs. The bones also are actively involved in calcium and phosphorus storage and use.

STRUCTURE & FUNCTION

The bones in the limbs can be separated into categories, based on their size, shape, location, and function. The four basic types of bones are:

- "longbones"—long, roughly cylinder-shaped bones, including the cannon bone, radius, humerus, tibia, and femur
- "cuboidal" bones—block-shaped bones of the knee and hock
- "sesamoid" bones—bones suspended at a joint by ligaments, including the navicular bone, sesamoid bones of the fetlock, and the patella
- "irregular" bones—pedal bone, pastern bones, splint bones, accessory carpal bone, ulna, shoulder blade, larger bones of the hock, and the pelvis

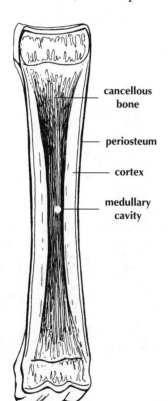

cancellous
bone

periosteum

cortex

medullary
cavity

Fig. 9–2. A typical longbone.

Problems associated with the bones of the spinal column (the vertebrae) can also cause lameness.

(The Appendix includes a diagram of the equine skeleton.)

Bones consist of:

Periosteum—meaning "around the bone." The periosteum is a thin, but very tough membrane that covers the outer surface of the bone. It consists of fibrous tissue, blood vessels, nerves, and osteoblasts (bone-forming cells).

Cortex—the outer layer of dense bone. It is the strength layer of the bone.

Cancellous bone—the lattice-like center of the bone. The fairly loose arrangement of cancellous bone absorbs concussion. It also contains most of the bone's blood vessels.

The longbones also have a relatively hollow interior, called the medullary cavity, which is more like honeycomb than a hollow space. In young horses this cavity contains bone marrow. In mature horses the bone marrow is mostly replaced with fat.

Functions

Bone is dynamic, living tissue; it only seems to be inactive because it has a very slow metabolic rate (cell activity). Although the main structure of the bone is made of solid calcium and phosphorus deposits, bone also contains blood vessels and specialized cells, called osteocytes. Like any other tissue in the body, bone is constantly active, replacing old cells with new ones, and laying down or absorbing mineral deposits. Calcium and phosphorus are required for many bodily functions, including muscle and nerve activity. So, one of bone's most important activities is the storage or release of these minerals, according to the body's requirements. Its other major activities are growth (in immature horses), and adapting to the stresses and strains of exercise.

BONE RESPONSES TO STRESS

Normal Responses

Bone is constantly responding to the forces placed on it. Regular exercise increases bone density by increasing the amount of mineral deposited in the bone. On the other hand, inactivity decreases bone density. This dynamic process is called bone remodeling, and it is part of the bone's normal response to the forces it experiences.

Exercise places large loads on the bones of the legs. The bones respond by laying down extra mineral in the areas where loading is greatest. This increases the strength, or loading capacity of the bones. The mineral is normally laid down in layers around the outside of the bones, beneath the periosteum. It can take several weeks for this process to adequately increase the bones' loading capacity in an untrained horse.

Inactivity or reduced weight bearing results in a loss of mineral (demineralization). Eventually, this process can result in a reduction in bone density, or osteoporosis. For example, several weeks of stall confinement can lead to mild osteoporosis in all of the bones. In a very lame horse, loss of mineral occurs in the

> **Terminology**
>
> The word "stress" can be used to mean normal, appropriate load on a bone, or it can mean abnormal or excessive load. To avoid confusion, the word "load" is used for normal forces on the bone, and the word "stress" is reserved for situations that overload the bone.

lame leg because the bones of that limb are not being loaded. Osteoporosis is reversed with regular exercise. However, after prolonged confinement the bones are not as strong as when the horse was in training. Therefore, the return to regular training should be very gradual.

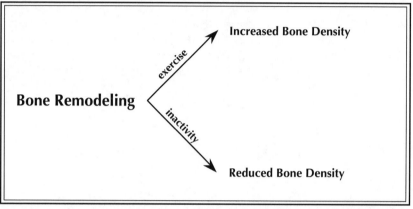

Fig. 9–3. Bone remodeling is a dynamic process: regular exercise results in an increase in bone density, whereas inactivity leads to a decrease in bone density.

Abnormal Responses

Excessive load, or stress on the bone can produce some unwanted bone responses:

- exostoses—areas of new bone production on the outside of the bone
- sclerosis—areas of increased density within the bone
- demineralization—loss of bone density
- fractures

The amount of stress which causes *excessive* load depends on the stage of bone remodeling and the bone's present loading capacity. The amount or intensity of exercise required to overload a bone at the beginning of training is less than when the horse has been in training for a couple of months.

The first three responses are discussed in the following sections. Because it is such a large topic, fractures are discussed later in the chapter.

Exostoses

Excessive tension on the periosteum or trauma to the bone surface (for example, a kick or knock) can cause inflammation of the periosteum. This results in new bone production at that location. The area of new bone formation is called an exostosis (literally, "outside the bone"). Another term is osteophyte.

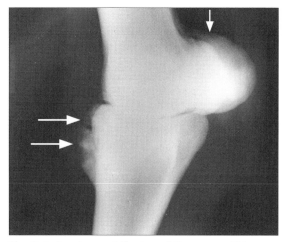

Fig. 9–4. Exostoses at the top of the sesamoid bone and at the front of the fetlock. (Note also the small chip fracture in the front of the joint.)

"Splints" are good examples of this process.

Exostoses can also develop where a tendon, ligament, or joint capsule attaches onto the bone. These exostoses are called enthesiophytes: new bone production at the site where soft tissue attaches onto bone. This process is the body's attempt to strengthen a stress point.

Exostosis around a joint is one of the bony changes that occur with osteoarthritis *(see Chapter 8)*. This is likely due to excessive tension on the joint capsule and/or uneven stresses on the edges of the bones. Ringbone is a good example of this abnormal bone response.

An exostosis at the site of a healed fracture is commonly called a callus. It is a normal response which increases the bone's strength at a point of weakness.

Terminology

For the sake of simplicity, enthesiophytes are called "exostoses" throughout the book.

Sclerosis

Sclerosis means hardening of a tissue. When discussing bones, sclerosis is an abnormal increase in bone density. On radiographs, this change is seen as areas of very white bone. The normal lattice-like pattern of the cancellous bone is replaced with dense bone.

While an increase in bone density can be a normal response to regular loading, this process can be counter-productive if it is excessive. The lattice-like structure of normal cancellous bone absorbs some of the ground impact forces during intense exercise. Increasing the density of cancellous bone reduces its shock-absorbing capacity, and the bone becomes brittle and more prone to fracture.

Demineralization

As discussed earlier, demineralization is a normal response to inactivity or a reduction in the load on a leg. However, mineral may also be absorbed from bone under some abnormal circumstances. Pressure is one of the most common causes of demineralization. For example, demineralization of the pedal bone is sometimes seen with

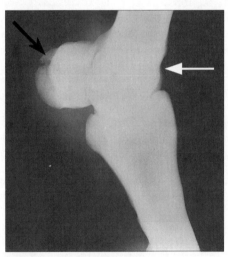

a chronic subsolar abscess or a keratoma *(both discussed in Chapter 15).* Also, demineralization of the cannon bone at the front of the fetlock is often seen with chronic proliferative synovitis. In this case, repeated overextension of the fetlock in a galloping horse compresses the synovial pad between the cannon bone and first pastern bone *(see Chapter 8).*

Bone infection (osteomyelitis; discussed later) is another major cause of demineralization. The infection and the body's response to it can actually dissolve the bone.

Fig. 9–5. Demineralization associated with chronic proliferative synovitis [white arrow]. Note also the fractured sesamoid bone [black arrow].

Dietary calcium-phosphorus imbalance (metabolic bone disease) can also result in a loss of bone mineral. This problem is discussed later in the section entitled *Nutritional Secondary Hyperparathyroidism.*

Factors That Influence Bone Quality

"Bone quality" is a combination of the thickness and density of the bone's cortex. There are several factors that can influence bone quality for better or for worse. Exercise improves bone quality, whereas disease processes, such as infection and metabolic bone disease, reduce it. Other factors that can influence bone quality and its responses to stress include:

- conditioning of the other musculoskeletal components (muscles, tendons, ligaments)
- conformation
- nutrition
- early history (mare and foal factors)

If the other musculoskeletal components are not sufficiently conditioned for training and competition, the bones may be more easily overloaded. Although the bones provide the main structural support, the soft tissues (in particular, the tendons and muscles) absorb much of the concussive forces on the limbs during exercise. Inadequate conditioning can indirectly add to the concussive load on the bones.

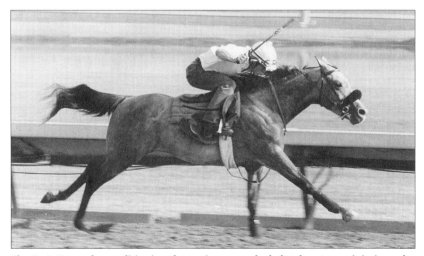

Fig. 9–6. Properly conditioning the entire musculoskeletal system minimizes abnormal stresses on the bones.

Poor conformation may add to the load by causing abnormal or uneven stresses on the bones. Because conformation is, in part, genetically determined, heredity may also play a role in determining bone quality.

An unbalanced or incomplete diet can affect all of the musculoskeletal components, including bone. The amount and ratio of calcium and phosphorus, and the amount of copper (in growing horses) are especially important with respect to bone quality.

The pregnant mare's diet and the foal's diet in the first 12 months are very important in determining growth, conformation, and bone quality *(discussed in more detail in Chapter 14)*. The other major factor that influences growth and development in young horses is exercise. Diet and exercise are the two most important factors which affect bone quality in any age group of horses. However, the relative importance of each factor changes over time. Foals and weanlings need regular exercise for their entire musculoskeletal systems to develop normally. Yet diet is more important in this age group. It is during this period of rapid growth that bone development can be affected the most. Once the young adult horse starts training, exercise is the more important factor.

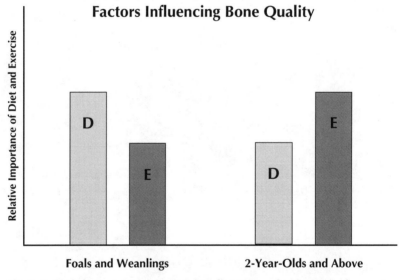

Fig. 9–7. Both factors are important, but diet (D) predominates in the growing horse, and exercise (E) predominates in the working horse.

Breeders and trainers should give serious thought to nutrition and exercise in all foals and young horses, because the consequences can affect the horse's entire working life. There are two extremes that are equally harmful to the young horse's development. The first involves the breeder or owner who pays strict attention to the foal's diet (or worse, overfeeds), yet keeps it in a stall or small paddock and does not allow it enough exercise. These "hothouse" foals often develop leg problems as they grow or once they begin training. At the other extreme is the breeder or owner who leaves a foal to fend for itself in a large acreage, with nothing but its mare and whatever pasture is present. Adjusting the amount of exercise and providing a balanced diet maximizes bone quality and reduces the risk of leg problems in each situation.

Training and Bone Quality

A basic knowledge of normal and abnormal bone responses to exercise can help trainers ensure that their horses make the necessary improvements in bone quality during training. This knowledge helps the trainer reduce the potential for bone problems, such as bucked shins and fractures.

Recent research on bone responses to exercise in young Thoroughbreds may be especially important for racehorse trainers. This information can also be used when training young or untrained mature horses for other sports which place large demands on the bones. Scientists have found that to significantly increase the thickness and density of the cortex, the bones must be loaded with fast work—that is, galloping. Moderate intensity exercise (trotting and cantering) does not result in a significant response in most horses, particularly if the young horse was active in the pasture during its growth period. Except for weanlings and yearlings that are raised in a barn and allowed little exercise, the bones of most young adult horses can cope with the load during moderate intensity exercise—that is, provided the other musculoskeletal structures have also adapted sufficiently. **Note:** It is assumed that bone quality is normal to begin with and not decreased by metabolic bone disease (discussed later), enforced inactivity, a fracture, etc.

Improving bone thickness and density takes as little as 5 or 6 strides at speed, although up to 30 strides appears to be safe in untrained young horses. Thirty strides is about 1 furlong (220 yards) at the gallop. Allowing more than about 30 strides can overload the bone and eventually cause damage, such as bucked shins or an incomplete ("stress") fracture. It takes about 10 days for bone quality to be significantly increased in response to an exercise session. Therefore, very short bouts of fast work every 7 – 10 days is the best way to produce an increase in bone quality without causing damage.

The distance of each bout of fast work can be gradually increased by 1 – 2 furlongs (or 30 – 60 strides) every 2 – 3 weeks. In between these "fast" days, the horse's fitness must be improved with the traditional "slow, distance work." This is important to ensure that the other musculoskeletal structures and the cardiovascular system also adapt well. If a racehorse must go around turns, it is important to include corners or turns in the "fast work" sessions. This ensures that the bones increase their strength and resilience in the direction of greatest load during a race.

The recommendations from this research include:

• begin galloping the horse earlier in the training program (within the first few weeks)
• limit the first few gallops to 15 – 30 strides (½ – 1 furlong)
• separate the "fast work" sessions by 7 – 10 days
• gradually increase the distance galloped over a period of several weeks

With this approach, the young horse can still be ready to race within the traditional 12 weeks of training, with far less risk of bone problems.

If the horse is large and growing rapidly during training, the trainer should take the horse along more slowly. These horses have relatively inferior bone quality because lengthwise bone growth is given a higher priority than increasing the bone's thickness and density. Therefore, it takes longer to sufficiently increase bone quality with exercise in these horses.

There is only a small difference between the workload that improves bone quality and that which overloads the bones. Longer or more frequent sessions of fast work in the first few weeks of training do not result in more or faster bone production. There is a limit to how quickly bone can increase its strength in response to exercise. Pushing the horse "too far, too soon" is likely to cause injury.

FRACTURES
Definitions

A fracture is a break or disruption in the bone. Complete fractures do not occur very often, but when they do, they are usually very serious. Fractures may be described in several ways, depending on their location, shape, and extent.

Complete or Incomplete

Complete fractures go through both sides of the bone, dividing it into two or more pieces. Incomplete fractures either do not penetrate the bone's dense outer cortex, or they involve only one side of the bone. Incomplete fractures are often called "stress" fractures. They are most common in the cannon bone and tibia. "Microfractures" are a type of incomplete fracture in which tiny cracks develop in the outer surface of the bone, just beneath the periosteum. They may or may not be large enough to see on radiographs.

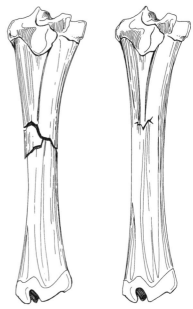

Simple or Comminuted

Simple fractures consist of a single fracture line which separates the bone into two pieces. Comminuted fractures involve multiple fracture lines which create several bone fragments.

Fig. 9–8. Left: Complete fracture. Right: Incomplete fracture.

Displaced or Non-displaced

When a fracture is displaced, the bone pieces are physically separated. With a non-displaced fracture, the bone pieces are in the cor-

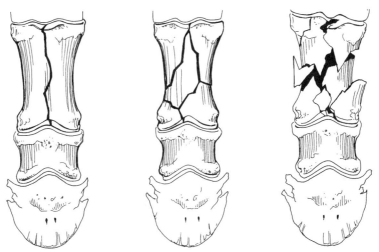

Fig. 9–9. Left: Simple fracture. Middle: Non-displaced, comminuted fracture. Right: Displaced comminuted fracture.

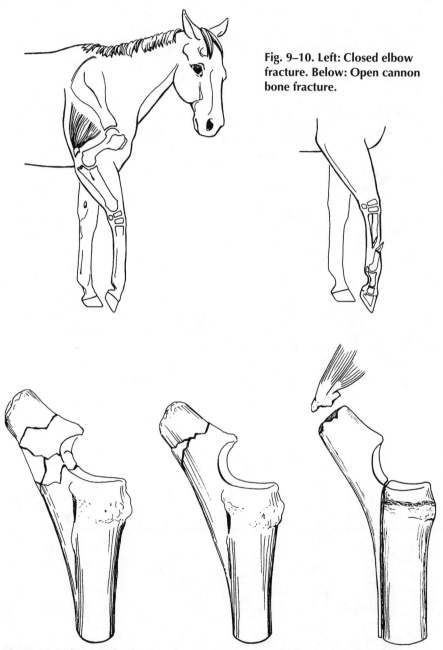

Fig. 9–10. Left: Closed elbow fracture. Below: Open cannon bone fracture.

Fig. 9–11. Left: Articular fracture in a mature horse. Middle: Non-articular fracture. Right: Physeal fracture in a foal.

rect position, but divided by a thin fracture line. Only complete fractures can be displaced. Weight-bearing, or tension from the attached muscles or tendons can displace even a simple fracture. These forces often cause the bone pieces to over-ride, or overlap.

Closed or Open

The fracture is closed if the skin over the fracture is intact. The fracture is open, or "compound" when there is a wound over the fracture or a piece of bone penetrating the skin. *(See Chapter 13 for first aid care of wounds that may involve a fracture.)*

Articular or Non-articular

Articular fractures extend into a joint, whereas non-articular fractures do not involve a joint surface.

Physeal

Physeal fractures involve or begin in a physis. These fractures are fairly common in foals and weanlings because the physes are still "open" or active. Fractures involve the physis because it consists of cartilage, so it is the weakest part of the developing bone. If the physis is badly damaged, it may "close" (stop producing bone) early. As a result, that limb may be slightly shorter than the other. If just one side of the physis closes early, an angular limb deformity may develop. Physeal fractures often are complete, displaced fractures that may or may not involve the nearby joint.

Definition
Physis: an area of specialized cartilage near the ends of the bones in young horses. It is commonly called the growth plate because it is responsible for bone growth.
(Chapter 14 contains more information on angular limb deformities, and on osteochondrosis, a defect of developing bone.)

Avulsion

An avulsion fracture is a type of complete, displaced fracture that occurs when a tendon or ligament pulls away a piece of bone from its point of attachment. For example, an avulsion fracture at the top of the sesamoid bone occurs when the suspensory ligament tears away, taking a piece of the bone with it.

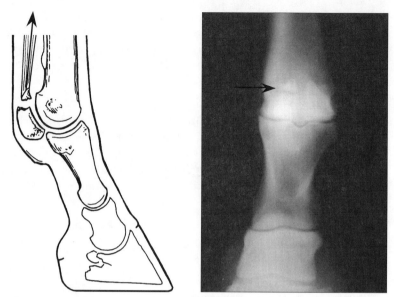

Fig. 9–12. Avulsion fracture of the sesamoid bone.

Chip, Slab, or Sagittal

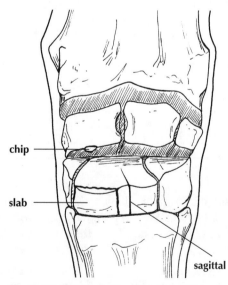

chip

slab

sagittal

Fig. 9–13. Types of carpal bone fracture.

Fractures within a joint can be described as "chip," "slab," or "sagittal" fractures. Chip fractures are generally small fragments of cartilage and bone that break off one edge of the bone. They can occur on any bone, in any joint. Slab fractures affect the cuboidal bones of the knee or hock. They usually take off the whole face of the bone, and therefore involve both the upper and lower joint surface. Sagittal fractures involve a vertical fracture line that extends into the center of the bone.

Causes of Fractures

Trauma

Fractures may be caused by direct trauma from external sources, such as a kick or a fall. Or, they may be caused by trauma from internal sources. For example, two bones impacting in the front of the joint during overextension is a common cause of chip fractures in the fetlock and knee.

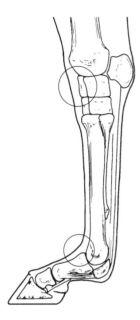

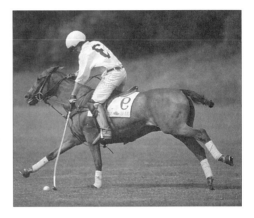

Fig. 9–14. Chip fractures are often caused by bones impacting during overextension (circled in the drawing on the left).

Excessive Loading

In many cases the bone is broken by excessive loading during exercise. The forces bones must withstand during exercise are:

- compression, or vertical loading—the primary cause of incomplete cannon bone fractures
- tension—e.g., the ligaments that attach to the sesamoid bones pull the bones in different directions
- rotational or "shearing" forces which wring (or torque) the bone—the pastern bones of polo ponies and Western performance horses experience this type of stress during sharp turns

A single bone may experience more than one type of stress. For example, the cannon bone bows backward slightly during the gallop,

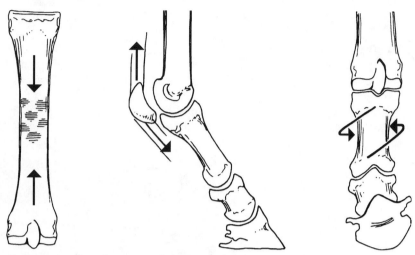

Fig. 9–15. Various forces on a bone. On the left, compression. In the middle, tension. On the right, rotation or shearing.

so it experiences compression at its front edge and tension at its back edge. In the pastern bones, all three forces (compression, tension, and rotation) can occur together during sharp turns and spins.

If any of these forces exceed the bone's loading capacity, microfractures, a "stress" fracture, or even a complete fracture may occur. Excessive loading can be a chronic event caused by repeated overloading (for example, daily rigorous exercise in an under-conditioned horse). Or it may be a single traumatic event during which the bone's loading capacity is suddenly and massively exceeded. In many cases, when a fracture occurs during

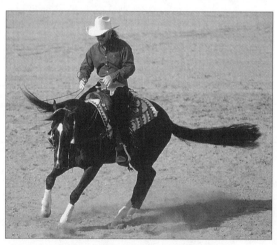

Fig. 9–16. In the pastern bones, compression, tension, and rotation can occur together.

exercise, the bone has withstood overloading for some time before finally giving way. Although the fracture may appear to be an isolated event, it is actually the result of the bone's chronically overstressed state.

The bones of young athletic horses are more prone to fracture under these extreme stresses if they are not given sufficient time to strengthen in response to the demands of exercise. This is a common scenario when young horses are worked up to peak intensity in only a few weeks.

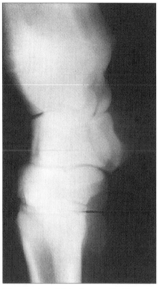

Fig. 9–17. This horse is "back at the knee."

Other Factors

Poor conformation can exaggerate these stresses. For example, rotational forces on the pasterns are greater in horses with long, sloping pasterns. As another example, horses that are "back at the knee" are more prone to knee chips than well conformed horses.

Foot conformation can also play a part, as can improper trimming and shoeing. For example, horses with the long toe–low heel foot shape are more prone to various exercise-related injuries. Using shoes with short branches or toe grabs can further increase the stresses on the lower leg in these horses. *(Foot conformation and shoeing are discussed in Chapter 7.)*

Lack of proper conditioning, and an uneven work surface (such as irregular track conditions) are other factors that can contribute to excessive stress on the bones. Osteochondrosis is another common cause of chip fractures, and possibly vertical cannon bone fractures (condylar fractures; *see Chapter 17*) in young athletic horses.

Signs of Fractures

The specific signs that indicate a fracture depend on the location, type, and extent of the fracture. As a general guide, the signs listed in the following sections are typically seen.

Complete, Displaced Longbone Fractures

• sudden, severe, nonweight-bearing lameness (grade 5 of 5); the leg may appear to dangle below the fracture site
• extensive swelling quickly develops around the fracture site (although swelling over the femur may be difficult to detect at first)
• crepitus (grinding or crunching of bone-on-bone) may be felt or heard when manipulating the leg
• extreme pain during palpation, manipulation, and movement; the horse may appear distressed if forced to move

If the fracture is open, there is a wound over the fracture site, whether or not a bone fragment protrudes through the skin.

These signs are also seen with complete, displaced fractures of the first or second pastern bone, and the shoulder blade.

Incomplete Longbone Fractures

• sudden, moderate to severe lameness (grade 3 – 4 of 5) during exercise; in some cases the lameness may only be mild to moderate (grade 2 – 3 of 5) and may not appear until the horse has cooled down
• some "stress" fractures may not cause sudden lameness, but the lameness is worsened by exercise
• slight to moderate swelling, confined to the fracture area or an associated joint (if the fracture is articular); e.g., the fetlock is swollen with an incomplete condylar fracture of the cannon bone
• pain during palpation, manipulation, and direct pressure
• positive flexion test in horses with an incomplete articular fracture

These signs may be seen with several other conditions that do not directly involve bone. For example, sudden lameness during exercise is a typical feature of exertional rhabdomyolysis ("tying up"; *see Chapter 10*). Lameness that worsens with exercise is often seen in horses with osteoarthritis. Also, slight to moderate swelling around a joint is typical of synovitis and degenerative joint disease *(see Chapter 8)*. As discussed later, incomplete fractures can be very difficult to diagnose from the signs.

Chip, Slab, and Sagittal Fractures

• the signs develop during or shortly after exercise
• chip and sagittal fractures may only cause mild to moderate lameness (grade 1 – 3 of 5) and effusion (accumulation of joint fluid); these signs are easily confused with acute synovitis

• slab fractures cause moderate to severe lameness (grade 3 – 4 of 5) and obvious joint effusion, heat, and pain during palpation and flexion

Signs of these and other types of fractures in specific locations are detailed in the relevant chapters of Section IV: Treatment of Specific Conditions.

Diagnosis of Fractures

History and Signs

Complete fractures can usually be diagnosed from the history and the signs. Most other types of fractures are usually less obvious. Physeal fractures should be suspected in any horse less than 12 months old with a sudden, severe lameness and obvious swelling around a joint.

> ## More Information
>
> The diagnostic tools mentioned in this section are discussed in Chapter 2.

Radiography

Radiography is important for identifying and classifying all types of fractures. Even if the leg is obviously fractured, radiographs are necessary to determine the extent of the fracture and the best course of action. (However, if the horse has an obviously untreatable, severe fracture, it may be inhumane to delay euthanasia simply to take radiographs.)

In some cases, special radiographic views may need to be taken. For example, slab and sagittal fractures in the knee may only be visible with a skyline view. This involves flexing the knee and directing the x-ray beam down over the front of the knee. Extra angles may be necessary when a suspected fracture is not found on the initial radiographs.

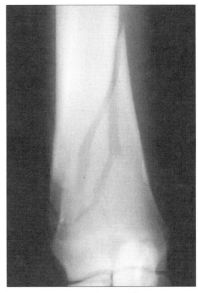

Fig. 9–18. Even obvious fractures require radiographs to determine the extent of the injury.

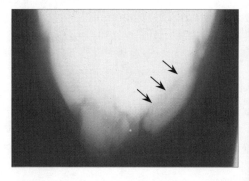 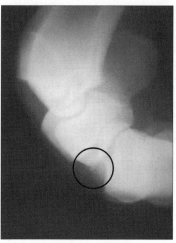

Fig. 9–19. Above, a slab fracture visible on a skyline view of the knee. On the right, this chip fracture was not visible when the knee was straight.

Non-displaced or incomplete fractures, and pedal bone fractures can be very difficult to diagnose. The history and signs often are inconclusive, and the fracture line may not be obvious on radiographs for several days after the injury. A fracture can be very difficult to see unless it is separated, even if only by a millimeter, and the exact radiographic view is taken. In non-displaced, complete fractures the fracture line often becomes obvious on radiographs a day or two after injury because the horse's weight and activity (even when restricted) displace the fracture a little.

With incomplete fractures and pedal bone fractures (which are prevented from displacing by the hoof wall) there is a loss of bone density around the fracture line as the bone remodels and begins to heal. This is sometimes the only radiographic evidence of the fracture. These cases are a diagnostic challenge, and it may first be necessary to localize the area of lameness with careful palpation, and possibly with nerve blocks. However, the veterinarian must be extremely cautious when blocking a horse that is suspected of having a fracture. Once the pain is temporarily resolved, the horse may completely fracture the bone by bearing full weight on the leg or being too active. A thick support bandage and strict stall confinement can help to prevent this devastating result in most cases. Some veterinarians do not take the risk, and will not block a horse suspected of having a fracture. Instead, they confine the horse to a stall and repeat the examination and radiographs in a few days.

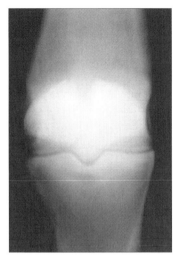 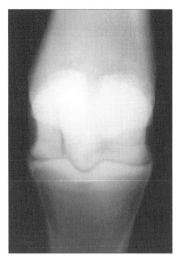

Fig. 9–20. Left: The initial radiograph. Right: A radiograph taken a few days later shows the cannon bone fracture behind the left sesamoid bone. Now that the fracture is obvious, it is easier to find on the initial radiograph.

Nuclear Scintigraphy

Nuclear scintigraphy is very useful for identifying the site of bone lesions. In many cases scintigraphy can reveal a problem days, and sometimes a week or more before the changes can be seen on radiographs. Where available, it is a valuable method of identifying incomplete fractures.

Treatment of Fractures

Horses with open fractures and complete, displaced fractures require first aid care until the veterinarian arrives. *Emergency management of these injuries is discussed in Chapter 13.*

Fracture Healing

For rapid and complete repair, the basic need of every fracture is *stability*, no matter which bone or fracture type is involved. It is very difficult for the bone to repair itself if the fracture pieces are allowed to move.

Fracture repair begins when the gap between the bone pieces is bridged with a blood clot, which then forms a fibrous union. This fibrous bridge provides a framework onto which bone cells (osteoblasts) migrate and begin depositing mineral to finally fill the defect with new bone.

As long as the fracture site is stabilized, most fractures heal within 6 – 8 weeks. This can be confirmed by repeating the radiographs and finding that the original fracture line has been replaced with bone. The fracture has essentially healed at this stage. But the new bone that bridges the fracture line requires at least another 2 months, and sometimes up to 6 months, to increase its density and strength enough to withstand vigorous exercise. So, when specific fractures are discussed in later chapters, the standard recommendation is an initial confinement period of at least 6 weeks, followed by a period of paddock or pasture rest.

It is important to note that these are only approximate times. They will vary with the circumstances and the individual horse's rate of healing. Also, fracture repair is severely compromised by loss of bone, instability, and infection.

Pain Relief

Complete fractures are very painful injuries. Stabilizing the fracture is the first and most important step in reducing the horse's pain. But in most cases NSAIDs are also necessary for pain relief in the first stage of healing. However, when a horse is facing a long convalescent period with a very painful injury, care must be taken to avoid the harmful effects of these drugs *(see Chapter 5)*.

Long-Term NSAID Use

It is very important to remember that NSAIDs can make the horse more comfortable, but they cannot completely resolve its pain, no matter how much of the drug is given. Just as aspirin or Tylenol cannot completely mask the pain of a fracture in people, no amount of "bute" can prevent fracture pain in horses. So there is nothing to be gained, and much to be lost by giving more than the recommended dose, or keeping the horse on a high dose for several days. These issues are even more important in foals because they are more sensitive to the harmful effects of NSAIDs.

Another point to consider is that pain is "nature's cast"—the body's way of ensuring that the injured area is protected. Removing the horse's pain can be harmful in some cases, particularly when it allows the horse to become more active. When NSAIDs are given but the horse is kept in training or allowed unrestricted activity, an incomplete, or "stress" fracture can become a complete fracture.

Repair Options

The owner and veterinarian must consider several factors when deciding how to treat a fracture:

- the location, type, and extent of the fracture
- the horse's age
- the horse's use, both current and potential
- the horse's value, both financial and emotional
- the chances of a successful outcome
- the owner's budget
- insurance company input

Because treatment varies with the location, type, and severity of the fracture, this section is an overview of the treatment options available. *Most of these options are discussed and illustrated in more detail in Section II: Principles of Therapy. Specific treatment recommendations are covered in later chapters.*

Confinement

No matter what method is used to stabilize the fracture, the horse must be confined to a stall or small pen to restrict its movement until the fracture has healed. In some cases, the veterinarian may also recommend that the horse stay cross-tied for the first couple of weeks. An example of a fracture which may require cross-tying is an incomplete tibial fracture *(see Chapter 21)*.

In most cases the best type of bedding for a horse with a serious fracture is deep sand or shavings. These materials are easier for the horse to move around in than straw. They provide more protection against pressure sores if the horse spends a lot of time lying down, and they help prevent or manage laminitis. Laminitis in the opposite, weight-bearing limb is a common consequence of severe lameness, no matter what the injury.

The veterinarian may recommend stall rest as the sole treatment for certain incomplete fractures, such as tibial "stress" fractures. Confinement as the primary treatment may also be advised for complete pedal bone fractures that do not involve the coffin joint, and for navicular bone fractures.

Shoeing

In most cases the type of shoeing should not be changed, other than to

> **More Information**
>
> Foot conditions are covered in Chapter 15. They include:
>
> - laminitis
> - pedal bone fractures
> - navicular fractures

restore and maintain correct hoof balance. Horses that are facing a prolonged recovery period may be left unshod, unless their hooves are prone to cracking and chipping, or they have a specific foot problem which requires shoes. Horses with pedal bone or navicular bone fractures often benefit from a bar shoe, with or without side clips or a raised rim to prevent hoof wall expansion.

In horses that cannot bear weight evenly on both limbs, a frog support (such as a Lily Pad) should be kept on the opposite, weight-bearing limb. This device can help support the pedal bone and prevent its rotation. *(Shoeing options and frog support are discussed in Chapter 7.)*

Non-surgical Options
Cast
A fiberglass cast provides good stability for some fractures of the lower leg. However, the cast does not provide much support against vertical loading forces when the horse puts weight on the leg. For this reason, a cast generally cannot provide enough stability for a complete, displaced fracture—for example, a comminuted pastern fracture *(see Figure 9–9)*. But casts are often used for extra support during post-operative recovery, after the fracture has been surgically repaired.

Support Bandage
A well-padded, firm bandage (with or without splints) may be used instead of a cast to treat some fractures, such as an incomplete condylar fracture of the cannon bone. No matter what treatment option is used on the fractured leg, a support bandage should be placed and maintained on the opposite, weight-bearing leg in horses that are very lame.

Euthanasia
While not a "therapeutic" option, euthanasia is sometimes the most humane course of action in adult horses that have comminuted longbone fractures, especially if the fracture is open. Often, there is not enough solid bone in which to anchor bone screws. Also, the pull of the attached muscles and tendons can cause the fracture to displace and the implants to loosen. Furthermore, the horse's weight often causes the implants to bend or break.

Surgical Options
Internal Fixation
Internal fixation is a surgical procedure which uses metal implants

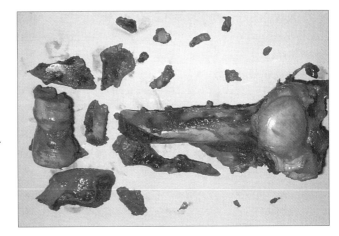

Fig. 9–21.
Sometimes a
bone breaks
into too many
pieces to be re-
paired.

(bone screws, plates, pins, and orthopedic wire) to firmly hold the
bone pieces together while the fracture heals. These implants help
counteract the distracting forces from the
attached muscles. Bone plates and long
bone pins can also take some of the vertical
load off the fracture site. Internal fixation
can speed up fracture repair. It can also
reduce the potential for arthritis to develop
with articular fractures.

Bone Grafts
Bone grafts can also speed repair by providing the fracture site with healthy osteoblasts—cells that are vital for bone
production. However, bone grafts do not
improve the stability of the fracture.

External Fixation Device
In young foals and small ponies, certain
fractures of the lower leg may be stabilized
with an external fixation device. This device
consists of horizontal bone pins inserted
through the bone above and below the fracture site. These pins are attached to two
vertical metal splints on the outside of the
leg. The splints are then fixed to a special
shoe. The device ensures that the fracture
site is stable, and the horse's weight is

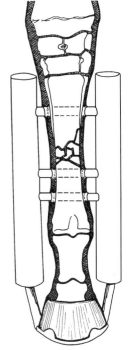

Fig. 9–22. An exter-
nal fixation device.

borne on the healthy bone above the fracture, and on the bone pins and splints. However, success is limited by the size of the horse relative to the strength of the bone pins.

Arthroscopic Surgery

Removing the bone fragment(s) with arthroscopic surgery is often the best treatment for chip fractures and OCD fragments *(see Chapter 14)*. Arthroscopy can also be used during internal fixation of an articular fracture to ensure that the fracture pieces are perfectly aligned at the joint surface. This is important in limiting the potential for degenerative joint disease to develop.

Amputation and Prosthesis

Until recently, amputation and replacement with a prosthetic limb (a "wooden leg") was very unsuccessful in horses. Problems with both the stump of the injured leg and the opposite, weight-bearing leg were very common. Humane considerations usually prevented this option from being tried in all but very valuable breeding animals. However, recent advances in prosthetic technology are meeting with better success in horses. In certain cases, horses with severe fractures of the lower limb may be candidates for limb amputation. Often, the severity of the soft tissue damage (for example, loss of blood supply to the foot) is a deciding factor.

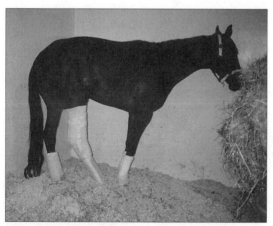
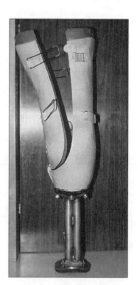

Fig. 9–23. Above: This horse's right hindleg has been amputated and fitted with a prosthesis. Right: The prosthetic limb.

The surgery is the simple part; it is fitting the metal prosthesis that requires the most attention and skill. To minimize pressure-related damage at the end of the stump, some surgeons graft frog tissue from the amputated foot onto the end of the stump. Once the frog tissue begins to grow, it creates a thick, insensitive, protective pad on the end of the stump. This minimizes pressure-related tissue damage and pain when weight is taken on the prosthetic limb. When all goes well, the horse may be able to move around freely in a paddock, once it gets used to its new limb.

Complications of Fractures

Other than metal implant failure, the complications that can develop with fractures in horses include:

- extension of the fracture
- non-union (delayed fracture healing)
- laminitis in the weight-bearing leg
- osteomyelitis (bone infection; discussed later)

Complications are more common in horses than in small animals and people. This is because of the horse's large size and the fact that it stands for most of the day. Also, it is impossible to keep a horse still, even when confined to a stall.

Extension of the fracture is most likely when the horse gets up from anesthesia, after surgical repair. To help prevent this, the surgeon usually applies a cast to the horse's leg to protect the repair site while the horse gets to its feet. In many cases, the cast is no longer necessary once the horse is steady. For fractures that do not require surgical repair, stabilizing the fracture and keeping the horse confined until it has healed usually prevents extension of the fracture. With some incomplete fractures, the veterinarian may also recommend cross-tying for the first couple of weeks.

Instability slows or prevents fracture healing—a situation called non-union. Stabilizing the fracture is the only way to prevent and manage non-union. Ensuring that the horse's diet contains enough calcium (in an ideal ratio with phosphorus; discussed later) may also improve the rate and quality of fracture healing.

Laminitis can be prevented by applying a frog support to the weight-bearing foot and bedding the horse on deep shavings or sand. Stabilizing the fracture also helps by allowing the horse to bear some weight on the fractured leg more comfortably.

Rehabilitation After Fracture Repair

Once the fracture has healed, and the horse has been rested in a paddock or pasture for the recommended time, a program of light, graded exercise should begin *(see Chapter 4)*. It is very important that the healed bone is gradually loaded with controlled exercise before the horse resumes regular training.

Graded Exercise Program

The exercise program should begin with just a few minutes of walking and jogging, either on a longe line or ridden/driven. The duration and intensity of each exercise session can then be gradually increased over several weeks.

The speed at which the exercise program progresses depends on:

- the type, location, and extent of the fracture
- the stage of training the horse was at when the fracture occurred
- the length of time the horse was confined

For example, if a mature horse that has been in training for several months develops an incomplete fracture, that horse will probably return to normal training more quickly than a younger horse that had been in work only a few weeks. The difference lies in the bone density at the time of the fracture.

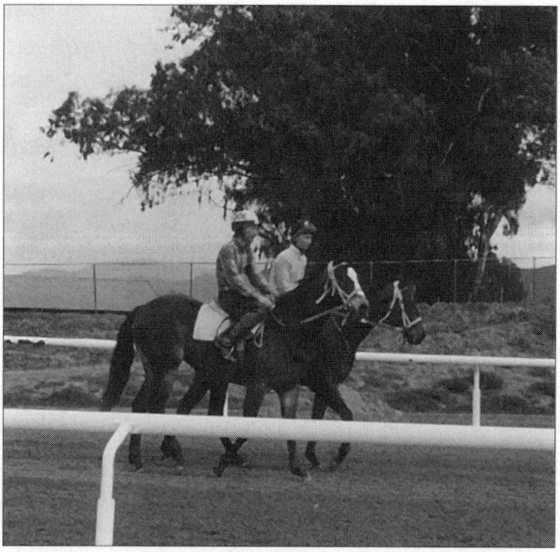

An important fact to keep in mind is that the fracture may have occurred as a result of chronic overloading of the bone. Consequently, the training program may need to be modified.

The horse's response to exercise is another factor which determines its progress. Lameness is an important sign that the fractured bone, although healed, may be overloaded. When

Fig. 9–24. A program of light, graded exercise is very important rehabilitation therapy for horses recovering from a fracture.

lameness develops, the workload (frequency, speed, and duration) should be reduced to a level the horse can tolerate, even if this means the horse is only walked. The goal of the graded exercise program is to gradually increase the load on the bone, stimulating it to strengthen. Overloading the bone by pushing the horse too quickly through this phase is counter-productive, if not harmful to the weakened bone.

Prognosis for Fractures

The prognosis for *survival* is guarded with comminuted longbone fractures in adult horses. Implant failure and bone infection are fairly common post-operative complications which often require euthanasia for humane reasons. However, surgical implants and procedures are being modified and improved all the time, and the prognosis will also likely improve.

The prognosis for *future usefulness* following other fractures depends on the location and type of fracture. There are some generalizations which can help determine the prognosis:

1. Fractures involving a "supporting" bone, such as the longbones, pastern bones, and shoulder blade, usually have a poorer prognosis than fractures of other bones.
2. Fractures involving a "non-supporting" bone, such as the splint bones, accessory carpal bone, and ulna (point of the elbow), usually heal well with proper treatment.
3. Bones under tension, such as the navicular bone, sesamoid bones, and patella, heal very slowly. Often the repair process is incomplete, and consists mostly of a fibrous union.

No matter which bone is involved, fractures that involve a joint have a guarded prognosis for continued athletic usefulness. This is because degenerative joint disease is a common result, especially if the repair procedure could not perfectly align the bone pieces at the joint surface.

The age and use of the horse may also influence the prognosis. Foals are lighter than adult horses, so there is less load on the metal implants, and less likelihood of implant failure. Also, young horses heal faster than older horses. Further, a horse that is simply

Definitions
Supporting bone: a bone that bears weight, or supports the body.
Non-supporting bone: a bone that does not bear much, if any weight.

used for pleasure riding is more likely to return to its usual activities than a racehorse or eventer.

(The prognoses for fractures in specific locations are given in Section IV: Treatment of Specific Conditions.)

OSTEOMYELITIS
Definition

Osteomyelitis is the bacterial infection, and resulting destruction, of bone. It is a potentially serious condition, and one that can be very difficult to resolve.

There are three situations in which osteomyelitis can occur:

- superficial damage to an otherwise healthy bone
- infection of a fracture site
- infection in young foals

The basic disease process is the same for all three situations, but the causes, amount of bone destruction, and prognoses are very different. Therefore, in this section, the three conditions are discussed separately.

Superficial Osteomyelitis
Causes

The periosteum, which is the bone's tough outer membrane, contains blood vessels that supply the outer few millimeters of the cortex. When a kick, a knock, or a wound crushes or tears away the periosteum, the bone surface at that location may lose its blood supply and die. This thin piece of bone becomes a *sequestrum*—an isolated fragment of dead bone. In some cases the force of the kick or knock actually breaks off a small piece of bone from the surface. This fragment usually loses its blood supply and becomes a sequestrum.

These traumatic incidents commonly result in a skin wound, which allows bacteria to invade the damaged bone. Devitalized bone and surrounding soft tissue bruising are excellent environments for bacterial growth. Even if the injury does not involve a skin wound, bacteria can invade the site through the bloodstream. The toxins produced by the bacteria, and the enzymes released by the responding white blood cells can further damage the bone. The processes the body uses to resolve the infection and rid itself of the sequestrum dissolves some of the surrounding bone; this is called *lysis*. Sequestrum formation and bone lysis are the hallmarks of osteomyelitis.

This type of injury is more common on the cannon bone, radius (in the forearm), and jaw. Infected wounds and deep abscesses can also lead to osteomyelitis of the bone surface if the bacteria spread and invade the bone nearby.

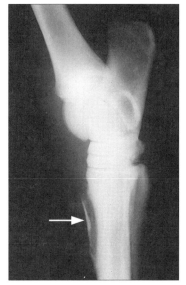

Fig. 9–25. Sequestrum formation and bone lysis are the hallmarks of osteomyelitis.

Signs

The signs of superficial osteomyelitis may be mild because the bone damage and infection are confined to a small area on the surface of the bone. Initial signs include:

- evidence of trauma; e.g. a wound (may only be small), abrasion, or bruising
- mild to moderate swelling just over the area
- pain during palpation of the affected area
- mild to moderate lameness (grade 1 – 3 of 5)

The wound may appear to heal, but it swells or breaks open and oozes pus after several days. In most cases, the horse does not develop a fever, or any other signs of generalized (systemic) infection.

Diagnosis

Osteomyelitis on the bone surface should be suspected if the history includes a traumatic incident, and the mild lameness, swelling, and pain persist or return despite treatment. A wound that oozes pus after several days should increase the suspicion of osteomyelitis in a horse with such a history.

Following is a common scenario. The wound is of little concern, so the owner or trainer treats the horse with a few days of rest, anti-inflammatory therapy, and bandaging. Some may also give the horse antibiotics, although this is not a good idea. The wound appears to heal, and the lameness disappears for a while. However, the condition cannot resolve while the sequestrum remains. The signs return a

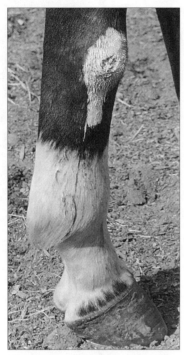

Fig. 9–26. With osteomyelitis, the signs may persist or return despite treatment.

week or so later, and the swelling, pain, and lameness are more obvious than before.

The diagnosis can be confirmed with radiography. It usually takes at least 10 days for a sequestrum to form or bone lysis to be seen on radiographs, unless the injury caused a piece of bone to be broken off the surface. Ultrasonography may also be useful in diagnosing superficial osteomyelitis. However, radiography provides a much more detailed view of the damaged bone. *(See Chapter 2 for more information on these two imaging procedures.)*

Radiographing these injuries is important for another reason—it can reveal an incomplete fracture radiating from the site of impact. If the kick or knock had enough force to break off a piece of bone, it may also have caused a more extensive but incomplete fracture. This possibility may not be obvious from the signs.

Treatment of Superficial Osteomyelitis

The bone heals faster when all dead or damaged bone is surgically removed. Liberally lavaging (flushing) the site is also important to reduce the amount of bacteria and the harmful inflammatory substances that can cause further bone destruction.

In most cases involving superficial damage to a healthy bone, surgically removing the sequestrum and surrounding diseased bone is a relatively minor procedure. Complete recovery usually takes a couple of weeks (unless a more extensive, incomplete fracture is present), and complications are uncommon. Most veterinarians prescribe broad-spectrum antibiotics to prevent infection of the surgery site in the 7 – 10 days after surgery. NSAIDs are also given for a few days to minimize post-operative swelling and pain. Tetanus toxoid should be given at the time of surgery, unless the horse was recently vaccinated. *(These medications are discussed in Chapter 5.)*

The surgery site should be kept bandaged, if possible, and the horse should be confined to a stall or small paddock until any sutures are removed (7 – 10 days after surgery). The veterinarian may recommend hand-walking the horse during this time. Once the surgery site has healed, which generally takes 1 – 2 more weeks, it is usually safe to resume regular training.

Note
Antibiotics alone are ineffective. For best results the sequestrum and other damaged bone should be removed.

Prognosis for Superficial Osteomyelitis

Osteomyelitis on the surface of an otherwise healthy bone generally has an excellent prognosis for return to full athletic function. Provided it is properly treated, this type of osteomyelitis usually resolves quickly and completely.

Osteomyelitis at a Fracture Site

Causes

Bacteria thrive in devitalized bone and damaged soft tissues, so fracture sites provide an excellent environment for bacteria. Osteomyelitis is inevitable with open fractures because bacteria from the skin surface quickly invade the damaged tissues. Although far less common, osteomyelitis can also occur after surgical repair of a closed fracture. This is more likely if the surgery was complicated and there was a lot of soft tissue trauma around the fracture site. Also, bacteria may invade the fracture from the bloodstream. The fracture itself can result in sequestra, particularly if there are small fragments that lose their blood supply.

This type of osteomyelitis in a longbone fracture can be a very severe condition. The bone destruc-

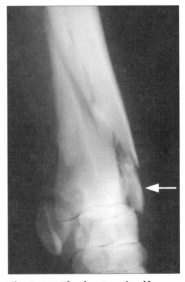

Fig. 9–27. The fracture itself can result in a sequestrum.

tion that occurs often is extensive. It seriously affects fracture healing because the bone is destroyed faster than new bone is produced. Osteomyelitis around bone screws causes them to loosen, resulting in an unstable fracture which further compromises healing. Moreover, new fractures may occur in the damaged, weakened bone.

Signs of Osteomyelitis at a Fracture Site

The signs of osteomyelitis at a fracture site depend on the location of the fracture. For example, an infected splint bone fracture causes much milder signs than an infected cannon bone fracture. The difference relates to the amount of bone affected. Also, the cannon bone is a major weight-bearing structure, whereas the splint bone is not. Conditions involving a "supporting" bone usually are more serious than those involving a "non-supporting" bone.

In general, osteomyelitis at a fracture site causes these signs:

- increased lameness (grade 3 – 5 of 5), depending on which bone is involved
- cellulitis—generalized soft tissue swelling caused by bacterial infection of the overlying soft tissues *(see Chapter 13)*
- heat and pain during palpation of the affected area
- a wound that oozes pus at the site of infection—**note:** this is not always present

A sudden increase in the degree of lameness may mean that a metal implant (bone screw, plate, or pin) has failed, or the diseased bone has re-fractured.

A wound that oozes pus may not be seen if the original skin wound or surgical incision has already healed, or if the infection did not enter through the skin. However, it is not uncommon for the infection to "break out" at a new site, or for pus to accumulate in the tissues over the infected bone, like an abscess. With this type of osteomyelitis the horse may have a fever.

Diagnosis of Osteomyelitis at a Fracture Site

The diagnosis of osteomyelitis is based, in part, on the history (such as an open fracture or surgical fracture repair), and the signs. Although the bacteria may have gained entry to the bone during the initial injury or surgery, it may be days before the signs are obvious.

This delay contributes to the poor success rate in longbones because the disease often is well advanced before it is diagnosed.

If there is a wound that is draining pus, bacterial culture and antibiotic sensitivity testing *(see Chapter 2)* can be used to identify the bacteria present. These tests are needed to determine which antibiotics will be most effective. A blood test may reveal an elevated white blood cell count, which is an indication of the body's response to the infection. Repeating the white blood cell count a few days after treatment began can help determine whether the treatment is effective. The cell count should be close to the normal range with appropriate treatment.

Radiography

In all cases radiography is very important for:

- confirming the diagnosis
- defining the extent of the bone damage
- determining whether affected bone screws need to be removed
- evaluating the stability of the fracture site
- identifying the presence and location of any sequestra or new fractures

This information is important for making decisions about treatment and for making an accurate prognosis.

Treatment of Osteomyelitis at a Fracture Site

Surgery

Treating osteomyelitis at a fracture site can be difficult, especially when it involves a "supporting" bone. The dead and diseased bone, including any small, devitalized fragments, must be surgically removed. These fragments cannot add to the stability of the fracture site, and they can become sequestra. If the fracture was surgically repaired, the infected bone screws may also need to be removed, and, if possible, the fracture site should be restabilized with new implants and/or a cast. Stability is essential for fracture repair, particularly when healing is compromised by infection.

Medications

Antibiotics are an important part of treating this type of osteomyelitis. The choice of drug(s) is based on the results of bacterial culture and antibiotic sensitivity tests. In most cases antibiotic therapy must continue for several weeks; but even then, the infection may persist or return. In some instances the veterinarian may treat the horse

Equine Lameness

with antibiotics for a few days (or longer) before surgically removing the damaged bone. This approach can reduce the amount of bacteria at the site, which helps slow further bone destruction and tip the balance in favor of bone repair.

Most of these horses are already receiving NSAIDs for the fracture pain. However, the issues discussed in the earlier section on *Fractures* regarding long-term NSAID use are very important when infection worsens the horse's pain.

More Information

Bandaging techniques are discussed in Chapter 4.

Using the frog for support is covered in Chapter 7.

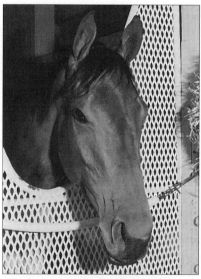

Fig. 9–28. The horse should be confined to a stall until the infection is resolved and the bone is healing well.

Other Treatment Recommendations

While the horse is very lame, the normal, weight-bearing limb should be supported with a firm bandage and frog support. The horse should be confined to a stall until the infection is resolved, and repeat radiographs show that the bone is healing well. Bones repair slowly in the best of circumstances. After osteomyelitis has destroyed part of the bone it may be months before the bone is strong enough for the risk of re-fracture to be reduced.

Rehabilitation of a horse that has recovered from osteomyelitis at a fracture site should involve a very gradual increase in the workload (as discussed earlier for fractures). Because the weakened bone is prone to re-fracture, rehabilitation should begin only after radiographs indicate the fracture(s) has healed and bone density in the surrounding area is normal.

Prognosis for Osteomyelitis at a Fracture Site

The prognosis for survival is guarded at best when osteomyelitis involves a fracture site in a "supporting" bone. If the diseased bone re-fractures, this further worsens the prognosis. In many cases the horse must be euthanized for humane reasons. Osteomyelitis in a "non-supporting" bone, although it can be difficult to resolve, usually has a much better outcome.

Osteomyelitis in Young Foals

Causes

In newborn foals, osteomyelitis is usually caused by bacteria that spread to the bone through the bloodstream. This is most common in foals that did not receive enough colostrum in the first 12 – 18 hours of life. (Colostrum is the antibody-rich milk the mare produces around the time of foaling.) Infected joints (septic arthritis; *see Chapter 8*) are more common than osteomyelitis in these foals. However, bacteria can spread from the infected joint to the epiphysis or physis and cause infection. Osteomyelitis in the epiphysis or physis of a young foal is a very serious condition. Infection of an epiphysis can cause malformation or collapse of the joint, and infection of a physis can result in arrested bone growth or angular limb deformity.

> ### Definitions
>
> **Epiphysis:** the end of the bone, between the physis and the joint surface.
> **Physis:** an area of specialized cartilage near the ends of the bones in young horses; "growth plate."
> **Angular Limb Deformity (ALD):** deviation in the angle of the limb when viewed from the front; "crooked legs."
>
> **(See Chapter 14 for more information.)**

Signs

The typical signs of osteomyelitis in young foals include:
- moderate to severe lameness (grade 3 – 4 of 5)
- heat and swelling, usually around a joint
- pain during palpation of the swollen area
- fever

It is often difficult to evaluate the degree of lameness in young foals, particularly in a well-bedded stall. It may be necessary to take the mare and foal out of the stall and watch the foal walk on a firm surface.

In addition to the fever, other common signs of generalized (systemic) infection may be present. They include sleeping more than normal, lack of interest in nursing, and lethargy (lack of energy). If

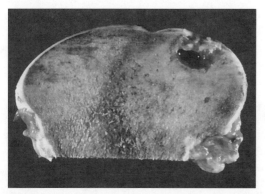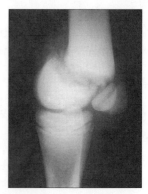

Fig. 9–29. On the left, a bone sliced lengthwise. Osteomyelitis of the epiphysis has led to collapse of part of the joint surface. On the right, osteomyelitis has so weakened the physis of this young foal that it has fractured.

the infection began in, or spread to other organs, the signs may also include abnormal breath sounds or breathing pattern, a hot, swollen umbilicus, or diarrhea.

Diagnosis of Osteomyelitis in Young Foals

The history (insufficient colostrum) and signs usually make it clear that the foal has an infectious condition. However, it is very difficult to distinguish between an infected joint and osteomyelitis based on the history and signs. In fact, many cases of osteomyelitis in young foals begin with an infected joint. It is necessary to take radiographs of the leg to diagnose osteomyelitis, and to determine the extent of bone destruction.

The veterinarian must either sample the joint fluid or take a blood sample (a blood culture) for bacterial culture and antibiotic sensitivity testing *(see Chapter 2)*. These tests identify which bacteria are causing the infection, and which antibiotics will be most effective. This information is vital for a successful outcome.

As with osteomyelitis involving a fracture site, monitoring the foal's white blood cell count can help the veterinarian determine how severe the infection is, and whether treatment is effective. In many of these foals the white blood cell count is lower than normal, especially if the infection is extensive and involves other organs. A low white blood cell count usually means that white blood cells are moving from the bloodstream into the site of infection faster than the body can replace them. As the condition improves, the white cell count should return to normal.

Treatment of Osteomyelitis in Young Foals

Osteomyelitis in a young foal can be very difficult to treat. In many cases the degree of bone damage is so great that removing the diseased bone would leave too little healthy bone remaining. In these foals antibiotic therapy or euthanasia are usually the only two realistic options. If radiographs show that there is extensive damage to the joint or physis, the foal should be euthanized.

Prognosis for Osteomyelitis in Young Foals

Osteomyelitis has a poor prognosis in young foals. It can result in malformation or collapse of the affected joint, or early closure of the physis. The prognosis is worse if more than one site is affected, and if fractures occur in the infected bone.

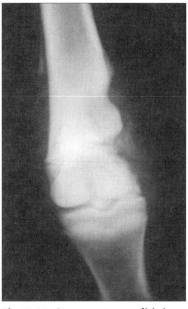

Fig. 9–30. Severe osteomyelitis in a young foal. Removing the damaged bone would not leave much healthy bone remaining.

OTHER BONE CONDITIONS

The conditions discussed in this section are relatively uncommon, and some are even rare. Nevertheless, they are included to complete the discussion on bone problems.

Nutritional Secondary Hyperparathyroidism

Definition

Nutritional secondary hyperparathyroidism (NSH) is a metabolic bone disease—a disease that affects bone metabolism (cell function).

In its more advanced stages, NSH is often called "big head" or "bran disease." It has also been called Miller's disease.

Causes of NSH

NSH is caused by a persistent increase in parathyroid hormone (PTH) production. PTH is produced by the parathyroid glands in response to a drop in the blood calcium concentration. When the blood calcium concentration drops, the body must extract calcium from the bones. PTH and vitamin D work together to increase calcium absorption from the bones and intestines, and reduce calcium excretion in the urine. At the same time, the kidneys increase the amount of phosphorus that is excreted in the urine.

> **Extra Information**
>
> The parathyroid glands are tiny glands located beside the thyroid glands in the throat.

As the name indicates, NSH develops as a result of a nutritional imbalance. There are three dietary situations that can lead to a drop in blood calcium, and hence to NSH:

- insufficient calcium intake
- excessive phosphorus intake (with either a low or normal amount of dietary calcium)
- eating plants which contain oxalates

An excess of phosphorus affects the body stores of calcium in a few ways:

1. High levels of dietary phosphorus reduce calcium absorption from the intestine. So, although the diet may contain enough calcium, the horse may not be absorbing it all.
2. Excessive intake of phosphorus results in an increase in the blood phosphate concentration. The phosphates bind to the calcium in the bloodstream, causing the blood calcium concentration to drop.
3. A high blood phosphate concentration also interferes with the conversion of inactive vitamin D to its active form. Vitamin D has an important role in calcium and bone metabolism in the body.

A typical high phosphorus, low calcium diet consists of unsupplemented grain, and grass hay of poor to average quality—a typical equine diet. Oats, for example, contain very little calcium (less than 0.1%), and the phosphorus content is at least three times that of calcium. Bran also contains very little calcium, but it is even more likely to cause NSH because its phosphorus content is about 10 times that of calcium (hence the common term, "bran disease"). Most grass hays contain about equal amounts of calcium and phosphorus, but the calcium content is still very low (around 0.3%). In comparison, alfalfa hay contains at least 1% calcium, and only about 0.2% phosphorus. *(Figure 9–33 gives the average calcium and phosphorus content and ratio of common hays and grains. For more information, read Feeding to Win II, published by Equine Research, Inc.)*

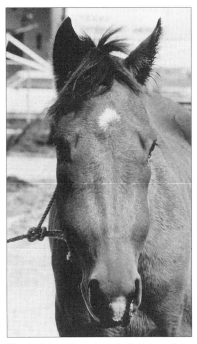

Oxalates are plant compounds that can bind to dietary calcium and prevent it from being absorbed from the intestine. So, even if the diet contains enough

Fig. 9–31. A horse with "big head," or NSH.

calcium, the horse eventually becomes calcium-deficient when grazing on plants which contain oxalates. Pasture grasses that contain oxalates include:

- setaria
- green or blue panic (*Panicum* species)
- argentine or dallis grass (*Paspalum* sp.)
- buffel grass (*Cenchrus* sp.)

(For more information on oxalate-containing plants, consult a regional agricultural agent.)

Effects

If the dietary imbalance continues for weeks or months, the persistent elevation in PTH can lead to substantial loss of calcium from the bones. This results in weaker, thinner bones, or osteoporosis. In growing horses it also slows growth and can affect bone development.

In severe, long-standing cases, the body lays down fibrous tissue beneath the periosteum in an effort to strengthen the bones. As a result, the bones may appear thickened. Tension on the periosteum and overloading of the weakened bone cause pain.

Signs of NSH

The classical form of the disease causes enlargement of the facial bones, which explains the common name "big head." This form is actually very uncommon, and represents severe, long-standing dietary imbalance. More often, affected horses have a vague, shifting, multiple-site lameness. Because bone pain affects more than one limb, the gait is stiff and stilted. Young horses may also have evidence of physitis *(see Chapter 14)* or pain when the physes are pressed with the fingers. They may also show signs of neck pain because all the bones in the body are affected, including the vertebrae.

When there is such a profound imbalance of one or two nutrients, it is common for there to be other dietary deficiencies. Thus, other signs may include poor body and/or coat condition, lethargy, and (in young horses) poor growth.

In severe cases, enforced exercise may result in joint problems, tearing (avulsion) of tendons and ligaments away from the bone surface, or fractures. These problems can cause obvious lameness.

Diagnosis of NSH

The horse's use or activity can help determine its potential for NSH. The horses most at risk of developing NSH are growing horses, hardworking mature horses, and lactating mares—horses with an increased calcium demand *(see Figure 9–34)*. However, it can occur in any horse if the dietary imbalance is profound and prolonged.

Dietary analysis is an important part of establishing that a horse is a candidate for NSH, and of correcting the condition. An experienced equine veterinarian or animal nutritionist can analyze the horse's diet and identify any imbalances.

The diagnosis can be confirmed by measuring the urinary fractional excretion (FE) of phosphorus. In horses with NSH, the FE of phosphorus is at least eight times the normal amount. If the diet appears to contain enough calcium and an appropriate ratio of calcium to phosphorus, the pasture should be inspected for oxalate-containing plants. Another way to detect poor calcium absorption is to measure the amount of calcium and phosphorus in the horse's manure. The calcium-phosphorus ratio in manure is normally less than 2:1.

Blood tests usually are not helpful in these cases because the primary aim of PTH is to maintain a normal blood calcium concentra-

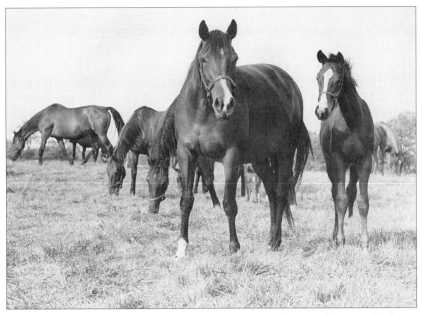

Fig. 9–32. Young, growing horses and lactating mares have an increased calcium demand, making them more at risk for NSH.

tion by absorbing calcium from the bones. In some horses the blood phosphate concentration may be slightly elevated, although it is rarely outside the normal range. Radiographs are also disappointing because osteoporosis is very difficult to confirm until it is severe. The facial swelling usually takes several weeks to develop, so it is not a reliable sign.

Treatment and Prevention of NSH

Because NSH is a condition that results from dietary imbalance, treatment and prevention must focus on correcting the diet. Some veterinarians suggest increasing the calcium intake to two to three times maintenance for a few weeks. Others simply add enough calcium to supply the horse's maintenance needs and restore an ideal calcium-phosphorus ratio. This latter approach is probably safest in growing horses because there is some

More Information

Urinary Fractional Excretion (FE): measurement of electrolytes or minerals excreted in the urine.

(An FE of phosphorus which is higher than normal occurs when the diet contains too much phosphorus or too little calcium. See Chapter 2 for more information on this test.)

evidence to suggest that too much calcium can be as harmful to bone development as too little *(see Chapter 14).*

<table>
<tr><td>

Extra Information

The least expensive form of calcium is ground limestone, or calcium carbonate. But it is not well absorbed from the intestine. The best-absorbed calcium supplements are those that are chelated— bound to particles that are well absorbed.

</td><td>

Calcium Supplements
Calcium can be provided through a variety of sources. But supplements that also contain phosphorus, such as dicalcium phosphate (DCP) and bone meal, should be avoided. Extra calcium—in excess of the horse's maintenance needs—should only be given for a few weeks. If the horse is to stay on a high-grain diet with a low quality grass hay as the only roughage source, calcium supplementation (to maintain a *balanced* diet) should continue indefinitely. Alfalfa is a very good natural source of calcium, and can be offered in place of,

</td></tr>
</table>

or in addition to grass hay.

If oxalate pastures are the cause of NSH, the horse should be removed from the pasture. Adding calcium to the diet will not help because the oxalates simply bind up the added calcium, making it unavailable to the horse. Because oxalates are not absorbed by the intestine and are eliminated in the manure, the condition is reversible once the horse is removed from the oxalate pasture.

Other Recommendations

In severe cases, affected horses should be confined to a stall or small paddock to prevent serious bone injury. NSAIDs *(see Chapter 5)* should be used with caution because reducing pain may inspire an increase in the horse's level of activity, which increases the risk of bone damage. Even if the signs resolve with a few weeks of rest and calcium supplementation, the horse should not be returned to vigorous training for a couple of months. Bone remodeling is a slow process, and it takes time for the bones to regain their former density and strength. Unlike the situation with "bucked shins"—in which bone density is normal, although inadequate for the load—exercise will not accelerate bone remodeling in horses with NSH. It is more likely to result in serious damage, until bone density is restored to normal by a balanced diet.

CALCIUM & PHOSPHORUS CONTENT

Type of Feed	Calcium g/kg (%)	Phosphorus g/kg (%)	Ca to P Ratio
HAY			
Alfalfa	11 – 14 (1.1% – 1.4%)	1.9 – 2.4 (0.2%)	5 : 1 – 7 : 1
Timothy	3.4 – 5.1 (0.3% – 0.5%)	1.3 – 2.9 (0.1% – 0.3%)	1.2 : 1 – 4 : 1
Orchard Grass	2.4 – 2.7 (0.2% – 0.3%)	2.7 – 3.4 (0.3%)	0.7 : 1 – 1 : 1
Fescue	3.7 – 4.3 (0.4%)	2.7 – 3.2 (0.3%)	1.2 : 1 – 1.6 : 1
Bermuda Grass	2.4 – 4.0 (0.2% – 0.4%)	1.7 – 2.7 (0.2% – 0.3%)	0.9 : 1 – 2.4 : 1
GRAIN			
Oats	0.5 – 1.1 (<0.1%)	3.1 – 3.8 (0.3% – 0.4%)	0.1 : 1 – 0.4 : 1
Barley	0.5 (<0.1%)	3.4 – 3.8 (0.3% – 0.4%)	0.1 : 1 – 0.4 : 1
Corn	0.5 (<0.1%)	2.7 – 3.1 (0.3%)	<0.2 : 1
Bran (wheat)	1.3 (0.1%)	11.3 – 12.7 (1.1% – 1.3%)	0.1 : 1

Fig. 9–33. The calcium and phosphorus content of common hays and grains.

CALCIUM & PHOSPHORUS REQUIREMENTS

Type of Horse	Calcium (grams/day)	Phosphorus (grams/day)	Ca to P Ratio
MAINTENANCE (ADULT)			
880 lb (400 kg) horse	16	11	1.4 : 1
1,100 lb (500 kg) horse	20	14	1.4 : 1
1,320 lb (600 kg) horse	24	17	1.4 : 1
BROODMARES (1,100 lb/500 kg)			
late pregnancy	35	27	1.3 : 1
nursing mares (foaling – 3 mos.)	56	36	1.6 : 1
nursing mares (3 mos. – weaning)	36	22	1.6 : 1
GROWTH (1,100 lb/500 kg Mature Weight)			
weanling (4 mos.)	34	19	1.8 : 1

weanling (6 mos., moderate growth)	29	16	1.8 : 1
weanling (6 mos., rapid growth)	36	20	1.8 : 1
yearling (12 – 18 mos., moderate growth)	29	16	1.8 : 1
yearling (12 – 18 mos., rapid growth)	34	19	1.8 : 1
2-year-old (not in training)	24	13	1.8 : 1
EXERCISE (1,100 lb/500 kg Mature Weight)			
2-year-old in training	34	19	1.8 : 1
mature horse, light work	25	18	1.4 : 1
mature horse, moderate work	30	21	1.4 : 1
mature horse, intense work	40	29	1.4 : 1

Fig. 9–34. The calcium and phosphorus requirements for various types of horses. For more information on feeding horses of different sizes, consult the tables in *Feeding To Win II*, published by Equine Research, Inc.

NSH becomes a herd problem when a group of young horses is fed a similar diet. In this situation, the dietary changes should be made for the whole group, even if only a few individuals are showing signs. In young horses other dietary requirements, especially energy and copper, should also be examined and corrected *(see Chapter 14).*

Prognosis for NSH

The prognosis for athletic use is fairly good, although it depends on the severity of the signs, and on the length of time the horse was fed the imbalanced diet. In most cases improvement is seen within a few weeks on the corrected diet. When facial swelling has developed, it may not resolve for months, if at all. The lameness may also take several weeks or months to resolve if there has been any bone, joint, tendon, or ligament damage.

Severe dietary imbalances in growing horses can cause permanent abnormalities of bone development, so correcting the diet is sometimes "too little, too late."

Rickets

Rickets is caused by either phosphorus or vitamin D deficiency in young animals. It is now very uncommon. Phosphorus deficiency can occur in orphan foals that are fed a milk or feed supplement that is grossly deficient in phosphorus. Vitamin D deficiency generally only occurs if the foal is totally deprived of sunlight (which is essential for the conversion of inactive vitamin D into its active form).

Insufficient phosphorus and/or vitamin D adversely affects bone development in the physes (growth plates). The cartilage in the physes cannot develop into normal, healthy bone. Also, the existing bone is weaker than normal because the body must remove phosphorus from the bone stores to supply its other phosphorus needs. The result is a foal that has enlarged physes, slow or arrested bone growth, and weak bones that tend to bow. Foals with rickets have a stiff gait, and are reluctant to move.

Treatment involves correcting the dietary calcium-phosphorus ratio by adding phosphorus. Dicalcium phosphate and bone meal are good sources of calcium and phosphorus. The foal should also be exposed to sunlight for a few hours each day. As long as the physes are not permanently affected, the foal should recover completely if treated early.

Chapter 9 – Bone Problems

As with many musculoskeletal conditions, rickets is easier to prevent than treat. Feeding mare's milk or a suitable commercial milk replacer to the orphan foal, and allowing the foal some exercise outdoors each day is all that is necessary to prevent rickets.

Hypertrophic Osteopathy

Hypertrophic osteopathy (HO) is a rare condition. It occurs in horses that have a chronic condition involving the chest cavity, such as an abscess, tumor, or even a rib fracture with adhesions (fibrous bands) to the lung. Some tumors of the ovary can also cause HO. For reasons that are not well understood, conditions involving the inside of the chest wall can cause new bone to be laid down beneath the periosteum on the bones of the lower legs, especially the pastern and cannon bones. This

> **Extra Information**
>
> Hypertrophic osteopathy is also called hypertrophic pulmonary osteoarthropathy. Another name is Marie's disease.

results in hard swellings, pain, and lameness. The swellings are identical in each leg (bilaterally symmetrical). If the new bone growth occurs near a joint capsule, joint swelling, reduced joint motion, and pain during flexion may also occur.

In some cases the bony changes and lameness are seen before the primary condition is obvious. So, it is very important that a thorough physical examination is performed on horses showing signs of HO. Once the primary problem is corrected, the extra bone may be absorbed and the lameness resolves. However, in some cases the primary condition is so advanced that successful treatment is not possible. Such cases have a very poor prognosis.

335

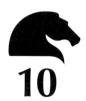

10

MUSCLE PROBLEMS

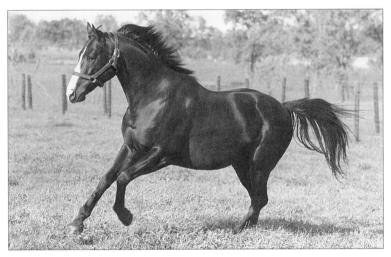

Fig. 10–1.

Muscle is the tissue that generates movement. The amount and type of muscle are what determine the horse's power, speed, and stamina. Thus, muscle problems are very important in athletic horses. This chapter covers a variety of muscle problems, focusing on the major muscles of locomotion—the muscles of the horse's limbs and back. These problems include exercise-related conditions and those caused by trauma or intramuscular injection reactions. Some other conditions, such as HPP and nutritional disorders, are also discussed.

STRUCTURE & FUNCTION

A locomotor muscle's primary purpose is to cause movement. To achieve this, the muscle is attached to the bone on each side of a joint. When the muscle contracts, one or both bones are moved in the direction of the muscle contraction.

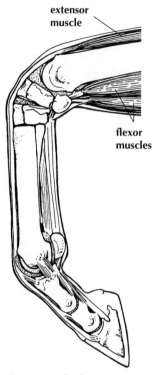

extensor muscle

flexor muscles

Basically, each joint has a pair of muscles: a flexor and an extensor. These muscles function in opposition to one another—one muscle flexes (closes) the joint and the other extends (opens) it. To function properly, the flexors must be relaxed while the extensors are contracting, and vice versa. The result of this coordinated muscle contraction is locomotion.

The entire muscle is covered with a whitish, fibrous membrane called fascia, which helps protect it from being overstretched. At each end of the muscle, tendonous tissue anchors the muscle to the bone. Some tendons are very long, and they attach to a bone that is a long way from the muscle. As a result, several joints are flexed or extended at once. The fascia and tendonous tissue are strong, but inelastic compared with muscle. These tis-

Fig. 10–2. The bones are moved in the direction of muscle contraction.

sues provide tensile strength—an ability to resist stretching and tearing.

Each muscle is made up of many small bundles of muscle cells, arranged lengthwise along the muscle. Each bundle is surrounded by a thin membrane of connective tissue. Within the bundle are many individual muscle cells, or fibers. The muscle fibers are long and narrow, and are arranged lengthwise. Each fiber contains many individual contracting units called myofibrils. Each myofibril

Extra Information

The muscle contracts when the myofilaments move past one another like a ratchet.
The muscle relaxes when the myofilaments slide back to their original position.

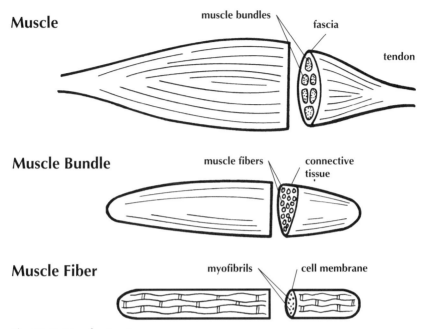

Fig. 10–3. Muscle structure.

contains hundreds of myofilaments, which are also arranged length-wise along the cell.

Muscle contraction is an active process that requires energy production within the muscle cell. But relaxation is a passive process. In addition to energy, normal muscle function requires the correct balance of electrolytes (particularly sodium and potassium) and calcium. Large shifts in the concentration of these elements, or depletion of the body stores can cause problems with muscle function, especially during exercise.

MUSCLE RESPONSES

Muscles have a limited number of responses: they can either contract or relax. If the contraction is excessive or prolonged, the muscle is in spasm. If the muscle is relaxed and unable to contract with normal strength, the result is weakness or paralysis, which is complete loss of function. Over time (usually a couple of weeks) weakness or paralysis can lead to atrophy: loss of muscle bulk and tone.

Muscle Spasms

A muscle spasm, or "cramp," is an area of intense and prolonged muscle contraction. It can occur within an otherwise normal muscle, forming a "knot," or it can involve the entire muscle. When the normally soft, pliable muscle is palpated, an area of tense, firm muscle is found. This area is painful when pressed with the fingers.

A spasm is a general response, not a specific condition. It can result from a variety of muscle "insults," including:

- overstretching (strain)
- fatigue
- metabolic conditions, especially exertional rhabdomyolysis ("tying up")
- a direct blow
- cold temperatures
- tension or anxiety
- an abnormal body position (e.g. holding up a sore foot for several hours)

Muscle spasms are painful. The connective tissues within and around the muscle (including the fascia and tendonous tissue) contain nerves that register stretching. Overstretching of these tissues and their nerve endings causes pain. When part of the muscle goes into spasm, the muscle bundles next to the contracted area are overstretched, which causes pain. To add to this, the nearby muscle bundles may themselves spasm in response to being overstretched. So, the spasm may spread to involve a larger area of the muscle, particularly if the muscle is forced to function.

A spasming muscle cannot contract properly. It also cannot relax to allow the opposing muscle to function normally. The result of this pain and restriction of movement is reluctance to exercise or perform specific maneuvers. In some cases it causes an obvious gait abnormality. The pain and loss of normal muscle function persist for as long as the muscle remains in spasm.

Treatment of Muscle Spasms

Muscle spasms respond well to deep massage, followed by light exercise. This approach appears to be the most effective method of resolving muscle spasms and preventing their return.

Although electrical muscle stimulation causes muscle contraction, the part of the muscle that is in spasm does not respond to this stimulus. Therefore, the spasm may not be relieved by this therapy.

Heat therapy is used to encourage muscle relaxation, but heat applied to the body surface may not effectively warm a thick or deep muscle. Also, the slight increase in muscle temperature does not persist for more than a few minutes.

Because muscle spasms often are due to another problem (such as overexertion in an under-conditioned horse), efforts should also be made to identify and correct the cause.

> **More Information**
>
> Massage, exercise, electrical muscle stimulation, and heat therapy are discussed in Chapter 4.

Muscle Atrophy

Muscle atrophy, or wasting, is a reduction in the size, tone, and strength of a muscle. It can be caused by a loss of muscle fibers (severe cell damage). But in most cases it is due to a reduction in the size of the existing muscle fibers—the normal number of fibers is present, but they are thinner or narrower than normal. Muscle atrophy can be mild and barely noticeable, or it can be severe, resulting in apparent loss of the entire muscle.

Atrophy is a symptom, not a disease. It may be the end result of several problems, including:

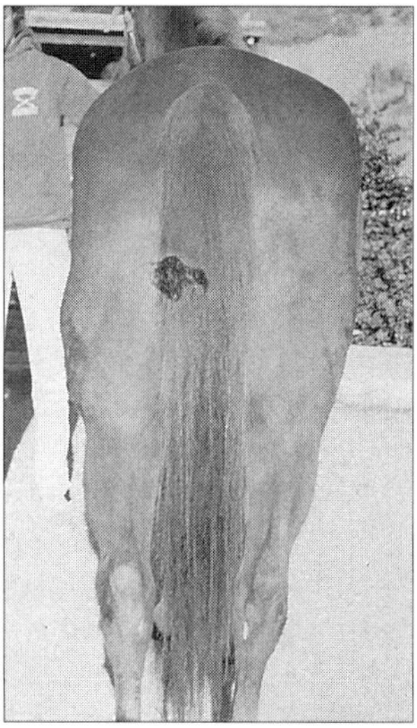

Fig. 10–4. Mild atrophy of the right rump muscles.

- loss of the muscle's nerve supply
- severe muscle damage
- damage to an associated bone or tendon
- disuse
- severe illness or malnutrition

Because atrophy is not a primary condition, treatment involves addressing the problem that led to it.

Neurogenic Atrophy

If the muscle's nerve supply is lost, the muscle cannot contract (unless artificially stimulated). As a result, the muscle wastes—a condition called neurogenic atrophy. It causes rapid, and often severe atrophy. In horses with neurogenic atrophy, the loss of muscle bulk may be minimized with electrical muscle stimulation, which replaces the nerve impulses to the muscle. However, if this therapy is not used regularly, or if it is discontinued, the atrophy will persist until the nerve supply is restored. This can take several months in some cases *(see Chapter 12).*

Severe Muscle Damage

When muscle damage is so severe that muscle fibers are completely destroyed, the muscle shrinks or wastes. Muscles have a set number of fibers. The total number of fibers is present at birth and generally cannot be increased. It can, however, be decreased if the muscle is severely damaged. When muscle fibers are lost they are replaced with fat and/or fibrous (scar) tissue, neither of which can contract. So, the result of severe muscle damage is a permanent reduction in muscle size and function.

Disuse Atrophy

Severe damage to the associated bones, joint, or tendon may lead to muscle atrophy. This is because pain or mechanical disruption prevents the muscle from functioning normally. Without regular stimulation, it wastes. Likewise, if the limb is not used regularly the muscles will atrophy. For example, disuse atrophy commonly occurs in a horse that has worn a cast for several weeks. Atrophy resulting from disuse or bone, joint, or tendon damage is reversible once the limb, and hence the muscle, can be used normally.

Severe Illness or Malnutrition

Severe illness or malnutrition causes another type of atrophy, in which all of the muscles shrink in size and strength. This happens because the body must use its own proteins—of which muscle is a prime source—for nourishment. This type of atrophy is reversible once the horse recovers from the illness or is fed properly, and begins to gain weight and exercise regularly.

Muscle Hypertrophy

Although the number of muscle fibers that are present at birth generally does not increase, the size of each fiber (and hence the entire muscle) increases with training. This normal response to regular exercise is called hypertrophy, and it results in an increase in the bulk,

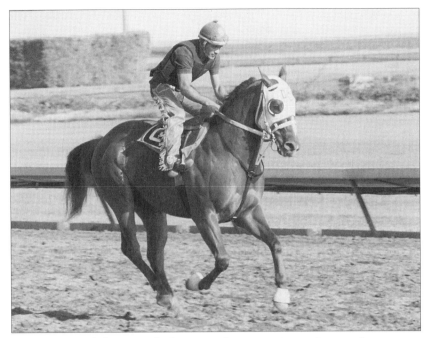

Fig. 10–5. Muscle hypertrophy is a normal response to regular exercise.

tone, strength, and stamina of the muscle. It is caused by an increase in the number of myofilaments within the muscle fiber, and an accumulation of fuel and enzymes the muscle cell needs to function efficiently. It takes a couple of weeks of regular exercise for hypertrophy to become obvious. It persists during training and for several weeks after training ends.

Myositis and Myopathy

The term "myositis" means inflammation of a muscle. It is a non-specific term that is often used (or rather, misused) as a label for muscle soreness. The soreness may have been caused by any number of insults. In many cases the pain is due to muscle spasms and overstretching (strain) of nearby muscle bundles. Inflammation may develop in the overstretched connective tissue, which causes the soreness to persist for a couple of days. But inflammation of the muscle fibers usually is not a major component. In this chapter the term myositis is reserved for conditions that involve muscle fiber damage, such as tearing, chemical irritation, and infection.

The word "myopathy" is used for conditions that adversely affect muscle function, but do not primarily involve inflammation. Examples include fibrotic myopathy, heat-related myopathy, and nutritional myopathy.

MUSCLE INJURIES
Strains and Tears

Muscle strain is a common reason why horses do not perform to their owners' or trainers' expectations. Most muscle strains are minor or low-grade, although they can be persistent or recurrent problems that are often difficult to identify and manage. A typical picture is the "muscle-sore" horse that is not exactly lame, but does not want to stride out. Its muscle enzymes are normal (discussed later in the section on *Exertional Rhabdomyolysis*), but when the muscles are palpated the horse is a little tense or sore in several places.

Muscle strain or tearing occurs when the muscle is overstretched. In most cases the strain or tear occurs in a muscle that is already contracted, particularly if it is in spasm. It is easy for the normal action of the opposing muscle (discussed earlier) to overstretch a spasming muscle. This is because the spasm shortens the muscle and prevents it from relaxing and lengthening normally. In contrast, a relaxed muscle has plenty of "give," so it can be stretched without pain or damage when its opposing muscle contracts.

There are various degrees of muscle injury, the severity depending on the extent of tissue damage:

> ## Of Interest
>
> A relaxed muscle can be overstretched by sudden, extreme contraction of its opposing muscle, or by abnormal activity, such as a fall, but this is uncommon.

Mild strain occurs when the limit of the muscle's normal "stretch" is reached, and the nerves in the connective tissue are stimulated. This causes sudden pain; if the muscle then spasms, the pain persists. Most people call this mild injury a "pulled muscle."

Moderate strain occurs when the muscle's normal "stretch" is exceeded and the connective tissue surrounding the muscle bundles and/or the fascia surrounding the entire muscle is overstretched. Small tears in the connective tissue can develop, although the muscle itself usually is undamaged.

Severe strain causes tearing, and sometimes complete rupture of the fascia or tendonous tissue that attaches the muscle onto the bone. In some cases the muscle tissue also is damaged. This injury truly is a muscle tear.

It can be difficult to tell the difference between mild and moderate muscle strain based on the degree of muscle soreness. The time it takes for the pain to resolve is usually the best indicator of the degree of muscle damage. If the pain is gone in a day or two, the strain was only mild. If, however, the pain and muscle tension persist for several days, the strain was moderately severe.

In many cases muscle strain results from overexertion during strenuous exercise, particularly if the horse is unused to the workload. In contrast, a muscle tear is generally caused by a single, massive overload, such as a fall over a jump. In general, strain occurs in the middle of the muscle, whereas tears tend to occur in the tendonous portion at either end.

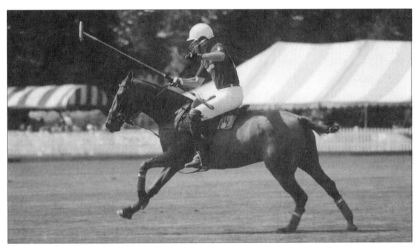

Fig. 10–6. Muscle strain may result from overexertion during strenuous exercise.

Muscle Strain

Causes

The common factors that can contribute to muscle strain include:
- insufficient conditioning, undertraining
- failure to warm up before more vigorous exercise
- sudden increase in workload, or very difficult terrain
- compensation for an orthopedic problem
- cold weather

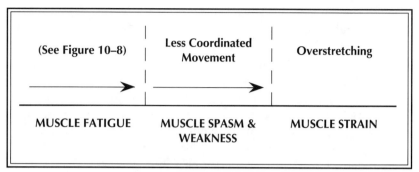

Fig. 10–7. Muscle fatigue can lead to muscle strain.

The common result with each factor is *muscle fatigue*—inability of the muscle cells to continue to contract efficiently. When there is not enough blood flow to supply the needs of the working muscles, less oxygen and fuel reach the muscle, and the cells' waste products are not efficiently removed. The net result is muscle fatigue.

Extra Information

Muscle fuels include glycogen, glucose, and fatty acids.

Muscle waste products include carbon dioxide and heat.

The outward signs of fatigue are muscle weakness and spasms. These problems cause less coordinated movement, which increases the potential for one or a whole group of muscles to be overstretched, and strained or torn if exercise continues.

Undertraining

Muscle fatigue is more likely, and occurs earlier in a horse that is improperly conditioned. Regular exercise (training) increases the concentration of enzymes and fuel within the muscle cells, and increases the number of blood vessels within the muscle. Each of these factors makes it possible for the muscle to contract more efficiently, and for longer.

Failure to Warm Up

Failing to warm up the horse before exercise can also lead to early muscle fatigue. Warming up—walking and slowly jogging the horse for at least 10 minutes—increases blood flow to the working muscles, and gently stretches them in preparation for further activity.

Sudden Increase in Workload

A sudden increase in workload means that the horse is no longer sufficiently conditioned for the activity. Exercising in muddy or icy conditions, or on steep hills also increases the horse's workload, making muscle fatigue occur sooner. It can also make the horse more likely to slip and overstretch a muscle.

Compensating for a painful condition, such as degenerative joint disease, can also cause fatigue in a specific muscle or group of muscles. These muscles must work harder than normal because of the uneven load.

Other Factors

Cold weather causes an increase in muscle tension. It also results in reduced blood flow to the superficial muscles as the body tries to conserve heat. If the horse is not warmed up before exercise, muscle tension and fatigue can lead to strain.

A traumatic incident, such as slipping or falling, may also strain a muscle by overstretching it. In fact, any sudden, "violent" movement, such as an evasive move, may strain a muscle. In these instances, fatigue is not the cause of muscle strain.

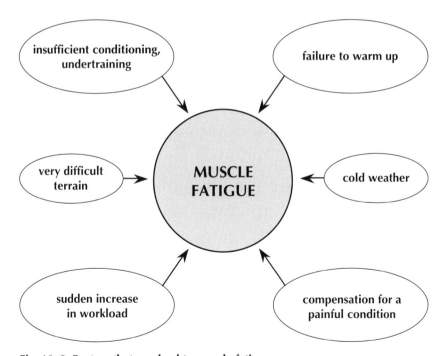

Fig. 10–8. Factors that can lead to muscle fatigue.

Each of these factors can add up. For example, muscle strain is more likely when exercising in cold, wet weather, particularly if the work surface is muddy or slippery. Also, fatigue is more likely to cause the horse to fall when jumping, which can suddenly over-stretch a muscle.

Diagnosing Muscle Strain

Diagnosing muscle strain can sometimes be difficult. Muscle spasms are easily identified with palpation as areas of pain and tension. However, the affected muscles may be deep, or on the inside of the leg (for example, on the inside of the thigh). Therefore, it is important that palpation is thorough and includes "deep" palpation, with pressure, of all the accessible muscles. It is also important to palpate the areas where the muscles attach onto bone, if possible. These sites are often a source of pain.

Most muscle strain involves the major muscles of the rump, thigh, or shoulder. The pectoral muscles that run across the front and underside of the chest can also be damaged. Pectoral muscle strain can result in resentment when the girth area is groomed or the girth is tightened, reluctance to have the forelegs pulled forward, and a shortened stride in the forelegs. In severe cases the horse minces along as if its forelegs are tied together.

When large muscle groups are strained, the signs can look like exertional rhabdomyolysis ("tying up"). The horse's history and measurement of muscle enzymes in a blood sample help the veterinarian distinguish between these two conditions.

Other causes of lameness or a stiff gait must also be ruled out. The veterinarian examines the horse for foot pain, joint swelling, and other obvious problems before deciding that muscle strain is the cause of the lameness.

Another useful sign is whether the gait improves as the horse is walked and jogged. Generally, foot, joint, and bone problems remain the same or worsen with exercise, whereas minor muscle problems often improve with light activity.

Managing Muscle Strain

Managing muscle strain is aimed at relieving the muscle spasms that may have preceded or contributed to it, and giving the muscle time to heal.

Activity

Complete rest is often counter-productive in resolving muscle strain; there must be a balance between rest and exercise. Confinement allows the spasm to persist and any small tears in the connective tissue to heal with fibrous (scar) tissue. Because fibrous tissue tends to contract a little as it matures, the result can be permanently restricted muscle function. However, it is important to remember that exercise most likely caused the muscle injury. So, while a little light exercise is good, vigorous or prolonged periods of forced exercise can be harmful to the injured muscle.

After warming up the horse with at least 10 minutes of walking, the horse should be longed or ridden/driven at the walk or jog for 15 – 20 minutes, once or twice per day. The horse should also be cooled down with at least 10 minutes of walking at the end of the exercise session.

The amount of time the horse must spend out of regular training depends on the severity of the injury. If the muscle strain was mild, the horse may only need to be kept from training for a few days. More severe muscle strain may take weeks to completely heal. When the horse is ready to resume regular training, the

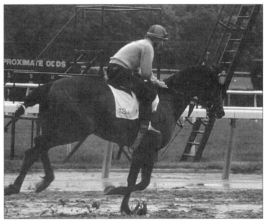

Fig. 10–9. The horse must be properly conditioned to prevent repeated muscle problems.

owner or trainer must make sure that the horse is properly conditioned to prevent repeated muscle problems.

Physical Therapies

Massage and passive motion (stretching) before exercise help relax the affected muscles and relieve muscle spasms. Other physical therapies, such as therapeutic ultrasound, magnetic field therapy, and electrical muscle stimulation, can also help to resolve the pain and promote healing with these injuries. These muscle problems are where physical therapies are of most benefit.

More Information

Physical therapies are discussed in Chapter 4.

NSAIDs and other medications are covered in Chapter 5.

NSAIDs

In some horses a low dose of an NSAID can make the horse more comfortable and willing to exercise during the healing phase. Provided a diagnosis is made, NSAIDs and controlled exercise will do no harm to a horse with muscle strain.

Muscle Tears

It takes a great deal of concentrated force to tear a muscle. In most cases the fascia or tendonous tissue tears first. This is how it should be; these tissues are meant to protect the muscle from overstretching. However, when the fascia or tendonous tissue tears, it heals with fibrous (scar) tissue. Fibrous tissue can permanently restrict muscle function. If the outer fascia of the muscle is torn, adhesions (bands of fibrous tissue) may further restrict muscle function by fixing the muscle to a neighboring muscle or to the skin.

A muscle can be partially or completely torn from the bone. When this occurs in one of the important locomotor muscles, it causes obvious lameness. There may also be a permanent gait defect once the pain and damage have resolved.

Treatment of muscle tears follows the same guidelines given for muscle strain: light exercise, physical therapy, and NSAIDs. If the muscle tear is severe or extensive, the veterinarian may recommend confining the horse for 1 – 2 weeks before gentle exercise (hand-walking and paddock turnout) begins. This approach allows the body to repair the damage and strengthen the torn tissue without the demands of activity. Muscle tears take longer to resolve than muscle strain, so the return to regular training should be gradual.

Fascial Tears

Small tears in the outer fascia of the superficial muscles can sometimes be seen or felt as a soft, non-painful swelling beneath the skin. These small swellings are most common on the side of the thigh. When the lump is palpated, the fibrous edges of the torn fascia can be felt as a ring around the protruding muscle. These minor injuries can be painful at first. But they generally do not cause persistent pain or restriction of movement once they have healed.

Lacerations

Lacerations involving muscle tissue can be awful looking injuries, although they usually heal well because muscle has such a good

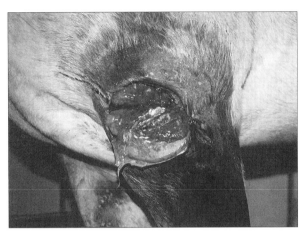

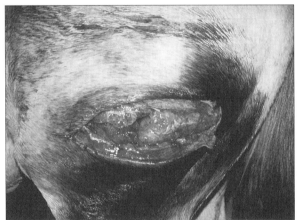

Fig. 10–10. Muscle lacerations can be awful looking injuries (top & middle), but they usually heal well (bottom).

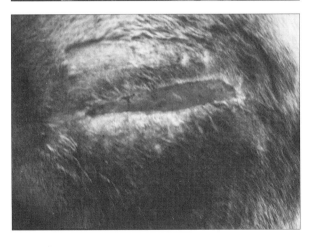

blood supply. The most common sites of muscle lacerations are the pectoral muscles (at the front of the chest), the muscles of the forearm, and the muscles at the side and the back of the thigh. In most cases the injury is caused by wire fencing, sheet metal, a fence nail, or a gate latch.

Where possible, the muscle and skin should be sutured closed within a few hours of the injury. However, even when they are sutured immediately, many of these wounds break down (the sutures fail to hold). This is due to the tension that swelling and movement place on the sutures. In many cases the veterinarian sutures whatever tissue can be closed with little or no tension, and leaves the rest of the wound open to heal by granulation *(see Chapter 13)*.

This approach may not be attractive, but suturing a wound that is under tension is usually a waste of time and effort. Nevertheless, sometimes the veterinarian sutures such a wound simply to narrow the gap between the skin edges. Even though the sutures will break down, it gives the body several days to fill the defect with granulation tissue. However, suturing a wound of this type can result in wound infection, which slows healing.

If the wound is sutured, the veterinarian may suture in a latex drainage tube (a Penrose drain). The drainage tube allows the serum that "weeps" into deep wounds to drain. If the serum cannot escape, it builds up and puts tension on the sutures. It also provides an ideal environment for bacterial growth.

The veterinarian may prescribe a course of antibiotics. If the wound is clean and is managed properly, antibiotics may not be necessary. But this is a decision for the veterinarian to make. The horse's tetanus status should be reviewed when the wound is first noticed *(see Chapter 5)*.

With skin wounds, restricting the horse's activity is necessary for rapid healing. But wounds that involve muscle often drain better and heal more quickly if the horse moves around a little. Gentle exercise improves blood flow and reduces adhesion formation in the damaged tissues. So depending on the location and extent of the wound, the veterinarian may recommend that the horse is hand-walked for 15 – 20 minutes twice per day or given an hour or two of pasture turnout.

In most cases muscle function and athletic performance are affected very little, if at all, once healing is completed. However, some restriction may result when a large piece of the muscle is lost at the time of the injury or if severe adhesions develop.

Fibrotic Myopathy

Fibrotic myopathy occurs when the normal function of a muscle is restricted by scar (fibrotic) tissue. This condition typically affects the muscles at the back of the thigh, although it could occur in any muscle. It is the end result of a muscle tear or some other type of muscle damage. The following situations could cause fibrotic myopathy:

Of Interest
The muscles at the back of the thigh are: • the semitendinosus • the semimembranosus • the biceps femoris

- sliding stops and quick turns on the haunches (e.g. Western performance and polo horses)
- a fall
- violently pulling back from a hitching rail
- sitting back suddenly on a butt chain or bar in the trailer
- intramuscular injection reactions in the thigh muscles

Adhesions (fibrous bands) within or between the muscles at the back of the thigh prevent the horse from bringing the hindleg as far forward as normal. In severe cases this results in a characteristic gait abnormality in which the hind foot is abruptly set down too soon at the walk. (This gait can be confused with mild stringhalt, which causes hyperflexion of the hock.) The fibrotic myopathy gait is an excellent example of non-painful mechanical restriction of normal

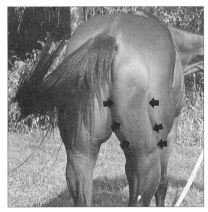

Fig. 10–11. Fibrotic myopathy typically affects the muscles at the back of the thigh.

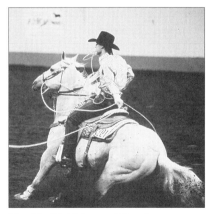

Fig. 10–12. This condition is common in horses that perform sliding stops.

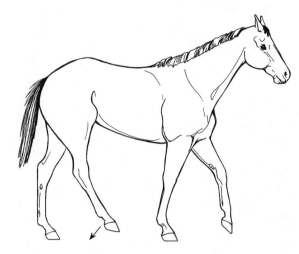

Fig. 10–13. With fibrotic myopathy the hindleg is abruptly set down too soon.

movement *(see Chapter 1).* However, not all horses with fibrosis in the thigh muscles have such an obvious gait abnormality. Many are able to trot, canter, and gallop relatively normally.

Diagnosis and Treatment of Fibrotic Myopathy

Fibrotic myopathy can usually be diagnosed by palpating the muscles at the back of the thigh. The affected muscles have an area of firm, fibrous tissue within them. In some cases this tissue is calcified, which feels hard and irregular.

Although the condition is unlikely to get worse, it is also unlikely to improve. If the gait abnormality is severe, surgery to break down the adhesions between the muscles may improve the horse's gait. However, this surgery is traumatic and it can cause more adhesions and persistence of the problem. As long as the horse's gait at the trot, canter, and gallop is unaffected, surgery probably is unnecessary in most horses.

Prevention of Fibrotic Myopathy

Owners and trainers can reduce the chances of fibrotic myopathy by warming up their horses before exercise, and regularly checking the commonly affected muscles for signs of strain. Daily exercise is necessary to prevent or limit adhesions in damaged muscles. So, even when muscle strain or tears at the back of the thigh temporarily halt training, the horse should be lightly exercised each day.

Intramuscular injections into the thigh muscles of athletic horses should be limited to small volumes (less than 10 ml) of non-irritant substances. (Consult a veterinarian for advice.)

Compartment Syndrome

The fascia surrounding the muscle is meant to protect it from injury. However, if pressure builds up within the muscle, the fascia can act like a restrictive casing around the muscle. For example, a direct blow can cause bleeding or edema within the muscle. This increases the pressure within the "compartment" formed by the muscle fascia. The pressure compresses the muscle fibers and reduces blood flow within the muscle. As a result, the muscle fibers begin to degenerate. This condition is called "compartment syndrome."

Definitions
Fascia: whitish, fibrous membrane. **Edema:** accumulation of tissue fluid

In horses, this problem is usually caused by severe muscle trauma, such as being hit by a car or tipped over in a trailer wreck, or by prolonged compression. When horses remain lying down for more than a couple of hours, blood flow to and from the muscles on the "down" side is severely reduced. Blood flow away from the muscle is affected first because veins are more easily compressed than arteries. So, blood builds up within the muscle and increases the pressure in the compartment. Situations in which the horse may remain down for too long include general anesthesia, severe illness, and certain neurologic diseases *(see Chapter 12)*.

Compartment syndrome due to general anesthesia can develop in as little as 1 – 2 hours because most anesthetic drugs lower the blood pressure, and hence blood flow to the tissues. This is most likely in large, heavily-muscled horses. It is not only the muscles on the "down" side of the body that are compressed. The muscles on the inside of the thigh in both hindlegs can be compressed by the weight of the upper hindleg.

Signs

The signs of compartment syndrome include heat, pain, and swelling of the affected muscles. Partial or complete loss of muscle function is also seen. The gait abnormality in the affected limb(s) can be severe, and in some cases, the horse cannot get up or stand. It sometimes appears as if the horse has nerve damage. In fact, nerve compression may also occur in some cases.

The pain can be so severe that the horse sweats and seems anxious—signs similar to those seen in a horse with exertional rhabdomyolysis ("tying up"). However, compartment syndrome is easily diagnosed from the history: severe muscle trauma, inability to stand, general anesthesia, etc.

Treatment of Compartment Syndrome

Treatment involves reducing pressure within the muscle by improving blood flow from the muscle. Massage and heat therapy can relieve some of the muscle swelling and pain in milder cases *(see Chapter 4)*. Gentle activity, such as slow hand-walking, can also help these horses. More serious cases may require intravenous fluids and vasodilator drugs (which cause blood vessel dilation). In some cases the veterinarian may need to surgically open the fascia to relieve the pressure on the swollen muscles. But surgery is usually reserved for extreme cases that do not respond to other measures.

Milder cases usually resolve with little or no permanent muscle damage, if treated early. Severe cases may result in loss of muscle fibers and permanently reduced muscle function.

Prevention of Compartment Syndrome

The veterinarian can help to prevent this problem in anesthetized horses by:

- providing thick padding beneath the horse
- separating the horse's hindlegs with padding
- ensuring that anesthesia is as short as possible
- using intravenous fluids and drugs to maintain the blood pressure close to normal

In horses that cannot stand due to illness or injury, providing deep bedding and rolling the horse from one side to the other every hour may help prevent serious muscle injury. Massaging the compressed muscles after the horse has been rolled over can also improve blood flow. However, nothing is as effective as getting the horse to its feet.

METABOLIC MUSCLE PROBLEMS

Metabolic muscle problems are abnormalities of muscle function (metabolism) rather than structure. The most common metabolic muscle disorder in horses, and one that has the greatest impact on performance, is exertional rhabdomyolysis. Although muscle cell damage can result from this condition, the primary problem is abnormal cell function, not physical injury.

Exertional Rhabdomyolysis ("Tying up")

Definition

There are several names that have been used for the syndrome of exercise-related muscle damage that is now called exertional rhabdomyolysis (ER). One of the oldest names is "Monday Morning Disease." This term dates back to the days when horses were used for transport and farm work. Affected horses became stiff and reluctant to move when they were put to work on Monday morning, after spending Sunday in the barn on full feed. "Black water" is another old term that takes its name from the dark urine many of these horses pass. "Azoturia" is a more modern (although now outdated) term that describes the excess of nitrogen-containing compounds, such as urea, in the urine of affected horses.

"Myositis" is another common term for this condition. However, it is a very general term, and it implies that the primary disease process is inflammation, which is not the case. Probably the most appropriate common term is "tying up." It graphically describes the short, stiff stride and tight muscles seen in these horses.

However, none of those names adequately define the syndrome. The term, exertional rhabdomyolysis, is now used because it defines the condition as one of skeletal muscle (rhabdomyo-) cell breakdown (lysis) due to exertion, or exercise.

Causes

No single cause has been identified to explain the development of ER in horses. The one common factor is exercise—the condition is seen during or immediately after exercise. However, exercise alone does not cause ER. Several other factors are known or suspected to contribute to the condition, although none are consistently found in each case. In all likelihood, ER is caused by a combination of factors, so it is actually a syndrome—a collection of symptoms with a variety of possible causes.

The known or suspected contributing factors that have been identified include:

- overfeeding carbohydrates—grain and grain products
- insufficient conditioning—lack of fitness

- exercise after a period of rest, while still on a high-grain diet
- dietary electrolyte and mineral imbalances—especially potassium
- vitamin E and/or selenium deficiency
- hormonal imbalances—reproductive hormones in "high-strung" fillies and mares; thyroid hormones in other horses
- weather conditions—especially cold, wet, or windy days
- heredity

These factors can add up; the more factors that are present, the more likely that ER will occur. For example, a nervous, excitable filly may develop ER if the weather conditions prevent the trainer from exercising her for a day or two, and she stays in the barn on full feed. An overfed, lightly worked show horse is also more prone to developing ER if its workload is suddenly increased. These two examples highlight an important point: *ER is commonly the result of an imbalance between diet and exercise,* in particular, carbohydrate excess in relation to the workload. In some horses it takes very little exercise to bring on an attack. Usually ER is a persistent or recurring problem in these horses.

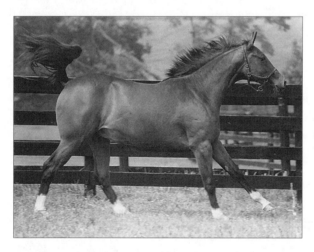

Fig. 10–14. A nervous, excitable filly may be more prone to developing ER.

Basic Process

No matter what the cause, the result is the same: dysfunction and possible breakdown of muscle cells in the working muscles of the rump, thigh, back, or shoulders. The problem is thought to begin with insufficient blood flow to the working muscles, for reasons that are still not well understood. When blood flow is inadequate, the muscle cells must function anaerobically, which results in the rapid buildup of heat, acidity, and waste products within the cells. This alters cell function by preventing the enzymes from working and the myofilaments from contracting efficiently. If the muscle is forced to continue functioning, the cell membranes may be damaged, allowing muscle enzymes and pigment (myoglobin) to leak out into the bloodstream.

One explanation for the role of dietary carbohydrate excess involves a buildup of glycogen within the muscle cells. Glycogen is a glucose-based fuel that muscles use during activity. The glycogen

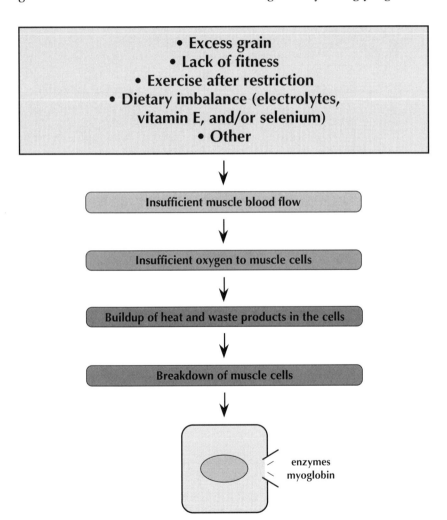

Fig. 10–15. The basic process of exertional rhabdomyolysis.

Definitions
Aerobic: using or requiring oxygen
Anaerobic: without, or lacking oxygen

stores are depleted during exercise and replenished during rest. Presumably, a horse that is fed a high-grain diet, but is exercised little can accumulate more muscle glycogen than it can efficiently use when exercise begins. So, although the muscle blood flow may be adequate under normal circumstances, it is not enough to rapidly metabolize (use) the large glycogen store. As a result, some glycogen is metabolized aerobically and the rest is metabolized anaerobically. Heat and waste products rapidly build up, and ER develops.

The concentration of enzymes needed for energy production in the muscle cells, and the number of capillaries in the muscle increase with training. These improvements take several weeks. This may help explain why ER is more often seen at the start of training, and in horses that are only lightly or occasionally exercised.

Note: ER is *not* caused by lactic acid buildup. Although lactate (lactic acid minus its hydrogen ions) does build up in a cell that must function anaerobically, lactate is a fuel—not a waste product. The muscle cells can use lactate as an energy source once the blood supply, and therefore the oxygen supply to the cells is adequate. The acidity of the lactic acid molecule is one of the factors that inhibits normal enzyme function and contractility within the muscle cell. But lactate does not damage the cell. It is the inadequate blood supply and the altered cell function that damage the cell (and cause lactate to build up). In normal horses, lactate builds up in the muscle cells and bloodstream during strenuous exercise, without causing muscle damage. It is metabolized within an hour of exercise, so sore muscles should not be blamed on "lactic acid buildup."

Lack of blood flow to any tissue causes pain, as does the inflammation that results from cell damage and the release of enzymes and other cell contents *(see Chapter 5)*. Insufficient blood flow to a muscle also causes painful muscle spasms, which further prevent normal muscle function.

Signs of ER

The signs of ER reflect pain and abnormal muscle function. They are usually seen shortly after the start of exercise. But in mild cases they may not be obvious until the horse has cooled down afterward. Most horses with ER exhibit the following signs:

- exercise intolerance; in many cases, the horse is reluctant to move at all
- stiffness or a short, stilted gait when forced to move
- muscle spasm (cramps)—the affected muscles are hard and painful when palpated

In general, the faster the signs develop, the more severe the episode.

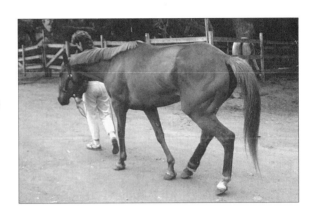

Fig. 10–16. ER often causes painful muscle cramps and a short, stilted gait.

Some or all of the following signs may be seen in a severe case of ER:

- sweating, elevated heart rate and respiratory rate due to pain
- distressed or anxious expression
- standing hunched and tense, and/or shifting weight from side to side
- passing red-brown colored urine
- dehydration or shock (circulatory collapse)
- going down and being unable to rise unassisted

Note: When any of these signs are seen, the horse should not be moved. When the signs develop some distance from the barn (such as on a trail ride), it is best to trailer the horse rather than walk it home. Exercise can cause further muscle degeneration.

Diagnosis of ER

The diagnosis is usually based on a history of recent exercise, and on the signs. Some of these signs can be confused with laminitis, colic, tetanus, pleu-

---

More Information

Laminitis: "founder"; *see Chapter 15.*
Tetanus: *see Chapter 12.*
Pleuritis: inflammation of the chest cavity, usually caused by infection; *see Chapter 1.*
Hypocalcemia: low blood calcium; *discussed later.*

ritis, or hypocalcemia. A thorough physical examination will rule out these conditions.

Measuring Muscle Enzymes

The veterinarian can confirm the diagnosis and determine the amount of muscle damage by measuring the blood concentration of muscle enzymes. These enzymes are CPK (creatine phosphokinase) and AST (aspartate aminotransferase). They are normally found in high concentrations in muscle cells. So, if there has been widespread or severe muscle damage, the enzyme concentrations in the bloodstream, which are normally quite low, rise.

In most cases the increase in enzyme concentration relates to the severity of muscle damage. In horses showing mild to moderate signs of ER, a modest increase is typically seen. In severe cases the AST may increase 10-fold, and elevations in the CPK can reach up to 250-fold.

The blood concentration of CPK usually peaks within about 6 hours of muscle damage, and returns to normal within the next 2 – 3 days. In contrast, AST takes at least 24 hours to peak, and does not return to normal for 7 – 14 days, sometimes longer. So if a blood sample is taken within a few hours of a bout of ER, the CPK may be greatly elevated, yet the AST may be normal or only slightly elevated. A blood sample taken a few days later would show the opposite: CPK near the normal range, and an elevated AST. The persistent increase

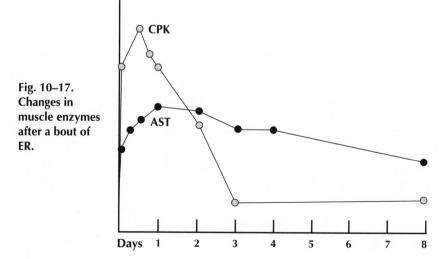

Fig. 10–17. Changes in muscle enzymes after a bout of ER.

in AST is not due to continued or repeated muscle damage. It is because this enzyme is slowly broken down and eliminated by the body.

The veterinarian must be careful to interpret the blood test results in light of the horse's signs and history. CPK is almost exclusively found in muscle cells. But AST is also found in other tissues, such as the liver, so an elevation in AST can occur with liver disease. When both the CPK and AST are elevated, muscle damage likely has occurred. However, ER is not the only muscle condition that causes a rise in these enzymes. Furthermore, regular vigorous exercise can result in a slight elevation of CPK, despite the fact that the horse may not have ER. It is common for normal horses in hard training to have CPK levels about twice that of inactive horses.

Investigating the Cause

An attempt should also be made to identify the contributing factors, especially in horses that suffer repeated attacks of ER. The horse's history—particularly its diet and exercise program—must be examined for recent changes, no matter how minor. ER often results from an upset in the diet and exercise schedule.

The veterinarian may also use some of the following tests to develop a long-term management plan:

• measuring the urinary fractional excretion (FE; *see Chapter 2*) of sodium, potassium, and phosphorus to determine the role of electrolyte and mineral imbalances
• measuring the blood vitamin E and selenium concentrations, and analyzing the horse's diet for deficiencies
• performing a reproductive examination on fillies and mares to check for ovarian problems
• testing thyroid function; this involves measuring the blood levels of the thyroid hormones, T3 and T4, before and after injection with Thyroid Stimulating Hormone (TSH)
• performing a muscle biopsy (seldom useful)

Treatment of ER
Mild to Moderate Cases

Mild to moderate cases are usually treated with rest from active training and a few days of NSAIDs. Also, grain and grain products, such as pellets, should be withheld. Heat therapy and gentle massage may relieve the muscle spasms and improve blood flow to the affected muscles. Slow hand-walking can also improve muscle blood flow. However, if the horse is reluctant or unwilling to walk, it should

Equine Lameness

not be forced. Turning the horse out into a grassy paddock or pasture encourages it to move around. In most mild to moderate cases the horse should be moving normally within 12 – 36 hours.

Severe Cases

Severe cases may also need oral or intravenous fluids, vasodilators, and other drugs. Fluids are very important if the horse is passing discolored urine because myoglobin can damage the kidneys, particularly if the horse is dehydrated and receiving NSAIDs. Fluid administration increases urine production, which helps to "flush out" the myoglobin from the kidneys. It also reduces the risk of NSAID-associated kidney damage *(see Chapter 5)*. It is usually necessary for the veterinarian to continue fluid therapy until the horse's urine is clear. This can take from a few hours to a couple of days.

> **Definitions**
>
> **Vasodilators:** drugs that cause the blood vessels to dilate.
> **Myoglobin:** muscle pigment.
> **Circulatory collapse:** shock.

Acepromazine ("ace") is a vasodilator that can improve muscle blood flow. However, it should only be given or prescribed by the veterinarian. Ace lowers the blood pressure, which can cause circulatory collapse in a severely dehydrated horse. Some veterinarians give the human drug dantrolene (Dantrium®) to relieve muscle spasms and prevent further muscle degeneration in horses with severe signs. Other muscle relaxants are also occasionally used.

Oral or injectable vitamin E may be of some value because it is an anti-oxidant, which may help prevent further cell injury in the affected muscles. However, vitamin E products that also contain selenium should not be used unless blood tests or dietary analysis confirm that the horse is low in selenium.

Although affected *muscle cells* may have high levels of lactic acid, these horses generally do not have greater than normal amounts of lactic acid in their *bloodstreams*. Therefore, giving the horse bicarbonate to counteract the effects of lactic acid does no good, and may actually worsen the problem.

Horses showing severe signs of ER should not be moved, except to get them to the closest stall. They should not be walked until they are comfortable enough to do so willingly. In some cases this may take several days. But as soon as the horse is able, hand-walking two or three times per day, or a few hours of paddock/pasture turnout each day should begin.

Return to Training

Once the signs have resolved and NSAIDs have been stopped, the horse should be lightly exercised (walked and jogged) for 10 – 15 minutes at least once per day. The duration and intensity of exercise can then be gradually increased, using the horse's comfort and willingness as a guide, until it can tolerate its normal work schedule. NSAIDs can mask the warning signs of another bout of ER, so they should not be used once regular exercise begins. If NSAIDs are necessary for the horse's comfort, it is not ready for more vigorous exercise.

The horse should not be returned to its regular training schedule until a repeat blood test shows that the CPK concentration is normal and the AST is returning to normal. This may take a couple of weeks in severe cases.

After recovery from a moderate to severe bout of ER, the return to vigorous exercise should be made gradually, over a period of 4 – 6 weeks. Returning the horse to regular training too quickly often causes a relapse. When this happens, the second episode is usually much more severe than the first, which means the horse is out of training for much longer (and may actually develop permanent muscle damage). It is not worth returning the horse to regular training too quickly.

Grain can be gradually reintroduced into the horse's diet once regular exercise resumes. However, it must be remembered that too much grain most likely contributed to the development of ER.

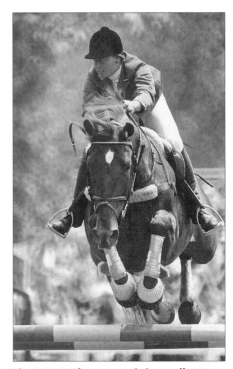

Prognosis for ER

The prognosis for return to the previous level of performance is excellent when ER is a mild and isolated event. However, after even one bout of ER the horse is at risk of repeat attacks, especially if the contributing factors are

Fig. 10–18. The prognosis is excellent when ER is a mild and isolated event.

not identified and controlled. But if the trainer follows the recommendations for preventing ER, both the chance of recurrence and the severity of the attacks can be reduced.

Horses recovering from a severe bout of ER, in which muscle degeneration was significant, may have some fibrosis (scarring) and loss of muscle function. This could permanently affect their exercise capacity. The prognosis for return to full athletic function at the previous level of performance is guarded in these horses.

Prevention of ER

Following are some management recommendations that can prevent ER in susceptible horses, and reduce its incidence in horse that suffer repeat episodes.

Diet

The horse should be fed a well-balanced diet that does not exceed its energy requirements. In many cases reducing the amount of carbohydrate in the ration, and increasing the amount of good quality hay or pasture is all that is necessary. In other cases, grain must be substantially decreased or eliminated all together. Adding fat, such as vegetable oil, to the diet can help meet the horse's energy needs. (For more information on feeding horses, read *Feeding to Win II*, by Equine Research, Inc.)

If, on any given day, the horse cannot be exercised, grain should be reduced or withheld until regular exercise resumes. Circumstances that might prevent the horse from being exercised include bad weather, illness, and injury.

Exercise and Housing

It is very important that the horse is suitably conditioned for the activity it must perform. Several weeks of "slow, distance work" is a good way to ensure that the horse's muscle function and cardiovascular fitness improve before more intense exercise is introduced.

Before the start of each exercise session the horse should be warmed up with at least 10 minutes of light work (walking and jogging) before more vigorous exercise begins. At the end of the training session the horse should be cooled down in the same way: at least 10 minutes of light exercise.

Breaks in the training schedule should be avoided. No matter what, the horse should have some exercise *every day* while in training. Some horses that suffer repeat episodes have problems unless they are exercised twice per day, every day. Minimizing stress and excitement is also important in these horses.

If training is suspended, the horse should be turned out onto pasture and longed or ridden/driven each day. Where possible, the horse should even be kept on pasture while it is in training. This is good for two reasons: the horse receives more roughage in its diet, and it can exercise freely throughout the day.

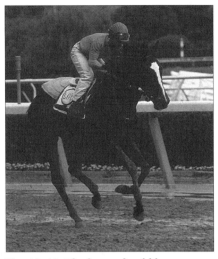

Fig. 10–19. The horse should be exercised every day.

Supplements and Drugs

Correcting the electrolyte and mineral balance of the horse's diet is an important part of managing many cases of recurrent ER. Potassium is vital for normal muscle function, and it also acts as a vasodilator. So, adding potassium to the diet of all horses with recurrent ER may be worthwhile. Adding salt (sodium chloride) also helps in some cases.

Horses that are deficient in vitamin E or selenium should be supplemented with a suitable feed additive. Even though most equine diets supply enough vitamin E for the horse's maintenance requirements, horses in hard training may need more than inactive horses or those in light work. Adding vitamin E to the diet can help horses with recurrent ER. Vitamin E may safely be given in greater than recommended amounts. However, selenium should only be supplemented if a blood test confirms a deficiency. *It is not safe to exceed the recommended amount of selenium.*

Caution
Vitamin E-selenium solutions occasionally cause a serious, potentially fatal reaction when injected intramuscularly.

Nervous fillies and mares may benefit from oral or injectable progesterone. Some veterinarians also prescribe small doses of tranquilizer (such as ace) for these horses. Ace has the added benefit of causing blood vessel dilation, which may be why it helps prevent ER in some horses. Herbal or nutritional calming products, such as thiamine, valerian root, and tryptophan, do not produce this effect.

Supplementation with thyroid hormones may help horses with low thyroid activity. However, this should not be done without a definite diagnosis of hypothyroidism (low thyroid hormone production).

Other drugs and nutritional supplements that have been used with some success include phenytoin (the human anti-convulsant drug, Dilantin®), dantrolene, and dimethyl glycine (DMG). Adding bicarbonate to the horse's ration does not prevent ER. NSAIDs are also of little use in preventing ER, and they may be counter-productive if they mask the early signs of muscle pain.

All of the drugs mentioned in this section should be withheld for at least 4 days before competition. More accurate withdrawal times are not available because clearance or excretion rates are not well documented and are highly variable.

Polysaccharide Storage Myopathy

Definition and Causes

Polysaccharides are complex carbohydrate molecules composed of many simple sugars; glycogen is an example. These substances are used by muscle cells as fuel. Polysaccharide storage myopathy is a disorder in which there is an abnormal accumulation of glycogen and other polysaccharides in the muscle cells. For some reason, the muscle cannot use much of this fuel, so signs similar to exertional rhabdomyolysis (ER) develop with exercise.

It is mostly seen in draft horses, especially Belgians and Percherons, but it is sometimes seen in draft/Lighthorse crosses, such as Shire-Thoroughbred crosses. Occasional cases have also been reported in Quarter Horses and their crosses. The cause is not known, but it may be an enzyme deficiency in the working muscles. There could be a hereditary link because it is seen more often in certain families.

Signs

The signs are quite variable. The most common signs include:
• poor performance
• lethargy or weakness
• mild muscle atrophy
• stiff gait

Some horses have a hindlimb gait abnormality that looks like shivers *(see Chapter 12)*. Others may also show colic-like discomfort, which is probably due to muscle cramps. In a few cases the signs are so severe that the horse is found lying down and unable to get up;

some of these horses die or must be euthanized.

In the Lighthorse crosses and Quarter Horses, the signs are typical of those seen with ER. In fact, the storage myopathy may be the cause of ER in these horses.

Diagnosis

The diagnosis may be suspected from the history, in particular, the horse's breed, and the signs. Measurement of muscle enzyme levels in a blood sample is not very useful, although it does help distinguish between this syndrome and ER. In most horses with polysaccharide storage myopathy, the enzymes are normal or only mildly elevated.

The diagnosis can be confirmed with a muscle biopsy, usually taken from the semitendinosus muscle at the back of the thigh.

Treatment and Prognosis

There is no specific treatment for this condition. Long-term management involves feeding a low carbohydrate diet, consisting mostly of pasture or grass hay. Grain should be severely restricted or removed from the diet altogether. The horse's energy requirements can be met by adding fat, such as vegetable oil, to the ration. Up to 25% of the horse's daily calorie needs can be supplied by fat. Many horses refuse feed containing large quantities of vegetable oil, so it should be introduced gradually, starting with ½ – 1 cup per feed.

The signs are usually brought on by exercise, so paddock or pasture rest is advisable for a couple of months. The dietary changes usually result in an improvement within 1 – 3 months. After this time, the horse should be managed like a horse with recurrent ER. Most horses respond well to these management changes and can eventually be used for light activities.

Heat-Related Myopathy

Any horse that is made to exercise in hot, humid weather is prone to heat-related myopathy. Horses with this syndrome show the following signs:

• muscle weakness
• muscle spasms
• short, stilted gait
• fatigue—inability to continue exercising

This problem is more common in endurance horses on hot, humid days, especially horses that are not conditioned for the distance and climate. In most cases the signs are seen toward the end of a ride, and probably relate to a combination of factors, including:

- high body temperature, especially within the muscle cells
- dehydration
- electrolyte and mineral losses in sweat, in particular, sodium, potassium, chloride, calcium, and magnesium
- depletion of muscle energy stores (glycogen)—like an engine running out of fuel

This condition does not just occur in endurance horses—any horse can develop this problem. For example, if a horse that is used to working for 30 – 40 minutes every few days in mild weather is made to exercise for 2 – 3 hours on a hot, humid day, it may develop this syndrome. Large, heavily muscled horses are especially vulnerable.

Signs of Heat-Related Myopathy

As well as muscle weakness, spasms, and a stiff gait, other common signs include high heart rate, respiratory rate, and rectal temperature (often over 103°F). The skin may stay "tented" when pinched, indicating that the horse is dehydrated. The horse may also appear distressed or exhausted.

Although the horse may have sweated heavily during exercise, it may sweat very little once its sweat glands are "exhausted" and it is dehydrated. An inability to sweat slows the drain of fluid and electrolytes from the body, but it also makes the horse far less efficient at lowering its body temperature.

Thumps

It is fairly common for horses with heat-related myopathy to have "thumps," or synchronous diaphragmatic flutter. "Thumps" is so-named because the sides of the flank twitch in time with the heart beat, which can be over 80 beats per minute in these horses. This looks as if something is tapping, or thumping on the inside of the flank. The abdominal wall twitches this way because the diaphragm (the large, sheet-like muscle that separates the abdominal and chest cavities) contracts at the same rate as the heart beat, instead of with every breath. The phrenic nerve, which activates the diaphragm, runs very close to the heart. When a horse has major upsets in its blood electrolyte and mineral concentra-

Extra Information
An adult horse's heart rate at rest is normally 30 – 40 beats per minute.

tions—especially calcium and magnesium—the phrenic nerve is more reactive than normal. Instead of stimulating the diaphragm to contract with every breath, it causes the diaphragm to contract with every heart beat.

"Thumps" does not cause a gait abnormality. However, it is a warning flag that the horse has developed serious electrolyte, mineral, and fluid imbalances.

Treatment of Heat-Related Myopathy

Treating heat-related myopathy involves:

- resting the horse
- cooling the horse—e.g., with cold hosing
- replacing the lost fluid and electrolytes

In most cases the veterinarian can replace the fluid and electrolytes orally, using a nasogastric ("stomach") tube. Adding glucose to the water/electrolyte mix provides an energy source to the depleted muscles. It may also aid electrolyte absorption from the intestines. If the horse is severely dehydrated or very weak, the fluid and electrolytes must be replaced intravenously.

Often these horses are not very thirsty, despite being very dehydrated. Thirst—the desire to drink—is stimulated by an increase in the sodium concentration in the bloodstream. The concentration is the number of molecules per liter of fluid: blood and tissue fluid. If fluid, but not sodium is lost, the sodium concentration rises. But with heavy sweating, both fluid and sodium are lost from the body, so the sodium concentration does not change much. This is because there are still approximately the same number of sodium molecules per liter of fluid. In other words, the ratio of sodium to fluid is roughly the same because both have been lost.

The desire to drink comes from the thirst center in the brain when the sodium concentration in the bloodstream rises. In horses that have sweated heavily, the sodium concentration may only rise slightly, if at all. As a result, the thirst center is not stimulated and the horse feels no desire to drink. *The horse will not voluntarily replace its fluid loss by drinking.* So, the fluid and electrolytes must be given through a nasogastric tube or intravenously.

When a large amount of chloride is lost in sweat, the bicarbonate concentration in the bloodstream increases to maintain the normal balance of positive and negative ions. Therefore, these horses have proportionately too much bicarbonate in their bloodstreams, so *electrolyte mixtures that contain bicarbonate should not be given.*

Sodium Concentration and Loss of Body Fluid

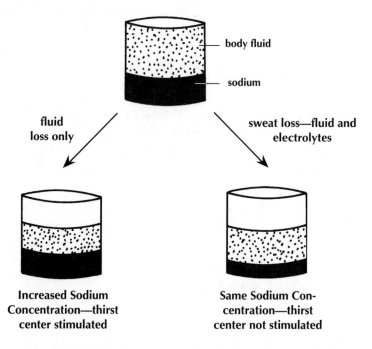

Fig. 10–20. When both fluid and sodium are lost, the horse does not feel the desire to drink.

In all but the severest cases, the horse usually responds to rest, cooling, and fluid therapy, and is relatively normal within a few hours. But it will probably seem tired for 3 – 5 days after such an episode. During this time the horse should be rested in a pasture or large paddock, and allowed time to replenish its muscle energy stores.

Prevention of Heat-Related Myopathy
Conditioning

The owner or trainer can prevent heat-related myopathy by ensuring that the horse is conditioned for the duration and intensity of the exercise. It also helps to reduce the amount of exercise in hot, humid weather, and work the horse in the early morning or late evening. These measures are especially important in horses that have recently been moved from a cooler climate.

Cooling

Cooling the horse with cold water baths, shade, and fans (or a natural breeze) is also important when training or competing in hot weather. It is not true that cooling a hot horse too quickly causes it to "tie up." In fact, it helps prevent muscle problems and fatigue by reducing the temperature within the overheated muscles. This has been proved by veterinarians conducting research on overheating in eventing and dressage horses in preparation for the Olympic Games in Atlanta.

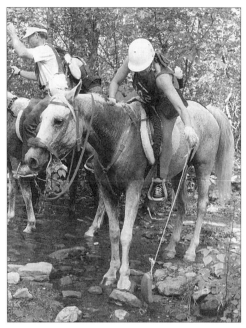

Fig. 10–21. Sponging the horse with cool water can help prevent heat-related myopathy.

Fluid and Electrolytes

When the horse must compete in hot weather, it should be offered both electrolyte-spiked and fresh water frequently throughout the day. Some horses will not drink water that has had anything added to it, no matter how thirsty they are. Horses that are sweating heavily need both fluid and electrolytes. But if the horse will not drink the spiked water, it is better that it drinks fresh water than nothing at all.

Adding electrolytes to the horse's feed on a regular basis may ensure that any previously depleted electrolytes are replaced. It also stimulates the horse to drink. Ensuring that the diet contains enough calcium and magnesium is also important.

Hypocalcemia

Hypocalcemia means low blood calcium concentration. The body maintains the blood calcium concentration in a very narrow range. It does this by moving calcium into or out of the bones, depending on its needs. If the horse is not receiving enough calcium in its diet, or if there is a large demand for calcium (for example, mares producing a lot of milk), absorption from the bones may not be enough to maintain the blood calcium concentration at the normal level. Muscles require calcium to function properly, so the most obvious sign of hypocalcemia is muscle dysfunction.

Signs of Hypocalcemia

There are two basic forms of hypocalcemia. The first occurs with a moderate drop in blood calcium, and causes:

• muscle stiffness and spasms
• stiff, stilted gait
• difficulty eating (the jaw muscles spasm)

These signs can look like tetanus *(see Chapter 12)*. In fact, when this form of hypocalcemia occurs in nursing mares it is called "lactation tetany." Horses with mild to moderate hypocalcemia may also develop "thumps" (discussed earlier).

The second form of hypocalcemia occurs with severe drops in the blood calcium concentration. The signs of this disorder are:

• generalized muscle weakness
• severe depression
• inability to stand
• rapid heart rate and weak heart beat (the pulse is also fast, weak, and "fluttery")

This form is extremely unusual in horses, but is common in high-producing dairy cows ("downer cow syndrome").

Diagnosis of Hypocalcemia

Hypocalcemia can sometimes be diagnosed just on the history and the signs. Neither form of hypocalcemia is very common in horses. But it is more likely in nursing mares on low calcium diets. A mare that is producing a lot of milk for a large, rapidly growing foal may become depleted in calcium if she is not fed a high calcium diet. When the demand exceeds the body's ability to extract calcium from the bones, the blood calcium concentration drops. Other adult horses on low calcium diets may show signs of hypocalcemia if they are stressed by prolonged transport ("transit tetany"), prolonged and strenuous exercise, or severe diarrhea.

Hypocalcemia is easily diagnosed by measuring the horse's blood calcium concentration. However, most of the time the veterinarian cannot get a result immediately. He or she must decide whether to treat the horse for hypocalcemia based on the signs and history. In theory, tetanus could occur in a vaccinated horse, but it is extremely unlikely. Therefore, if a horse that is currently vaccinated against tetanus suddenly (in a few hours) develops these signs, it is usually safe to assume that it has hypocalcemia and not tetanus.

Treatment of Hypocalcemia

Treatment involves giving calcium to return the blood cal-

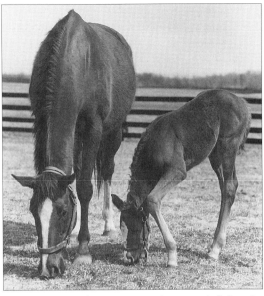

Fig. 10–22. Nursing mares can become deficient in calcium.

cium concentration to normal and replenish the horse's depleted calcium stores. Calcium solution can be given intravenously (IV), but it must be infused slowly. Giving IV calcium too rapidly can cause cardiac arrest, so only a veterinarian should administer IV calcium.

Calcium can also be given orally. But hypocalcemia can cause muscle spasms that prevent the horse from eating or drinking. So, the veterinarian must give the calcium by nasogastric ("stomach") tube. This method of calcium therapy is very safe, but it takes a little longer to work than intravenous calcium. Nevertheless, once the calcium is absorbed into the bloodstream the signs disappear quickly.

Caution
Injecting the calcium solution subcutaneously is common practice in cows, but it should not be performed in horses.

If the foal is older than about 1 week (which is usually the case in mares with hypocalcemia), it is best to prevent the foal from nursing for the next 6 – 8 hours. This does not affect the mare's milk production in the long term, but it temporarily halts the drain of calcium from her system. The foal can go this long without milk, although it should be provided with water and some source of feed, such as milk replacer pellets or alfalfa hay.

Treatment should not stop at resolving the signs. This condition only arises after the body's calcium stores have been depleted by weeks or months of insufficient dietary calcium. The horse must be placed on a diet that meets or slightly exceeds its maintenance requirements, while keeping the calcium-phosphorus ratio at the recommended level. Nursing mares must receive extra calcium for as long as they are producing milk because the drain on their calcium stores will continue until the foal is weaned. *(Figure 9–34 in Chapter 9 gives the calcium and phosphorus requirements and ratio for foals, mature horses, and pregnant or nursing mares.)*

MISCELLANEOUS CONDITIONS
Intramuscular Injection Reactions

Intramuscular (IM) injections can cause little or no muscle inflammation, or they can result in:

- volume-related muscle disruption
- chemical myositis
- vaccine-related myositis
- nerve dysfunction

Reminder
"Myositis" means muscle inflammation.

These effects are usually mild and self-limiting. But in some cases fibrotic myopathy (discussed earlier) may be the end result of severe muscle damage following an IM injection.

Two more serious conditions are discussed in the later section on *Bacterial Myositis:*

- abscessation
- clostridial myositis

Generalized allergic (anaphylactic) reactions are possible with any drug injected, whether IM, intravenous, or subcutaneous. Reactions are rare, but when they happen, they can be fatal. Another type of drug reaction may occur after IM injection with procaine penicillin, although this is not a true allergic reaction *(see Chapter 5)*. Neither of these reactions primarily cause lameness, but they are serious conditions.

Possible Consequences of IM Injection
Volume-Related Muscle Disruption

Muscle damage can occur when more than about 20 ml (cc) is injected into one site in an adult horse. Less is needed to cause the same problem in ponies and foals. It can also occur with smaller volumes in any size animal when the drug is injected too quickly. Unlike the center of a vein or the potential space beneath the skin (the subcutaneous space), there is no space or cavity in a normal muscle into which the drug can be deposited. Muscle is solid tissue, and the injected substance must diffuse among the muscle fibers. When a large volume is given, or the substance is injected too quickly, it can create a cavity in the muscle.

In most cases actual muscle fiber damage is minimal. The drug mostly disrupts the individual muscle bundles, causing local inflammation. The swelling and pain usually disappear once the drug is absorbed and the inflammation has subsided, which typically takes 2 – 3 days.

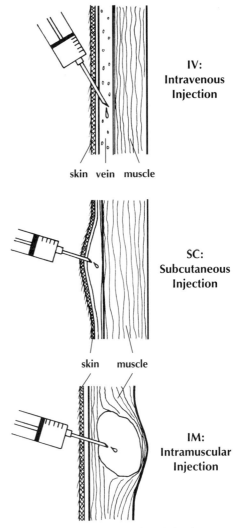

IV:
Intravenous
Injection

skin vein muscle

SC:
Subcutaneous
Injection

skin   muscle

IM:
Intramuscular
Injection

Fig. 10–23. Unlike IV and SC injections, a drug that is given IM is injected into solid tissue. It can create a cavity if injected too quickly.

Chemical Myositis

Chemical myositis is caused by irritant drugs: substances that are too concentrated, acidic, or alkaline, and so cause muscle damage and inflammation. In many cases chemical myositis results when someone mistakenly injects a drug that is not designed for IM use. Phenylbutazone (PBZ, or "bute") is a good example. There is an oral formulation and an intravenous formulation. The IV solution causes no irritation when properly injected IV, but when given IM it can cause severe inflammation.

This type of myositis can also occur with a drug that is approved for IM use if it is chemically altered by:

Caution
Do not inject "bute" IM.   Oral formulation—paste or tablet   IV formulation—clear solution   IM formulation—NONE

- adding another drug
- exposing it to light or air
- storing it too long (exceeding the expiration date)

Even drugs that are approved for IM use, and stored and administered correctly can cause chemical myositis in some horses. However, in most cases the inflammation is very mild. For some reason, certain horses are more sensitive than others, and react to drugs that would not normally be a problem.

Chemical myositis can be very painful, even though the swelling may not be great. If the inflammation and muscle damage are severe, an abscess may develop at the site. Damaged muscle is an excellent environment for bacteria, which can enter the muscle when the needle is inserted through the skin. Bacteria may also invade the damaged muscle through the bloodstream.

Vaccine-Related Myositis

IM vaccines can cause inflammation at the injection site by stimulating an immune system reaction. Most vaccines contain an adjuvant, which is a chemical that causes a mild inflammatory reaction for the specific purpose of attracting white blood cells to the injection site. The white blood cells engulf the foreign particles (vaccine) and the immune system then makes antibodies against the "invading organism." That is how vaccines stimulate a protective immune response (immunity). But sometimes the muscle inflammation is greater than expected, and a short-lived myositis results. Strangles vaccines often cause this type of myositis, although any vaccine can cause it. In most cases, pain and swelling develop at the injection site each time that vaccine is given. In some horses the reaction is a little worse each time.

Nerve Dysfunction

Temporary nerve dysfunction may occur when an IM injection is given too close to a nerve. For example, weakness or paralysis in a hindleg may occur if an IM injection in the rump is given too close to the sciatic nerve *(see Chapter 12)*. Nerve dysfunction is more common in foals and ponies because they have less muscle overlying the nerve than adult horses. In most cases the nerve dysfunction resolves once the drug is completely absorbed, usually within a few hours. However, if chemical myositis results from the injection, nerve function may not return to normal until the surrounding muscle inflammation subsides (which usually takes a couple of days). Rarely, if ever, is the paralysis permanent.

Signs of IM Injection Reactions

The typical signs of IM injection reactions are muscle pain and mild swelling at the injection site. Injection reactions on the side of the neck often make the horse reluctant to lower or turn its head. The horse may also walk stiffly. If the injection was given in the pectoral muscles (at the front of the chest), or in the rump or thigh, the horse may be stiff or lame in that leg. *(The common IM injection sites are illustrated in Figure 10–25.)*

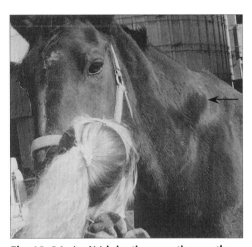

Fig. 10–24. An IM injection reaction on the neck, just in front of the withers.

Often the signs are noticed within the first 24 hours after injection, sometimes within the first hour. Any time a horse is lame within about 3 days of an IM injection, the injection site should be palpated for signs of pain and swelling. There may be little or no swelling at the site, but when it is present, the size of swelling usually reflects the degree of inflammation and muscle damage. Injections given into the pectoral muscles can also cause edema (accumulation of tissue fluid), which gravitates under the skin to the lowest point on the front of the chest. This soft, fluidy swelling is not painful. Edema can develop with injection reactions in other muscles, but because of their location it is not as obvious.

Fever, depression, and loss of appetite do not normally occur as a result of these IM injection reactions. If these signs are present, some other process, such as bacterial myositis or an infection unrelated to the muscle or the injection, is the most likely cause.

The primary sign of nerve dysfunction is temporary weakness or paralysis in the limb. With the commonly used IM sites, only the sciatic nerve is at risk. Even then, the chances of nerve dysfunction are very low.

Treatment of IM Injection Reactions

Treatment is aimed at increasing the absorption of the drug and relieving inflammation. These goals can be achieved with:

• heat therapy, or alternating hot and cold
• gentle massage
• light exercise at least twice per day
• NSAIDs

(These therapies are discussed in Section II: Principles of Therapy.) Corticosteroids should not be used for treating IM injection reactions. Bacterial infection is a possibility after every injection. Corticosteroids may encourage bacterial myositis by inhibiting the immune system response. Corticosteroids can also mask the early signs of abscessation by suppressing inflammation. Further, they may prevent a protective immune response if they are given to treat a vaccine-related IM injection reaction. In other words, they may make the vaccine ineffective.

Unless infection develops, the signs should resolve within 2 – 3 days. Any IM injection reaction that has not resolved in 4 – 5 days should be examined by a veterinarian. If the swelling and pain worsen, or disappear and then return, this may mean that an abscess is developing.

If possible, no more injections should be given into that muscle for 2 – 3 weeks after a reaction. Occasionally, a small "knot" of scar tissue may be left at the injection site, but this usually does not affect muscle function or cause an obvious blemish.

> **Note**
>
> Corticosteroids are potent anti-inflammatory drugs. But they also inhibit the immune response. The body may not be able to control infection when these drugs are given.
>
> (See Chapter 5 for more information.)

Prevention of IM Injection Reactions
These problems can usually be prevented by:
- using a sterile injection technique
- using only products specifically formulated for IM injection
- limiting the injection volume to 15 – 20 ml per site for adult horses (less in foals and small ponies), and using two or more sites for larger volumes
- injecting the drug very slowly
- ensuring correct needle placement in the recommended injection sites
- rotating the injection sites when giving a course of IM injections; e.g. alternating between the left and right sides of the neck and the left and right pectoral muscles
- giving an NSAID (either orally or intravenously) before vaccinating sensitive horses

Sterile Injection Technique
Sterile injection technique involves using a sterile needle, syringe, and drug. Although it can be acceptable to reuse a syringe for antibiotics (provided the syringe is kept in a clean container between uses), *needles should never be reused.* Not only are they contaminated once they have penetrated the skin, they also become blunt. Needles are so inexpensive and readily available that there is never a good excuse for reusing a needle.

Once the top of a vial or bottle is pierced with a needle and some of the solution is withdrawn, the remaining solution may no longer be sterile. The unused portion should be kept refrigerated, and thrown out if it is not used within a few weeks. Also, if the solution has changed in any way it should be thrown out. For example, the drug may have changed color, or produced a sediment or floating particles. All bottles, whether opened or not, should be discarded once their expiration date has passed.

The skin should be cleaned before each injection, using alcohol or an antiseptic solution. No amount of scrubbing or disinfecting will rid the skin of all bacteria, but it is important to remove as much dirt as possible. It is essential that the injection site is free of manure. *If the site is soiled with manure, it should not be used, no matter how much cleaning is done.* The risk of serious infection with the harmful bacteria normally found in manure is too great.

Recommended Injection Sites
The commonly recommended sites for IM injection in horses are:
- the front of the chest—pectoral muscles
- the side of the neck—cervical muscles
- the back of the thigh—semimembranosus and semitendinosus muscles
- the top of the rump—gluteal muscles

There are a few important landmarks to identify and avoid when giving IM injections into these areas.

Chest
The pectoral muscles are the bulky muscles on either side of the breastbone at the front of the chest. The two sites to identify and avoid when giving injections into these muscles are the breastbone and the point of the shoulder. The injection should be given between these two sites into the thickest part of the muscle, with the needle inserted horizontally.

Neck
The "safe" area on the side of the neck is bordered by three structures that must be avoided:
- the spinal column, easily felt directly above the jugular groove
- the front of the shoulder blade
- the nuchal ligament, which is the large ligament that runs from the poll to the withers underneath the mane

These three structures form a roughly triangular area on the side of the neck, with the shoulder blade as the base of the triangle. In an average sized adult horse a good rule of thumb is to insert the needle into the muscle in a place that is at least one hand's width away from each of these structures: one hand's width in front of the shoulder blade, above the spinal column, and below the mane. The needle should be inserted horizontally.

Thigh
When giving an IM injection into the thigh muscles, the needle should be placed at the back of the thigh, several inches below the point of the buttock. The needle should be inserted horizontally.

Rump
The gluteal muscles are the large muscles that cover the top of the rump, on each side of the spinal column. The landmarks to identify and avoid are:

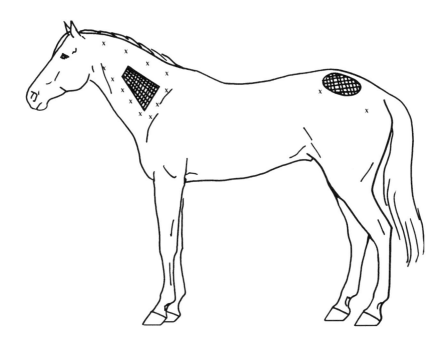

Fig. 10–25. The recommended sites for IM injection (shaded) and the landmarks to avoid (x).

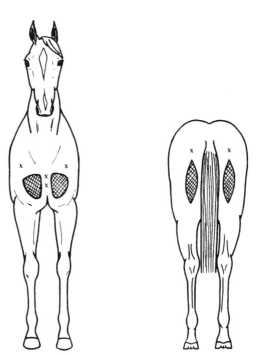

- the spine
- the point of the hip
- the hip joint

The hip joint is several inches behind, and a couple of inches lower than the point of the hip. Ensuring that the needle is placed at least one hand's width away from each of these structures is a good rule of thumb. The needle should be inserted almost vertically, so that it is at right angles to the skin surface.

Because an abscess in the gluteal muscles cannot easily be drained (discussed later), some veterinarians avoid giving injections there.

Other Recommendations

In adult horses the drug should be injected into the muscle using a needle that is 1 – 1½ inches (25 – 38 mm) long. Shorter needles can be used in foals and ponies. In every age and size of horse, the smallest diameter (gauge) needle possible should be used so that pain and muscle damage are minimized. When injecting thick substances, a large-gauge needle (such as an 18-gauge) is necessary. However, using a large-gauge needle for a thinner solution allows rapid injection, which increases the potential for muscle disruption and damage. *In every case, IM injections should be given very slowly.*

To minimize volume-related muscle disruption when giving injections over about 10 ml, some veterinarians recommend injecting about 5 ml, then sliding the needle back (but not all the way out) and redirecting it before injecting another 5 ml in the new site. The needle can be redirected two or three times if necessary until the entire volume is injected. This technique, which should not be attempted without advice from a veterinarian, saves injecting the horse in two or more locations because the redirection can be done without removing the needle from the skin.

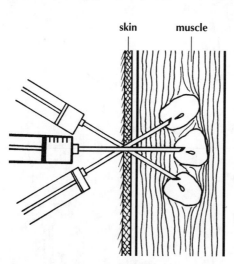

skin   muscle

Fig. 10–26. Redirection can be done without removing the needle from the skin.

Bacterial Myositis

Bacteria may enter a muscle through an IM injection, a wound, or the bloodstream. (Bacterial infection through the bloodstream is very uncommon and generally occurs in a muscle that is already damaged.) The infection may be localized, and confined to an abscess, or it may involve large areas of muscle. Fortunately, IM abscesses and the more extensive type of bacterial myositis are uncommon, given the frequency with which horses receive IM injections and injure themselves.

Abscessation

An abscess is a specific area of tissue damage and pus. This area usually is surrounded by a fibrous tissue reaction. The fibrous tissue is the body's attempt to "wall off" the infection, and prevent it from spreading. Some bacteria cause a severe fibrous reaction, which results in a thick capsule around the abscess. But others cause very little reaction.

In most cases the abscess is the result of an IM injection. An abscess may develop if a contaminated needle or syringe

Definition
Pus: accumulation of tissue fluid, white blood cells, cell debris, and bacteria.

is used, or if the injected solution is unsterile. However, in many cases the person giving the injection did use a sterile needle, syringe, and solution—the bacteria were introduced into the muscle from the skin surface. Bacteria are inevitably taken into the muscle with the needle because it is impossible to remove all bacteria from the skin, no matter how well it was scrubbed with disinfectant.

Although every IM injection introduces bacteria into the muscle, the conditions must be suited to bacterial growth for an abscess to form. Muscle has a very good blood supply, which ensures that plenty of white blood cells and antibodies are available to combat bacterial invasion. In most cases there must be an area of muscle damage for the bacteria to survive and multiply within the muscle. As discussed earlier, large volumes and irritating drugs can cause muscle damage. Abscessation is more likely when giving non-antibiotic drugs, particularly long-acting (depot) substances such as oil-based hormones, including progesterone and anabolic steroids. These substances are not immediately absorbed from the muscle, so they provide the bacteria with a good environment for growth.

When an IM abscess is the result of a puncture wound, the penetrating object both causes muscle damage and "seeds" the muscle with bacteria. An abscess is even more likely, and develops more quickly, if a piece of wood or metal breaks off within the muscle.

Signs of Abscessation

The most consistent sign of an IM abscess is a painful swelling within the muscle. If the injection was given deep into the muscle, there may be little or no swelling at the site until the abscess is well advanced (although the site is painful when palpated with any pressure). An IM abscess does not usually break out through the skin; it is far easier for it to spread within the muscle. Depending on the location of the abscess, the horse may be obviously lame, or just a little stiff.

Because the infection is contained within the abscess, fever, depression, and loss of appetite are uncommon. Although, if the injection was given into the muscles of the neck, pain and stiffness may make the horse reluctant to lower its head to eat or drink. In a few cases infection in this area may spread to involve the nerves as they exit the spinal column, or even the vertebrae themselves. When this happens, the signs are more severe *(see the section on Vertebral Osteomyelitis in Chapter 12)*.

Diagnosis of Abscessation

Diagnosis usually is based on the history of an IM injection (or wound), and on the signs. However, the signs of an IM abscess usually take several days to become obvious. It is common for the owner or trainer to forget that an injection was given, and not associate the signs of muscle pain and lameness with an injection given a week or more earlier.

Sometimes ultrasonography is used to confirm the presence of an abscess *(see Chapter 2)*. It can also determine how deep it is, how thick its wall is, and whether it is a single, large cavity or several small pockets. Ultrasonography may also identify the presence of a "foreign" object, such as a piece of wood or wire. This information can help the veterinarian decide how to manage the problem.

Treatment of Abscessation
Drainage

Treatment must involve draining the abscess. This can be difficult if the abscess is in the gluteal muscles at the top of the rump because gravity works against drainage in this area. But opening the abscess and flushing it with large volumes of sterile saline or very dilute antiseptic solution are essential to completely resolve any abscess.

Some veterinarians prefer to make a small hole through the skin and muscle, and insert a Foley catheter into the abscess. The abscess can be flushed several times per day through the catheter until the infection is resolved. This technique minimizes muscle damage and scarring because it uses a small incision. It is the best way to effectively drain a deep abscess, especially on the top of the rump.

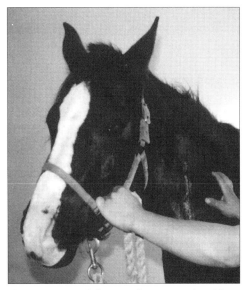

Fig. 10–27. Draining an abscess on the side of the horse's neck.

Antibiotics

Antibiotics are important in resolving the infection, but they are not effective if the abscess has not been drained, and any "foreign" material removed. In most cases the bacteria causing the abscess are those normally found on the skin. However, if the harmful bacteria commonly found in manure are introduced into the muscle, they can cause severe muscle damage and illness. Thus, it is usually worthwhile for the veterinarian to take a sample of pus and submit it to the laboratory for culture and sensitivity *(see Chapter 2)*, to be sure the organism(s) is sensitive to the antibiotic chosen.

Other Recommendations

Heat therapy (or alternating hot and cold) and gentle exercise can help resolve the drained abscess by improving blood supply to, and drainage from, the area. Giving NSAIDs for a couple of days after drainage makes the horse more comfortable and more willing to move around. An infected muscle should not be massaged because this could spread bacteria throughout the muscle. However, once the abscess is drained, the

---

Definition

A Foley catheter is a plastic or rubber tube about the width of the little finger. It has a small, inflatable cuff just behind the tip. When the catheter is inserted into the cavity and the cuff is inflated, it remains in place until the cuff is deflated.

surrounding muscle can be "kneaded" to work the pus and flush fluid out of the cavity. *(These therapies are discussed in Section II: Principles of Therapy.)*

Prognosis and Prevention of Abscessation

The prognosis for complete recovery and return to full athletic function usually is good, provided proper treatment is continued until the infection is completely resolved. These abscesses can usually be prevented by following the guidelines for IM injection discussed in the previous section. Depot (long-lasting) substances should not be injected into the gluteal muscles because it is very difficult to drain an abscess in this area.

Pigeon Breast

"Pigeon breast" or "pigeon fever" is a type of muscle abscessation that is caused by the bacteria *Corynebacterium pseudotuberculosis.* It is more often seen in the western and southwestern U.S. Occasional cases are also seen in the southeastern states. The bacteria enter through a small wound, and then spread to the surrounding muscles. The most common sites of abscessation are:

- the front of the chest
- the underside of the chest and abdomen
- around the point of the hip

These bacteria cause deep, thick-walled abscesses within the muscles. In some sites there may be many small abscesses, while in

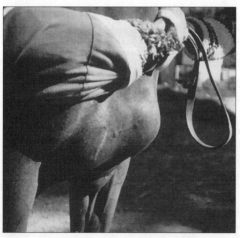

others there are a couple of large abscesses. The outward signs—painful swelling in the affected muscles and lameness—reflect the location and size of the abscesses. Fever is also a common sign. If the infection invades the lymphatic system of the leg, ulcerative lymphangitis may develop.

This infection can be spread to other horses. When the veterinarian

Fig. 10–28. A horse with "pigeon breast."

suspects "pigeon breast" a definite diag-nosis should be made by sampling the pus and submitting it to a laboratory. Ultrasonography is useful because it can locate the deep, thick-walled abscesses, and identify other small abscesses. It is also useful for guiding a needle into the center of an abscess to sample the pus. When multiple abscesses with thick, fi-brous walls are found, it is safe to assume the horse has a *C. pseudotuberculosis* infection. Appropriate precautions should then be taken when treating the horse.

More Information

The lymphatic system is a network of small vessels that collect excess tissue fluid and return it to the blood-stream.

(See Chapter 13 for in-formation on ulcerative lymphangitis.)

Treatment

Effective treatment requires drainage of the abscesses. The Foley catheter technique mentioned earlier is very useful for draining and flushing these deep abscesses. Prolonged antibiotic therapy (2 – 3 weeks) is also necessary to resolve this infection. Because the disease is contagious, draining and flushing the abscesses should only be performed in an area that can be thoroughly cleaned and disinfected afterward, such as a concrete wash stall. The people handling the horse and treating the abscesses should wear latex or rubber gloves, wash their hands, and clean their boots thoroughly after each treat-ment. If necessary, they should also change their clothes. *(Hygiene and disinfection measures are discussed in more detail in Chapter 4.)*

Recovery from this condition can be slow, and abscesses can de-velop in other sites even after the infection is apparently resolved.

Clostridial Myositis

Clostridial bacteria (typically *Clostridium perfringens*) may invade the muscle through an intramuscular injection or a puncture wound. They can rapidly cause severe muscle damage, serious illness, and even death. These bacteria produce toxins that damage the muscle. When absorbed into the bloodstream they can cause fever, depres-sion, and circulatory collapse (shock) in a matter of hours. *Veterinary attention is urgently needed for these horses.*

The bacteria also produce gas, which further disrupts the muscle and spreads underneath the skin and between other muscles. Gas beneath the skin causes a crackling sound and sensation when the skin is palpated. In medical terms, this is called subcutaneous emphysema.

To be successful, veterinary treatment must begin as soon as the signs of muscle swelling, pain, and depression are first noticed. Intravenous fluids are often necessary to support the horse's failing circulation, and intravenous penicillin must be given to kill the bacteria. The clostridial organisms are very sensitive to penicillin, so if started early, this treatment usually saves the horse's life.

The gas and fluid must be drained from the infected muscle if further muscle damage is to be avoided. These bacteria are anaerobic, and need a low-oxygen environment to survive. They are very sensitive to oxygen, so making a large hole in the infected muscle, or many small holes if the area is extensive, and flushing oxygen or air into the muscle can be very effective. (Hydrogen peroxide, although it supplies oxygen, can further damage the tissues, so it should not be used.)

The prognosis for survival is guarded, unless the condition is diagnosed and treated early. The prognosis for return to full athletic function is also guarded because the bacterial toxins can cause extensive muscle damage.

Strep. equi Myopathy

Streptococcus equi is the bacteria that causes strangles, a respiratory disease that results in abscesses under the jaw and in the throat. Occasionally, secondary problems develop, sometimes weeks after the infection has apparently resolved. One problem is limb edema (purpura; *see Chapter 13*). Another is muscle damage, or myopathy.

Myopathy seen in these horses is caused by the body's immune response to the bacteria. Immune complexes—bacteria plus antibodies—in the bloodstream damage the blood vessel walls, a condition called vasculitis. This interrupts the blood supply to the muscles and can lead to severe muscle degeneration. In some cases the immune complexes also damage the muscle fibers directly.

The diagnosis is made on the history of exposure to strangles, and elevated muscle enzymes in a blood sample. The severity of the muscle damage, and therefore the prognosis, is determined with a muscle biopsy.

Severe myopathy is seen in horses showing typical signs of strangles or purpura. Myopathy causes muscle stiffness and moderate lameness; colic may also be seen in some horses. The muscle damage is extensive, and the response to treatment is poor. Most of these horses are euthanized for humane reasons.

Less serious myopathy occurs in horses that were exposed to strangles, yet did not develop obvious signs. The muscle damage in these horses is mild to moderate, and usually is reversible with proper treatment. Signs include mild depression and loss of appetite, a short, stilted gait, and rapid muscle atrophy along the back and rump. Treatment includes antibiotics, corticosteroids, and rest. The prognosis for complete recovery is good, and in most cases the muscle mass returns to normal in about 2 months.

Hyperkalemic Periodic Paralysis (HPP)

Hyperkalemic Periodic Paralysis (HPP) is an inherited condition. It is seen in heavily muscled, purebred and cross-bred Quarter Horses related to the Quarter Horse stallion, Impressive. Some publications refer to this condition as "HYPP." However, as the three-word title has no word beginning with "Y," the correct abbreviation is "HPP." Human medical texts use "HPP" for the similar condition in people, and some veterinary texts also are now using this term.

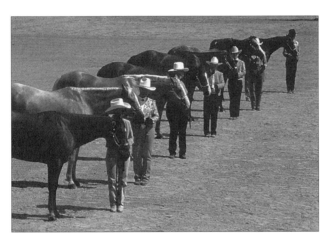

Fig. 10–29. HPP is seen in well-muscled Quarter Horses.

The condition involves a defect in the muscle cell membrane. The mechanism that keeps potassium inside the cell and sodium outside the cell does not function properly. As a result potassium leaks from the cell into the surrounding tissue, and from there into the blood-stream. This leakage of potassium from the muscle cells causes abnormally excitable muscles.

So, the name reflects the primary features of this condition:

Episodes — periodic incidents
of **Elevated blood potassium concentration** — hyperkalemia
leading to **Muscle weakness and collapse** — paralysis

Signs of HPP

The signs can be as mild as weakness and small muscle tremors in only a few muscle groups. But during a severe attack, the signs may include:

- generalized weakness
- widespread muscle tremors
- collapse
- difficulty breathing
- cardiac arrest and death—this is very uncommon

During an episode, which can last as little as a few minutes or as long as a few hours, the horse is weak and walks with a very stiff, unsteady gait—if it is able to walk at all. Exertional rhabdomyolysis ("tying up") can cause some of the same signs. But with HPP the horse is normal within minutes after the episode, and has no elevation in the blood concentration of muscle enzymes.

Diagnosis of HPP

HPP is occasionally seen in foals, but it is usually first noticed in young horses between 1 and 3 years old, when the horse begins showing or training. In most cases the attacks are brought on by excitement or stress, for example:

- exercise
- cold temperatures
- general anesthesia
- transport
- hospitalization for veterinary treatment
- breeding

However, some attacks occur for no apparent reason while the horse is at rest. The episodes are more common in horses fed potassium-rich feeds, such as alfalfa or other legume hays, and molasses.

Blood taken during an attack would usually reveal an elevated blood potassium concentration. However, the episodes may last only a few minutes, and the blood potassium concentration is normal between episodes, so it is a matter of luck if the veterinarian can definitely diagnose the condition this way. The best way to make the diagnosis is with DNA testing, which determines whether the horse carries the HPP gene.

Management of HPP

There is no cure or definite treatment for this condition. However, changing some management practices often reduces the incidence and severity of the episodes. Such changes include:

- feeding a low-potassium diet, with grass hay as the main fiber source
- avoiding potassium-rich feeds
- keeping the diet and feeding schedule constant
- reducing stress as much as possible
- exercising the horse every day
- keeping the exercise schedule constant

At the beginning and end of the training and competition season it is best to increase or decrease the amount of daily exercise gradually, over a period of weeks. Training should not begin or end abruptly for these horses.

Drugs that cause the kidney to "dump" potassium into the urine (such as acetazolamide and hydrochlorothiazide) may also help reduce the frequency and severity of the attacks. However, these drugs deplete the body stores of potassium, which can in itself cause weakness and muscle tremors. So they should probably only be used while the horse is under stress.

The American Quarter Horse Association (AQHA) now considers HPP to be a genetic defect—an undesirable trait. The organization has taken steps to control this problem. As of January 1, 1998, all foals whose bloodlines can be traced back to a known carrier of the HPP gene will have that fact written on their registration papers. This allows owners to select breeding stock that do not carry the gene.

White Muscle Disease

"White muscle disease," or nutritional myopathy, is occasionally seen in horses less than 1 year old in selenium-deficient regions. The condition is called white muscle disease because at postmortem examination the muscles of affected foals are pale.

Selenium is a trace mineral—a mineral that is essential to the body, but in very small amounts. It is needed for the normal function of an enzyme that destroys oxidants: cell by-products that can damage other cell membranes. When selenium is deficient, whether in the pregnant mare's diet or the foal's diet, the "anti-oxidant" enzyme cannot function efficiently and oxidant-induced muscle damage can occur.

Signs of White Muscle Disease

In some foals the signs are restricted to the head and neck. The more obvious ones are swelling under the throat and difficulty swallowing. Milk may dribble from the nostrils when these foals nurse. In other foals the signs are more generalized and include sudden episodes of weakness and stiff, painful muscles. In severe cases the heart muscle may also be affected, which could lead to cardiac arrest and death if the foal is stressed.

Diagnosis of White Muscle Disease

The diagnosis usually is based on the signs, the age of the foal, and a knowledge of the selenium status of the region. Other causes of these signs (such as botulism; *see Chapter 12*) must be ruled out if possible. A blood sample can be taken to check the foal's blood selenium concentration. Finding high blood levels of the muscle enzymes CPK and AST (discussed earlier in the section on *Exertional Rhabdomyolysis*) can also help confirm the diagnosis of white muscle disease.

Treatment of White Muscle Disease

Treatment involves intramuscular injection with selenium and vitamin E. These substances work together, so it is best to give both. The veterinarian's recommendations should be followed closely if toxicity is to be avoided. Signs of selenium overdose include "blind staggers" (apparent blindness, aimless wandering), colic, diarrhea, sweating, and increased heart and respiratory rates.

Another caution: injection with selenium-vitamin E products occasionally causes sudden death from a generalized hypersensitivity (anaphylactic) reaction. Nevertheless, most veterinarians prefer to give selenium by injection. Giving oral selenium and vitamin E to a foal with obvious signs of white muscle disease is not as effective in preventing further muscle damage and reversing the signs.

The diets of all foals and pregnant mares on the farm should be analyzed, and any selenium deficiency corrected with a selenium-containing supplement.

> **Caution**
>
> It is not safe to give selenium in greater than recommended amounts—*more is not better with this mineral.*

11

TENDON & LIGAMENT INJURIES

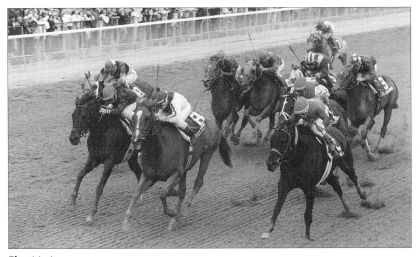

Fig. 11–1.

Tendons and ligaments are important parts of the musculoskeletal system. Although the energy of movement is generated
by muscle activity, that energy is transmitted to the bones
through tendons. Therefore, the primary role of a tendon is to transmit muscle activity to a bone, such that a joint is moved when the

muscle contracts. Some tendons attach to more than one bone, and move more than one joint.

Ligaments play a more passive role. Whereas tendons run from muscle to bone, ligaments run from bone to bone, over at least one joint. The primary role of a ligament is to provide structural support for a joint.

The basic structure, function, disease conditions, and healing processes are similar for all tendons or all ligaments. This chapter focuses on the tendons and ligaments that run down the cannon. Problems with these structures are among the most common conditions that temporarily or permanently halt training and competition in athletic horses.

STRUCTURE & FUNCTION

The tendons in the legs can be divided into two types: flexors and extensors. There are two major flexor tendons—the superficial digital flexor tendon (SDFT) and the deep digital flexor tendon (DDFT). There is one major extensor tendon—the common digital extensor tendon. These tendons attach to muscles in the upper leg, just above the knee or hock. They then run down the leg and attach onto the pastern or pedal bone.

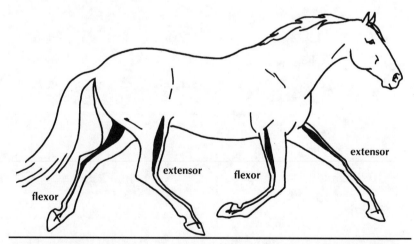

Fig. 11–2. Forelimb: The extensor muscle extends (straightens) the knee, fetlock, pastern, and coffin joint. The flexor muscles flex (bend) these joints. Hindlimb: The extensor muscle extends the fetlock, pastern, and coffin joint, but flexes the hock. The flexor muscles flex the fetlock, pastern, and coffin joint, but extend the hock.

In the foreleg, the flexor tendons flex (bend) the knee, fetlock, pastern, and coffin joint. The extensor tendon extends (straightens) these joints. In the hindlimb the flexor tendons flex the fetlock, pastern, and coffin joint, but they extend the hock. The extensor tendon does the opposite: extends the fetlock, pastern, and coffin joint, but flexes the hock. This is because the knee flexes backward, in the same direction as the fetlock, pastern, and coffin joint, whereas the hock flexes forward.

The other structures discussed in this chapter are the superior and inferior check ligaments and the suspensory ligament.

When looking at the cannon from the side, the order of structures, from front to back, is:

- extensor tendon
- cannon bone and splint bones
- suspensory ligament
- inferior check ligament
- deep digital flexor tendon
- superficial digital flexor tendon

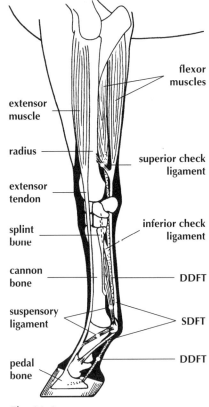

Fig. 11–3.

Ext. = extensor tendon
S = splint bone
SL = suspensory ligament
ICL = inferior check ligament
DDFT = deep digital flexor tendon
SDFT = superficial digital flexor tendon

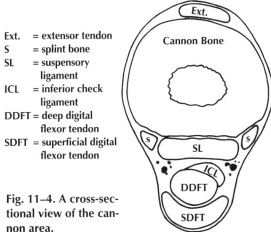

Fig. 11–4. A cross-sectional view of the cannon area.

Digital Flexor Tendons

For most of their path down the cannon, the SDFT and DDFT are oval-shaped when viewed in cross-section. But just above the fetlock the SDFT flattens and wraps around the sides of the DDFT. At the base of the sesamoid bones the SDFT then splits into two branches, which attach onto the sides of the pastern a little further down. The DDFT runs over the back of the sesamoids and continues down the pastern, where it flattens out. It runs over the back of the navicular bone before attaching onto the bottom of the pedal bone.

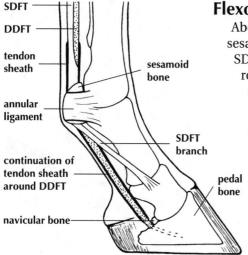

Fig. 11–5. The flexor tendon sheath (in black).

Flexor Tendon Sheath

About 2 – 3 inches above the sesamoid bones, both the SDFT and DDFT are surrounded by the flexor tendon sheath. The sheath is similar to a joint capsule *(see Chapter 8)* in that the lining secretes fluid into the sheath. The fluid lubricates the tendons, allowing them to glide smoothly over the back of the sesamoid bones. Ordinarily, the sheath contains only a very small quantity of fluid.

When the SDFT splits at the base of the sesamoid bones, it leaves the tendon sheath. The sheath continues down the back of the pastern, surrounding the DDFT, until just above the navicular bone. The DDFT is protected by the navicular bursa (a small sac of fluid; *see Chapter 15*) as it runs over the back of the navicular bone.

Terminology

The superior check ligament is also called the radial check ligament.

The inferior check ligament is also called the carpal check ligament.

Check Ligaments

In the forelimb each flexor tendon has a check ligament that anchors the top of the tendon onto the bone at the back of the leg. Check ligaments are also called accessory ligaments. They help prevent the flexor unit—flexor muscle and tendon—from being overstretched. The superior check ligament anchors the SDFT to the back of the radius at the point where the flexor muscle and tendon fuse, about level with the chestnut. The inferior check ligament begins at the back of the knee and attaches onto the DDFT about halfway down the cannon. *(The check ligaments are illustrated in Figure 11–3.)*

In the hindlimb there is no superior check ligament, and only some horses have an inferior check ligament, which usually is small and thin.

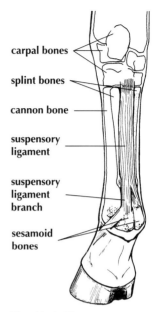

carpal bones

splint bones

cannon bone

suspensory ligament

suspensory ligament branch

sesamoid bones

Fig. 11–6. The suspensory ligament of the forelimb (flexor tendons removed).

Suspensory Ligament

The suspensory ligament begins at the back of the knee or hock, where it is attached to the lower row of carpal (forelimb) or tarsal (hindlimb) bones and the top of the cannon bone. It runs down the back of the cannon bone, in between the splint bones, and between the cannon bone and the inferior check ligament/DDFT. About two-thirds of the way down the cannon, the suspensory ligament splits into two branches. These branches attach onto the top and outer surface of the sesamoid bones at the back of the fetlock. Some of the fibers then continue across the side of the fetlock and attach onto the extensor tendon at the front of the pastern.

The suspensory ligament's role is to support the fetlock by "slinging" the back of the joint. It is an essential component of the "stay apparatus" (discussed later).

Extensor Tendon

The long or common digital extensor tendon is usually just called the extensor tendon. It attaches to an extensor muscle at the front of the forearm or thigh, and then travels down the front of the leg. It is anchored at several places along its length. But its final point of attachment is the extensor process on the top of the pedal bone *(see Chapter 15)*. When the extensor muscle contracts, the joints of the lower leg are extended (straightened). In the forelimb the knee is also extended, but in the hindlimb contraction of the extensor muscle flexes (bends) the hock. *(This concept is illustrated in Figure 11–2.)*

There are other smaller extensor tendons, including the lateral digital extensor tendon and the extensor carpi radialis tendon (in the forelimb). But only the common digital extensor tendon is discussed in this chapter.

TENDONITIS (BOWED TENDON)
Definition

Tendonitis is inflammation of a tendon; usually it includes disruption of some tendon fibers. The most common type of tendonitis involves the flexor tendons (SDFT or DDFT). In most cases it is the

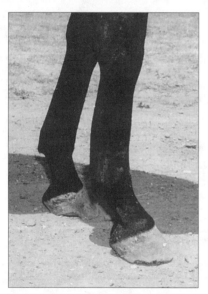

Fig. 11–7. A severe bowed tendon.

SDFT of a foreleg that is damaged. It is relatively uncommon for the DDFT of a foreleg, or either tendon in a hindleg, to be damaged. Tendonitis involving the SDFT of a foreleg is the focus of this section.

Damage in the SDFT causes thickening of the tendon. When viewed from the side this swelling gives the back of the leg a bowed-out appearance, hence the term, "bowed tendon." Most "bows" occur in the middle third of the tendon. When they develop closer to the knee or hock they are called "high bows"; when they occur just above the fetlock, they are called "low bows."

Causes

Tendons are made of thousands of collagen fibers. The fibers are arranged lengthwise along the tendon, like the fibers of a rope (although the collagen fibers do not spiral down the tendon). The collagen fibers are connected to neighboring fibers with short "bridging" molecules that cross-link the fibers, keeping them together and in alignment. A thin fibrous membrane, called the peritendon, surrounds the tendon for most of its length.

As with a rope, there is a point at which excessive stretching of the tendon results in fiber damage. This is the basic cause of tendonitis in athletic horses. Strenuous exercise, such as galloping or jumping, generates loading forces that cause the fetlock and knee to overextend. When overextension is extreme, the back of the fetlock actually touches the ground.

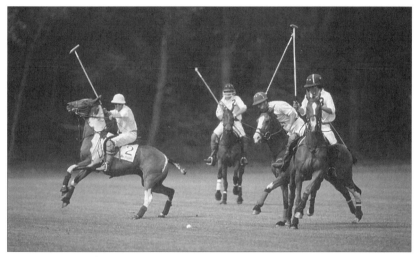

Fig. 11–8. Strenuous exercise creates extreme loading forces that may overstretch the tendons.

Overextension of the fetlock and knee leads to overstretching of the flexor tendons, which can cause individual tendon fibers to break. Repeated bouts of intense exercise, especially in unfit or improperly conditioned horses, can lead to disruption of a large number of fibers. This disruption may be gradual, over a period of weeks or months, or it may be sudden. The result is hemorrhage and edema (accumulation of tissue fluid) within the tendon, which causes obvious swelling in the injured area. The pressure that builds up can further damage the tendon by disrupting the cross-links between undamaged collagen fibers, and obstructing blood flow to the damaged area.

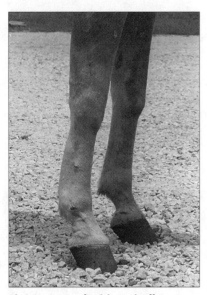

Fig. 11–9. Tendonitis typically occurs in the middle third of the SDFT.

Structural Factors

Most cases of tendonitis occur in the middle third of the SDFT. This tendon is narrower in the middle than it is at the top, and it becomes broader and flatter as it nears the fetlock. So, the middle third of the tendon is the weaker area. Also, because it branches and ends just below the fetlock, the SDFT forms a sling for the back of the fetlock. Fetlock over-extension stretches the SDFT more than the DDFT, which continues straight down the back of the fetlock and pastern.

The tendon's blood supply may also play a part in the development of tendonitis. The top third of the tendon is supplied with blood vessels from the back of the knee, and the bottom third with vessels from the back of the fetlock. The fibers in the middle third of the tendon are relatively poorly supplied with blood, especially in the core of the tendon. This part of the tendon must rely on the tiny vessels that infiltrate from the outer covering (peritendon). Compromise of this meager blood supply can cause the collagen-producing cells to die. This weakens the tendon's structure and makes fiber damage more likely at this location. The poor blood supply is also one of the main reasons why tendons heal slowly.

Other Factors

Tendonitis is an intensity-related condition. It is seen more often in horses that gallop or jump: activities that put a lot of strain on the flexor tendons. However, there are other factors that may increase the likelihood of tendonitis in any horse, including:

- faulty conformation—e.g. long, sloping pasterns and the long toe–low heel foot shape *(see Chapter 7)*
- improper trimming and shoeing
- toe grabs *(see Chapter 7)*
- lack of fitness, leading to flexor muscle fatigue
- poor work surface—e.g. very uneven or slippery footing

Each of these factors can contribute to tendonitis because they encourage overextension of the fetlock and knee during strenuous exercise. These factors can add up to increase the chance of tendon injury. For example, an under-conditioned racehorse with the long toe–low heel foot shape is more likely to bow a tendon than a fit horse with normal feet.

Direct trauma to the tendon can cause a small area of hemorrhage and inflammation within the tendon, but it generally does not cause fiber disruption. Examples include interference from a hindfoot, and being struck with a polo mallet.

A tight bandage can cause swelling around the tendon that may be mistaken for a bowed tendon. This problem, which is called a "bandage bow," is the result of pressure-related damage. Usually it just involves the skin and tissue beneath, not the tendon. *(Managing "bandage bows" is discussed in Chapter 13.)*

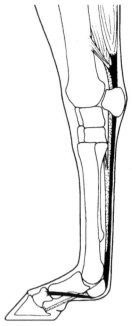

Fig. 11–10. Overextension of the fetlock and knee can overstretch the SDFT (in black).

Signs of Tendonitis

The signs of acute tendonitis include swelling, heat, and pain during palpation of the tendon. Mild or early cases of tendonitis may not have obvious swelling, although heat and pain during palpation are usually found on careful examination. In these cases the lameness is generally mild (grade 1 – 2 of 5). More severe cases have obvious swelling of the tendon and a moderate lameness (grade 2 – 3 of 5). The damaged tendon feels a little more firm than normal, and light pressure causes pain.

Sometimes it is difficult to determine which structure is involved just by looking at, or running a hand down the leg. The leg must be lifted and each tendon carefully palpated from the base of the knee to the bottom of the fetlock. The branches of the SDFT should not be overlooked. One or both may have been damaged as well as the body of the tendon. It is also worth palpating the DDFT as it runs down the back of the pastern, until it disappears between the heel bulbs. The inferior check ligament and suspensory ligament should also be

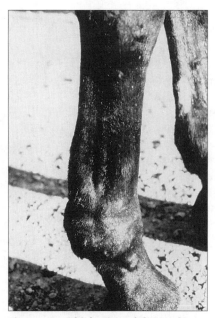

Fig. 11–11. Thickening of the tendon often remains after it has healed.

palpated. The forces that damaged the SDFT may also have caused less obvious damage in these other structures.

It is important to thoroughly examine the tendons of both legs to compare the size, temperature, and texture of the tendons. Tendonitis usually occurs in only one leg, but it is always worth checking both legs.

Thickening of the tendon often remains after it has healed, although there is generally no lameness, heat, or pain during palpation. The thickened tendon feels firm and fibrous (even "woody"), in contrast to the more elastic texture of normal tendon.

Diagnosis of Tendonitis

Diagnosing tendonitis begins with the history—especially the stage of training and recent activity—and the signs. If the history is inconclusive, it is important to inspect the skin over the swollen area. There may be a small mark on the skin if the inflammation is due to direct trauma.

It is easy to miss or disregard the early signs of tendonitis, so examination of the tendons must be thorough. It is important to note that *the amount of tendon damage is usually greater than the lameness indicates.* That means the degree of lameness is not a reliable way to determine the severity of the tendon injury. Extensive fiber disruption may have occurred, yet the horse may only be grade 2 of 5 lame. It is also easy to be deceived by the small amount (or absence) of swelling and heat if the horse has been treated with anti-inflammatory medications or cold therapy.

Ultrasonography

Wherever possible, ultrasonography *(see Chapter 2)* should be used to determine whether fiber disruption has occurred, and if so, to what extent. This is important in deciding how to manage the condition. Without the ultrasound image the veterinarian can only guess as to the presence and extent of fiber damage.

If ultrasonography is not available, the severity of the signs must be used to determine whether fiber disruption is a possibility. The more severe the swelling, heat, pain, and lameness, the more likely that tendon fibers have been damaged.

Although the collagen fibers are microscopic, areas of fiber disruption can be seen on ultrasound as dark patches within the white, speckled substance of the tendon. The dark area occurs because some tendon fibers are broken and the remaining fibers are separated by the blood and tissue fluid that builds up in the defect. Veterinarians usually grade tendon lesions from 1 to 4, based on the lesion's darkness. A grade 1 lesion is a very faint, darker area within the tendon. Most of the tendon fibers are intact, and only separated by a small amount of fluid. At the other extreme, a grade 4 lesion is a solid black area. Most or all of the tendon fibers are torn and the defect is filled with blood and tissue fluid. In most cases there is also obvious thickening of the tendon at that location.

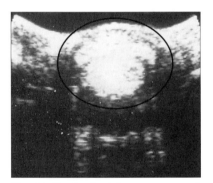 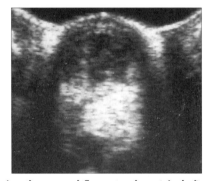

Fig. 11–12. On the left, a sonogram showing the normal flexor tendons (circled) at the back of the cannon. On the right, a grade 3 lesion in the SDFT.

The veterinarian also estimates how much of the tendon's width and length are affected. For example, the tendon injury may be defined as a grade 3 lesion, which takes up about 40% of the tendon's width, and runs for about 2 inches (5 cm). Basically, the more extensive the lesion (in width or length), the worse the prognosis. The lesion's location is recorded, and pictures of the ultrasound image are taken for later reference.

Unfortunately, ultrasonography is not 100% accurate at identifying

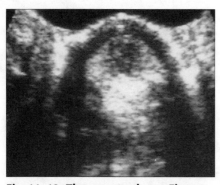

Fig. 11–13. The same tendon as Figure 11–12, right. As the tendon heals, the defect fills in with collagen fibers.

very small areas of fiber breakage, or areas in which only a few fibers are damaged. That is, it cannot always identify mild or early tendonitis. Nevertheless, it is the most useful diagnostic tool available. A trainer's fingers may be very sensitive at detecting the early signs of pain, heat, and mild swelling. However, it is impossible to tell whether there is any fiber disruption. Ultrasonography is needed to obtain this information.

Ultrasonography is also valuable for monitoring healing and determining when the horse is ready to return to training. As it heals, the defect fills in with collagen fibers. Over time it begins to look more like the surrounding tendon.

Treatment of Tendonitis

Healing Process

Tendon injuries heal slowly because tendons have a relatively poor blood supply, especially in the most commonly damaged area. Also, there is constant tension on them while the horse is standing and moving. With moderate to severe injuries it takes several months for the "repair" tissue to fill in the defect and reach maximum strength.

The tendon heals by replacing the damaged fibers with new collagen fibers. However, if left to itself, the healed tendon is not as strong as an undamaged tendon, for two reasons. First, the new collagen fibers are slightly different from the original tendon collagen. The new collagen is more like fibrous tissue, which is not as strong or "elastic" as healthy tendon tissue. Second, the new collagen fibers are laid down in a crisscross pattern. Although this effectively fills in the defect, the tendon is not as strong or resilient as when the fibers are aligned lengthwise, along the line of greatest tension. So, even though the lesion seems to disappear on ultrasound, the healed area is weaker than before the injury. As a result, the tendon is more vulnerable to re-injury.

Because of these factors, time and rest from training and competition are essential for a successful outcome. The length of time the horse must spend out of training, and the amount of activity it is allowed during that time, depend on the severity of the injury and how quickly the tendon heals.

Mild Tendonitis

When ultrasonography does not reveal obvious fiber disruption, conservative management is usually recommended. It involves:

- rest in a stall or small paddock
- hand-walking twice per day
- anti-inflammatory treatment for 3 – 5 days
- support bandage for 3 – 5 days, unless the swelling was caused by a "bandage bow"

Any swelling, heat, or pain—no matter how mild it is—should be taken as a sign that there has been excessive strain on the tendon, whether or not the horse is lame. (That is, unless the tendon swelling was simply caused by a knock.) Ultrasonography cannot detect small areas of fiber disruption, so if there is any doubt about the integrity of the tendon, the horse should be rested from regular training.

Note
The following therapeutic options are covered in more detail in Section II: Principles of Therapy.

Rest

The veterinarian may specify a rest period from 1 to 8 weeks, depending on the history and the injury. The horse can be gradually returned to regular training after the veterinarian has re-examined the tendon and found it to be normal. It is not worth returning the horse to training any sooner. Impatience is usually rewarded with more serious injury to the tendon.

Hand-walking for 20 – 30 minutes twice per day is very good for a healing tendon. It improves blood flow and limits adhesions (fibrous bands) between the tendon and surrounding tissues. Hand-walking can begin the day after injury, and should continue for as long as the horse is confined.

Anti-inflammatory Therapy

Anti-inflammatory therapies are usually only of value, and in fact should only be necessary for the first 3 – 5 days. These therapies include ice packs, cold hosing, NSAIDs, DMSO, and "sweats." Corticosteroids should not be used to treat tendonitis because they slow the rate of tendon repair. They may also mask the signs of inflammation once work resumes.

A firm, but not tight bandage can also reduce swelling in the first few days after injury. If pressure from a tight bandage caused a "bandage bow," any further bandaging should be left to the veterinarian, especially if pressure sores have developed *(see Chapter 13).*

Return to Training

Unless the tendon was merely bruised, the return to full training should be gradual, rather than simply resuming the horse's previous level of exercise. It is usually safe to use the length of time the horse was rested as a general guide. For example, if the horse was rested for 2 weeks, it should then receive at least 2 weeks of gradually increasing exercise before resuming its normal activities. If the horse was rested for 8 weeks, the return to normal activities should take at least 8 weeks. This period not only allows the newly-healed tendon to strengthen, it ensures that the horse's fitness improves before strenuous exercise resumes.

These tendons must be monitored closely once regular exercise begins. Any amount of heat, swelling, or pain is a sign that the tendon is being overloaded. If any of these signs are seen, the horse should be rested and the veterinarian called to re-evaluate the tendon. The trainer may also need to review the training program and modify the amount of fast work or jumping accordingly.

Moderate to Severe Tendonitis

The management of moderate to severe tendonitis depends on the degree of fiber disruption, and on the horse's use. Small areas of complete fiber disruption may heal well with conservative management: rest, anti-inflammatory therapy, and the rehabilitation program described below. This approach is more likely to be successful in a pleasure horse than a racehorse.

But conservative management of a tendon with more extensive fiber disruption is often disappointing in athletic horses. Even 12 months of pasture rest (a traditional recommendation) may not result in a tendon that can withstand athletic training and competition. When fiber disruption is suspected or is seen on ultrasound, surgery is the best option.

Surgery

Two different procedures may be used; some veterinarians recommend both at the same time.

Tendon Splitting

Tendon splitting involves making several small incisions into the tendon with a scalpel blade. This must be done either under local or general anesthesia. The procedure has three benefits:

1. It drains the blood and tissue fluid that has accumulated within the lesion, relieving pressure in the tendon. If the pressure is not relieved, the cross-links between the undamaged fibers may be broken, which further weakens the tendon.
2. The hole fills in much more quickly if the fluid-filled lesion is "deflated."
3. The small incisions cause mild inflammation, which may improve blood supply from the edge of the tendon into the damaged area.

This procedure does the most good in the first 3 – 5 days. After this time the fluid in the lesion forms a clot that does not drain through the small incisions. Nevertheless, the procedure may still be of some benefit in older lesions because it stimulates blood flow to the damaged area.

After surgery, a sterile dressing is placed over the incisions (which are too small to require sutures). The leg is kept bandaged for about a week, and the bandage is changed as needed. Antibiotics may or may not be given, but NSAIDs are usually prescribed for a few days, for the horse's comfort. The horse's tetanus status should be checked before surgery *(see Chapter 5)*.

It is often remarkable how quickly the tendon's appearance on ultrasound improves in the days and weeks after tendon splitting. Although there has been little scientific research on this procedure, most veterinarians who routinely use it agree that it can significantly speed up tendon healing.

Check Desmotomy

The other common surgical procedure involves cutting the check ligament that stabilizes the affected flexor tendon. This procedure is called a desmotomy ("cutting a ligament"), and it is performed under general anesthesia. The check ligament's role is to protect the tendon and muscle from being overstretched. However, once the damaged tendon has healed with inelastic fibrous tissue, the check ligament can reduce the amount the muscle-tendon unit can lengthen during exercise. As a result, the vulnerable tendon is more likely to be overstretched again.

After the desmotomy, the check ligament heals and rejoins, although it is a little longer than before the surgery. This small increase

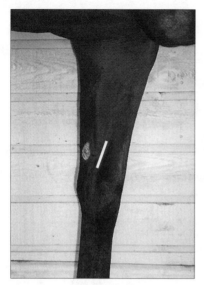

Fig. 11–14. The site for superior check desmotomy.

in length gives the muscle-tendon unit an extra ¾ inch or so of "give" before the fibers are overstretched.

For horses with SDF tendonitis, the superior check ligament is cut a few inches above the knee, on the inside of the leg. Some surgeons cut the superior check ligament in both forelegs, even though only one leg may have tendonitis. The reasoning behind this is that even after the tendon has healed, the horse shifts some of its weight onto the "good" leg, making it more prone to tendonitis. So, the desmotomy is therapeutic in one leg and preventive in the other leg.

The check desmotomy can be performed at the same time as the tendon splitting procedure, although some surgeons prefer not to perform the desmotomy until the tendon lesion has healed and the horse has started light work. The reason is that if the tendon cannot stand up to light work on its own, the desmotomy is unlikely to prevent re-injury during strenuous exercise.

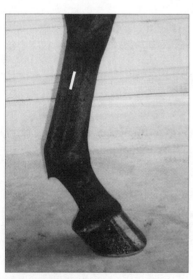

Fig. 11–15. The site for inferior check desmotomy.

Horses with DDF tendonitis may benefit from an inferior check desmotomy. The inferior check ligament can be cut anywhere along its length, although it is usually safest to perform the desmotomy about one-third of the way down the cannon, just before the ligament attaches onto the DDFT.

Post-Operative Care. After either procedure the leg is kept bandaged until the sutures are removed, usually about 7 – 10 days after surgery. NSAIDs are usually given for at least 4 – 5 days after surgery, and antibiotics are also prescribed for a few days. The horse's tetanus status should be checked before surgery.

Swelling may develop around the surgery site, and a seroma may form beneath the suture line after the superior check desmotomy. It takes quite a bit of tissue dissection to expose the check ligament, and the space that is created in the tissues fills with serum after the surgery. This is usually not a major problem;

Definitions
Seroma: collection of serum beneath the skin or within the tissues. **Serum:** clear, yellow, liquid portion of the blood.

the body absorbs the fluid in about 4 – 5 days, and the final cosmetic result generally is excellent. To prevent or limit seroma formation, some surgeons apply a thick pad or roll of gauze directly over the incision. The pad is then bandaged firmly in place for a few days.

Most surgeons recommend keeping the horse confined for at least a week after surgery, or longer if there are problems with the surgical site. During that time the horse should be hand-walked for 10 – 15 minutes twice per day, beginning 1 – 2 days after surgery.

Rehabilitation

Phase I: Light Exercise

The tendon will not heal without rest from *vigorous* exercise. However, *light* exercise, such as hand-walking, is very important during healing. The collagen fibers that repair the defect tend to be laid down in a crisscross pattern. Gentle exercise puts light tension on the healing tendon, which encourages the body to lay down the new collagen fibers in the direction of tension (lengthwise). This improves the strength and resilience of the healed tendon, making re-injury less likely.

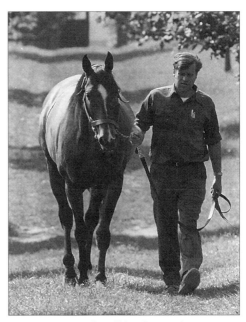

Fig. 11–16. Hand-walking is very important while the tendon is healing.

Activity has some other benefits. It improves blood flow to the injured tendon, and reduces the potential for adhesions to form. It also prevents the tendon from shortening as it heals. Fibrous tissue contracts a little as it matures. After a SDFT injury, this can shorten the tendon, causing the horse to become "over at the knee" or "tied in at the knee."

The amount of exercise a horse gets in a pasture can vary; sometimes it is too little, other times too much. Stall or small paddock rest combined with daily hand-walking usually has far better results than pasture turnout. As the tendon heals, the duration of each walking session can be gradually increased to 30 – 40 minutes twice per day.

Hand-walking should continue for at least 12 weeks—the minimum time it takes for the repair tissue to fill in the defect and reach peak strength. Healing is best monitored with ultrasonography. If the defect is still visible at 12 weeks post-injury, hand-walking should continue until the lesion has completely resolved.

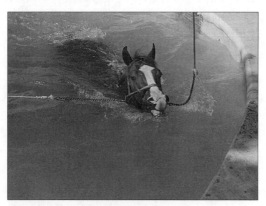

Swimming gently stretches the tendon without overloading it. However, it should not begin until after 4 weeks post-injury or -surgery because it can be too strenuous for the healing tendon. Also, bacteria from the water can infect the surgical wound if it is not completely healed before swimming is started.

Fig. 11–17. Swimming gently stretches the tendon without overloading it.

Phase II: Gradual Return to Normal Activities

Once physical examination and ultrasonography indicate that the tendon lesion has healed, then ridden/driven exercise can begin. The exercise program should start with only 10 – 15 minutes of walking and slow jogging, and very gradually build up to normal training activities. *It is essential that the load on the damaged tendon is increased slowly,* over at least 3 months. The tendon must be allowed to strengthen before high-speed work or jumping is introduced.

Damaged tendons often bow again. Another common occurrence is tendonitis in the other leg because the horse protects the injured leg by transferring more of its weight to the "good" leg. Slowly returning the

Graded Exercise Program for Horses With Tendonitis

Phase I

Amount   Start with 10 – 15 minutes of hand-walking twice per day.
Gradually increase to 30 – 40 minutes twice per day.

Duration   Until the tendon lesion has filled in on ultrasound.
Usually takes 3 – 4 months.

Purpose   Allows the lesion to fill in with new collagen fibers.
Improves blood flow and prevents adhesions.
Aligns the new fibers lengthwise for greatest strength.

Phase II

Amount   Start with walking and jogging for 10 – 15 minutes once
or twice per day.
Gradually increase to trotting and cantering.

Duration   Minimum of 3 months.

Purpose   Allows the healed tendon to strengthen before more
strenuous activities are resumed.
Improves the horse's fitness.

Fig. 11–18.

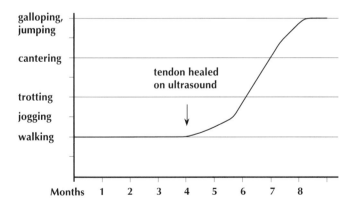

Fig. 11–19. The return to strenuous exercise must be gradual.

horse to full work reduces the chance of these problems occurring.

Before and after each exercise session the tendons should be carefully palpated for signs of pain, heat, or swelling. If any of these signs are noticed, or if the horse feels a little "off," the exercise program should be suspended. Hand-walking should be resumed until the veterinarian can re-examine and re-ultrasound the tendon.

Other Treatments

Several other treatments have been tried to improve the rate and quality of tendon healing.

Hyaluronic Acid

Some veterinarians inject hyaluronic acid into or around the tendon to reduce inflammation, promote healing, and limit adhesion formation. It is moderately successful in some horses.

Physical Therapies

Physical therapies, including "cold" laser, therapeutic ultrasound, and magnetic field therapy, are used to treat acute and chronic tendon injuries. These techniques may speed healing by improving blood flow to the injured tendon. However, because of this effect, they should not be started until 3 – 4 days after injury. Improving blood flow can increase bleeding into the damaged area. These therapies are more successful on mild, acute tendon injuries than on severe tendonitis or old, fibrous lesions.

Shoeing

In the past, veterinarians and farriers recommended raised heel shoes or wedge pads to relieve tension on the flexor tendons. However, it has now been proven that raising the heels does not reduce tension on the superficial flexor tendon unless they are raised several inches. But raising the heels this much can result in a shortened tendon. It is usually best just to aim for a normal hoof-pastern angle in horses with tendonitis, particularly in those with the long toe–low heel foot shape. A shoe that adequately supports the heels is best once training resumes. *(Shoeing options are discussed in Chapter 7.)*

BAPN-F

An experimental drug, called BAPN-F, has been studied in horses with acute tendonitis. When injected into the tendon lesion, it prevents new collagen fibers from cross-linking with other fibers for a couple of weeks. If combined with hand-walking, the drug gives the new collagen fibers a chance to align themselves lengthwise along the tendon before they cross-link with other fibers. As a result, the defect in the tendon fills in with correctly-aligned fibers. This drug is showing promise in improving the quality of tendon healing.

Prognosis for Tendonitis

The prognosis for long-term athletic usefulness is good for tendonitis that does not involve obvious fiber disruption. It is also fairly good for small defects that heal rapidly and completely. However, in every case of tendonitis that involves fiber disruption there is always the potential for the tendon to "bow" again, particularly if the horse is returned to training too quickly.

The long-term prognosis for moderate to severe tendonitis depends on the injury and the treatment method used. In most cases that are managed conservatively, 50% – 60% return to full function. This figure rises to 70% – 80% with surgery and proper rehabilitation.

The prognosis depends to some degree on the horse's use. For example, tendonitis is less likely to limit a medium level dressage horse than a three-day-eventer. The difference lies in the amount of stress the tendon must withstand during training and competition.

Although surgery can reduce the risk of re-injury, the most important factor in returning the horse to full function is daily light exercise as the tendon heals. The time spent rehabilitating the tendon is the best investment the owner/trainer makes in the horse's future.

Prevention of Tendonitis

Tendonitis may be prevented, and the chances of re-injury reduced by:

- regular trimming and shoeing by an experienced farrier so that a normal hoof-pastern angle is maintained and the heels are always well supported
- using exercise bandages that restrict fetlock overextension *(see Chapter 8)*
- feeling the tendons for swelling, pain, or heat before and after each training session or competition
- suspending training at the first sign of swelling, pain, or heat in a tendon
- ensuring that "slow, distance work" is the basis of the horse's training schedule, no matter what the sport or activity

TENDON LACERATIONS & RUPTURE
Flexor Tendons

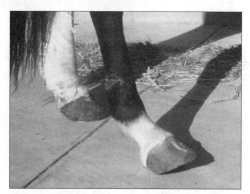

Fig. 11–20. This laceration has severed the flexor tendons.

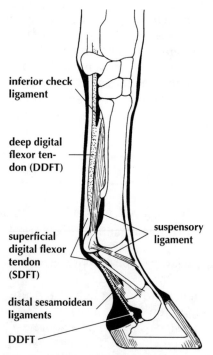

inferior check ligament

deep digital flexor tendon (DDFT)

superficial digital flexor tendon (SDFT)

suspensory ligament

distal sesamoidean ligaments

DDFT

Fig. 11–21. The fetlock's support structures.

Because of their relatively exposed location at the back of the leg, the flexor tendons may be partially or completely severed with wounds that involve the lower leg. The most common offending objects are fencing wire and sheet metal. The wound may look small, but it only takes a cut about ¾ inch (1.8 cm) wide to sever the flexor tendons. Any wound that completely cuts through the skin at the back of the cannon should be looked at carefully. If there is any question whether the tendons are damaged, the veterinarian should be called immediately. *(First-aid for a wound that exposes or involves the flexor tendons is covered in Chapter 13.)*

Although it is uncommon, the flexor tendons can be ruptured by extreme overstretching. This injury can occur during strenuous exercise if the tendon is already weakened by tendonitis.

Flexor tendon lacerations or rupture are very serious injuries. Not only are these tendons essential for normal movement, they also make up part of the "stay apparatus" of the leg—they support the fetlock and pastern joints. If one or both tendons is completely severed or ruptured, excess strain is placed on the other major structures that support the fetlock: the suspensory ligament and the distal sesamoidean ligaments. When these structures are overloaded, the stay apparatus of the fetlock can completely break down. The fetlock drops and the horse is unable to bear weight on the leg. *(The fetlock's support structures and "break-down" injuries are discussed further in Chapter 16.)*

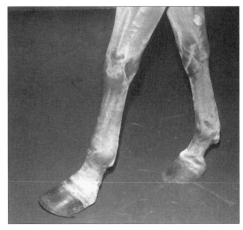

Fig. 11–22. Lacerated DDFT: the toe has tipped up, but the fetlock has not sunk because the other support structures are intact.

If only the SDFT is severed or ruptured, the normal fetlock angle and foot position may be maintained (although the pastern may knuckle forward). However, this injury increases the burden on the other structures. If the DDFT is also disrupted, the toe tips up and the fetlock sinks when weight is placed on the leg.

Treatment
Surgical Repair

If the ends of the severed tendon can be located the veterinarian may attempt to rejoin them. Non-dissolving suture material is used in a pattern that causes little or no pressure on the outer layer of the tendon, in which the blood vessels run. Suturing a severed tendon is best done under general anesthesia so there is no tension on

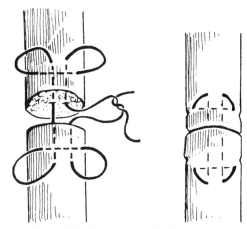

Fig. 11–23. Surgical repair of a severed tendon.

the tendon. Even then, it is sometimes difficult to join the ends because the upper end is pulled upward an inch or two by the flexor muscle. If the tendon is not completely severed, the veterinarian may still reinforce it with sutures. Wherever possible the skin is sutured closed, unless the wound is badly contaminated.

Bacterial infection is a common and serious complication of open wounds involving the tendons. Infection of the repair site reduces the chances of a successful outcome. Therefore, broad-spectrum antibiotics are important in managing tendon lacerations. NSAIDs are usually given to relieve some of the horse's discomfort. Also, the horse's tetanus status should be checked. *(These medications are discussed in Chapter 5.)*

The results of surgical tendon repair are often disappointing. While the horse is bearing weight on the leg, the ends of the severed tendon are being pulled apart. This constant tension on the sutures often causes the surgical repair to fail. Another contributing factor is the relatively poor blood supply to the tendon.

Surgical repair of a ruptured flexor tendon usually is impossible. When a tendon ruptures under extreme tension, the ends fray like a piece of rope. It is very difficult to make sutures hold in such damaged tissue. Also, the blood vessels to that part of the tendon usually are destroyed. These serious injuries are managed with a support bandage or cast, special shoes, and several months of rest.

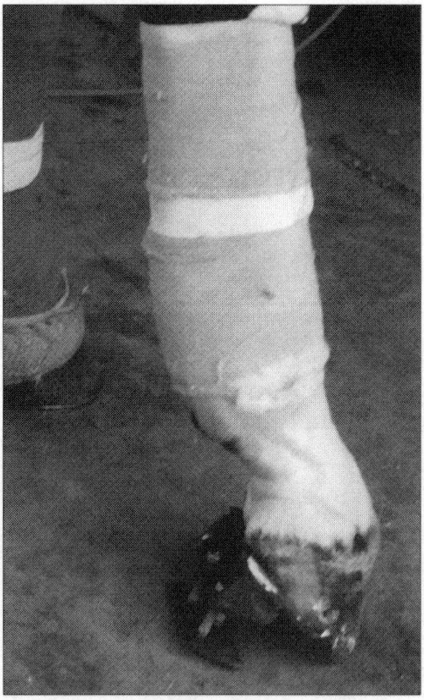

When the stay apparatus breaks down completely, surgical fusion (arthrodesis) of the fetlock has a better outcome than casting.

Bandaging and Shoeing

To support the repaired tendon and reduce tension on the sutures, and in horses with a ruptured tendon, the veterinarian may apply a fiberglass cast for a few weeks *(see Chapter 6)*. If a thick bandage is used instead of a cast, the horse's heels should be raised at least 2 inches (5 cm) with a special shoe. This measure reduces tension on

Fig. 11–24. A raised heel shoe reduces tension on the tendon.

the tendon, and therefore on the suture line. Even if the tendon was not completely severed or ruptured, a thick bandage and raised heel shoe are good precautions. For injuries just to the DDFT, a level shoe with a long heel extension can stop the toe from tipping up and pulling on the tendon.

The length of time the leg must remain cast or bandaged depends on the severity of the injury and how quickly the tendon is healing. The veterinarian re-evaluates the tendon every 3 – 4 weeks and bases further treatment decisions on this information. In most cases the raised heel shoe is lowered by about an inch each time the horse is reshod (every 4 – 6 weeks). It is very important that the heels are lowered gradually. Suddenly lowering the heels to normal can place excessive tension on the healing tendon, which may result in tendon rupture.

> **More Information**
>
> Raised heel shoes, heel extensions, and other shoeing options are covered in Chapter 7.

Rest and Rehabilitation

The horse should be confined to a stall for at least 3 months after complete tendon laceration or rupture. This is the minimum time it takes for the "repair" tissue to fill in the defect and reach peak strength. Unlike horses with tendonitis, in which most of the tendon fibers are intact, *hand-walking is not recommended* for the first 2 – 3 months following a complete tendon laceration or rupture. The tendon needs this time to bridge the gap with collagen fibers. Although hand-walking may help align the fibers properly, the direction in which the fibers are aligned is of little importance if the repair site is not strong enough to resist being pulled apart.

Tendon healing can be monitored with ultrasonography. This is the best way to determine when the horse is ready to begin exercising. Once the tendon has healed, the rehabilitation program outlined earlier for horses with tendonitis can begin. As an alternative, the horse can be turned out into a large paddock or pasture for a further 6 – 9 months, depending on the severity of the injury and the horse's intended use. However, as with tendonitis, daily hand-walking generally has a better outcome than pasture turnout.

The same preventive measures outlined earlier for horses recovering from tendonitis also apply to horses returning to light exercise after a flexor tendon laceration or rupture.

Prognosis for Flexor Tendon Lacerations and Rupture

In every case where both flexor tendons are completely severed or ruptured, the prognosis for future athletic function is poor. For all the care the surgeon takes with placing the sutures, the suture material can pull through the tendon because of the tension on the repair site. Also, the collagen that crosses the defect is never as strong or elastic as undamaged tendon fibers, so tendon rupture is always a risk. If there is complete breakdown of the fetlock's stay apparatus, the best that can be achieved is a "pasture-sound" horse.

If just the SDFT is damaged, the prognosis is a little better, provided the DDFT and other supporting structures are intact and the wound heals without infection or other complications. Nevertheless, the chances of a horse performing very athletic activities, such as racing or show jumping, are not good.

Extensor Tendon Lacerations

Wounds anywhere along the front of the leg can sever the extensor tendon. The most frequent location is at the front of the hock—a very common wound site in pastured horses. Horses can usually walk fairly well with a severed extensor tendon, although they land toe-first and tend to knuckle over onto front of the fetlock. Once they learn that they have to lift the leg a little higher to bring the foot forward, they can walk almost normally. This injury does not prevent them from bearing weight on the leg.

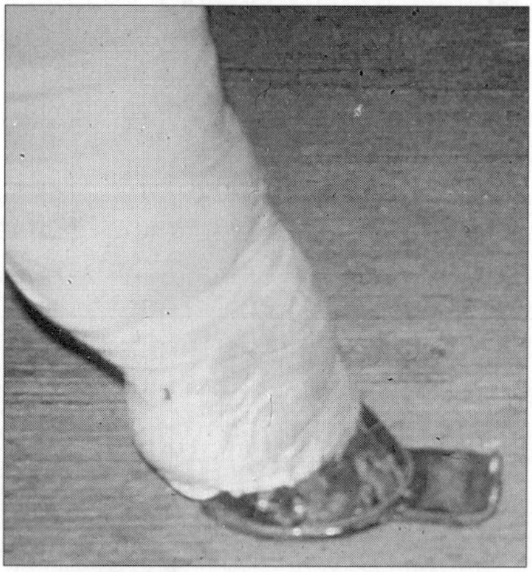

Fig. 11–25. Treating an extensor tendon laceration with a toe extension and a thick support bandage.

Extensor tendon lacerations generally heal well without surgery. In fact, suturing the severed tendon is usually unsuccessful because of the tension on the sutures whenever the horse flexes its leg. So treatment simply involves managing the primary wound *(see Chapter 13)*. If the horse is having trouble bringing the foot forward and placing it flat, a shoe with a toe extension can help prevent knuckling and tripping. But if the horse knuckles over with this shoe on, it is even more difficult for it to bring the foot forward. For this reason, some veterinarians prefer simply to keep a thick support bandage on the lower leg (from the base of the knee or hock down to the hoof) until the horse learns to compensate. The bandage acts like a cast to restrict fetlock flexion. As the primary wound heals, the ends of the tendon may rejoin to some extent, so normal function can be regained.

In most cases the prognosis for a return to full athletic function is very good, provided the primary wound heals uneventfully and does not involve any other important structures, such as a joint or bone.

TENOSYNOVITIS
Definition

Reminder
Tendon sheath: thin sheath that surrounds and lubricates a tendon as it travels over a joint; it has a lining that produces fluid.

Tenosynovitis is inflammation of a tendon sheath. Inflammation of the sheath (or its contents) results in effusion—fluid accumulation—within the tendon sheath. When this fluidy swelling occurs at the back of the fetlock, it is often called a "wind puff" or "wind gall." A similar swelling can occur over the front of the knee and at the back of the hock (where it is called thoroughpin).

Although tenosynovitis can occur in any tendon sheath, this discussion is limited to tenosynovitis of the flexor tendon sheath at the back of the fetlock. The same treatment principles also apply to other tendon sheaths.

Causes

Tenosynovitis can be acute—it first developed a few hours or days ago. Or it can be chronic—it has been present for weeks, months, or even years.

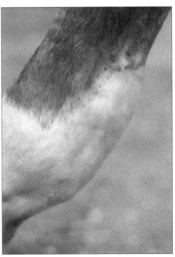

Fig. 11–26. Tenosynovitis of the flexor tendon sheath at the back of the fetlock.

Acute Tenosynovitis

Acute tenosynovitis may be further classified as either primary or secondary. Primary tenosynovitis occurs alone, whereas secondary tenosynovitis occurs as a result of another problem.

Primary tenosynovitis is the result of strain and inflammation of the tendon sheath itself. In the flexor tendon sheath it is due to over-extension of the fetlock during strenuous exercise. Suddenly wrenching the fetlock by stepping in a hole, for example, can also strain the tendon sheath.

Secondary tenosynovitis (or simply tendon sheath effusion) is usually caused by one of two conditions:

1. **Tendonitis of the SDFT or DDFT** in the part of the tendon that is within the sheath (a "low bow"). Inflammation of the tendon can cause secondary inflammation of the sheath lining. Or, it may simply cause the lining to produce more fluid in an effort to dilute the harmful inflammatory substances *(see Chapter 5).*

2. **Inflammation and thickening of the annular ligament** that wraps around the back of the fetlock. The thickened annular ligament may cause effusion simply by restricting the normal flow of fluid down the tendon sheath and forcing it to accumulate above the site of restriction. However, inflammation of the ligament may also cause inflammation of the tendon sheath. *Annular ligament damage (annular desmitis) is discussed in Chapter 16.*

(Infection of the sheath—septic tenosynovitis—also causes effusion. This condition is discussed later.)

Chronic Tenosynovitis

Most owners and trainers think of "wind puffs" or "wind galls" as mere blemishes. However, *effusion in a tendon sheath is not normal.* It may just be the result of an episode of acute tenosynovitis that occurred in the past. When acute tenosynovitis is untreated, the effusion may persist and the tendon sheath may become stretched. From then on the sheath remains filled to its new capacity.

However, chronic tenosynovitis may also be due to repeated strain of the tendon sheath or persistence of the primary problem—tendonitis or annular ligament constriction. So, it should not be assumed that all cases of chronic tenosynovitis are unimportant.

Signs of Tenosynovitis

Tendon sheath effusion causes a well-defined, soft, fluid-filled swelling at the back of the fetlock. It extends about 2 – 3 inches (5 – 7.5 cm) above the sesamoid bones. It is important to distinguish between fetlock joint effusion and tendon sheath effusion. The location of the swelling helps determine which structure is involved. Fetlock joint effusion pouches out between the back of the cannon bone and the suspensory ligament branches. Tendon sheath effusion pouches out between the suspensory branches and the flexor tendons. In some cases there is also a small pouch of fluid at the back of the pastern, over the deep flexor tendon.

In primary acute tenosynovitis, there may be heat and mild pain detected during palpation, particularly at the

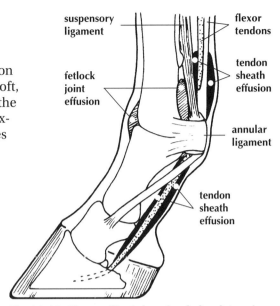

Fig. 11–27. The swelling's location helps determine which structure is involved.

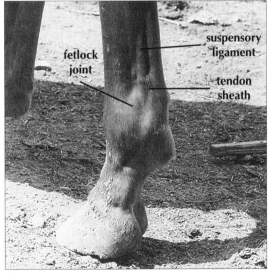

Fig. 11–28. Locations where fetlock joint and tendon sheath effusion are seen.

top of the sheath where it attaches onto the flexor tendons. The lameness is usually mild (grade 1 – 2 of 5). If tendon sheath effusion is caused by tendonitis or annular desmitis, the swollen sheath may not be hot or painful. However, careful palpation of the tendons or annular ligament may reveal thickening, heat, and pain. Lameness usually is mild to moderate (grade 2 – 3 of 5), depending on the severity of the injury.

In many cases of chronic tenosynovitis there is no pain, heat, or lameness. But if any of these signs are seen, it means that there is active inflammation involving the sheath, flexor tendons, or annular ligament.

Diagnosis of Tenosynovitis

Diagnosis is based on the history (especially the stage of training and recent activity) and the signs. The length of time the effusion has been present separates acute from chronic tenosynovitis.

Ultrasonography is useful for identifying flexor tendon or annular ligament damage. Also, the veterinarian can assess the nature of the fluid and check for adhesions between the tendons and the lining of the sheath.

Definition
Fibrin: blood-clotting protein that can form fibrous bands, or adhesions.

Severe inflammation of the tendon sheath lining can allow fibrin to leak into the sheath. Bands of fibrin can then cause adhesions between the sheath and the tendons. Normally, the tendon sheath fluid forms a thin, black halo around the flexor tendons. Adhesions or other debris within the inflamed sheath appear as white bands or flecks within an enlarged area of black fluid.

Unless the horse is very lame and the swelling is hot and very painful (signs of septic tenosynovitis), there is little to be gained by analyzing the tendon sheath fluid.

Treatment of Tenosynovitis
Acute Tenosynovitis

For the first few days after injury, treatment should involve:

• confinement
• hand-walking
• anti-inflammatory therapy
• bandaging

These treatments are discussed in the earlier section on *Mild Tendonitis.*

After the first few days the horse can either be hand-walked twice per day or simply rested in a large paddock or pasture (unless the tenosynovitis is secondary to tendon or annular ligament injury). Horses with primary tenosynovitis can be returned to regular exercise after about 6 weeks of rest. More vigorous exercise before this time may result in persistence of the problem.

Some veterinarians drain the fluid from the sheath and then apply a firm bandage to the leg. This procedure can improve the cosmetic appearance of the leg, although if the inflammation persists, the effusion will return once bandaging stops. Injecting corticosteroids *(see Chapter 5)* into the sheath after drainage can reduce inflammation and prevent adhesions. However, these drugs slow healing, so they should not be used if there is tendon damage. They should also not be used if there is any risk of infection within or around the sheath (for example, if there is a wound near the sheath).

Hyaluronic acid *(see Chapter 5)* can be injected into the sheath to help reduce inflammation and prevent adhesions. This drug is not as effective as corticosteroids in reducing inflammation, but neither does it have the drawbacks of slowed healing and the potential for infection. *(Treating annular desmitis is discussed in Chapter 16.)*

Chronic Tenosynovitis

If the horse is lame, treatment of chronic tenosynovitis should follow the same guidelines as acute tenosynovitis: rest, hand-walking, and anti-inflammatory therapy. If tendonitis or annular desmitis is part of the problem, the specific treatment recommendations given in the relevant sections should be followed.

Annular ligament constriction can cause persistent tendon sheath effusion and low-grade lameness. However, these signs may also be caused by adhesions between the sheath and the tendons cause. Arthroscopic surgery may be necessary to break down the adhesions and remove any damaged tissue within the sheath. After surgery, hyaluronic acid and controlled exercise may help prevent adhesions from reforming.

If a good cosmetic result (no swelling) is important, chronic tenosynovitis can be very difficult, if not impossible to resolve. Even draining and injecting corticosteroids into the sheath, and bandaging the leg usually cannot permanently resolve the effusion.

Prognosis for Tenosynovitis

The prognosis for future athletic usefulness is very good if the tenosynovitis is acute and there is no tendon or annular ligament damage. However, if the condition is not managed properly and the horse is returned to training too soon, the signs may return and the condition could become chronic.

The prognosis for athletic function with chronic tenosynovitis varies. Many of these horses are no longer lame, so the swelling is only of cosmetic importance. But if the horse is lame, or becomes lame with exercise, the prognosis depends on which other tissues (flexor tendons or annular ligament) are damaged.

SEPTIC TENOSYNOVITIS
Definition and Causes

Septic tenosynovitis is bacterial infection of a tendon sheath. In most cases the bacteria enter the sheath through a wound—either traumatic or surgical—or by injection into the sheath. The sheath that surrounds the flexor tendons can also be infected if a nail or piece of wire penetrates the frog and extends into the deeper tissues of the foot *(see Chapter 15)*.

Although any tendon sheath may become infected, this section focuses on the flexor tendon sheath. Managing septic tenosynovitis in other sheaths follows the same principles.

Signs

Septic tenosynovitis causes severe lameness (grade 4 – 5 of 5), particularly if it was caused by a puncture wound in the foot. The fluid is confined within the sheath, and the pressure builds up, causing extreme pain.

There is obvious swelling of the tendon sheath. But because cellulitis is commonly present, the entire lower leg may be swollen. In most cases the swelling is worst at the back of the fetlock and pastern—where the tendon sheath is located. This swelling is hot and very painful during palpation. When the in-

> **More Information**
>
> Cellulitis is bacterial infection of the superficial tissues. It causes a soft, warm, mildly painful swelling. *See Chapter 13 for more information.*

fection begins in the upper part of the sheath, the swelling extends from the heel bulbs to above the fetlock. But when the infection begins in the foot, the swelling may at first only be obvious at the back of the pastern. It may take a few days to progress further up the sheath.

Some horses also have a fever, depression, and loss of appetite—signs of generalized (systemic) infection. But the pain alone may affect the horse's appetite.

> ### More Information
>
> Septic tenosynovitis is very similar to septic arthritis. They share many of the same signs, diagnostic methods, and treatments.
>
> The information in this section is an overview of the more complete section in Chapter 8 on Septic Arthritis.

Diagnosis

The diagnosis is obvious if there is a wound involving the tendon sheath or frog, or if an injection had been given into the sheath in the past 1 – 2 weeks. Otherwise, the signs may be a little confusing unless the swelling is confined to the tendon sheath. Generalized swelling and severe pain can easily be taken for signs of a fracture, so the veterinarian may radiograph the leg. Ultrasonography is often not very helpful, unless there are large, fibrous strands and clumps of debris within the fluid. These horses are usually in so much pain that they cannot tolerate even slight pressure from the ultrasound probe anyway.

If possible, the veterinarian should sample the tendon sheath fluid. The appearance and white cell count are important for diagnosing infection. Some of the fluid should also be submitted for bacterial culture and antibiotic sensitivity testing *(see Chapter 2)*. This test is important for determining which antibiotic(s) will be most effective.

For puncture wounds of the frog, contrast radiography *(see Chapter 2)* of the foot is often used to determine the depth and path of the wound. It is very important to know whether the navicular bone or bursa, the deep flexor tendon and its sheath, or the coffin joint are involved. *(Diagnosing and managing puncture wounds in the foot are discussed in Chapter 15.)*

Treatment
Drainage and Lavage

Treatment involves draining and lavaging (flushing) the sheath with sterile saline solution. It is sometimes best for the veterinarian to make a small incision into the tendon sheath above and below the fetlock to allow the infected material to drain. Two incisions are usually necessary because the annular ligament, which wraps around the back of the fetlock, can prevent the flow of lavage fluid below the fetlock. Also, the infected material in the lower part of the sheath cannot drain from an incision several inches above it. The sheath can be flushed through these incisions as often as necessary until the infection is resolved. A sterile dressing must be kept over the incisions until lavage is no longer necessary and they begin to heal.

Medications

In every case injectable antibiotics are necessary, although giving antibiotics without drainage and lavage is ineffective. The choice of antibiotic should be based on the bacterial culture and antibiotic sensitivity test. But while waiting for the results the veterinarian usually prescribes a broad-spectrum antibiotic combination. The horse's tetanus status must also be checked.

NSAIDs are given to relieve some of the pain, but because these horses are often very lame for several days, the concerns regarding long-term NSAIDs use in horses with serious fractures also apply here. *(This issue is discussed in Chapter 9.)*

Discontinuing the NSAIDs for a few days can be a useful way to gauge the horse's response to therapy. If the signs are reduced 1 – 2 days after the NSAIDs were stopped, conditions within the sheath are improving. However, if the horse is more lame and the sheath is more painful than when it was receiving NSAIDs, treatment must be re-evaluated.

More Information
Medications are discussed in Chapter 5.
Frog support is covered in Chapter 7.
Bandaging is discussed in Chapter 4.

Other Recommendations

The horse should be confined to a well-bedded stall. A frog support and supportive bandage should be kept on the opposite, weight-bearing leg until the horse can bear weight more evenly on both legs.

Activity is important for improving drainage, increasing blood flow, and limiting adhesion formation within the sheath. As soon as the horse is able, it should be hand-walked for short periods (5 –10 minutes) several times per day. Passive flexion and extension of the fetlock can also be performed *(see Chapter 4)*.

Prognosis for Septic Tenosynovitis

The prognosis for athletic usefulness is guarded at best. The infection can be very difficult to control, and adhesions between the sheath and the tendons are likely. Also, the infection may spread to the tendons, further compromising the success of therapy and the horse's career. In some cases the severe pain may necessitate euthanasia for humane reasons. In surviving horses, chronic lameness is a common result.

As with other infectious conditions, the sooner proper treatment begins, the better the result will be.

CHECK LIGAMENT INJURIES

The inferior check ligament (ICL) on the foreleg begins at the back of the knee, runs down the back of the cannon, and attaches onto the DDFT *(see Figure 11–3)*. Its role is to protect the DDFT from excessive strain. But in doing so, the ICL itself is sometimes strained or torn. This produces mild to moderate lameness (grade 1 – 3 of 5) and slight swelling at the back of the cannon, a few inches below the knee. However, this swelling can be difficult to detect.

By carefully palpating the flexor tendons, ICL, and suspensory ligament it may be possible to tell the difference between ICL strain and damage to these other structures. However, a definite diagnosis can only be made with ultrasonography. When the ICL is damaged, it is important to evaluate the origin of the suspensory ligament and the DDFT for signs of fiber disruption. The suspensory ligament often is damaged along with the ICL.

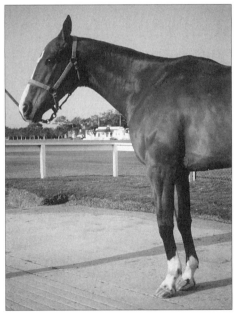

Fig. 11–29. The inferior check ligament may shorten as it heals, causing the horse to become "over at the knee."

Treatment involves rest from regular training, as well as hand-walking and anti-inflammatory therapy. The details are given earlier in the section on *Mild Tendonitis.* If the horse is not hand-walked every day, the fibrous tissue that repairs the damage may shorten the ligament, causing the horse to become "over at the knee" or "tied in at the knee."

Rehabilitation should also follow the guidelines given for horses with tendonitis *(see Figure 11–18).* As with other tendons and ligaments, the ICL heals slowly, especially if fiber disruption occurred. If the lameness persists, the veterinarian may recommend an inferior check desmotomy (discussed earlier), particularly if the DDFT was also damaged.

Definitions
Desmitis: inflammation of a ligament. **Desmotomy:** surgically cutting a ligament.

The prognosis for full return to athletic function is usually good after ICL strain, although the recovery period may be several months. The prognosis is worsened if the DDFT or other structures are also damaged.

SUSPENSORY LIGAMENT DAMAGE

Definition

Damage to the suspensory ligament or its branches is called suspensory desmitis. Fiber disruption is a common feature of suspensory desmitis.

There are two distinct types of suspensory ligament injury:

1. Desmitis of the suspensory branches or body of the ligament.
2. Desmitis at the top of the ligament, just below the knee or hock. This condition has several similar names, including suspensory origin desmitis, proximal suspensory desmitis, and high suspensory disease.

Causes

Suspensory desmitis is caused by excessive strain on the ligament during strenuous exercise. Extreme loading forces on the fetlock during intense exercise, along with fatigue of the flexor muscles, cause the fetlock to overextend. This overloads the supporting structures, including the suspensory ligament. Overstretching of the suspensory ligament can cause fiber damage at the origin, or in the body or

branches. The branches are more vulnerable to damage than the body because
they are narrower.

Overstretching may also cause the ligament to tear away from its origin at the
back of the cannon bone or from its attachment onto the sesamoid bones. This
is called an avulsion. When avulsion occurs, the ligament sometimes pulls away
a fragment of bone. Other times it causes
a bony reaction: loss of bone density (lysis) at the top of the cannon bone, or new
bone production (exostosis) on the top
or outer edge of the sesamoid bone.
*(These bony changes are discussed in
Chapter 9.)*

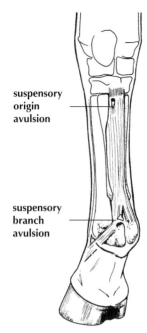

Fig. 11–30. Sites of
suspensory ligament
avulsion.

Like tendonitis, faulty conformation
and improper shoeing can contribute to
the development of suspensory desmitis.
Horses training or racing on tracks with
tight turns or steep slopes are more
prone to suspensory branch desmitis.
This is because excessive load is placed
on one side of the fetlock and its sup-
porting structures. Suspensory branch desmitis is also more common in horses that make sharp turns at speed, such as polo ponies.

The signs, diagnosis, treatment, and prognosis vary with the location of the damage. So from this point suspensory branch and suspensory origin desmitis are discussed separately.

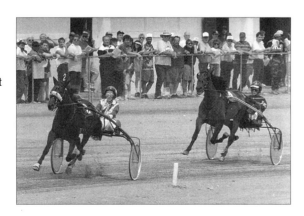

Fig. 11–31. Horses that
train or race on tracks
with tight turns are
more prone to suspen-
sory branch desmitis.

Suspensory Branch Desmitis

Signs

Most cases of suspensory desmitis occur in the suspensory branches of the forelegs. Common signs include:

- thickening of one or both branches
- heat
- pain during palpation
- mild to moderate lameness (grade 1 – 3 of 5) which typically is worsened by trotting the horse in a circle

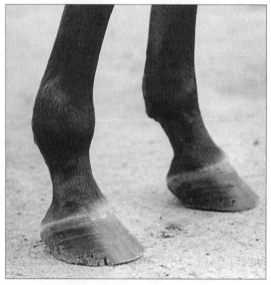

Fig. 11–32. Damage to the suspensory branches causes swelling at the back of the fetlock.

The horse may also have a positive fetlock flexion test *(see Chapter 2)*, which can be confusing.

In severe cases the entire back of the fetlock may be swollen. Careful palpation, both with weight on and off the leg, is required to identify which structure is affected. Although it may be obvious that the damage occurred in the suspensory branches, the following structures should be carefully palpated:

- suspensory ligament body and origin
- flexor tendons and inferior check ligament
- splint bones
- sesamoid bones and distal sesamoidean ligaments

Any of these structures may also have been damaged to some degree.

Although an avulsion fracture from the surface of the sesamoid bone is usually impossible to feel, the horse may show more pain during pressure over the sesamoid bone at the site of avulsion.

Suspensory branch desmitis may occur in both legs, so the examination should include a careful evaluation of the opposite leg.

Diagnosis

The history, specifically the stage of training and recent activity, and the signs are usually enough to diagnose suspensory branch desmitis. However, the diagnosis should be confirmed and the degree of fiber disruption determined with ultrasonography. If only a few fibers are damaged a defect may not be obvious, although the inflamed suspensory branch is clearly thicker than the other branch or those on the opposite leg. It is always worth ultrasounding the rest of the suspensory ligament, including the narrow band of fibers that run across the side of the fetlock and attach onto the extensor tendon at the front of the pastern *(see Figure 11–3)*. The flexor tendons and inferior check ligament should also be ultrasounded in case they too have been damaged.

The veterinarian may radiograph the fetlock and splint bones, particularly if ultrasound indicated that small fragments of bone may have been pulled away from the sesamoid bones. Even if an avulsion fragment is not found, roughening or exostoses along the upper or outer edges of the sesamoids indicates chronic suspensory ligament strain. It is fairly common for horses with suspensory branch desmitis to also have a splint bone fracture. This is a good reason why radiographs should be taken in every horse with suspensory branch desmitis.

> **More Information**
>
> Suspensory ligament damage and splint bone fractures often occur together. Managing splint bone fractures is covered in Chapter 17.

Treatment

Management of suspensory branch desmitis is similar to the conservative management of tendonitis. Initially, treatment includes rest from regular training as well as, anti-inflammatory therapy, bandaging, and hand-walking.

If the strain was mild, regular exercise can resume after a few weeks of daily hand-walking. But if ultrasound showed fiber damage or radiographs revealed abnormalities on the sesamoid bones, the rest period must be much longer. Ligaments can take several months to heal because they have a relatively poor blood supply. Also, there is constant tension on the ligament while the horse is bearing weight on the leg. If the horse is to remain in a stall or small paddock during the rest period, daily hand-walking should be continued. As an alternative, the horse can be turned out onto pasture for 4 – 6 months once the acute inflammation has subsided (usually 1 – 2 weeks after injury).

Shoeing changes should be limited to restoring the hoof balance and a normal hoof-pastern angle. Raising the horse's heels greater than that required to achieve a normal hoof-pastern angle increases tension on the suspensory ligament. *(Foot shape and shoeing options are discussed in Chapter 7.)*

Some people have found that laser therapy *(see Chapter 4)* can speed ligament healing in the first few weeks after injury. However, it does not appear to be of much use in chronic injuries. Splitting the affected suspensory branch, a similar procedure to tendon splitting (discussed earlier), has also been tried in an attempt to improve blood supply and speed healing. However, this surgery is usually only moderately successful.

If avulsion of the suspensory branch has torn away a fragment of the sesamoid bone, the veterinarian may recommend surgical removal of the fragment. However, the fragment can be very difficult to find, so in most cases, the veterinarian simply prescribes several months of rest. *(See Sesamoid Fractures in Chapter 16.)*

Rehabilitation

Training should not resume until physical examination, lameness evaluation, and ultrasonography indicate the ligament has completely healed. This can take over 4 months in some cases.

The guidelines given for rehabilitating horses with tendonitis also apply to horses returning to training after suspensory branch desmitis. To prevent re-injury, *it is important that the return to regular training is very gradual,* slowly building up to speed work over a 2 – 3 month period. If at any time there is heat, pain, further swelling in the ligament, or lameness, training should be suspended. In many cases the thickening in the damaged branch(es) remains once healing is completed, although the healed ligament should not be hot or painful, and the horse should not be lame.

The risk of re-injury can be reduced by following the management strategies outlined earlier for preventing tendonitis.

Prognosis for Suspensory Branch Desmitis

The prognosis for long-term athletic usefulness is fairly good in mild cases of suspensory branch desmitis, in which only one branch is involved and the sesamoid bones are normal on radiographs. However, all cases of suspensory desmitis have the potential to recur—a second episode substantially worsens the prognosis.

Avulsion of a piece of sesamoid bone often results in chronic, low-grade lameness. However, removing the fragment of bone does not guarantee that the horse will remain problem-free. The suspensory branch remains weakened because there is a smaller area of attachment onto the bone.

Suspensory Origin Desmitis

Signs

Suspensory origin desmitis usually occurs in the forelimbs, although in Standardbreds it develops just as commonly in the hindlimbs. This condition can be difficult to detect because the swollen ligament is hidden beneath the flexor tendons and inferior check ligament, and between the splint bones. In fact, the swelling usually cannot be seen. Moderate lameness (grade 2 – 3 of 5) is generally the only outward sign of this problem.

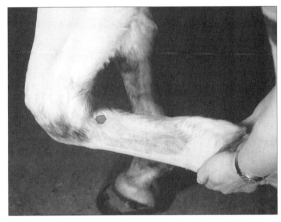

Fig. 11–33. The dot indicates the location of the suspensory origin.

Pain may sometimes be produced by lifting the leg, pushing the flexor tendons over, and pressing down on the back of the cannon (just below the knee or hock) with the thumb. However, this procedure is not specific enough to confirm suspensory origin desmitis. Pain in the inferior check ligament may also cause the horse to react.

Diagnosis

Suspensory origin desmitis can be very difficult to diagnose based on the history and signs. Typically, the site of lameness cannot be identified with physical examination and gait evaluation. The veterinarian must first rule out the possibility of foot, pastern, or fetlock problems. This is done by systematically nerve blocking up the leg, at least to the level of the fetlock.

More Information

Structures Near the Suspensory Origin

In the foreleg, the suspensory ligament lies very close to the Palmar Metacarpal nerves, which supply the cannon and fetlock.

Also, the origin of the ligament lies up against a pouch of the intercarpal joint (the middle knee joint). The pouch extends for 1 – 2 inches below the joint at the back of the knee.

(See Chapter 2 for more information on diagnostic procedures.)

Local anesthetic injected into the area around the suspensory origin temporarily improves the lameness in many of these horses. However, this technique is not foolproof. Even with careful needle placement and small volumes of local anesthetic, it can be difficult not to block nearby structures. So, although the lameness is improved or resolved, the veterinarian still cannot be certain that the suspensory origin is the site of pain.

Ultrasonography of the suspensory origin can also be difficult to interpret. This part of the suspensory ligament commonly has a few muscle fibers within it. In fact, this structure's older name was the interosseous muscle. Muscle is less dense than ligament, so the muscle fibers can easily be mistaken for an area of fiber disruption within the suspensory ligament. Radiography can sometimes identify an area of bone avulsion or lysis at the top of the cannon bone. But these changes are not present in every horse with suspensory origin desmitis.

Nuclear scintigraphy can help to pinpoint the site of injury when ultrasonography and radiography are inconclusive or show no abnormalities. Whether or not there has been an avulsion, there is usually a "hot spot" at the top of the cannon bone. The "hot spot" is present because the strained ligament stresses the bone surface where it attaches.

Treatment of Suspensory Origin Desmitis

Because of its obscure signs, suspensory origin desmitis often goes undiagnosed for weeks, or even months. So, the injury is no longer acute when the diagnosis is made. Nevertheless, rest from training and a few days of anti-inflammatory therapy are important in the initial management of this condition. If the horse has continued in training despite the lameness, there is probably still some active inflammation in the ligament.

The only successful treatment has been an extended rest period, either in a pasture or large paddock. The length of time the horse must be rested varies. In most cases at least 4 months is required. If there is bone avulsion, the rest period must be longer. Although the lameness may subside in a shorter period of time, it will return as soon as the horse is put back into work if the ligament has not completely healed. Therefore, it is best to rest the horse for the entire time the veterinarian specifies. As with tendon injuries, impatience is usually rewarded with re-injury or persistent lameness.

Corticosteroids injected into the suspensory origin can improve or resolve the lameness for a few weeks. But this procedure is not a good idea for a few reasons:

1. Corticosteroids slow healing, which is not good in a structure that is already slow to heal.
2. Inflammation is an important part of the healing process, particularly in structures that do not have a very good blood supply. It improves blood flow and stimulates repair in the damaged tissue.
3. These drugs block the signs of inflammation, including pain and lameness. If the horse is exercised after this treatment, any lameness—which would normally signal further ligament damage—is masked.

Because of the location of the suspensory origin, neither surgically splitting the ligament nor removing any bone fragments is possible.

Rehabilitation following suspensory origin injury should follow the same guidelines given for suspensory branch desmitis. Repeat nuclear scintigraphy before training resumes can be valuable in determining whether the suspensory origin injury has healed.

Prognosis for Suspensory Origin Desmitis

Suspensory origin desmitis that involves a large area of torn fibers or avulsion of a bone fragment carries a guarded prognosis for long-term athletic function. Chronic lameness, even after an extended rest period, is a common result of this injury.

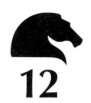

12

NEUROLOGIC CAUSES
OF LAMENESS

A healthy nervous system is essential for normal function of the musculoskeletal system. Aside from the obvious action of making muscles contract, which enables the horse to move, the nervous system controls balance, coordination, and fine-tuning of movement. The nervous system also alerts the horse to the pain of over-

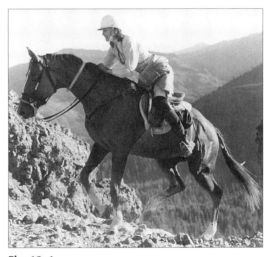

Fig. 12–1.

stretching, tissue damage, and inflammation.

Neurologic problems cause gait abnormalities because they affect muscle control and the horse's perception of how it is moving. Pain is a component of these gait abnormalities in only a few neurologic conditions.

The nervous system is complex, both in structure and function. Therefore, an overview of this system is given before the neurologic conditions that can cause gait abnormalities are discussed.

STRUCTURE & FUNCTION

The nervous system can be divided into two basic parts:

1. **The Central Nervous System, or CNS,** which consists of the brain and spinal cord.
2. **The Peripheral Nervous System,** which consists of the nerves that exit the brain or spinal cord, and supply the muscles and other tissues.

The brain and spinal cord are surrounded and protected by the bones of the skull and spinal (vertebral) column. The spinal column can be divided into five sections: the cervical (neck), thoracic (body), lumbar (loins), sacral (rump), and coccygeal (tail) segments. The

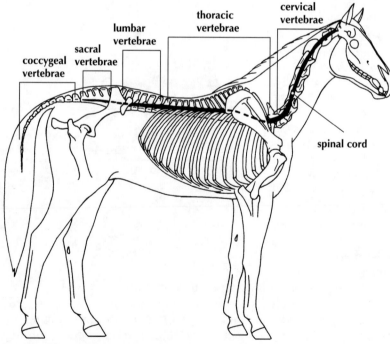

Fig. 12–2. The spinal column and cord.

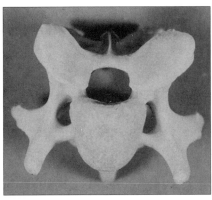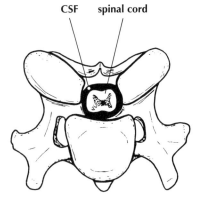

Fig. 12–3. A cervical vertebra. The spinal cord runs through the center hole. The smaller holes are for blood vessels and nerves.

spinal column continues to the tip of the tail dock, but the spinal cord ends in the sacral segment, just ahead of the tail base.

The brain and spinal cord are covered by protective membranes called meninges. Infection of these tissues results in meningitis. The meninges produce and contain cerebrospinal fluid, or CSF, which surrounds the brain and spinal cord. This fluid acts as a buffer between the CNS tissues and their bony casings.

Neurons

The basic component of the nervous system is the nerve cell, or neuron. Neurons are different from most other cells in the body in that they have a rounded or star-shaped cell body and a very long, narrow projection called an axon. The axon connects the neuron with other neurons or with the tissue that is supplied by that nerve (muscle cells, skin cells, etc.). It is the part of the neuron that is commonly called the nerve fiber. These fibers are microscopic—they

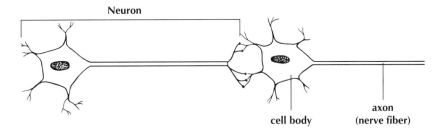

Fig. 12–4. Neurons have a star-shaped cell body and a very long axon.

441

cannot be seen without the aid of a microscope. What is visible as a nerve is actually a bundle of many microscopic axons, traveling together in the same protective outer sheath.

Neurons are divided into two categories:

- "motor"—taking signals from the brain to the tissues, which stimulates activity, or "motor function"
- "sensory"—taking messages, or sensations, such as temperature, pressure, tension, and pain, from the tissues to the brain

The motor neurons can be further divided into two types: upper and lower motor neurons. The cell bodies and axons of the upper motor neurons remain completely within the brain and spinal cord. They are part of the "internal wiring" of the CNS. The upper motor neurons connect different parts of the brain and spinal cord so that the activities of the nervous system are coordinated.

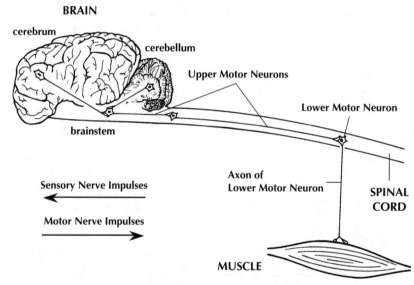

Fig. 12–5. Location of the upper and lower motor neurons, and the direction of nerve impulses.

The upper motor neurons in the spinal cord connect the lower motor neurons (and sensory neurons) with the brain, relaying the nerve impulses up and down the cord. The lower motor neurons are the nerves of the Peripheral Nervous System. Their cell bodies are located in the brain or spinal cord, but their axons exit the skull or spinal column and supply the tissues. Because of the horse's size, some axons are several feet long. Even in a small pony, the nerves in the feet are a long way from their cell bodies in the spinal cord.

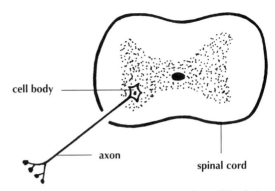

Fig. 12–6. A lower motor neuron. The cell body is within the spinal cord, but the axon (nerve fiber) leaves the cord and travels to the tissues.

The sensory neurons have a similar arrangement to the lower motor neurons. Their cell bodies are in the brain or spinal cord, and their axons travel to the tissues. The difference between lower motor and sensory neurons is the direction in which nerve impulses travel. Lower motor neurons carry messages from the brain or spinal cord to the tissues, whereas sensory neurons carry messages from the tissues to the brain.

(In some parts of the spinal cord the nerve cell bodies of the lower motor and sensory neurons are located just outside the spinal column, in a collection of neurons called a ganglion. However, for simplicity, only those neurons that have cell bodies within the brain or spinal cord are discussed and illustrated here.)

This information about upper and lower motor neurons, although technical, is important for understanding some of the neurologic conditions.

Responses to Injury or Disease

The nervous system can be damaged in many ways, including trauma, infection, toxins (plants, chemicals, etc.), and tumors. But no matter what the cause, the nervous system has a limited number of responses:

- loss of nerve function
- uncontrolled activity
- exaggerated nerve function
- "spinal shock"

Nerve function may be temporarily or permanently lost if the nerve is compressed, crushed, or severed. If a sensory nerve is damaged, the result is loss of skin sensation. If a motor nerve is damaged, the result is loss of function in the muscle supplied by that nerve. Over time, that muscle begins to atrophy (waste) because it is not being stimulated by the nerve. As long as the cell body of the neuron is not damaged, the axon can regenerate, although very slowly.

Upper motor neurons control and refine lower motor neuron activity, so damage to an upper motor neuron can result in exaggerated or uncontrolled motor nerve function. As a result, muscle contraction may be greater than needed. In some cases the muscle activity is excessive and repeated. The stringhalt gait is a classic example of exaggerated nerve function. Instead of movement being smooth and controlled, the hock is suddenly overflexed when the horse takes a step. Another example of exaggerated nerve function is seen with cervical vertebral malformation (CVM, or "wobbler" syndrome). In these horses, loss of upper motor neuron control of muscle activity results in either a stiff-legged, "toy soldier" walk or a poorly-coordinated, high-stepping, "spastic" gait.

Uncontrolled nervous system activity can result in widespread muscle tremors, spasms (a classic sign in horses with tetanus), or seizures. Spinal shock is the term used to describe total but temporary loss of function in the spinal cord, as a result of trauma. Although it may seem as though the spinal cord has been severed, function usually returns after a few days. Spinal shock is very uncommon in horses.

TERMINOLOGY

Prefix	Tissue Involved	Example
encephalo-	brain	encephalitis
myelo-	spinal cord	myelitis
myeloencephalo-	spinal cord and brain	myeloencephalitis
neuro-	peripheral nerves	neuritis, neuropathy

Fig. 12–7. Terms used to describe neurologic problems.

ASSESSING THE NERVOUS SYSTEM
History and Physical Examination

A comprehensive history and a thorough physical examination often are essential for an accurate diagnosis. With neurologic problems, important information from the history includes:

- age, breed, and use of the horse
- onset, duration, and progression of the signs
- known or suspected traumatic incidents
- vaccination history
- exposure to strange horses
- potential exposure to wildlife
- geographic location
- diet

The physical examination findings that are especially important in horses with a neurologic condition include:

- demeanor, or attitude
- head and neck posture, and general stance (the way the horse chooses to stand)
- muscle symmetry (or asymmetry)
- muscle tone, including tail tone
- evidence of trauma, such as skin abrasions, swellings, localized pain, etc.

During the physical examination the veterinarian should thoroughly evaluate the musculoskeletal system. It must be ruled out as the cause of the gait abnormality before focusing on the nervous system.

> **More Information**
>
> History and physical examination are covered in Chapter 2.

Neurologic Examination

The neurologic examination is a specific type of physical examination of the nervous system. It is aimed at identifying the location and nature of the neurologic problem. A common approach used by many veterinarians is to start at the head and work back along the horse, assessing the brain, the spinal cord, and finally the nerves. *(The signs typically associated with problems in these areas are summarized in Figure 12–44 at the end of the chapter.)*

Brain

Cerebrum

The front part of the brain, the cerebrum, has some important functions with respect to locomotion. The cerebrum processes information from other parts of the CNS and integrates the messages from the rest of the body. These messages include sight, sound, smell, touch, pain, heat, cold, and pressure. Using this information, the cerebrum directs the horse's behavior and conscious (voluntary) movements. It also processes the information which lets the horse know where its limbs are in relation to each other and to the ground. This sense is called proprioception.

The cerebrum's control over the horse's attitude, behavior, and voluntary movement results in some obvious signs when cerebral function is altered:

- depression
- compulsive wandering or circling
- continual yawning
- aggression
- head-pressing (pressing the head against solid objects)

The cerebrum is also responsible for vision. Even though the eyes are normal, the horse may be totally blind if the part of the cerebrum that processes images is damaged.

Gait defects are not the most consistent feature of cerebral damage. However, when these other signs of cerebral dysfunction are present, they signal serious neurologic disease.

Cerebellum

The cerebellum is located toward the back of the brain. It is responsible for balance, coordination, and fine-tuning of movements. Abnormalities in this part of the brain may cause:

- head tilt—the head is held tilted at an abnormal angle
- loss of balance
- jerky head movements
- "intention" tremors—head tremors during voluntary movements

Incoordination (ataxia) and a high-stepping, poorly-controlled gait (hypermetria) may also be seen in horses with cerebellar disease. However, these horses do not show signs of muscle weakness. Ataxia, hyper- or hypometria, and weakness are common signs of spinal cord problems, and are discussed later.

Brainstem and Cranial Nerves

The base of the brain, called the brainstem, is responsible for consciousness. Severe abnormalities in this part of the brain can cause unconsciousness. The brainstem is also where some of the cranial nerves exit the brain. These nerves provide sensory and motor nerve function to the head and neck, and one of them (the vagus nerve) supplies several internal organs. The cranial nerves are responsible for the senses of smell, sight, taste, and hearing. They also control sensation and movement of the eyeballs, eyelids, ears, jaw, and tongue, and direct the function of the muscles in the face and throat. One of the cranial nerves is also responsible for transmitting signals from the inner ear to the brain, giving the horse its sense of balance.

Except for the nerves involved in balance and vision, the cranial nerves do not affect the horse's gait. However, cranial nerve defects, such as paralysis of one side of the face or the tongue, may be seen with some of the neurologic conditions that do cause gait abnormalities. One good example is Equine Protozoal Myeloencephalitis, or EPM. So, the function of these nerves should be thoroughly assessed in every horse with neurologic disease.

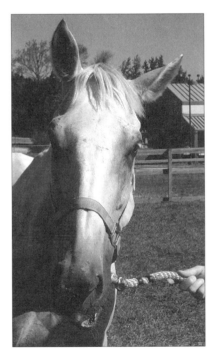 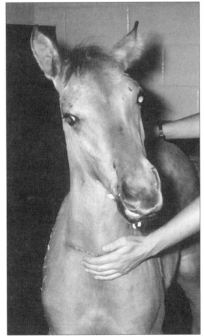

Fig. 12–8. Various neurologic defects. Left: Adult horse with a droopy left ear and paralysis on the left side of the face. Right: Foal with a head tilt, abnormal eyeball position, and paralysis of the right side of the muzzle.

Spinal Cord

The spinal cord contains upper motor neurons that transmit messages from the brain to the lower motor neurons, and from the sensory neurons to the brain. Any condition that interrupts the nerve impulses in the spinal cord can cause varying degrees of:

- ataxia
- hypometria or hypermetria
- muscle weakness

These abnormalities are seen when the horse is moving, although ataxia may be suspected in the standing horse if its stance is abnormal. Severe weakness may be obvious at rest as buckling of the affected limb(s).

Ataxia

Ataxia is abnormal, uncoordinated limb motion, such as swinging the leg out widely as it is brought forward, crossing one leg over the other, or stepping on the other foot. Normally, the signals from the

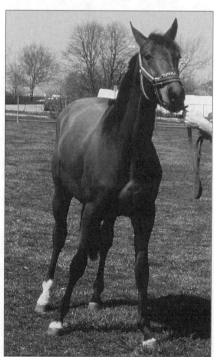

sensory nerves in the muscles, tendons, joint capsules, and hoof walls give the horse an awareness of where its limbs are placed in relation to each other and to the ground surface. This sense is called proprioception. If the signals from the sensory nerves to the brain are interrupted by a spinal cord problem, the horse loses its perception of where its legs are. As a result, horses with proprioceptive defects are unsteady and make mistakes when placing their feet.

Assessment at Rest

Ataxic horses may stand normally; that is, they do not necessarily have a problem with balance. But often they

Fig. 12–9. Ataxic horses may stand with their feet widely apart.

stand with their feet widely apart or in unusual positions.

The veterinarian can assess proprioception by lifting one of the horse's legs and crossing it over the other, or placing it widely apart from the other. A normal horse is aware that this is abnormal and immediately replaces the foot in the normal position. But an ataxic horse leaves the leg in that position.

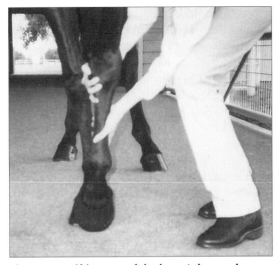

Fig. 12–10. Lifting one of the horse's legs and crossing it over the other assesses proprioception.

However, this test can be misleading in a well-trained or complaisant horse. These horses often leave the leg where it was placed. But the horse can sometimes be tricked into responding appropriately. The veterinarian places one of the horse's feet on a sack and slowly draws the sack (and the foot) out to the side. A normal horse will move its foot and place the leg back underneath itself once the sack is moved to the side 12 inches (30 cm) or so. This is an automatic response, so even a complaisant horse will usually move its foot.

Assessment While Moving

There are many methods the veterinarian may use to detect subtle ataxia in a moving horse. One way is to turn the horse in a tight circle and stop suddenly. An ataxic horse will usually stop with its legs in an abnormal position and leave them that way until walked forward. Another way is to longe the horse and suddenly turn it in toward the center of the circle, making it do a 90° turn. Ataxic horses often stagger slightly, swing their hindquarters too wide when making the turn, and stand with the feet placed widely apart. Another method is to jog the horse in a straight line, stop it suddenly, then immediately trot it off again. Ataxic horses have trouble with this maneuver.

Hypometria or Hypermetria

When an upper motor neuron is damaged, the control or fine-tuning of the connected lower motor neuron is lost, and muscle activity is affected. Which muscles are affected depends on which nerve pathways are damaged. The horse may have exaggerated flexor muscle activity and increased joint flexion (hypermetria). Or it may have exaggerated extensor muscle activity and reduced joint flexion (hypometria). A horse with a hypermetric gait takes high and poorly-controlled steps. A horse with a hypometric gait appears stiff-legged, and walks like a toy soldier.

Weakness

Muscle weakness is another sign of abnormal spinal cord function. It means that the nerve impulses to the lower motor neurons and the muscle(s) they activate have been interrupted. The degree of weakness can be assessed by pushing against the horse or pulling on its tail, either while the horse is standing or while it is walking. A normal horse resists the pressure and maintains its position. But a weak horse is easily pushed or pulled to one side.

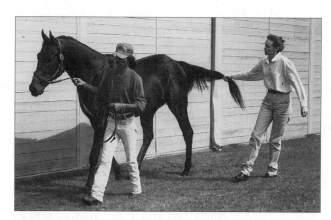

Fig. 12–11. Muscle weakness can be assessed by pulling on the horse's tail.

Weak horses commonly drag their toes as they walk. But this is also true of lazy horses, horses with musculoskeletal problems, and horses that are ill, dehydrated, or in poor condition. Severe muscle weakness may cause the affected limb(s) to buckle. This is because the muscles cannot stabilize the joints.

Nerves

Damage to an individual nerve may result in loss of skin sensation and/or muscle function, depending on the nerve and the degree of damage. Occasionally, loss of local nerve function may be seen as a small patch of sweat on a cool horse.

Lack of nerve supply to a muscle eventually results in atrophy—loss of muscle tone and bulk *(see Chapter 10)*. Complete loss of muscle function may also cause an abnormal limb position, or stance. For example, radial nerve paralysis results in an inability to extend the fetlock and knee, so the horse stands with the fetlock and knee flexed and the front of the hoof wall on the ground.

Sometimes nerve damage can cause signs similar to spinal cord dysfunction. For example, when a large muscle group loses its nerve supply, the horse may show signs of weakness in that leg. If an extensor muscle loses its nerve supply, the corresponding flexor muscle functions unopposed. With tibial nerve paralysis, for example, this can result in exaggerated hock flexion, or hypermetria. A thorough history and physical examination are necessary to tell the difference between local nerve damage and spinal cord damage in some cases.

Gait Evaluation

Gait evaluation is a very important part of the neurologic examination. To thoroughly evaluate the horse's gait, the veterinarian observes the horse as it:

- walks and trots (if it is safe) on a level surface
- walks up and down a slope
- turns in a tight circle (pivots)
- backs up

The veterinarian may also ask the handler to raise the horse's head or blindfold the horse and repeat some of these procedures. These maneuvers often make neurologic defects more obvious and easier to classify.

The ideal place to safely perform this evaluation is a level, even area with a non-slip surface, such as grass or dirt. (Asphalt and concrete are not safe surfaces for examining a horse with a severe neurologic problem.) A nearby area with a moderate

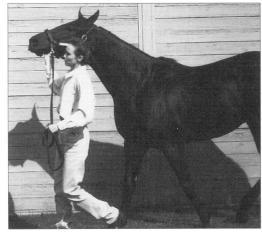

Fig. 12–12. Walking the horse with its head up.

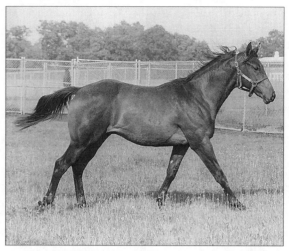

Fig. 12–13. Mistakes are sometimes easier to see when the horse is exercising freely.

slope is also good. The examination area should be large enough that the horse is unlikely to injure itself (or the handler) if it becomes more ataxic when blindfolded. A small paddock or round pen should also be available because mistakes (proprioceptive deficits) are sometimes easier to see when the horse is exercising freely.

Grading the Abnormalities

Veterinarians grade gait defects on a scale between 1+ and 4+ (that is, "+" to "++++"), with 1+ being mild and 4+ being severe. This scale is not to be confused with the lameness grading system described in Chapter 2. The horse may have a grade 1 of 5 lameness, but have a grade 3+ proprioceptive deficit, or grade 2+ weakness. Also, the horse may have a 3+ deficit in the hindlegs, but only a 1+ deficit in the forelegs, depending on the location of the problem. Even more specifically, the horse may have a 3+ defect in the left hindleg, but only a 1+ defect in the right hindleg. These examples raise an important point: differences between the forelegs and hindlegs, and between the left and right sides of the body can help locate and classify the abnormality.

Diagnostic Tests

Radiography, with or without myelography, can be useful in identifying abnormalities in the cervical (neck) vertebrae, but it is very difficult to take good quality radiographs of the rest of the spinal column. (The coccygeal vertebrae in the tail are easily radiographed, but abnormalities involving these vertebrae do not cause neurologic problems.) Even if a fracture or other abnormality is found in the vertebrae, radiography cannot determine how severely the spinal cord is affected. Nuclear scintigraphy is also limited in its ability to evaluate nervous system function, although it can locate subtle bone problems in the spinal column in areas that are hard to radiograph.

Electromyography (EMG) can be useful in some cases because it assesses the function of the lower motor neurons and the muscles they supply. CT and MRI may be able to identify specific lesions within the nervous system, but the availability of these sophisticated tools for use in horses is very limited.

More Information

The diagnostic techniques mentioned in this section are detailed in Chapter 2:

- radiography
- myelography
- nuclear scintigraphy
- electromyography
- computerized tomography (CT)
- magnetic resonance imaging (MRI)

Cerebrospinal Fluid Collection

Because cerebrospinal fluid (CSF) surrounds the brain and spinal cord, analysis of this fluid can provide information about the presence of disease in the central nervous system. CSF can be collected with a specialized spinal needle from two sites in the horse. One is the atlanto-occipital (A-O) joint, located just behind the poll. The other is the lumbosacral joint, which is located at the top of the rump, just behind the loins.

Wherever possible, CSF is collected from the site closest to the presumed site of damage. If the horse shows neurologic signs that indicate brain or upper spinal cord problems, the sample should be taken at the atlanto-occipital space. If the neurologic signs are more likely due to a problem lower down in the spinal cord, a lumbosacral tap usually provides more information.

Precautions and Limitations

There are several things the veterinarian considers before collecting CSF.

A-O Tap

The atlanto-occipital joint is the larger of the two joint spaces, and it is closer to the skin surface. So the A-O tap is easier to perform, and there is less risk of blood contamination of the sample. However, this tap can generally be safely performed only while the horse is anesthetized (although a very short intravenous anesthetic is usually all that is necessary). If the horse is down and unable to get up or move

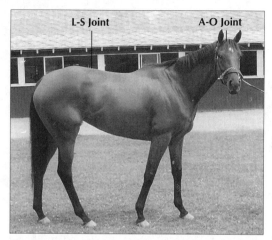

L-S Joint   A-O Joint

Fig. 12–14. Locations of the A-O and L-S joints.

its head, it may only need to be sedated. However, if the horse is still standing, but is ataxic or weak, many veterinarians feel there is more risk of the horse injuring itself trying to get up after anesthesia than there is benefit from the information provided by the tap.

Lumbosacral Tap

The lumbosacral (L-S) space is small and it is buried beneath at least 5 inches (13 cm) of muscle and connective tissue. Even with experience, this tap can be difficult to perform. To improve the chances of success, most veterinarians have the horse restrained in stocks, or at least against a wall. Often the veterinarian must stand on a box or small stepladder in order to lean over the horse's rump to position the needle precisely.

Most veterinarians tranquilize and/or twitch the horse for this procedure. Often, when the needle penetrates the tough, but sensitive membrane surrounding the spinal cord (the dura mater), the horse flinches. Occasionally, this response is instantaneous and explosive. The veterinarian, handler, and assistants should be alert and ready for the horse to crouch, jump, or kick. Once the needle is through the dura, the horse usually stands quietly while the CSF sample is collected.

No matter which site is used, the veterinarian must use strictly aseptic techniques to avoid infection of the spinal canal. The veterinarian must also be very careful not to damage the spinal cord with the needle. This is particularly important when performing the A-O tap.

> **Note**
>
> Sterile, or "aseptic" techniques include:
> • clipping the hair
> • scrubbing the skin with disinfectant
> • using sterile gloves
> • using sterile equipment and materials
>
> (See Chapter 2 for more information.)

Because of all the risks involved, CSF collection is not something the veterinarian performs or repeats without very good cause.

Testing the CSF
Fluid Analysis

Normal CSF looks like water and it has a very low cell count and protein concentration. If either of these are elevated, it can indicate a disease process, such as inflammation or infection. Discoloration of the fluid can also be a useful finding. The fluid may be red- or orange-tinged if there has been bleeding into the CSF. Trauma is the most common cause of red-colored CSF. But even with extreme care, CSF collection can cause bleeding into the spinal canal and leakage of blood into the CSF sample. If the CSF is cloudy, infection should be suspected, and the fluid should be submitted for bacterial culture and antibiotic sensitivity testing *(see Chapter 2)*.

Serology

Blood and CSF can be tested for the presence of antibodies against specific micro-organisms (bacteria, viruses, protozoa, etc.). The procedure of measuring antibodies in the bloodstream to establish a diagnosis is called serology ("study of serum"), and the result is called a titer. Although CSF is not blood, measuring antibody levels in the CSF is also called serology. Serologic testing of CSF is one of only two tests available to definitely diagnose some neurologic diseases while the horse is alive. Polymerase chain reaction (PCR) is the other test; it is discussed in the next section.

Whenever micro-organisms enter the body, the immune system is activated to destroy and remove them. To do this, the body produces specific antibodies, which are specialized protein molecules. Antibodies help rid the body of the invading organisms by either killing them or attaching to their outer surface and making it easier for the white blood cells to recognize, engulf, and destroy them. (White blood cells are another essential part of the body's defense system.)

Once antibodies are produced, they remain in the circulation for weeks or months after the infection has been resolved. These antibodies, which generally are very specific for the particular organism, can be measured in the bloodstream and other body fluids, including CSF. Their presence indicates that the horse has been exposed to a particular organism some time in the past few months.

Importance of the Blood-Brain Barrier

The blood vessels in the brain and spinal cord are specialized. The cells that line the vessel walls are much closer together in the CNS than in all other tissues and organs. This arrangement is called the blood-brain barrier. Normally, it prevents large protein molecules, including antibodies, from leaving the bloodstream and entering the nervous system tissues. So, whenever antibodies are detected in the CSF, the assumption is that they were produced within the nervous system tissues, rather than being delivered by the bloodstream. This means that the organisms that stimulated antibody production are (or were) actually within the CNS tissues.

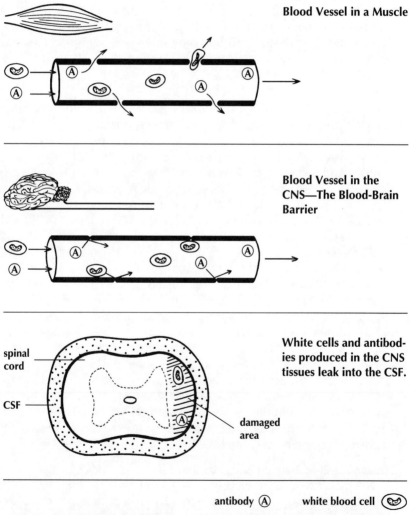

Blood Vessel in a Muscle

Blood Vessel in the CNS—The Blood-Brain Barrier

White cells and antibodies produced in the CNS tissues leak into the CSF.

spinal cord

CSF

damaged area

antibody Ⓐ   white blood cell

Fig. 12–15. Antibodies cannot enter the CNS from the bloodstream. They are produced within the CNS, and may leak into the cerebrospinal fluid (CSF).

This function of the blood-brain barrier can make serology more accurate. Detecting antibodies in the bloodstream means only that the horse has been exposed to a particular micro-organism at some time. The organism may not have caused disease. In fact, it may no longer be present in the body. The body retains these antibodies in the bloodstream for some time after exposure to the organism. But when antibodies are detected in the CSF, it generally means that the antibodies were produced within the central nervous system as a response to the presence of the organism *in* the nervous system tissues. In other words, when a positive titer is found in a CSF sample, it is generally safe to assume that infection with the particular organism caused the neurologic disease.

However, there are two instances when this assumption is not reliable. The first is when bleeding occurs during collection and blood mixes with the CSF. If the horse has antibodies in its bloodstream against the particular organism, bleeding during CSF collection can result in a positive CSF titer. Usually this situation is obvious because the CSF sample is discolored. The other instance is when the lesion in the brain or spinal cord is so severe that blood vessels are damaged. As a result, antibodies leak from the bloodstream into the nervous system tissues. This situation may be suspected when 1) the neurologic signs indicate that the damage is severe, and 2) the protein content (or specific antibody level) of the CSF is similar to that of the horse's blood. By comparing the CSF and a blood sample, it is usually possible to determine that blood (with antibodies) has leaked into the nervous system tissues. Therefore, in most cases it is best for the veterinarian to submit both blood and CSF to the laboratory.

Polymerase Chain Reaction (PCR)

Polymerase chain reaction (PCR) is a newer test that can be conducted on the CSF. PCR is designed to detect the invading organism's DNA—its genetic material—in the sample. For this reason, it can be more accurate than serology. PCR confirms the *presence of the organism* in the CNS, rather than measuring the *body's response to an organism* that may no longer be active, or even present in the body. PCR is sometimes used to diagnose Equine Protozoal Myeloencephalitis (EPM). Its advantages and limitations are discussed in the later section on EPM.

Blood and CSF samples for serology and PCR must be sent to a diagnostic laboratory. There are no simple, stall-side tests for neurologic diseases in horses. It can take from 2 days to 2 weeks to get the results, depending on the laboratory.

BRAIN & SPINAL CORD CONDITIONS
Trauma

Trauma means physical damage caused by an incident, such as a kick, fall, or trailer wreck. Traumatic injuries to the brain or spinal cord are fairly common in young horses, especially during breaking and training. A frequent cause of injury is flipping over backward and injuring the head, neck, withers, or tail base *(see Chapter 22)*. Other causes of head trauma include running into a solid object, or being kicked by another horse. Sometimes the horse is injured during exercise. Falling over a jump or colliding with another horse are two examples. Injuries of this type are more likely to damage the spinal cord than the brain. Occasionally, trauma may result from neurologic disease because ataxia and weakness make the horse more prone to falling and injuring itself.

Trauma to the brain or spinal cord can cause a variety of neurologic abnormalities, depending on the location and severity of the damage. Severe damage to the brain can result in coma (unconsciousness) or death. Severe damage to the spinal cord can result in paralysis. Injury to the front or side of the head can cause damage to the cerebral area of the brain. Injury to the poll can damage the cerebellar area, the brainstem, or the first part of the spinal cord. Common signs of CNS damage are listed in Figure 12–44 at the end of the chapter.

The damage to the nervous system tissues may be direct or indirect. Direct damage may be caused by a fragment of bone tearing or crushing the tissues. Dislocation of a vertebra can also crush the spinal cord. When nervous system tissue is damaged in this way, the nerve impulses can no longer travel between the CNS and the rest of the body past that point. In many cases this damage is permanent.

Indirect damage can result from bleeding into the tissues, and the inflammatory response that accompanies tissue damage. This includes fluid leakage from the blood vessels into the tissue, causing edema (swelling). These changes increase the pressure within the skull or spinal canal. Although the rigid bony casing around the CNS protects it, it also restricts the tissues from expanding. So, increased pressure within the skull or spinal canal compresses the brain or spinal cord. This interrupts nerve impulse transmission between the CNS and the rest of the body. But as long as the horse is appropriately treated within a few hours of injury, indirect damage usually is reversible.

Treatment of Traumatic CNS Injuries

Treatment varies with the location and severity of the signs. In all cases anti-inflammatory therapy is necessary to reduce edema within the nervous system tissues. Corticosteroids *(see Chapter 5)* are much more effective than NSAIDs in managing inflammation and edema in the central nervous system. However, corticosteroids reduce the body's ability to fight infection and repair itself. Thus, most veterinarians give only one or two doses of corticosteroids, and keep the horse on antibiotics.

Many veterinarians also give DMSO intravenously when treating central nervous system injuries. DMSO rapidly enters the CNS and it is a very good anti-inflammatory (and antibacterial) agent. Also, because it is fairly concentrated, it draws fluid out of the tissues, reducing edema and pressure within the CNS. DMSO is usually given once or twice per day for about 3 days.

If the damage is severe, the brain or spinal cord must be decompressed. This may involve surgery to remove bone fragments from a depressed skull fracture or stabilize a vertebral fracture or dislocation.

Diligent nursing care is essential if the horse is unable to stand, or if it has difficulty eating, drinking, or emptying its bladder and rectum. The veterinarian will either give detailed instructions on the horse's care, or attend to some of these matters directly. For example, the veterinarian may tube feed a horse that cannot eat, give intravenous fluids to a horse that cannot drink, and catheterize the horse's bladder to aid urination. Turning the horse from one side to the other every 1 – 2 hours is very important in reducing the potential for pneumonia, pressure sores, and muscle problems on the "down" side. However, if the horse has a fracture involving a cervical vertebra, extreme care should be taken when moving the horse's head or neck—if the fracture is unstable, further spinal cord damage can result.

More Information

A horse that is unable to stand needs good nursing care. Preventing and managing pressure sores are discussed in Chapter 13. Muscle problems that may occur are covered in Chapter 10.

Prognosis for Traumatic CNS Injuries

If the horse is showing severe signs, such as unconsciousness or complete paralysis, the chances of a successful outcome are poor. If the signs are less severe and the horse responds to anti-inflammatory therapy, the chance of recovery is better. In some cases the signs are more severe than would be expected from the degree of physical damage (bruising, abrasions, etc.). So, recovery can be rapid and remarkable. However, in other cases the horse's condition may deteriorate after a few days, particularly if degeneration or infection within the CNS occurs secondary to the initial trauma. Thus, horses with CNS trauma must be monitored closely for several days after the injury.

It is common for horses with moderate to severe CNS damage to have some permanent neurologic abnormalities once they have recovered from the injury.

Cervical Vertebral Malformation ("Wobbler" Syndrome)

Definition and Causes

Cervical vertebral malformation (CVM) is a condition in which abnormalities of the vertebrae in the neck cause compression of the spinal cord. It mostly affects horses less than 4 years old. Horses with CVM are often called "wobblers." There are a few other terms for this condition, including cervical stenotic myelopathy and cervical vertebral instability.

> **Definitions**
>
> **Osteochondrosis:** an abnormality of developing bone.
> **Physis:** area of specialized cartilage near the end of the bone; "growth plate."
> **Epiphysis:** end of the bone, between the physis and joint surface.
>
> (See Chapter 14 for more information.)

In some cases, CVM is caused by osteochondrosis. Osteochondrosis of the cervical vertebrae can result in enlarged physes and abnormal epiphyses. In other cases, thickening of the soft tissues and bony proliferation around the affected intervertebral joints contribute to the neurologic signs. This is actually a form of degenerative joint disease.

These changes can cause narrowing, or stenosis of the vertebral canal and compression of the spinal cord at the affected intervertebral joints. Compression of the spinal cord may occur only when the horse flexes or extends its neck. This is called dynamic compression. But in some cases the compression is constant, or static. Dynamic compression usually occurs as a result of abnormal bone development in the first four vertebrae. It is found more

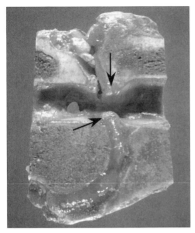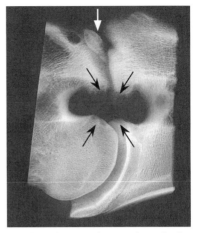

Fig. 12–16. Left: The soft tissues are thickened, and protrude into the spinal canal [black arrows]. Right: A radiograph of the same vertebrae, showing similar bony proliferation. Note also the bone chip in the upper intervertebral joint [white arrow].

often in younger horses, between 6 months and 2 years old. Static compression more commonly affects the fifth to seventh cervical vertebrae, at the base of the neck. It usually is the result of bone and soft tissue proliferation around the joints. It is more common in horses between 2 and 4 years old.

In many cases the neurologic signs *appear* to be caused by a traumatic incident, such as a fall or collision. But most often the trauma simply causes inflammation in the already abnormal joints and soft tissues. In other words, trauma aggravates the pre-existing problem, making the signs of spinal cord compression more obvious. Thinking

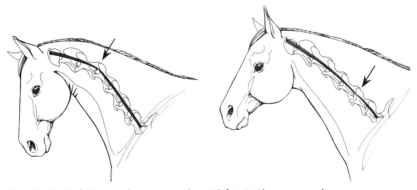

Fig. 12–17. Left: Dynamic compression. Right: Static compression.

back, the owner or trainer often realizes that the horse was always a little awkward. This indicates that the horse was most likely showing mild or subtle neurologic signs before the accident. Because ataxic horses are more prone to stumble or fall, the neurologic signs may actually have caused the accident, instead of the accident causing the neurologic signs.

Signs of CVM

The typical signs of CVM are the classic signs of spinal cord disease:
- ataxia
- hypometria or hypermetria
- muscle weakness

Reminder
Ataxia: incoordination
Hypometria: stiff-legged gait
Hypermetria: high-stepping gait
These signs are discussed in the earlier section on *Neurologic Examination.*

Horses with CVM are called "wobblers" because of the ataxia that is typical of this condition. The severity of the signs depends on the degree of spinal cord compression. In some horses the signs are obvious. In others they may be mild, sometimes being misinterpreted as vague lameness. These neurologic abnormalities are often more obvious when the horse is made to walk up or down a slope, over a low obstacle, up and down a curb, and with its head raised and neck extended.

When compression of the spinal cord occurs at the first few cervical vertebrae, all four legs are affected. However, the abnormalities are usually worse in the hindlegs. When compression occurs further down the neck, there may only be obvious neurologic abnormalities in the hindlegs. Cord compression at the last two cervical vertebrae can cause neurologic signs that are worse in the forelegs. This is because some of the nerves that supply the forelegs leave the spinal column at this point.

In almost all cases the signs are *symmetrical.* Whether or not the hindlegs are worse than the forelegs, the grade of abnormality is identical on the left and right sides.

There are few, if any, physical signs of CVM. Muscle atrophy is generally not seen in these horses. If the horse has poor muscle tone along its neck, there may be thickening and pain when pressure is applied to the affected intervertebral joints. However, these changes are not exclusive to CVM.

Ataxic horses sometimes have skin abrasions, or even "splints" on the insides of their legs. Minor interference wounds anywhere between the coronet and the knee or hock are fairly common in horses with CVM. These injuries usually occur while the horse is turned out, rather than during ridden exercise. In the pasture, the horse is free to move as it wants, but when ridden it is steadied or controlled by the rider. Wearing ("dubbing") of the hoof wall at the toe may also be seen.

Diagnosis of CVM

Diagnosis is based on the history, especially the horse's age, breed, growth rate, and level of activity, and on the signs. CVM is more often seen in large, rapidly growing horses between 6 months and 2 years of age. Thoroughbreds seem to be especially vulnerable. The condition is more common in colts than fillies, probably because colts are usually a little larger for their age. In most cases the signs become more obvious when breaking or training begins.

The signs may appear suddenly, or they may begin subtly and progress slowly. Although trauma may seem to cause or worsen the signs in the beginning, the signs generally stabilize to a point where no further change, for better or for worse, is seen.

Some horses with CVM have signs of osteochondrosis in the legs, in particular, joint effusion *(see Chapter 14)*. Physitis is also fairly common. Farms with a high incidence of osteochondrosis tend to have a higher incidence of CVM, so this condition should be considered a herd problem. Every horse with signs of CVM should be thoroughly examined for other signs of osteochondrosis. (Likewise, every horse with osteochondrosis in the limbs should probably be carefully observed for neurologic abnormalities.)

It is important for the veterinarian to perform a complete neurologic examination because there are several conditions that can cause similar signs in this age group. A cerebrospinal fluid (CSF) sample can help rule out infectious conditions. However, most horses with CVM have normal CSF, so this test cannot confirm the diagnosis.

The diagnosis of CVM can sometimes be confirmed with plain radiographs. The width of the spinal canal, relative to the outer width of the vertebrae, can be measured from the radio-

> **Note**
>
> Other problems that may cause similar signs include:
> • Equine Degenerative Myelopathy (EDM)
> • EHV-1 myeloencephalitis
> • Equine Protozoal Myeloencephalitis (EPM)
> • trauma to cervical vertebrae

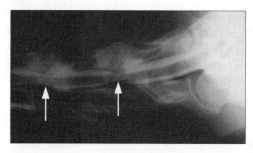

Fig. 12–18. Left: Myelogram from a horse with CVM. Note how the dye column narrows at the intervertebral joints [arrows].

Below: The spinal cord is compressed by a bony abnormality.

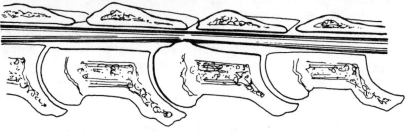

graphs. This measurement can be used to determine whether the horse is a candidate for CVM. Obvious abnormalities of the vertebrae are much more conclusive evidence. But in many cases spinal cord compression can only be confirmed with a myelogram *(see Chapter 2)*. Myelography is an involved and risky procedure, so it is not often recommended. However, it should be performed if surgery is being considered.

Treatment of CVM
Conservative Management
In horses less than 2 years old, conservative management is almost always the best treatment for CVM. This approach involves 1) changing the diet as discussed in Chapter 14 for managing osteochondrosis, and 2) confining the horse to a stall or small pen.

Some veterinarians recommend a low energy diet that consists only of grass hay and a vitamin and mineral supplement during the confinement period. This slows the horse's growth without any long-term effects on its size or build. The horse may become thin and poorly-muscled during this period. But poor body condition can be remedied, and it is a small price to pay for a safe and usable horse. In general, the younger the horse and the sooner the low energy diet is begun, the greater the potential for complete recovery.

Stall confinement reduces the risk that trauma or excessive movement will worsen the problem. Foals with signs of CVM should be confined for the rest of their rapid growth phase, at least until 12 months of age. Older horses should be confined until the neurologic signs stabilize. As long as the diet does not supply too much energy, confinement generally does not result in flexural limb deformities *(see Chapter 14)*. These problems are fairly common consequences of stall confinement in young, rapidly growing horses.

Compression of the spinal cord can cause inflammation within and around the cord, which can worsen the neurologic signs. So, most veterinarians prescribe anti-inflammatory therapy for a few days. This usually involves a combination of NSAIDs or corticosteroids, and intravenous DMSO *(see Chapter 5)*. In many cases these drugs improve the condition, when combined with stall confinement. However, they generally are of little use after the first week of treatment, and they do not result in a complete or permanent cure.

Surgical Options

Surgery is sometimes recommended for horses over 2 years old with severe CVM. However, it is very involved, "invasive," painful, and expensive. Dynamic compression of the spinal cord is managed by surgically fusing the affected intervertebral joint with a metal "basket" or another type of implant. Static compression is sometimes managed by removing the top part of the affected vertebrae. (This procedure is called a dorsal laminectomy.)

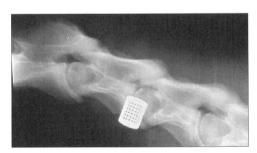

Fig. 12–19. A Bagby basket fuses the affected vertebrae and prevents dynamic compression of the spinal cord.

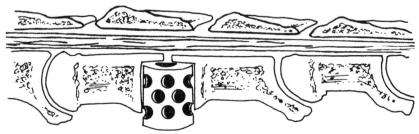

Few surgeons routinely perform these procedures, which require special equipment, considerable experience, and intensive post-operative care. Complications include:

- fractured vertebrae—usually necessitates euthanasia
- wound infection
- osteomyelitis—bone infection *(see Chapter 9)*
- inability to stand after anesthesia

If the horse has shown signs of CVM for months before the surgery, neurologic problems may persist because of permanent spinal cord damage. In most cases surgery only *improves* the neurologic abnormalities; it does not resolve them completely.

Rehabilitation

Whether treated conservatively or surgically, the horse should be started on a program of daily light exercise as soon as the signs have stabilized and no further improvement is anticipated. Daily exercise improves muscle tone and strength. It also helps to "retrain" or re-establish coordination and fine-tuning of movements through repetition. This is because exercise may stimulate other, unaffected nerve pathways to become involved in fine motor control.

It usually takes months before an improvement is obvious. But if the result is a serviceable horse, it is worth the effort. In some cases the ground that is gained through this exercise program may be lost if it is stopped.

Prognosis for CVM

The prognosis depends on:

- the horse's age
- the location and number of vertebrae involved
- the severity of the signs
- the length of time between the beginning of neurologic signs and the start of treatment

In general, the younger the horse, the better the response to conservative management. This is because there is a longer period in which growth can be manipulated. The more severe the signs and the greater the length of time between the onset of signs and treatment, the poorer the outcome is in most cases. Treatment may improve the grade of the neurologic abnormalities. But it is common for a horse with moderate to severe CVM to have some neurologic problems for the rest of its life. Nevertheless, if the horse learns to compensate well it may be able to safely perform some basic activities, such as pleasure riding.

Some horses have raced or competed in other athletic activities with CVM, after either conservative or surgical treatment. In many of these horses, subtle neurologic signs are apparent to the astute observer. This often raises questions about the safety of the rider/driver and other competitors if the horse takes a false step during competition. The decision to compete such a horse should be made only after discussion with the veterinarian who has been treating the horse.

Prevention of CVM

CVM sometimes is a herd or management problem. The methods discussed in Chapter 14 for preventing osteochondrosis should be used to prevent CVM or reduce its incidence and severity.

Equine Protozoal Myeloencephalitis (EPM)
Definition and Cause

Equine Protozoal Myeloencephalitis (EPM) is a disease that affects the horse's spinal cord and brain. It is caused by a protozoa that until recently was called *Sarcocystis neurona*. Researchers have discovered that this organism is virtually identical to a parasite called *Sarcocystis falcatula*, which is a protozoa that infests several bird species, including cowbirds and grackles. Opossums are the normal host animals, although the parasite must pass through a bird before completing its lifecycle in the opossum.

> **Definitions**
>
> **Protozoa:** single-cell, bacteria-like organism.
> **Parasite:** organism that lives off of, and at the expense of, its host organism.

Presumably, the parasite is spread to the horse in opossum droppings on the pasture. The horse is the wrong host—the parasite cannot complete its lifecycle in the horse's body. It also cannot be spread from horse to horse, or from the horse to other animals (or people).

Once the parasite enters the horse's body, it travels to the spinal cord and brain. There it enters the nerve cells and eventually destroys them. The horse's immune response to the parasite causes inflammation and further damage to the nervous system tissues. These destructive changes can occur anywhere in the CNS, often at multiple sites.

The disease has been reported in virtually all breeds of horses. It is seen in most states in the U.S., although it appears to be more common in the northeastern and northern Midwest states. All age groups of horses can be affected, but the disease is most often seen in young adult horses. The amount of stress the horse is under and its immune status probably have much to do with the incidence of this disease. Young horses in training are often under stress, and they are exposed to many infectious organisms that continually challenge their immune systems. Mature horses that are ill are more prone to developing EPM because their immune systems are compromised. Pregnant mares may be more prone to developing EPM in the second half of the pregnancy because of the demands on their systems.

In most cases, only one or two horses in a group are affected at any one time. Outbreaks of EPM are uncommon. Many people feel that this disease is on the increase. However, the apparent increase in the incidence of EPM is probably due to an increased awareness of its existence and improved diagnostic techniques.

Signs of EPM

The type, severity, and progression of the neurologic abnormalities vary widely among horses. This is because the parasite can cause damage anywhere within the CNS, and usually at more than one site. The signs may begin subtly and progress gradually, or they may appear suddenly and worsen rapidly.

Several neurologic abnormalities may be seen with EPM. Although highly variable, the most common signs are:

- ataxia and weakness
- muscle atrophy
- cranial nerve deficits

These signs are discussed in the earlier section on *Neurologic Examination.*

Ataxia and weakness—typical signs of spinal cord disease—are common findings in horses with EPM. The signs are usually *asymmetrical.* In many horses the only initial sign may be slight ataxia or weakness in one leg. This is often mistaken for low-grade lameness. Although the signs may at first be mild, it is common for them to worsen if left untreated. In severe cases the horse may be so unsteady that it falls and is unable to get up.

> **Warning**
>
> Any horse that suddenly shows neurologic signs that rapidly worsen should be treated as a rabies suspect until a specific diagnosis is known, or rabies is definitely ruled out.

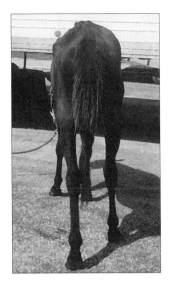
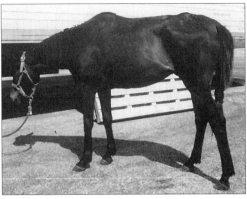

Fig. 12–20. A common symptom of EPM is asymmetric muscle atrophy, particularly over the hindquarters.

The muscle atrophy that is commonly seen with EPM is also asymmetrical. It is usually most obvious over the hindquarters. Muscle atrophy takes a couple of weeks to become obvious, so this sign may not be apparent at first.

Horses with EPM may also show evidence of brain involvement, in particular, cranial nerve deficits. These signs include facial paralysis, drooping ear, lazy eyelid, and difficulty eating and swallowing. As with the other signs, cranial nerve deficits are usually asymmetrical and highly variable. In some cases the signs reflect cerebral or cerebellar disease. Horses with EPM usually do not have a fever, depression, or loss of appetite, even though they may have difficulty eating. *(Cerebral, cerebellar, and cranial nerve signs are listed in Figure 12–44.)*

Diagnosis of EPM

In many cases the veterinarian suspects EPM simply on the signs, although there are several other neurologic diseases that can cause similar signs. In a horse with very mild signs, musculoskeletal causes of vague lameness or gait abnormalities should be ruled out before concentrating on the nervous system. Nuclear scintigraphy *(see Chapter 2)* often helps to pin-

Note

Other problems that may cause similar signs include:
- E/W/VEE (mostly brain signs)
- trauma, infection, or tumors at multiple sites
- rabies

469

More Information

CSF collection, serology, and PCR are discussed in the earlier section on *Diagnostic Tests*.

point the site(s) of low-grade lameness when physical examination and other tests cannot.

At present the only way to confirm the diagnosis of EPM in the live horse is by taking a sample of cerebrospinal fluid. This is usually done with a lumbosacral tap. The CSF sample is tested for antibodies against the parasite (serology), or for protozoal DNA using PCR. The serology test, called Western blot immunoassay, is used more often than PCR.

If the veterinarian cannot collect CSF from the horse, he or she may treat the horse based on the signs. This approach is reasonable; however, without a definite diagnosis it is impossible to know whether the horse actually has EPM. Treating the horse for EPM when it has another neurologic condition delays appropriate treatment. Also, the treatment for EPM can be expensive. So wherever possible the diagnosis should be confirmed.

Interpreting the Results

According to recent research, up to 50% of all horses (both normal horses and those with neurologic signs) have been exposed to this *Sarcocystis* and so have detectable antibodies in their bloodstreams. But detecting antibodies in the bloodstream only proves that the horse has been exposed to the parasite in the past. It does not mean that the parasite caused, or will cause disease, or even is still present in the body. *Therefore, testing for antibodies in a blood sample is usually a waste of time and can even be misleading if it is the only test performed.* (This is why requesting a blood test for EPM during a prepurchase examination is discouraged by most veterinarians, especially when there are no suspicions of neurologic disease.)

Treating a horse for EPM because it had a positive blood test is an even bigger waste of time and money in most cases. Nevertheless, in attempting to diagnose EPM, it is often useful for the veterinarian to submit *both* blood and CSF samples to the laboratory, especially if the CSF sample was contaminated with blood. Some veterinarians use the blood test as a "screen." If the blood test is negative, it is unlikely that the horse has EPM. However, if the blood test is positive, the CSF should be tested to determine whether the horse has the disease.

Serology on the CSF generally is accurate. However, there are a couple of situations in which false positive or false negative results may occur.

False Positives

A false positive result means that antibodies against the parasite were found in the CSF, yet the horse does not have EPM. This situation is possible if the horse was exposed to the parasite and has antibodies in the bloodstream. The CSF may be positive if inflammation or blood vessel damage allowed the antibodies to leak from the bloodstream into the nervous system tissues, or if the sample was contaminated with blood during collection.

Another possible explanation is that the horse may have had EPM in the past and resolved the infection on its own. If the infection caused significant damage to the nervous system tissues, the horse may have permanent neurologic defects, despite resolution of the infection. Antibodies may be detected in the CSF for weeks or months after the infection has resolved, so this horse with permanent neurologic signs may have a positive CSF titer for EPM.

These possibilities are not included to add to the confusion that surrounds EPM. However, it is important to realize that *not every horse with a positive CSF test has EPM.*

False Negatives

A false negative result means that antibodies against the parasite were not found in the CSF, yet the horse does have EPM. This situation could occur in the very early stages of EPM, perhaps because the horse has not had time to produce antibodies against the parasite. (Measurable antibody production usually takes at least 2 weeks after initial exposure.) It could also occur in horses with seriously compromised immune function because they are producing few or no antibodies. Severe illness or corticosteroid therapy are two examples in which this latter situation could occur.

Polymerase Chain Reaction (PCR)

In theory, PCR is more accurate than serology because it tests for the presence of the parasite in the central nervous system, rather than relying on the body's response to the parasite. It can give a true positive result even in horses with a compromised immune system, and in early cases that have not yet produced detectable levels of antibody. Also, PCR is unlikely to produce a false positive result if there has been bleeding into the CSF during collection.

However, no test is 100% accurate. PCR can give false negative results. The parasites invade the nerve cells, rather than floating free in the CSF. They are found in the CSF only when there has been extensive nerve cell damage. So trying to find them in a CSF sample can be like looking for a needle in a haystack. This is especially true when the damaged area is small or a long way from the CSF collection site (usually the lumbosacral space). In other words, when there are few free organisms, diluted in a large volume of fluid, they can be impossible to find. Another limiting factor is that in very severe cases white blood cells destroy and remove the parasites, including their DNA.

Some veterinarians request both serology and PCR when they submit CSF samples to the laboratory. This approach can improve the chances of making a correct diagnosis, especially if serology is negative yet PCR is positive.

Treatment of EPM

The aims of treatment for EPM are 1) to reduce inflammation and subsequent damage in the central nervous system, and 2) to destroy the parasites.

Anti-inflammatory Therapy

NSAIDs and DMSO are the drugs most commonly used to reduce inflammation in horses with EPM. Corticosteroids should be used with extreme caution. These drugs effectively suppress inflammation. But they also inhibit the body's immune response, and a fully functional immune system is essential for resolving the infection. Nevertheless, the veterinarian will give corticosteroids if he or she believes that the benefit of minimizing permanent neurologic damage outweighs the risk of allowing the parasite to spread. This risk can be reduced by starting the horse on anti-protozoal drugs immediately.

More Information
The process of inflammation and anti-inflammatory therapies are detailed in Chapter 5.

Anti-inflammatory therapy helps the most in the first week of treatment. After that, it probably is of limited benefit.

Anti-protozoal Drugs

The most effective anti-protozoal drugs are trimethoprim-sulfonamide combinations and pyrimethamine. Trimethoprim-sulfonamide is an antibiotic combination that is commonly called "trim-sulfa," TMPS, or SMZ. Pyrimethamine is a human anti-malaria drug with the brand name, Daraprim®. The usual recommendation is daily treatment with both drugs for as long as the horse is showing neurologic signs. Treatment is continued for at least 30 days after the signs have resolved. In severe cases the signs may never completely resolve because there is permanent damage in the spinal cord or brain. In these horses treatment should continue until there is a plateau in the horse's recovery, and then be extended at least 30 days past that point.

Continuing the anti-protozoal drugs at least a month after the signs have resolved or stabilized is very important if a relapse is to be avoided. These drugs only suppress the parasite and prevent it from multiplying—they do not kill it outright—so treatment must be prolonged. If the signs are mild, and the condition is diagnosed and treated early, the horse may require only 2 – 3 months of treatment. Others may need the drugs for 6 months or more. This is more likely if the horse is showing severe signs, or if there was a delay between when the signs first appeared and when treatment began.

Relapse of the disease can occur, particularly during periods of stress or illness, even in horses that received proper treatment. When relapse occurs the entire course of treatment must be started again, and continued for at least 30 days after the signs resolve or stabilize. There appears to be very little benefit to giving the drugs for only a month at a time, or only during stressful periods.

Side Effects

These anti-protozoal drugs work by preventing the protozoa from using folic acid, which is essential for protozoal reproduction. Unfortunately, the drugs also block folic acid use in the horse. Folic acid is required for red blood cell production, so the horse may become mildly anemic after several weeks on these drugs. Some veterinarians recommend a blood test to measure the red blood cell count every 3 – 4 weeks in horses being treated with these drugs. If the red cell count is low, a folic acid supplement can be given to the horse. This is more important in pregnant mares than in other horses.

Trim-sulfa can cause diarrhea in horses *(see Chapter 5)*. If the horse's manure merely becomes soft like a "cow-pattie," it is usually safe to continue treatment. The problems created by stopping treatment in a horse with EPM are usually worse than mild diarrhea. However, some horses develop profuse, watery diarrhea, which can be very serious and even life-threatening. Therefore, if there is *any* change in the horse's manure the veterinarian should be notified. He or she can then decide whether it is safe to continue treatment.

Nursing Care and Rehabilitation

Diligent nursing care is very important in all horses with neurologic disease. The feeder and the water container should be placed at

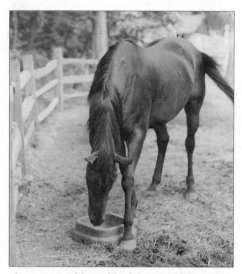

Fig. 12–21. This paddock has good fencing for an ataxic horse. However, it would be best to place the feeder at chest height.

about chest height, and the horse should be watched closely to ensure that it can eat and drink. Ataxic horses often injure themselves, so they should be confined to a well-bedded stall or a small, cleared paddock with good fencing. Whenever a very ataxic horse is moved from its stall or paddock, it is safest to use two people—one to lead the horse and stabilize the front end, and the other to keep a hand on the horse's rump or tail to stabilize the hind end.

Physical therapies, especially electrical muscle stimulation *(see Chapter 4),* can help minimize or reverse muscle atrophy. Once the neurologic signs have stabilized, most horses benefit from a program of daily light exercise. The benefits of such a program are discussed in the earlier section on *Cervical Vertebral Malformation.*

Prognosis for EPM

The prognosis for complete recovery from EPM depends on the severity of the signs. It also depends on the time between the onset of disease and the start of treatment. Horses that are diagnosed and treated early, and respond within days of beginning treatment have a good chance of returning to normal. Although, the disease can recur during periods of stress or illness if treatment was stopped too soon.

Horses that are slower to respond, and still have neurologic signs after about 3 months of treatment have a poor prognosis for complete recovery. In many cases the damage in the CNS is permanent, so these horses have some neurologic defects—although much milder than before treatment—for the rest of their lives.

Prevention of EPM

Currently there is no sure way to prevent exposure to the parasite.

Because it is apparently spread to the horse through the pasture, some people may think that keeping the horse off the pasture could prevent EPM. However, there are a few flaws in this theory. First, there is some evidence that the time between when the parasite enters the body and when the signs are first seen (the incubation period) is highly variable. It can range from a couple of weeks to a couple of years. So, the horse may already have the parasite when it is removed from the pasture. A period of stress or illness may allow the parasite to multiply and cause disease even though the horse has been removed from the pasture. Second, prohibiting all access to pasture is an unhealthy way for a horse to live, and probably does not prevent exposure to the parasite. It could be carried from the pasture to the barn or feed room by flies, rodents, and birds.

Another concern is whether the parasite can be spread in hay. It is not very hardy outside its host animal, so it probably cannot withstand the hay drying and curing processes.

Research is presently aimed at developing a vaccine that results in rapid destruction of the parasite as soon as it enters the horse's body, or at least prevents it from invading the CNS. However, developing a vaccine against EPM is difficult because the parasite is quite complex, and may be able to modify its structure slightly to adapt to its "environment."

Equine Herpesvirus type 1 Myeloencephalitis
Definition and Cause

Equine Herpesvirus type 1 (EHV-1) myeloencephalitis is a disease that affects the spinal cord and brain. It is caused by one of the herpesviruses that infect horses.

There are at least four types of herpesvirus that can cause disease in horses:

EHV-1 can cause three conditions: mild respiratory disease, abortion in pregnant mares, and neurologic disease.

EHV-2 can cause mild respiratory and eye disease in foals.

EHV-3 causes venereal disease (Equine Coital Exanthema).

EHV-4 causes respiratory disease, most often in horses less than about 4 years old. It is one of the leading causes of "colds" in horses.

EHV-1 is spread from one horse to another in secretions, particularly nasal discharges. After being inhaled, the virus invades the nasal passage and throat, causing very mild symptoms of upper airway infection. It then enters the bloodstream. In order to multiply, viruses must invade cells. EHV-1 prefers the cells that line blood vessels (endothelial cells). When the virus invades the arteries and veins in the CNS, damage to the walls of the blood vessels (and leakage of fluid from the damaged vessels) can obstruct blood flow to the tissues supplied by those vessels. However, direct damage by the virus is not what causes the most damage to the central nervous system—it is the body's response to the virus.

Neurologic signs usually begin 1 – 2 weeks after a mild respiratory infection. (In a mature horse the signs of respiratory disease may be so mild and short-lived that they are overlooked or disregarded.) As

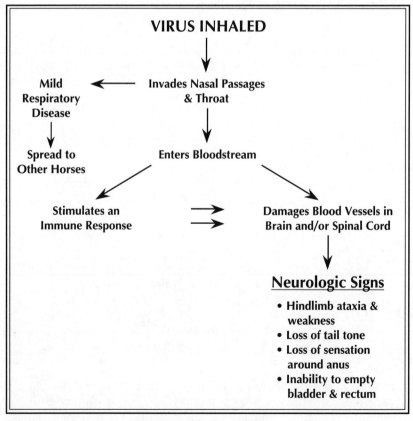

Fig. 12–22. The process of EHV-1 myeloencephalitis.

soon as the virus enters the body, the immune system begins producing antibodies to destroy it, although it takes at least 2 weeks for antibody production to peak. When the antibodies encounter the virus in the blood vessels of the CNS they combine to form an immune complex: antigen plus antibody. It is these immune complexes that cause the most damage. This is the reason for the time lag between viral invasion (seen as mild respiratory disease) and the signs of neurologic disease.

The immune complexes can cause damage anywhere in the CNS, often at multiple sites. However, the damage mainly occurs in the lower half of the spinal cord: the last part of the thoracic segment, and the lumbar and sacral segments.

Signs of EHV-1 Myeloencephalitis

Typical signs of EHV-1 myeloencephalitis include:
- ataxia and weakness in the hindlimbs
- weak or paralyzed tail
- loss of skin sensation around the tail and anus
- inability to urinate and pass manure

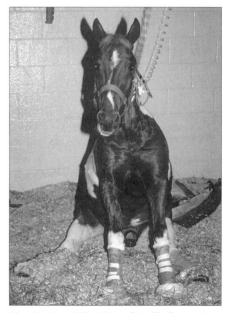

The signs generally are *symmetrical*—the same on both sides of the body. The ataxia and weakness affect both hindlimbs, and can be so severe that the horse is unable to remain standing. In some cases the horse sits like a dog; in others the horse cannot even sit up.

The signs of severe lower spinal cord damage often include a weak or paralyzed tail and paralysis of the bladder and rectal muscles. The penis may also be paralyzed. Often affected horses dribble urine because the bladder cannot be emptied and so it fills to overflowing. Impaction colic is also fairly com-

Fig. 12–23. With EHV-1, hindlimb ataxia and weakness can be so severe that the horse sits like a dog. This horse's penis is also paralyzed.

mon because they are unable to pass manure. The manure builds up in the rectum and lower part of the colon, causing an obstruction. Because the brain may also be affected, cranial nerve deficits *(see Figure 12–44)* are occasionally seen in horses with EHV-1 myeloencephalitis. In a small percentage of horses, the neurologic damage or complications may be so severe that the horse dies or must be euthanized for humane reasons.

Warning
Any horse that suddenly shows neurologic signs that rapidly worsen should be treated as a rabies suspect until a specific diagnosis is known, or rabies is definitely ruled out.

In most cases the first signs are an abnormal gait: mild ataxia, dragging the toes, etc. The signs then progress rapidly (often within hours), becoming most severe by about 48 hours after the first signs are noticed. Horses with EHV-1 myeloencephalitis generally do not have a fever, depression, or loss of appetite.

Diagnosis of EHV-1 Myeloencephalitis

The veterinarian may use several pieces of information to arrive at the diagnosis. The history is very important, as are the signs. But a definite diagnosis generally cannot be made without laboratory tests.

History

Incidents such as recent respiratory disease or abortion in the affected horse, a recently introduced horse, or other horses at the facility are important in determining whether EHV-1 infection is likely. Horses that develop EHV-1 myeloencephalitis often have had, or have been exposed to, a mild respiratory tract infection 1 – 2 weeks before the neurologic signs begin.

The horse's (and the herd's) vaccination status can also be important. Although vaccination will not prevent the neurologic form of the disease, it can reduce the incidence of respiratory tract infection and subsequent viral invasion of the CNS vessels. On the other hand, some veterinarians have observed that EHV-1 myeloencephalitis may be more likely to affect vaccinated horses than unvaccinated horses *(see the section on Prevention of EHV-1)*.

EHV-1 myeloencephalitis can occur as a single, isolated case (sporadic). However, because the virus is easily spread in nasal secretions, epidemics of EHV-1 myeloencephalitis can occur, affecting up to 90% of all horses in a group. Although any age group can be af-

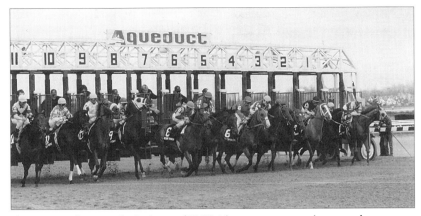

Fig. 12–24. The neurologic form of EHV-1 is more common in young horses under the stress of training and racing.

fected, the neurologic form of the disease is more common in young adult horses under stress, such as race or show training.

Signs

The signs of EHV-1 myeloencephalitis are fairly distinctive, so diagnosis is sometimes possible just from the signs. However, it is important to rule out other causes of hindlimb ataxia, tail weakness, and bladder dysfunction, such as:

- cauda equina neuritis
- sorghum/Sudan grass toxicity
- fracture or osteomyelitis in the lower thoracic or lumbar vertebrae

Laboratory Tests

Blood

There are a couple of laboratory tests that can be performed on a blood sample to help determine that the horse is infected with EHV-1. Serology can detect antibodies against the virus. However, detecting antibodies in the bloodstream simply means the horse was exposed to the virus at some time—it does not necessarily mean the horse has the disease. Also, if the horse has been vaccinated against EHV-1, it will have a positive antibody titer.

To be sure the horse is infected with the virus, it is necessary to take two blood samples, at least 2 weeks apart. It can take this long for a rise in antibody production to be detectable. If the antibody level is higher in the second sample, it is safe to assume that the horse had an active infection at the first sampling. However, this is not a useful method for immediate diagnosis.

The virus can be detected in a sample of blood or nasal secretions for up to 3 weeks after infection. This procedure, called virus isolation, is fairly accurate, but it usually takes several days to get a result. Even then, it does not conclusively prove that the horse has EHV-1 myeloencephalitis.

Cerebrospinal Fluid (CSF)

Performing serology on a CSF sample is the most accurate diagnostic test available. A high antibody titer in the CSF usually means that the horse has EHV-1 myeloencephalitis.

Treatment of EHV-1 Myeloencephalitis

Medications

Anti-viral drugs are not commonly used in horses, although there has been some research that indicates they may have some value in treating EHV-1 infection. However, the virus is only one part of the destructive team—the body's immune response does more harm than the virus.

Managing horses with this condition involves anti-inflammatory therapy, such as corticosteroids, NSAIDs, and/or DMSO *(see Chapter 5)*. Corticosteroids control the inflammatory response and limit further neurologic damage. However, they compromise the body's defense against other organisms, and slow healing. Therefore, the veterinarian may give only one or two doses of corticosteroids and follow up with NSAIDs or DMSO, and antibiotics.

Other Management

Diligent nursing care is important for horses with EHV-1 myeloencephalitis. If the horse is unable to empty its bladder, the veterinarian must insert a catheter into the horse's bladder to allow it to urinate. The catheter can either be sutured in place or reinserted at least twice per day. This procedure must be done very carefully to prevent damage to the urethra, and to minimize the chances of cystitis. Horses with bladder dysfunction commonly develop cystitis, although it can usually

> **Definitions**
>
> **Urethra:** passage between the bladder and the outside of the body.
> **Cystitis:** bacterial infection of the bladder.

be controlled with antibiotics. Vaseline® or Desitin® should be liberally smeared below the vulva and down the backs of the thighs to prevent urine scalding of the skin in mares that are dribbling urine.

If the horse is unable to pass manure, the veterinarian must gently remove all of the manure from the rectum at least once per day. Adding stool softeners, such as Metamucil™, to the horse's feed, or giving mineral oil and fluids through a nasogastric ("stomach") tube can also help prevent impaction colic. If the horse is able, light exercise can assist in emptying both the bladder and the rectum.

Deep, dry bedding is essential for horses that are unable to stand. These horses must be turned frequently to prevent pneumonia, pressure sores, muscle damage, and urine scalding on the "down" side.

Prognosis for EHV-1 Myeloencephalitis

In most epidemics the infection rate may be as high as 90%. Fortunately, the mortality rate is less than 30%.

The prognosis for full recovery is good if the infection is diagnosed and treated early. Recovery may take only a few days in some horses. But complete resolution of the signs may take a couple of months, if the signs are severe. Horses that are unable to stand have a poorer prognosis. They are also more likely to have lasting gait abnormalities or bladder dysfunction because of permanent CNS damage.

Prevention of EHV-1 Myeloencephalitis

Preventing the Disease

Preventing the spread of the respiratory infection is probably the only effective way to reduce the incidence of the neurologic disease. Restricting horse-to-horse contact in large barns and at competitions and shows is important to control the spread of the virus. Other control measures for preventing the spread of infectious diseases are discussed in Chapter 4.

Managing an Epidemic

Horses that develop this disease were probably infected with the virus 1 – 2 weeks earlier, so there is little that can be done to prevent the spread of the neurologic disease during an epidemic. The best plan is to watch all in-contact horses closely for the early signs, and have them examined and treated as soon as neurologic signs are seen. There is no value in vaccinating horses during an outbreak.

Vaccination

There are vaccines available against EHV-1; some just contain EHV-1, while others are combined with EHV-4. However, it is important to realize that *no vaccine is effective in preventing EHV-1 myeloencephalitis.* The EHV-1 vaccine may reduce the incidence of the respiratory disease, and therefore viral invasion of the CNS. However, some veterinarians have observed that EHV-1 myeloencephalitis may be more likely in vaccinated horses than in unvaccinated horses.

There are two possible explanations for this observation. Vaccination causes the body to produce antibodies against the virus. If the virus invades the body around the time of vaccination, immune complexes (virus and antibody) may form and cause CNS damage. Alternatively, if a recently-vaccinated horse encounters the virus, the "primed" immune system may rapidly form immune complexes with the virus, and damage the CNS. These explanations are mere speculation; however, the observation is valid. Because EHV-1 myeloencephalitis is primarily an immune complex disease, vaccination against this virus should not be taken lightly.

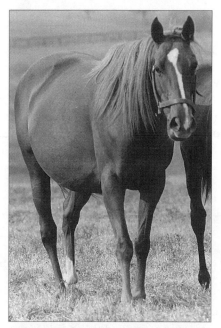

The respiratory disease caused by EHV-1 (or EHV-4, for that matter) is generally very mild in mature horses, compared with another common respiratory disease, influenza. So, the decision to vaccinate a particular adult horse or group of horses against EHV-1 is best made by the veterinarian who regularly attends that horse or facility. The veterinarian can also advise on the specific vaccination schedule(s) for the horse or herd. In pregnant mares, the risk of abortion from EHV-1 infection appears to be much greater than the risk of neurologic disease, so there is real merit in vaccinating mares against EHV-1 during the second half of the pregnancy.

Fig. 12–25. Mares in the second half of pregnancy should be vaccinated against EHV-1.

Equine Degenerative Myelopathy (EDM)

Definition and Causes

Equine Degenerative Myelopathy (EDM) is an uncommon degenerative condition that affects the spinal cord of horses less than about 12 months old. The cause(s) is still unknown, although one study identified several risk factors, including:

- vitamin E deficiency
- using insecticides on foals
- using wood preservers on fencing
- feeding pelleted feeds and hay, with no regular access to pasture
- keeping foals in dirt pens or paddocks, rather than on pasture
- heredity

The fact that many affected foals are deficient in vitamin E has led scientists to assume that vitamin E deficiency plays a key role in the development of EDM. Vitamin E is an antioxidant—it can prevent or minimize cell damage from oxidation. Perhaps insecticides and wood preservers contain compounds that cause oxidation, or cell damage by other means. Combating the effects of these chemicals may use up the foal's body stores of vitamin E, causing vitamin E deficiency. (However, this is just speculation.)

Definitions
Oxidation: destructive chemical reaction within the tissues. **Antioxidant:** prevents or limits cell damage from oxidation.

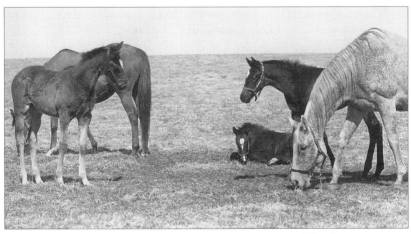

Fig. 12–26. Foals kept on pasture have a much lower risk of developing EDM.

483

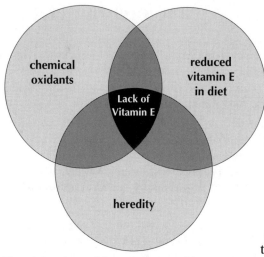

chemical oxidants

reduced vitamin E in diet

Lack of Vitamin E

heredity

Fig. 12–27. Several factors may combine to increase the likelihood of EDM.

Pelleted feeds and cured hays are low in vitamin E. This fact may explain why diets based on these feeds increase the risk of EDM. Foals kept in dirt pens or paddocks generally are fed a ration that contains little or no fresh feed materials, so their diet is likely to be vitamin E-deficient. In contrast, foals kept on pasture have a much lower risk of developing EDM.

Foals born to mares that have already produced a foal that developed EDM are more likely to develop the disease than foals born to mares with healthy foals. This fact has led scientists to believe that there may be a hereditary component to the disease, although this remains to be proved. It may be that some horses have an inherently greater need for vitamin E, or they are less efficient at absorbing it from the intestine or using it within their cells.

These factors tend to add up. On farms where many or all of these factors exist, EDM is more likely to occur. That is, the more factors present, the more likely the foal will develop EDM.

Signs of EDM

The signs of EDM are very similar to those of Cervical Vertebral Malformation ("wobbler" syndrome): symmetrical ataxia and weakness that often involves all four limbs, but is usually worse in the hindlimbs. There are no cranial nerve deficits or muscle atrophy, and the disease generally does not progress to the point of paralysis.

At first, the condition is usually subtle, being little more than a "clumsy" foal. However, the signs slowly progress until the foal shows obvious signs. In general, the younger the foal when the signs first appear, the worse the signs and the more rapid their progression.

Diagnosis of EDM

There is no diagnostic test that confirms EDM. A definite diagnosis cannot be made unless the foal is euthanized and sections of the spinal cord are examined under a microscope. The diagnosis in the live foal must be made by a process of elimination: ruling out other potential causes of the signs, including:

- Cervical Vertebral Malformation
- trauma
- Equine Herpesvirus type 1 (EHV-1) myeloencephalitis
- Equine Protozoal Myeloencephalitis (EPM)
- other developmental abnormalities

Careful physical and neurologic examinations, radiography, and CSF analysis can help eliminate most of these conditions from the list. Evaluating the foal's environment and diet can also help in making the diagnosis, especially if several of the risk factors are present.

Measuring the amount of vitamin E in the blood may indicate vitamin E deficiency, although this does not confirm the disease. The blood vitamin E concentration varies widely among horses, and it even fluctuates in the same horse in the course of a day. So, a single measurement of vitamin E in one foal is not very helpful. Either several foals should be tested (whether or not they are showing signs), or several blood samples should be taken from the affected foal over a 24-hour period. Young horses usually have a lower blood vitamin E concentration than mature horses, so this fact should also be taken into account when interpreting the test results.

In many cases the diagnosis is made "retrospectively." That is, if the foal responds to treatment, it can be assumed that it has EDM.

Treatment and Prevention of EDM

This condition does not resolve spontaneously. Long-term supplementation with large doses of vitamin E is necessary. Oral vitamin E is probably as effective as injectable products; also it is easier and less traumatic to administer. Vitamin E supplements that also contain selenium should not be used because, at the dose required to treat EDM, selenium toxicity can occur. Furthermore, these foals generally are not selenium-deficient.

> **More Information**
>
> Signs of selenium toxicity are given in the section on *White Muscle Disease* in Chapter 10.

Once vitamin E supplementation is begun, an improvement is usually seen in 3 – 4 weeks if EDM is the problem. The foal should continue to slowly improve over the next few months, but treatment should probably continue until the horse is at least 18 months old.

Vitamin E can also be given to the foal's herdmates to prevent EDM, although the protective value of this treatment remains to be determined. The benefits of vitamin E as an antioxidant may help horses with other neurologic diseases. So, even if EDM is never confirmed, or the foal proves to have another condition, vitamin E supplementation will do no harm, and may even be worthwhile.

Anti-inflammatory therapy is of little benefit in this condition, although some veterinarians give corticosteroids to limit further cell degeneration. The known risk factors for EDM should be avoided or corrected where possible. Also, the breeder should seriously consider not breeding from the affected foal's mare again.

Prognosis for EDM

It can take several months for the foal to recover, and the prognosis for future athletic usefulness is guarded. The younger the foal at the onset of the signs and the more severe the signs, the worse the prognosis. Older foals seem to stand a better chance than younger foals.

Rabies

Definition and Cause

Rabies is a deadly viral disease that can affect all warm-blooded animals and people. The virus is usually spread in the saliva of an infected (rabid) animal. In most cases transmission occurs via a bite, although the virus may also be spread if infected saliva contacts a wound on another animal or person. Because this disease is easily transmitted and highly fatal, a rabid (or even

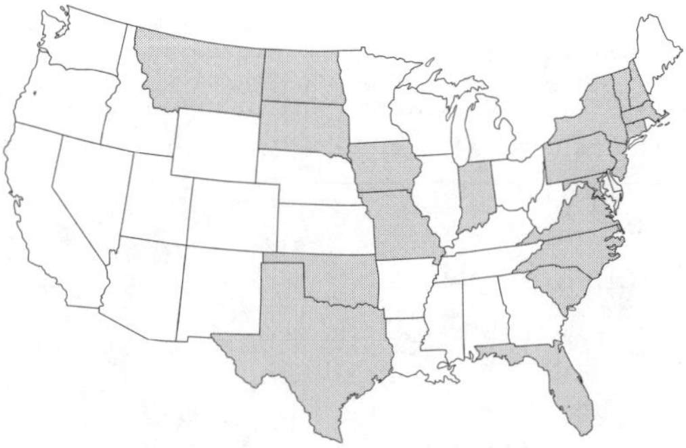

Fig. 12–28. States where rabies has been recently reported in horses. (Puerto Rico, not shown, has also reported cases.)

suspect) animal is a significant public health risk.

Rabies fluctuates in prevalence from year to year. It has been on the increase in several states in the U.S., particularly the Mid-Atlantic and northeast states. The disease has reached epidemic proportions in the wildlife populations in those states. Skunks and raccoons currently are most likely to spread rabies on the east coast, although foxes, coyotes, bats, bobcats, and other wild animals can also carry the disease. The risk of rabies is therefore increased on properties that are heavily wooded, or close to a wooded area.

Rabies is very uncommon in horses, so much so that the public health authorities consider the

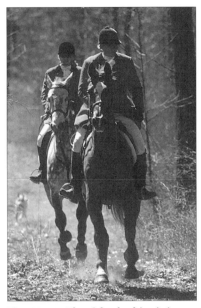

Fig. 12–29. The risk of rabies is increased in horses that live in or near wooded areas.

horse to be a "sentinel" animal. This means that when rabies is diagnosed in a horse, the disease has reached epidemic proportions in that area.

Signs

The signs of rabies in horses can be highly variable, although the most consistent signs are altered behavior and abnormal cranial nerve function *(see Figure 12–44)*. The incubation period—the time between infection and the first signs of disease—is also highly variable, ranging from several days to a few months. But once the signs develop they rapidly progress to recumbency (an inability to get up), seizures or coma, and death. In most cases death occurs within 3 – 7 days of the first signs.

Rabies should be seriously considered whenever a horse suddenly develops rapidly progressing neurologic abnormalities. Sometimes the first signs in horses are vague lameness or ataxia and weakness—that is, spinal cord signs. These symptoms rapidly worsen until the horse is unable to stand. In some cases the horse does not show behavioral abnormalities until just before death.

Hydrophobia ("fear of water," or refusal to drink) is a very uncom-

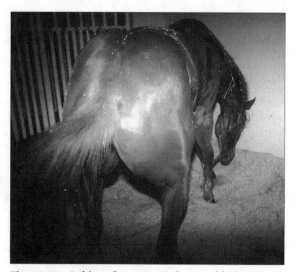

Fig. 12–30. Rabies often causes abnormal behavior, such as head-pressing.

mon sign of rabies in horses. More common signs include vision problems (apparent blindness), hyperreactivity, colic, and erratic behavior; the horse may also have a slight fever. Because the incubation period can be quite long, it is rare to find the original bite wound from the rabid animal.

Diagnosis of Rabies

It is usually impossible to definitely diagnose rabies before the horse dies. A thorough history, and comprehensive physical and neurologic examinations may raise a suspicion of rabies. But because the early signs are so variable, it is very difficult to be certain of the diagnosis. The veterinarian should be highly suspicious of any horse that suddenly develops neurologic signs which rapidly progress to recumbency and death in a few days. On the other hand, if the neurologic signs stabilize or improve after a few days, the veterinarian can be fairly confident the horse does not have rabies.

There is no laboratory test that can reliably confirm the diagnosis in a live animal. After the rabid animal bites the horse, the virus invades the nearest nerve fibers, travels up them, and spreads to the spinal cord and brain. So, the immune system may be unaware of the virus until it is too late. This is why taking a blood sample for serology is usually not useful. The disease progresses too rapidly for antibody production to help form the diagnosis. Also, prior vaccination against rabies results in a positive titer, which can be confusing. Is the test positive because the horse was vaccinated, or because it had rabies?

Virus isolation from the CSF or saliva takes too long to be of any use. Because of the potential human health risk, most veterinarians will not risk exposure to rabies by performing CSF collection on a suspect horse. It is sometimes possible to detect antibodies from the surface of the eye or the base of a hair follicle, although as with serology this test frequently is negative early in the course of the disease.

In almost all cases the diagnosis can only be confirmed by submitting the horse's brain to the state diagnostic laboratory. To be safe, every horse that died or was euthanized after a rapidly progressive neurologic disease should be tested for rabies. The veterinarian must remove the horse's brain and submit it to the state pathologist. The veterinarian should then arrange for the safe, immediate disposal of the rest of the carcass. This is necessary to identify a potential human health risk and to control the spread of this deadly disease. In most cases, the state pathologist will report the results in 1 – 3 days.

Management of Rabies

There is no cure for rabies—it is a fatal disease. It is also a disease that spreads readily to other animals and people in secretions, especially saliva. So, extreme care should be taken when working with any horse suspected of having rabies—that is, any horse with sudden onset of unexplained neurologic signs. Such precautions should include the following:

1. Avoid all contact with saliva from a suspect horse. Wear rubber or latex gloves at all times when handling the horse.
2. Isolate the horse, and limit access to only the one or two people directly involved with its care. If possible, the horse should be cared for only by people who have been vaccinated against rabies. The horse should be handled as infrequently as its medical condition allows.
3. Follow standard procedures for hygiene and disinfection of feed and water utensils, and other in-contact equipment *(see Chapter 4)*.
4. Keep all dogs, cats, other animals, and children away from the immediate area.

The law varies from place to place as to the procedure that must be followed when a horse is definitely diagnosed with rabies. All other horses on that farm or at that barn are considered to be potentially exposed to the disease. In some areas regulations require that "exposed" horses that have been vaccinated within the past year must be revaccinated within 72 hours. They may also need to be quarantined for up to 45 days. Unvaccinated "exposed" horses may either be euthanized immediately (by law), or strictly quarantined for up to

8 months. For specific regulations in the U.S., contact the State Department of Agriculture.

Prevention of Rabies

Annual vaccination against the rabies virus generally prevents the disease. It is recommended for all horses living in, or traveling to areas where rabies has been recently reported. Given that the vaccine is effective, inexpensive, and very safe, it is well worth protecting all horses against rabies.

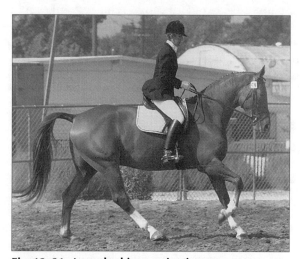

Fig. 12–31. Annual rabies vaccinations are recommended for horses traveling to areas where rabies has been recently reported.

Most veterinarians have themselves vaccinated against rabies, and it is a good idea for horse owners and trainers living in areas where rabies is always a threat to consult with their physicians about rabies vaccination for themselves. People can be vaccinated after exposure to a rabid animal. However, this involves a course of injections, which can be painful and expensive. Post-exposure vaccination is not practiced in animals because of the potential human health risk an exposed animal poses.

Other Conditions

The following conditions of the brain and spinal cord are uncommon in horses (and some are even rare). But they have been included because they can cause lameness or more vague gait abnormalities.

Bacterial Infections

Bacteria can enter the central nervous system in several ways:

• penetrating wounds that directly involve the CNS
• spread from a nearby abscess or infected bone
• through the bloodstream (more common in young foals)
• cosmetic tail surgery
• injecting substances into the tail base
• CSF collection

The results of infection within the CNS depend on which structures are affected, and the location.

Abscesses

Abscesses can develop anywhere in the brain or spinal cord, although they are more likely in the front of the brain (the cerebrum). The bacteria that cause strangles *(Streptococcus equi)* are the organisms most commonly cultured from brain abscesses in horses. The bacteria probably spread to the brain from infection in the throat or sinuses.

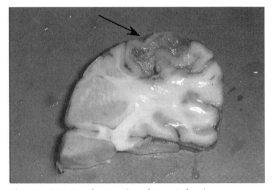

Fig. 12–32. An abscess in a horse's brain.

The signs of an abscess in the CNS depend on its location. When the abscess is located in the cerebrum the signs can rapidly progress to coma or seizures, and death. *(Figure 12–44 lists the more common signs of neurologic dysfunction in other parts of the CNS.)*

Treatment is often unrewarding because by the time the signs are obvious, the abscess and destruction of the nervous system tissues are well advanced. In all cases the prognosis for recovery is poor.

Meningitis

Meningitis is inflammation of the meninges, the membranes that cover the brain and spinal cord. Bacterial meningitis is most common in newborn foals that developed systemic infection (septicemia) because of inadequate intake of colostrum. Colostrum is the antibody-rich milk the mare produces around the time of foaling.

Bacterial infection of the meninges causes inflammation of the membranes and an accumulation of pus between the membrane and the brain or spinal cord. This increases the pressure within the

CNS. The infection can also spread to the nervous system tissues.

The initial signs are nonspecific and quite variable. Depression, loss of appetite, fever, and weakness are common at first. Neurologic signs, such as altered behavior or gait abnormalities (depending on the location of the infection) then develop and rapidly progress. Bacterial culture and antibiotic sensitivity tests *(see Chapter 2)* on the CSF are necessary to confirm the diagnosis, identify the bacteria responsible, and choose the most appropriate antibiotic.

Treatment involves antibiotics and anti-inflammatory drugs. Antibiotics are a very important part of treatment. They must be started early and continued for at least 7 days after the signs have resolved. DMSO is commonly used to treat meningitis in foals and adult horses. It is an effective anti-inflammatory drug, and it improves antibiotic penetration into the CNS—a problem for many antibiotics because of the blood-brain barrier (discussed earlier). But despite appropriate therapy and diligent nursing care, the prognosis is poor.

Fungal meningitis is even more serious than bacterial meningitis because fungal infection of the CNS usually only occurs in horses with a compromised immune system. Fungal infections can be very difficult to control at the best of times, but they are even more difficult to resolve if the horse's immune system is not functioning normally. Furthermore, many antifungal drugs have toxic side effects.

Vertebral Osteomyelitis

Osteomyelitis (bone infection; *see Chapter 9)* of the vertebrae occasionally occurs in foals. Several bacteria have been known to cause vertebral osteomyelitis. *Rhodococcus equi,* a common cause of pneumonia in older foals, is the bacteria that most often causes this condition. In adult horses vertebral osteomyelitis may develop as the result of a wound, either traumatic or surgical.

The signs of vertebral osteomyelitis include:

- fever
- stiffness
- reluctance to move
- neck or back pain
- weakness

Neurologic signs can develop if the diseased bone or pus compresses the spinal cord.

Radiography is helpful in establishing the diagnosis, but only after significant bone destruction has occurred. CSF analysis may confirm the diagnosis, but if the infection is confined to the bone, the CSF may be normal. In many cases bacterial culture of a blood sample (a blood culture) must be performed. This test identifies the bacteria responsible, and determines the most appropriate antibiotic for treatment.

In all cases the prognosis for full recovery is poor, particularly if substantial bone destruction has occurred.

Equine Encephalitis Viruses (E/W/VEE)

Eastern, Western, and Venezuelan Equine Encephalitis viruses cause neurologic disease in horses. The viruses are spread by mosquitoes, so these diseases are more common in the warmer months, and in warmer areas. As the names indicate, Eastern Equine Encephalitis (EEE) is more prevalent in the eastern United States, and Western (WEE) in the western United States. Venezuelan Equine Encephalitis (VEE) is more common in South America, but occasional cases are reported in the southern U.S. These diseases can affect people, although they are not caught from an infected horse. The disease is spread to people the same way it is spread to horses: by an infected mosquito.

The first signs of infection include fever, depression, and loss of appetite. Neurologic signs develop 1 – 5 days later. These viruses primarily affect the brain, especially the cerebrum. So altered behavior is the most consistent feature of these diseases. Occasionally ataxia (incoordination) and weakness are also seen. The severity of the signs and the mortality rate vary, depending on which virus is causing the disease. EEE and VEE usually cause more severe disease than WEE, and are more likely to be fatal. The diagnosis can be confirmed with serology (discussed in the earlier section on *Diagnostic Tests*).

There is no specific treatment for these diseases. At present all that can be done is anti-inflammatory therapy to reduce inflammation in the brain and spinal cord, and diligent nursing care. Anti-viral drugs are not commonly used in horses, but as newer drugs are developed and found to be effective, they may become important in the treatment of these diseases.

The prognosis for survival is guarded for WEE, and poor for EEE and VEE. If the horse recovers, neurologic abnormalities commonly persist.

These diseases can be prevented by annual vaccination. Booster injections should be given every 6 months in areas where the disease is prevalent. It is also worthwhile attempting to control the mosquito population in the area.

> **Of Interest**
>
> One way to control mosquitoes is to eliminate their breeding areas. For example, rain barrels, old tires, and soaks could be removed or filled in with dirt.

Tetanus

Tetanus is a highly fatal disease in horses. It is caused by a toxin that is produced by *Clostridium tetani* bacteria. The spores (the dormant form) of these bacteria are commonly found in the horse's environment, including normal horse manure. They can enter the tissues through any wound. These bacteria need an environment that is low in oxygen. Wounds that are deep or that do not have a good blood supply are perfect sites for these organisms to multiply and release their toxin. The toxin travels along the nerves to the central nervous system, where it prevents the normal control of lower motor neuron function (discussed earlier). The result is uncontrolled muscle spasms.

Signs and Diagnosis

The incubation period (the time between entry of the bacteria and the development of signs) can be as short as a few days, or as long as several weeks. The first signs of tetanus usually are subtle: mild stiffness or a reluctance to lower the head to eat or drink. The signs then progress over the next 2 – 4 days to generalized muscle spasms, which causes the classic "sawhorse" stance. Other signs associated with tetanus include an anxious facial expression, protrusion of the third eyelid (the small, pink flap of tissue in the inner corner of the eye), and an inability to relax the jaw muscles ("lockjaw").

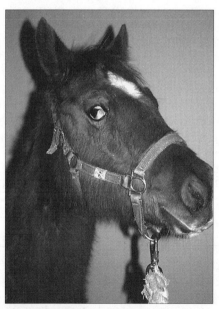

Fig. 12–33. A horse with tetanus.

Once the horse is showing obvious signs of tetanus the disease quickly progresses to the point where the horse is unable to eat, drink, or stand. Death is caused by paralysis of the respiratory muscles.

The diagnosis is based on the signs. However, early on the signs can be confused with laminitis, exertional rhabdomyolysis ("tying up"), and, in nursing mares, hypocalcemia. *(The latter two conditions are discussed in Chapter 10.)*

Treatment and Prognosis

Treatment involves giving large doses of tetanus antitoxin, either intravenously or into the CSF. This is usually done at the atlanto-occipital space. If the initial wound is still present, it should be opened and thoroughly cleaned. The horse should also be given a course of penicillin because the tetanus bacteria are very sensitive to this antibiotic. Most veterinarians prefer to use an intravenous form of penicillin, giving it through an intravenous catheter. This is because overstimulation and worsening of the muscle spasms can occur with IM injections.

In some cases the horse must be tranquilized or anesthetized to control the painful muscle spasms. Sudden movements or noise can cause the muscle spasms to worsen, so the horse must be kept in a quiet, dark, well-bedded stall. Handling and noise should be kept to a minimum. Diligent nursing care is essential, particularly if the horse is unable to stand, eat, or drink.

Of all the animals that are susceptible to tetanus, horses are by far the most sensitive to the toxin. For this reason, tetanus carries a guarded to poor prognosis in all cases. The prognosis is worse if the horse is unable to stand. If the horse does survive, it usually takes at least 6 weeks for it to fully recover. Fortunately, most horses that survive tetanus do not have any lasting neurologic defects.

Prevention

Tetanus is a preventable disease. It cannot be emphasized too strongly that *every horse should be regularly vaccinated against tetanus.* Vaccination involves an initial course of two injections, given 2 – 4 weeks apart, followed by a single "booster" injection every year for the rest of the horse's life. The tetanus vaccine (tetanus toxoid) is very effective, so in theory, a responsible owner should never lose a horse to tetanus. *(See Chapter 5 for more information on tetanus prevention.)*

Plant and Fungal Toxins
Locoweed

Locoweed is a plant that is found in the western part of the U.S. and Canada. Horses that graze this plant develop the following signs:

• progressive weight loss
• jerky head movements
• altered behavior (depression or hyper-excitability)
• ataxia

There is no treatment for this condition. Even if the horse is re-moved from the contaminated pasture, recovery can take a long time, and there may be some persistent gait abnormalities. If the horse is stressed the signs can return or worsen.

Sorghum/Sudan Grass

Sorghum species, such as Sudan and Johnson grass, can cause a syndrome of hindlimb ataxia and an inability to empty the bladder. This condition is occasionally seen in the southwestern U.S. during periods of high rainfall and rapid plant growth. The toxin causes degenera-tion of the lower part of the spinal cord (the lumbosacral region). There is no specific treatment. Most horses improve slowly once they are removed from the pasture. The more severely affected horses may have some persis-tent neurologic abnormalities.

Note
Other problems that may cause similar signs include: • EHV-1 myeloencephalitis • cauda equina neuritis • trauma to lumbar or sacral vertebrae

Bracken Fern

Bracken fern and horsetail fern both contain the enzyme thiami-nase. This enzyme breaks down thiamine, an essential B vitamin. After eating bracken or horsetail fern for several weeks, the horse may develop signs of thiamine deficiency, which include ataxia in all four limbs. Treatment involves removing the horse from the pasture (or removing the ferns from the pasture), and giving the horse oral or injectable thiamine until the signs resolve. Recovery is usually rapid and complete.

Leukoencephalomalacia (LEM)

Leukoencephalomalacia (LEM) is a fatal disease of the brain that is caused by eating corn that is infested with a fungus. "Moldy corn poisoning," "corn stalk disease," and "blind staggers" are common names for this condition. The fungus infests the corn before harvest, and when the horse eats the dried corn, fungal toxins cause severe brain damage which rapidly ends in death. The early signs of LEM are highly variable, and may include ataxia, weakness, and muscle tremors, in addition to cerebral and cranial nerve signs *(see Figure 12–44)*. There is no treatment for this condition, other than support-ive care. The prognosis is grave because large areas of the brain can be permanently damaged in a very short period.

"Ryegrass Staggers"

Perennial ryegrass, Dallis grass, and Bermuda grass may be infested with a fungus that can produce CNS disease. The signs indicate cerebellar and spinal cord involvement: jerky head movements, ataxia, stumbling, and muscle tremors or spasms. Horses usually recover within a few weeks of being removed from the pasture or fed a different type of hay.

Parasitic Migration

Occasionally, internal parasites migrate through the central nervous system, causing massive tissue damage and hemorrhage. This condition is called verminous encephalomyelitis. One parasite that has been known to invade the CNS is *Strongylus vulgaris* (redworms, or bloodworms). Another is warble fly larvae ("cattle grubs"). The neurologic signs vary with the site and severity of the damage, although they typically develop and worsen rapidly. Diagnosis is difficult while the horse is alive. It is often based on the horse's poor deworming history. In the case of the warble fly, evidence of skin infestation can be seen. Treatment, which involves deworming and anti-inflammatory therapy, is seldom successful because of the amount of tissue destruction the parasites cause.

Developmental Abnormalities

Abnormalities of the brain, spinal cord, or spinal column can develop before birth, although these conditions are rare in horses. Two of the conditions that are more likely to cause gait abnormalities in foals are described below.

Atlanto-Occipital Malformation

Inherited abnormalities of the first two cervical vertebrae (the atlas and the axis) are occasionally seen in Arabian foals. In atlanto-occipital malformation, the atlas and the occipital bone at the back of the skull are malformed or fused. In atlanto-axial malformation, the atlas and the axis are malformed or fused. In some cases the atlas or axis is underdeveloped, which can cause dislocation of the affected vertebrae. Malformation, fusion, or dislocation can compress the spinal cord, causing ataxia and weakness from birth.

In many cases the diagnosis is obvious because the foal's head and neck posture are abnormal, the range of head motion is reduced, and the vertebrae are obviously abnormal when palpated. The diagnosis is confirmed with radiography. Some foals improve with surgical stabilization of the vertebrae, although surgery may not make the foal completely normal.

Cerebellar Abiotrophy/Hypoplasia

Cerebellar abiotrophy is a congenital, degenerative disease of the cerebellum that is also found in Arabian foals. The first signs, which reflect cerebellar disease *(see Figure 12–44)*, may be seen within a few days of birth. But usually they are not noticed until about 2 – 4 months of age. The diagnosis is based on the history, particularly the breed and age of the foal, and on the signs. There is no treatment for this disease. The signs improve in some horses as they mature, perhaps because they learn to compensate for the condition. This condition may be hereditary, so the foal's dam and sire should probably not be bred together again.

Definitions
Congenital: present at birth. **Hereditary:** passed down from the sire or dam through the genes.

Cerebellar hypoplasia is underdevelopment of the cerebellum. It is a rare condition that has been reported in Thoroughbreds, Paso Finos, and Haflingers. The signs of cerebellar disease are present from birth. The cause(s) is unknown, and there is no treatment for the condition.

Tumors

Tumors that begin in, or spread to the brain or spinal cord are rare in horses. Of the possible tumor types, melanomas and lymphosarcomas are more likely to spread to the CNS and cause gait abnormalities, as well as other signs of CNS disease. The type and severity of the signs depend on the location and size of the tumor. Treatment is difficult and almost always unsuccessful. The prognosis is poor because the tumor is usually quite advanced before the diagnosis is made.

CONDITIONS INVOLVING NERVES
Trauma

Trauma involving the nerves can occur at any location. However, some nerves are more at risk, and are damaged more often than others. In most cases it is the superficial nerves that run over a bone surface that are damaged. Nerve function may be interrupted if the nerve is:

- bruised
- compressed by soft tissue swelling or fibrosis (scar tissue)
- crushed
- severed by a laceration, surgical incision, or bone fragment
- stretched or torn

The severity of nerve damage determines the outcome. Bruising and swelling within or around the nerve usually resolve, and nerve function returns within days or weeks of injury. (Although signs of nerve dysfunction may persist if fibrosis compresses the nerve.) For example, radial nerve paralysis is occasionally seen after general anesthesia, as a result of the horse lying on its side for a long time. Although the paralysis may be severe, nerve function usually returns within 2 – 3 days with appropriate treatment.

In contrast, when nerve fibers are completely crushed, severed, or torn, they take several months to regenerate. Unless the nerve is surgically reconstructed, the part of the nerve fiber that is no longer connected to the nerve cell body dies. For nerve supply to be restored to the area, the nerve fibers must regrow between the site of damage and the tissues they are meant to supply. Nerve fibers regrow at a rate of about 1 mm per day, or an inch per month. So, it can take several months for function to be restored to a tissue that is some distance from the site of nerve injury. In some cases the loss of nerve function is permanent.

General Management of Nerve Injuries
Anti-Inflammatory Therapy

Unless it is clear that the nerve has been completely severed, anti-inflammatory therapies (cold, corticosteroids, NSAIDs, and DMSO; *see Chapter 5*) are very important for the first week after injury. These therapies are most effective in limiting inflammation and swelling (which can cause further nerve compression) in the first few hours after injury. As long as there is no potential for infection, corticosteroids are often the best anti-inflammatory drugs for nerve injuries. However, the harmful effects of corticosteroid use must be considered.

If the nerve has been severed it is sometimes possible to surgically reconnect the two ends. However, it is usually very difficult to find the ends of the nerve with all the tissue trauma that can occur with such an injury.

It is often impossible to know how severely the nerve has been damaged at first. Compression of a nerve can cause temporary loss of skin sensation or muscle function that is just as complete as if the nerve was crushed or severed. For this reason, the response to anti-inflammatory therapy is important in determining how the condition should be managed in the weeks and months following injury. It can also help determine the long-term prognosis. Based on the response to treatment, nerve injuries can be divided into three categories:

1. **Mild damage,** such as bruising and compression, responds in 2 – 3 days. Nerve function usually returns to normal within a week.
2. **Moderate damage,** such as crushing or stretching that does not completely disrupt the nerve fibers, improves in the 2 – 3 weeks following injury. Full function usually is restored in the following weeks or months.
3. **Severe damage,** such as a severed or torn nerve, shows no change in the 2 – 3 weeks following injury, and may not even improve in the following few months. If nerve function returns, it usually takes at least 6 months.

After 2 – 3 weeks, whatever nerve function has returned to the area is usually all that will be present for the next few months.

Other Recommendations

If the horse cannot bear weight on the affected leg, the veterinarian may recommend confining the horse to a stall or small paddock until it is able to use the leg more normally. Confinement may last for as little as a couple of weeks, or as long as several months. The length of time depends on the severity of nerve damage and the rate at which nerve function is restored. Splinting the lower leg can help the horse place the foot and bear weight on the leg. It also helps prevent flexor contracture in young horses *(see Chapter 14)*. A firm support bandage and frog support should be kept on the opposite, weight-bearing limb until the horse can use the affected limb. The frog support helps prevent laminitis in the weight-bearing limb. Bedding the horse's stall with deep shavings or sand can also reduce the risk of laminitis.

As soon as the condition allows, a program of daily light exercise should be started. Exercise (longeing or riding, if safe) can help minimize muscle atrophy. It is also important for retraining the nerve and muscle as function is restored.

Physical therapies *(see Chapter 4)*, in particular electrical muscle stimulation, can also help minimize muscle atrophy. Low-level laser therapy may promote nerve regeneration in some cases, although it is difficult to objectively evaluate the success of this treatment. Some veterinarians have used injections of Rubeola virus (an immune system stimu- lant) in an effort to speed the return of nerve function. However, the results are highly variable, and claims of its effec- tiveness are often made within 2 – 3 weeks of injury. This is about when mod- erate nerve injuries substantially im- prove anyway. Attributing the improvement to the Rubeola injection probably is giving it too much credit.

More Information
Bandaging and splinting techniques are dis- cussed in Chapter 4.
Using the frog to sup- port the foot is covered in Chapter 7.

Prognosis for Nerve Injuries

The long-term prognosis depends on the degree of nerve damage. For mild injuries, the prognosis for rapid and complete return of nerve function and a normal gait is excellent. Moderate injuries take longer to resolve. But in most cases partial or complete return of nerve function results in a serviceable horse within a few months. When severe damage results in complete disruption of the nerve, the prognosis for return of nerve function is guarded at best. Patience and persistence with these cases are sometimes rewarded. However, there is always the possibility that the horse will have a permanent gait abnormality after such severe nerve damage.

Specific Nerve Injuries

The nerves that are more commonly damaged in horses, and the associated gait abnormalities that are typical of such damage, are discussed below.

Radial Nerve Paralysis

The radial nerve supplies:

- the extensor muscles at the front of the forearm *(see Chapter 11)*
- the triceps muscles at the side of the shoulder
- the skin on the outside and front of the forearm

Radial nerve damage usually occurs where the nerve runs across the side of the humerus, midway between the elbow and the shoulder. A blow to the side of the shoulder or a humeral fracture can damage the radial nerve as it tracks across the humerus *(see Chapter 19)*.

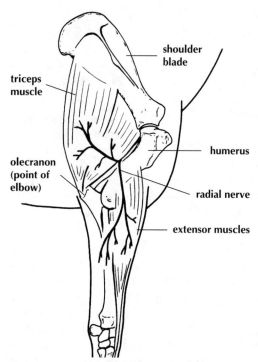

triceps muscle

shoulder blade

humerus

olecranon (point of elbow)

radial nerve

extensor muscles

Fig. 12–34. The path of the radial nerve.

Some of the more common incidents that can cause radial nerve paralysis are collision with a solid object (such as a tree, stall door, or fence post), a kick, and a fall. The nerve can also be stretched or torn if the horse slips and its leg slides out sideways. Temporary radial nerve paralysis is also occasionally seen after general anesthesia, if the horse has been lying on its side during a long procedure.

Signs and Diagnosis

Radial nerve paralysis prevents the horse from extending (straightening) its fetlock and knee, and bringing the lower leg forward. If only the extensor branch is damaged, the horse may be able to bear weight when the leg is manually placed in the normal position. However, the horse cannot bring the foot forward or place it flat on its own. Typically, the horse stands with its knee and fetlock flexed, and the front of the hoof on the ground. When it walks it drags the foot and hops on three legs. With practice, the horse may be able to pull its leg forward a little using its shoulder muscles, although it cannot place or stand on the foot without assistance.

If the triceps branch of the nerve is also damaged, the elbow appears "dropped," which makes the leg appear longer. It also prevents the horse from bearing weight on the leg, even when placed manually, because it cannot fix its elbow in the standing position.

Pinching or lightly pricking the skin over the front and side of the forearm reveals loss of skin sensation in this area. Over time, usually a couple of weeks, the muscles supplied by the radial nerve begin to atrophy from lack of stimulation. Muscle atrophy is usually reversible, if nerve function returns.

In horses showing these signs the shoulder and elbow should be carefully palpated for evidence of a humeral or olecranon fracture.

Signs of a fracture include pain, swelling, and crepitus *(see Chapter 9)*. At first glance these fractures can cause signs similar to radial nerve paralysis. In fact, if a humeral fracture also directly damages the radial nerve, signs of both fracture and nerve damage will be present.

Specific Treatment

The management of radial nerve paralysis is similar to that discussed in the section on *General Management of Nerve Injuries*. Splinting the lower leg is especially useful in horses with radial nerve paralysis. If a splint is not applied, the affected leg should be bandaged to prevent abrasions on the front of the coronet, pastern, and fetlock.

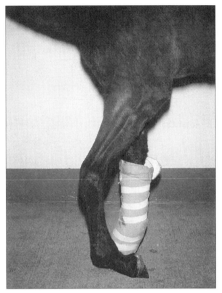

Fig. 12–35. A horse with radial nerve paralysis. Note the flexed lower leg and dropped elbow.

If a humeral fracture compresses the radial nerve, surgery to free the nerve of the bone fragment, callus, or scar tissue may promote the return of radial nerve function. However, this surgery is usually not attempted for at least 2 months after injury. This delay allows the fracture to heal, and gives the nerve a chance to regenerate on its own. A major concern is that, because most humeral fractures cannot be stabilized or reinforced with bone pins or plates, anesthetizing the horse to surgically free the radial nerve may cause the humerus to refracture as the horse gets up from anesthesia. Even if the surgery is successful, full recovery of nerve function may still take several months.

> **More Information**
>
> Olecranon and humeral fractures, and how they compare with radial nerve paralysis, are discussed and illustrated in Chapter 19.

"Sweeney"

"Sweeney" is a condition in which the suprascapular nerve is compressed, crushed, or stretched as it runs around the front of the shoulder blade. In most cases sweeney is the result of trauma to the

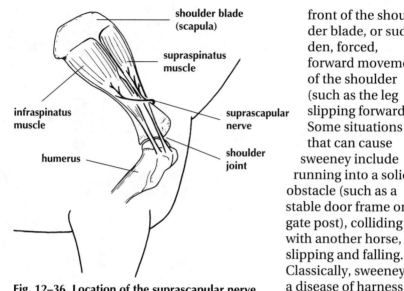

shoulder blade (scapula)

supraspinatus muscle

infraspinatus muscle

suprascapular nerve

humerus

shoulder joint

Fig. 12–36. Location of the suprascapular nerve.

front of the shoulder blade, or sudden, forced, forward movement of the shoulder (such as the leg slipping forward). Some situations that can cause sweeney include running into a solid obstacle (such as a stable door frame or a gate post), colliding with another horse, or slipping and falling. Classically, sweeney is a disease of harness horses. The heavy collar worn by cart horses would compress the nerve, particularly when the horse was pulling a very heavy load.

The suprascapular nerve supplies the muscles over the shoulder blade. These muscles attach onto the top of the humerus and support the side of the shoulder joint. Once the nerve supply to these muscles is interrupted, the shoulder joint can slip sideways, causing subluxation (partial dislocation; *see Chapter 8*). This results in a distinctive gait abnormality in which the shoulder "pops" to the side when weight is placed on the leg. It occurs because the muscles that

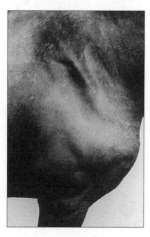
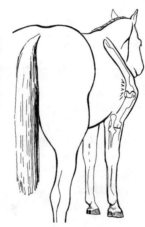

Fig. 12–37. Left: Sweeney results in atrophy of the muscles over the shoulder blade. Right: Once the nerve supply to the muscles is interrupted, the shoulder joint slips sideways, causing subluxation.

normally support the shoulder joint lose their tone and are no longer stimulated to function. After a few weeks these muscles atrophy, which makes the bony spine of the shoulder blade more prominent. Because this condition only affects the muscles on the side of the shoulder, horses with sweeney can bear weight on, and move the leg normally.

Specific Treatment of Sweeney

The initial management of sweeney should follow the guidelines in the earlier section on *General Management of Nerve Injuries*. It is important to confine horses with sweeney to a stall or small paddock to prevent further stretching of the nerve (and joint capsule) as the shoulder slips to the side.

Horses that do not improve after 2 – 3 months may be treated surgically. Surgery involves freeing the suprascapular nerve as it runs across the front of the shoulder blade. Any scar tissue is removed from around the nerve, then a small piece of bone at the front edge of the shoulder blade is cut away directly beneath the nerve. This procedure can relieve some of the tension on the nerve, and enable it to regenerate and return to normal function in some horses. However, this surgery does not produce immediate results in most cases. Neither is it always successful in restoring nerve function in the long-term.

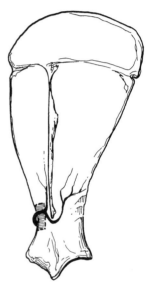

Fig. 12–38. Surgical treatment for sweeney: a small piece of bone is removed directly beneath the nerve.

Brachial Plexus Damage

The brachial plexus is a collection of "nerve roots"—bundles of nerves that have just left the spinal column. It is located beneath the shoulder blade. A hard blow to the side of the shoulder can compress the nerves between the shoulder blade and the ribcage. Brachial plexus damage can also occur when the horse slips and the leg slides out to the side. This can stretch or tear the nerves from their "roots," a condition called brachial plexus avulsion.

The brachial plexus includes "nerve roots" of the radial and suprascapular nerves. Therefore, damage to this area can cause signs of both radial and suprascapular nerve paralysis. It also contains the nerves that supply the rest of the forelimb, so severe damage can result in complete paralysis of the affected limb.

The treatment for brachial plexus damage is stall confinement, anti-inflammatory therapy, and physical therapy, as discussed in the earlier section on *General Management of Nerve Injuries*. The prognosis depends on the severity of the damage, but in most cases it is guarded.

Nerve Damage in the Hindlimb

The following conditions involving the nerves of the hindlimb result in varying degrees of dysfunction in the muscles that stabilize, flex, or extend the joints. In many cases damage to one or more of these nerves prevents the horse from bearing weight on the affected leg. Treatment should follow the guidelines discussed in the earlier section on *General Management of Nerve Injuries*.

Femoral Nerve Paralysis

The femoral nerve can be damaged by a blow to the side of the hip or thigh. It occasionally occurs in mares after a difficult foaling if the sacro-iliac joint *(see Chapter 22)* is damaged. When the femoral nerve is damaged the horse cannot bear weight on the leg because it cannot fix (or stabilize) the joints, particularly the stifle. As a result the stifle, hock, and fetlock remain flexed, and the horse cannot bring the leg forward. Femoral nerve damage also results in loss of skin sensation on the inside of the thigh.

Sciatic Nerve Paralysis

The sciatic nerve leaves the spinal column in the sacral section (at the top of the rump). It runs across the side of the pelvis, underneath the large rump muscles, and down the outside of the leg. The nerve may be damaged by an intramuscular injection into the rump in foals and small ponies *(see Chapter 10)*. Unless the injection is given near the hip joint, adult horses usually have too much muscle for the sciatic nerve to be damaged in this way. Pelvic fractures *(see Chapter 21)* can cause sciatic nerve damage in any age group or breed.

When the sciatic nerve is damaged, the horse cannot bring the leg forward and place it because the stifle and hock are extended and the fetlock is flexed. The horse can only bear weight on the leg if it is manually brought forward and the foot is placed in the normal position. Skin sensation is lost from the stifle down, except on the inside of the thigh, which is supplied by the femoral nerve.

Tibial and Peroneal Nerve Paralysis

The tibial and peroneal nerves are major branches of the sciatic nerve. A kick or other injury to the stifle or thigh can damage one or both of these nerves. A tibial fracture *(see Chapter 21)* can also cause nerve damage. Temporary peroneal nerve paralysis may also occur after general anesthesia, if the horse was lying on its side for a long time.

Tibial nerve damage results in a hypermetric (high-stepping), stringhalt-like gait because the flexor muscles of the hock are unopposed by the inactivated extensor muscles. At rest the hock remains flexed. There may be loss of skin sensation on the back of the cannon and pastern.

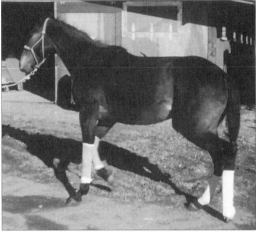

Fig. 12–39. A horse with peroneal nerve damage.

Peroneal nerve damage prevents the horse from flexing its hock or extending its fetlock. Skin sensation may be lost on the front and outside of the limb.

Obturator ("Foaling") Paralysis

The obturator nerve supplies the muscles on the inside of the thigh. These muscles function to keep the leg under the horse: when they contract, the leg is brought in toward the horse's body. The obturator nerves pass through holes in the floor of the pelvis (the obturator foramen) before reaching the thigh muscles.

One or both of the mare's obturator nerves can be damaged during a difficult foaling if the nerves are compressed between the foal and the mare's pelvis. This causes temporary paralysis of the muscles on the inside of the thigh. As a result, the mare cannot prevent her hindlegs from splaying out when she attempts to stand. In severe cases the mare cannot even get to her feet. In mild cases, she can rise either with or without assistance, but cannot prevent her legs from splaying as she stands or walks.

Nursing care includes keeping the stall well-bedded and the floor dry. If the mare is able to stand, attaching hobbles to her hind pasterns and connecting them with a short piece of rope (about 2 feet, or 60 cm long) helps to prevent her legs from sliding out from underneath her. The mare can still walk around the stall to reach her food and water. In most cases obturator nerve function returns in a few days, although the nerve may not function normally for weeks, or even months.

Stringhalt

Stringhalt is a gait abnormality that consists of involuntary, exaggerated flexion (hyperflexion) of the hock. Mild cases have slightly exaggerated hock flexion when walking. In severe cases the hyperflexion may be so extreme that the horse kicks its belly each time it takes a step.

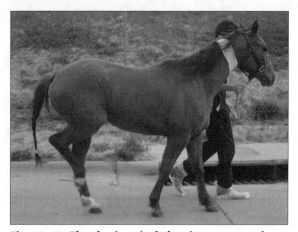

In the northern hemisphere, only occasional cases of stringhalt are usually seen. Until recently, the problem was thought to be due to a structural problem in the hock, such as bone spavin. But some scientists question this assumption. In Australia and New Zealand stringhalt can occur in outbreaks, in which most of the horses on a farm or in a particular pasture are affected. Although the cause(s) is not known, a plant or fungal toxin is thought to be involved. Similar outbreaks of stringhalt have been reported in the northwestern U.S. (northern California and Washington). The toxic plant suspected in those cases was smooth catsear, or flatweed, a pasture plant that looks like a dandelion. This fact has led some scientists to rethink the hock problem theory. They speculate that most cases of stringhalt, whether isolated or an outbreak, may be caused by a toxin.

In the Australian stringhalt cases the underlying problem is degeneration of the nerves that supply the extensor muscles of the hock. This allows the flexor muscles of the hock to function unopposed *(see*

Fig. 12–40. The classic stringhalt gait: exaggerated hock flexion.

Chapter 10). Local spinal cord damage (loss of upper motor neuron control; discussed earlier) may also be involved. The damage is reversible in most cases, provided the horse is removed from the pasture containing the weeds.

There is no definite treatment for stringhalt. Traditionally, veterinarians have removed a section of the lateral digital extensor tendon at the side of the hock. This is one of the structures that flexes the hock (while it extends the fetlock and pastern). The surgery, called a lateral digital extensor tenectomy, may provide relief in some horses. Various drugs have been tried to suppress excessive muscle activity. Phenytoin (Dilantin®) and baclofen (Lioresal®) are effective in many horses.

In the cases involving a plant toxin, the prognosis for full recovery is very good. However, in very severe cases improvement is all that can be expected. Even in mild cases, complete recovery can take from several months to 2 years.

> **Extra Information**
>
> Phenytoin (Dilantin®) is used to control epilepsy in people and small animals.
>
> Baclofen (Lioresal®) is used to help manage Parkinson's disease in people.

Cauda Equina Neuritis

The spinal cord ends in the sacral segment of the spinal column (at the top of the rump). The remaining bundle of nerves travel within the spinal canal before leaving the spinal column further down. This

Fig. 12–41. The cauda equina, as seen when looking down onto the spinal column from above the horse, with the tops of the vertebrae removed.

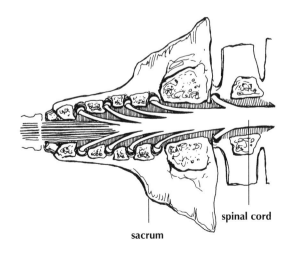

spinal cord

sacrum

<table>
<tr><td>

Terminology

Cauda equina literally means "end of the horse."
Cauda equina neuritis is also called polyneuritis equi.

</td></tr>
</table>

collection of nerves is called the cauda equina because it looks a little like the hairs of a horse's tail.

Cauda equina neuritis is a syndrome that involves inflammation and degeneration of the cauda equina nerves. The cause(s) is unknown, although it may be due to a viral infection and/or an immune system reaction.

Whatever the cause, the result is inflammation and fibrosis (scarring) around the "nerve roots," and degeneration of the nerve fibers. In most cases only the nerves and "nerve roots" are affected. But in severe cases the last part of the spinal cord may also be involved.

Signs and Diagnosis of Cauda Equina Neuritis

The signs of cauda equina neuritis may develop slowly or suddenly. They include:

- progressive tail paralysis
- loss of anal tone (inability to constrict the anus)
- bladder paralysis

Hindlimb ataxia (incoordination) and muscle atrophy may also develop if the end of the spinal cord is affected. The horse dribbles urine when its bladder fills to overflowing; in male horses the penis also may be paralyzed. The signs can include areas of decreased or absent sensation (anesthesia), surrounded by an area of increased sensitivity (hyperesthesia) around the tail base.

<table>
<tr><td>

Note

Other problems that may cause similar signs include:
- EHV-1 myeloencephalitis
- sorghum/Sudan grass toxicity
- trauma to lumbar or sacral vertebrae

</td></tr>
</table>

There is no specific diagnostic test for cauda equina neuritis. In most cases the diagnosis can be made only when all other likely causes of these signs are ruled out.

Treatment and Prognosis for Cauda Equina Neuritis

There is no specific treatment for this condition. Supportive care is similar to that described for horses with EHV-1 myeloencephalitis: anti-inflammatory therapy and diligent nursing care, particularly if the horse cannot urinate or pass manure normally. Because of the possible link between an immune system reaction and this disease, the horse may need anti-inflammatory therapy for a long time. The prognosis is poor in all cases of cauda equina neuritis; recovery, if it occurs, is usually slow and incomplete.

Equine Motor Neuron Disease (EMND)

Equine motor neuron disease (EMND) is a degenerative condition that affects the lower motor neurons (discussed at the beginning of the chapter). It has only recently been recognized and studied in horses. In many respects EMND is similar to Lou Gehrig's disease in people. The cause of EMND is unknown, although the following factors have been suggested:

- vitamin E deficiency
- heavy metal poisoning
- dietary mineral deficiencies, especially copper and zinc
- plant or fungal toxins
- viral infection
- auto-immune disease, where the body is attacked by its own immune system

Researchers have found a possible link between EMND and horses without access to pasture or other fresh feed materials. They speculate that vitamin E deficiency plays a key role, much like it does with Equine Degenerative Myelopathy (EDM) in foals.

The disease is more commonly seen in the northeastern U.S. and mostly affects mature Quarter Horses. It has also been seen in Thoroughbreds, Standardbreds, and Morgans. There may be an inherited predisposition to developing the disease because only one horse in a group usually is affected. Outbreaks have not been reported in the U.S.

Signs and Diagnosis

The signs of EMND include:

- muscle tremors, trembling limbs
- standing "camped under"
- tendency to lie down a lot
- severe weight loss and muscle atrophy despite a good appetite
- weakness, inability to hold the head up
- pain in the affected muscles
- sweating (presumably due to pain)
- abnormal tail carriage

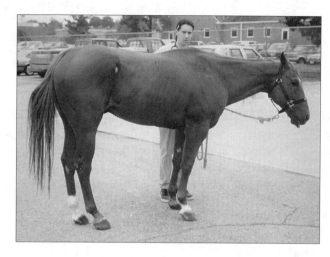

**Fig. 12–42.
Horses with
EMND often
stand "camped
under" with their
head lowered.**

Horses with EMND also have a short, stilted gait, and some are also ataxic, although this can be difficult to determine in a very weak horse. The signs may begin suddenly, but they progress slowly. Sometimes they stabilize for weeks or months, but they almost always worsen over time.

EMND can be definitely diagnosed by surgically removing a small section of nerve and submitting it to a laboratory for microscopic examination. The spinal accessory nerve on the side of the neck is the nerve that is usually biopsied. It is easy to get to and is not vitally important. The biopsy is performed under general anesthesia, and the results usually take 2 – 3 weeks.

There is another test that is quicker and simpler, and can be done under local anesthetic. It involves taking a biopsy of the muscles at the top of the tail. Nerve degeneration leads to muscle atrophy and replacement with fibrous tissue (fibrosis). These changes, and the abnormal tail carriage they cause, are very common in horses with EMND. The diagnosis is strengthened if a degenerated nerve is also found in the biopsy sample. **Note:** Similar abnormalities may be found in normal horses that have had a tail block for showing.

Treatment and Prognosis for EMND

Until the cause(s) is known, treatment can only address the symptoms and possible factors. Supplementing the horse's diet with vitamin E and allowing the horse access to pasture or fresh feeds stabilizes or improves the signs in some horses. Anti-inflammatory therapy, a balanced diet that supplies the horse's mineral requirements (particularly copper), and physical therapy may also help prolong the horse's life. But unfortunately, euthanasia is inevitable in most cases.

Other Conditions

"Shivers"

"Shivers" is a condition that mostly affects draft breeds. The cause(s) is unknown, but viral infection or an immune system reaction to a virus has been suggested. The possibility that it is hereditary cannot be ruled out.

The signs primarily involve the hindlimbs. Typically, the horse holds the affected limb up and out, and the muscles of the upper limb quiver. These signs are worsened by backing or turning the horse, or making it step over an obstacle. In between episodes, the horse appears normal. The frequency of the episodes lessens with rest, but it usually increases once the horse is returned to regular exercise. The long-term prognosis for athletic usefulness is poor.

There is a similar condition that is occasionally seen in Lighthorse (non-draft) breeds. However, it is generally mild, non-progressive, and does not affect the horse's athletic ability. The cause is unknown, although joint or bone pain in the back or upper hindlimbs could be responsible in some cases.

Botulism

Botulism is a disease that affects the neuromuscular junction—the connection between the nerve end and the muscle cell. The nerve impulses cannot cross the junction so the muscle is not stimulated to contract. Botulism is caused by toxins released from *Clostridium botulinum* bacteria. These bacteria grow best in decaying carcasses. It is fairly common for a dead snake or other small animal to be baled with the hay, or a mouse or rat to die in a grain bin. A dead bird in a water trough can also provide an ideal environment for these bacteria. Botulism bacteria can survive in rotting vegetation, such as spoiled or discarded hay, in soil that is rich in organic matter, and in silage. They have also been found to grow in wounds and ulcerated areas of the bowel (for example, stomach ulcers in foals).

The disease appears to be more prevalent in the Ohio River valley and the northern Mid-Atlantic states. When just a single, isolated case is seen, the source of the toxin is usually impossible to pinpoint. However, in most outbreaks the source is eventually found.

Signs of Botulism

Any age group of horse can develop botulism, but the disease most often affects either foals between 2 and 8 weeks of age, or adult

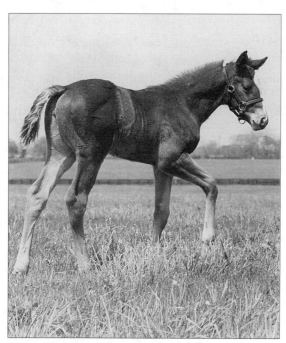

horses. In foals, the toxins cause generalized muscle weakness and tremors. The common term for these foals is "shaker foal." The signs progress over a period of hours or days until the foal is too weak to stand. Despite this, the foal usually remains alert and has a normal temperature and appetite. The toxin also affects the muscles necessary for eating and swallowing, so the foal may dribble saliva from its mouth. Often

Fig. 12–43. Botulism is more common in foals between 2 and 8 weeks old.

the tongue is paralyzed and hangs limply from the lips. Dribbling milk from the nostrils is also a fairly common sign in foals. As the disease worsens, the respiratory muscles are paralyzed, and death follows quickly.

In adult horses, the early signs can be variable and confusing. Occasionally, colic and/or vague lameness are noticed before the more typical signs of muscle weakness, difficulty swallowing, etc. As with foals, death is caused by respiratory paralysis. In some outbreaks the first—and only—sign is sudden death.

Diagnosis of Botulism

The botulism toxins are some of the most potent toxins known; minute quantities are deadly. So, it is often impossible to detect either the toxins or the organism in the affected animal's manure or in the contaminated feed or water source. For this reason, botulism is almost always diagnosed by the signs and the response to treatment.

Treatment of Botulism

Treatment includes botulism antitoxin (antiserum), intravenous penicillin, and diligent nursing care. If the antitoxin is given early, it can result in a dramatic (and lifesaving) improvement in the animal's condition—this is the single most important and effective therapy.

In severe cases, it may take up to a week before a definite improvement is seen. But during that time the signs should not get any worse. Until recently, botulism antiserum was very expensive, and veterinarians were reluctant to even order it until they were certain the foal (or horse) had botulism. By that time, it was often too late for the antitoxin to save the animal. However, the cost of the antitoxin is now much more reasonable. Because it can result in such a profound turnaround in the animal's condition, it should probably be used as soon as the suspicion of botulism arises.

Prognosis for Botulism

The prognosis is guarded in all cases—this is a highly fatal disease in horses and foals, particularly when the signs progress rapidly. If the horse or foal survives, it may have muscle weakness for several weeks.

Prevention of Botulism

Botulism in foals can be prevented by vaccinating mares in the last trimester of pregnancy. Vaccinating non-pregnant adult horses in areas where botulism is common may also be of value. However, vaccinating during an outbreak is probably useless. Careful inspection of hay, grain, and all water sources for decaying materials, especially dead animals, may also help prevent botulism.

(The signs of nervous system injury are listed in the chart on pages 516 – 517. For comparison, similar signs of muscle disorders are also included.)

SIGNS OF NERVOUS SYSTEM INJURY

Location	Typical Signs
BRAIN	
Cerebrum (front of brain)	Altered Behavior: depression/aggression compulsive wandering bizarre appetite circling head-pressing continual yawning etc. Blindness
Cerebellum	Loss of Balance Head Tilt (head held at an abnormal angle) Jerky Head Movements "Intention Tremors" During Voluntary Movements Ataxia Without Weakness Hypermetria
Brainstem (base of brain)	Lack of Awareness: severe depression unconsciousness (coma)
Cranial Nerves	facial paralysis drooping ear drooping eyelid unresponsive pupils abnormal eyeball position blindness tongue paralysis difficulty chewing difficulty swallowing loss of balance deafness etc.

SIGNS OF NERVOUS SYSTEM INJURY, Cont.

Location	Typical Signs
SPINAL CORD (General)	Ataxia Hypometria or Hypermetria Weakness
Cervical	all four limbs affected, but signs worse in hindlimbs
Cervical-Thoracic Junction	all four limbs affected, but signs worse in forelimbs
Thoracic	hindlimbs only
Lumbar	hindlimbs only may also affect bladder, rectum, and tail
Sacral	loss of muscle tone and sensation around anus and tail may also affect bladder and rectum
PERIPHERAL NERVES	Loss of Muscle Function and/or Skin Sensation at a Specific Location Weakness Without Ataxia

Fig. 12–44. The signs seen when specific areas of the nervous system are damaged.

SIGNS OF MUSCLE DISORDERS

Loss of Muscle Function Only

Weakness Confined to Specific Muscle

Fig. 12–45. Some signs of muscle disorders are similar to those of nervous system injury.

13

LAMENESS CAUSED BY SKIN PROBLEMS

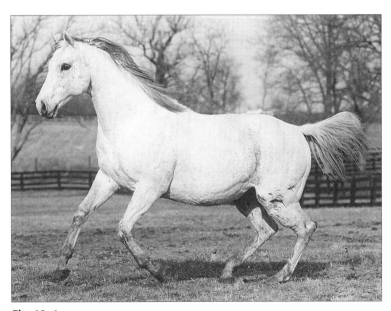

Fig. 13–1.

Strictly speaking, the skin is not part of the musculoskeletal system. But certain skin problems do cause lameness. The skin is well supplied with sensory nerves—nerves that report sensations, including pain, to the horse's central nervous system. So, injuries or conditions that damage the skin can cause pain and lameness, particularly if they occur on a limb, the lower part of the chest wall, or the hindquarters.

Some skin problems, such as large wounds, may be obvious causes of lameness. However, others, such as bacterial dermatitis, or "scratches," are often overlooked as possible causes of lameness.

This chapter is divided into three sections: wounds, dermatitis, and limb edema (swelling).

WOUNDS

Wounds can simply involve the skin, or they can also damage the structures underneath: joints, bones, muscles, tendons, or ligaments. Deeper wounds are more likely to cause lameness. Superficial wounds cause lameness if they are very large or involve an area of skin that is stretched during activity, such as the skin over a joint.

The following section is an overview of how wounds heal, and which factors or management practices can slow or speed up wound healing.

Wound Healing

All wounds heal by the same basic process. The following description of wound healing involves a fresh skin wound that is managed properly.

Phases of Wound Healing

Inflammation

Inflammation is the first phase of wound healing. During the injury, blood vessels in the skin and underlying tissue are damaged, which causes bleeding. A blood clot forms within a few minutes, sealing the blood vessels and preventing further bleeding. (When larger blood vessels—particularly arteries—are damaged, bleeding may continue and pressure must be applied to the wound; this is discussed later.)

Within a few minutes of injury, inflammation in the damaged tissue causes heat, redness, and swelling around the wound. Inflammation is an important part of the healing process because it increases blood flow and stimulates the migration and activation of white blood cells into the damaged area. This process removes bacteria and debris from the wound, and begins tissue repair. *(The process of inflammation is detailed in the Anti-Inflammatory Therapy section of Chapter 5.)*

Repair

The inflammatory phase of wound healing starts the repair phase as fibroblasts migrate into the wound. Fibroblasts are cells that produce collagen, the substance that gives the tissues strength and resilience. The blood clot that formed earlier now acts as a framework in which the fibroblasts lay down collagen fibers to repair the defect. As healing continues, new capillaries extend into this area from the edges of the wound. This bed of fibroblasts, collagen, and new blood vessels is called granulation tissue. The reddish-pink granulation tissue fills in the defect within a few days of injury (a little longer in very large or deep wounds).

Definition
Granulation tissue is: • fibroblasts • collagen fibers • new capillaries

The other major process that begins during the repair phase is the re-covering of the wound surface with skin. This is called epithelialization. Skin (epithelial) cells must migrate across the wound from the skin edges, so this process lags behind the development of the granulation bed.

Remodeling

The final phase of wound healing is the remodeling phase. During this phase, the collagen bundles within the defect are reorganized, and some may even be removed. This causes the wound to contract a little. Also, skin cell migration over the wound surface is completed. The whole remodeling process can take several weeks, and in very large wounds, up to 12 months to be completed.

A scar consists of fibrous tissue and hairless skin. The final size of the scar depends on the wound's initial size and depth, the amount of tension on the tissues, and the blood supply. The smaller the

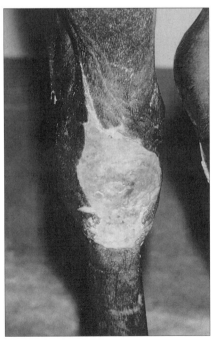

Fig. 13–2. This wound has a healthy granulation bed.

wound, the less the movement and tension on the skin edges, and the better the blood supply, the smaller the scar will be. Nevertheless, some large wounds heal with remarkably little scarring.

Second Intention Wound Healing

Wound healing can be divided into three categories, based on the amount of intervention the wound receives.

1. **First Intention Healing**—wounds that are sutured closed. The healing process follows the same lines as those described above, but the whole process is shortened because the sutures hold the skin edges together while the collagen fibers and skin cells bridge the narrow gap.
2. **Second Intention Healing**—wounds that are not sutured, or that are sutured but break open. The defect must fill in with granulation tissue before the wound can be covered with skin.
3. **Third Intention Healing**—wounds that are left open for a few days and then debrided (trimmed) and sutured once they have begun a healthy granulation bed. This is a compromise between first and second intention healing.

Some wounds cannot or should not be sutured, and so must heal by second intention. Such wounds have one or more of the following characteristics:

- loss of skin—not just a gaping wound, but actual loss of a piece of skin
- gross contamination with dirt, gravel, manure, etc.
- excessive swelling, such that the skin edges cannot be brought together without a lot of tension
- severely traumatized and devitalized tissue, particularly at the skin edges
- a deep cavity beneath the skin, such that serum can build up in the "dead space"

Definition
Serum: clear, yellow, liquid portion of the blood.

Management of these wounds is aimed at encouraging:

- rapid filling of the defect with granulation tissue
- uninterrupted migration of skin cells across the granulation bed
- early wound contraction

The speed of healing, and the final functional and cosmetic result depend in part on the wound's location. Wounds on the head, neck, body, and upper legs heal best because these areas have ample loose skin and underlying soft tissue (usually muscle). Loose skin is important because it minimizes tension on the wound. It also allows maximum contraction of the scar tissue during the remodeling phase. The underlying soft tissue is important because it provides a base for the developing granulation bed.

Proud Flesh

Wounds on the lower legs often develop excess granulation tissue, or "proud flesh." The granulation bed proliferates so much that it rises above the skin edges. This prevents migration of the skin cells across the wound, and it also limits wound contraction.

Research has shown that wounds on horses produce collagen earlier and in greater amounts than other animals. Other factors that make proud flesh a common problem in wounds on the lower legs of horses include:

- lack of loose skin to relieve the tension on the skin edges
- lack of an even soft tissue base for the granulation bed
- continual disruption of the wound by joint and tendon movement

Proud flesh is the body's attempt to stabilize and repair the wound. But in the process it slows comple-

> ### Note
>
> Healing in any wound may be slowed or complicated by one or more of the following factors:
>
> - contamination with hair, dirt, manure, etc.
> - "foreign" objects, such as a piece of wood or metal, or even a piece of bone or other devitalized tissue
> - bacterial infection from human or environmental sources

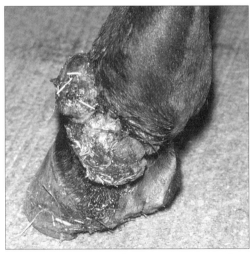

Fig. 13–3. Excess granulation tissue, or proud flesh in a pastern wound.

tion of the remodeling phase. A wound with proud flesh eventually heals, but it often leaves a large, unsightly scar, even if the granulation bed is trimmed. As well as affecting the cosmetic result, a fibrous scar over a joint can restrict normal joint mobility.

Preventing or Managing Proud Flesh

Proud flesh can be prevented or limited by:

- stabilizing the wound with a firm bandage *(see Chapter 4)*, where possible
- restricting excessive movement (if necessary, confining the horse to a stall or small paddock)

The aim of wound management is to encourage the wound to fill in with granulation tissue and be re-covered with skin as quickly as possible. Irritant or caustic medications on the wound can slow this process. In particular, strong disinfectants and lotions or powders that "cut back" excessive granulation tissue should be avoided in the early stages of wound healing.

Some veterinarians recommend using ointments that contain corticosteroids (such as Panolog® or Dermalone™ Ointment) beneath the bandage. Corticosteroids slow collagen production, so these ointments can prevent excessive granulation tissue if they are used when the granulation bed is forming. However, corticosteroids also inhibit skin cell migration across the wound surface, so they can delay wound healing if overused. Corticosteroids also interfere with the body's normal immune response to bacterial invasion. Even if the ointment also contains antibiotics, it should not be used on a deep or contaminated wound.

On parts of the lower leg where a bandage cannot effectively stabilize the wound, a fiberglass cast may be necessary to prevent proud flesh and encourage wound healing *(see Chapter 6)*. Lacerations at the back of the pastern or on the heel bulbs are examples of wounds that may require a cast. Casting the lower leg (to just above or below the fetlock) may sound excessive for a wound, but it speeds wound healing and ensures the best functional and cosmetic result. A wound that is just bandaged (or left uncovered) may take several weeks to heal. But that same wound may heal in 2 – 3 weeks if the leg is cast. The horse can return to training much sooner, and the scar will be much smaller.

On some parts of the leg a firm bandage is difficult to maintain and a cast is impractical. The front of the hock is a good example. With wounds in these areas, proud flesh may be controlled by cleaning the granulation bed and applying a corticosteroid ointment every day. In a normal wound, disrupting the granulation bed by vigorous cleaning or scouring slows down healing. However, in a wound with proud flesh, vigorous cleaning with a toothbrush or gauze pad can help control the excessive granulation tissue. It can also stimulate a static wound, in which skin cell migration has slowed or stopped. Granulation tissue is not well supplied with nerves, so scrubbing the protruding tissue usually does not cause the horse pain. Confining the horse is even more important when the wound cannot be bandaged or cast. Movement at the wound site must be kept to a minimum if healing is to proceed as quickly as possible.

Proud flesh that is older than about 2 weeks often must be trimmed back with a scalpel blade. (This is a job for the veterinarian; trimming too much or too little tissue, or damaging the wound edges can further slow wound healing.) Over the years various caustic preparations have been used to control proud flesh, including copper sulfate ("bluestone"), calcium carbonate (ground limestone), and "black powder." However, these products can damage the granulation bed and slow skin cell migration across the wound surface. For rapid healing and the best functional and cosmetic result, it is far better to put the time and effort into preventing or controlling proud flesh early in the course of wound healing.

Note: Infestation of a wound by certain parasites can cause excess granulation tissue. One example is infestation with fly larvae, a condition called habronemiasis. Another example is infection with a fungus-like organism, a disease called pythiosis. The veterinarian should be consulted for wounds that will not heal, or that continue to produce granulation tissue despite proper management.

Wound Infection

The skin is an important barrier to bacteria, so any break or disruption of the skin permits bacterial invasion. Normal skin has bacteria on its surface, and these organisms grow well in a wound. Other, more pathogenic (disease-causing) bacteria can also thrive in a wound. For example, the bacteria that are commonly found in horse manure can cause serious wound infection.

However, the body has a powerful defense mechanism to combat invading bacteria within or around a wound. Local antibodies kill the bacteria or attach to their outer surface so they can be engulfed and destroyed by the white blood cells. Dead or dying white blood cells give the normally clear, yellow tissue fluid a thicker, whitish appearance. This is pus: an accumulation of tissue fluid, bacteria, dead white cells, and cell debris.

Sometimes a deep wound oozes pus for a few days, although this should resolve with the routine wound care described later. However, if an otherwise healthy-looking wound becomes swollen, reddened, or painful, and begins to ooze pus, it requires veterinary attention.

Antibiotics

An infected wound may require antibiotics, but these drugs should not be given without consulting the veterinarian. Some antibiotics are better than others for treating wound infections. Also, a bacterial culture and antibiotic sensitivity test *(see Chapter 2)* may be necessary to determine which bacteria are causing the infection, and which antibiotic will be most effective. This test is often compromised if antibiotics are given before the sample is taken.

Most important, *a reason for the infection should be sought.* A common cause of wound infection is foreign material, such as wood, metal, gravel, etc. Another common cause is devitalized tissue, including bone fragments. In such wounds, antibiotics are of little use unless the foreign object or devitalized tissue is removed.

Managing Specific Types of Wounds

Note

With every wound, no matter how minor, the horse's tetanus status must be checked. *Every wound is a risk for tetanus.* Reviewing the horse's vaccination record is essential.

(Tetanus vaccination is discussed in Chapter 5.)

When deciding how to manage a wound, the factors that must be considered are:

• the type of wound
• the location of the wound
• the amount of contamination in the wound
• the age of the wound

This section gives practical advice on how certain types of wounds may be managed. However, a veterinarian should be consulted if there is any doubt about how a particular wound should be treated.

Lacerations

A laceration is a very common type of wound that damages the full thickness of the skin and possibly also the tissues beneath. The wound could be a simple cut, with fairly neat edges, or it may be a jagged tear. Some lacerations create a skin flap, where the skin is pulled back from the tissue beneath.

Initial Wound Care for Lacerations

When a laceration is found, the following steps should be carried out, in order:

1. Control the bleeding.
2. Call the veterinarian, if necessary.
3. Clean the wound.

Control the Bleeding

If the wound is bleeding freely, the first priority is to stop the bleeding. This is best done by applying a sterile dressing over the wound and bandaging it firmly in place, if possible. *(Applying a pressure bandage is described in Chapter 4.)* If blood seeps through the bandage, hand pressure can be applied or a second bandage placed over the first one.

For wounds in locations where bandaging is not possible, the wound should be covered with a sterile dressing, and firm pressure applied. Unless a large artery has been severed, the bleeding usually slows or stops within 3 – 5 minutes.

On all wounds it is best to use a sterile dressing, or at least a clean cloth. But if the wound is bleeding heavily and there is no suitable material nearby, pressure should be applied directly over the wound with the hand. Sometimes the tip of the damaged blood vessel is visible. It is best not to touch it; instead, pressure should be applied directly over the vessel until the veterinarian can tie it off.

Call the Veterinarian

The earlier a laceration is sutured, the better the outcome will be. Wounds should be sutured within 6 hours for the best results. So if there is a chance that the wound could be sutured, the veterinarian should be called as soon as the wound is discovered and any bleeding is controlled. The veterinarian should be informed of the location, depth, and probable age of the wound.

It may be necessary to clean the wound (see below) to determine its depth, particularly if there is a lot of dirt, mud, or dried blood in and around the wound. However, the wound should not be cleaned if it is still oozing blood, or it has only just stopped bleeding. If there is dirt in it, the wound is already contaminated. Waiting awhile longer to clean it will not make much difference to the amount of bacteria in the wound, whereas that time makes a big difference to the state of the blood clot.

The horse should be kept quiet and confined until the veterinarian arrives. It is important not to give anti-inflammatory drugs, antibiotics, or tranquilizers to the horse, unless instructed to do so by the veterinarian. These drugs may be necessary, but the decision to give them and the choice of drug should be left up to the veterinarian.

Clean the Wound

While waiting for the veterinarian to arrive, and with lacerations that do not require veterinary attention, the wound should be gently bathed to remove any hair, dirt, mud, and other debris. The wound can be cleaned with saline solution or dilute antiseptic. If there is a chance that the wound can be sutured, only saline solution should be used—some antiseptics irritate exposed tissues.

> **Note**
>
> To make saline solution, add 1 heaped teaspoon of salt to 1 quart of warm water.

Fresh wounds should not be hosed for two reasons: 1) the water pressure, even if not very strong, may disrupt the blood clot and cause more bleeding, and 2) tap water is much more dilute than tissue fluid. Using tap water to clean a fresh wound causes the skin edges and deeper tissues to swell, which can make suturing difficult.

After removing as much dirt and debris as possible, a sterile, non-stick dressing (or antiseptic ointment and gauze pad) and a standard bandage should be applied *(see Chapter 4)*. If the wound can possibly be sutured, no ointments or wound medications should be applied until the veterinarian has examined it. The wound should simply be covered with a sterile dressing and bandage. If there is a skin flap, the underside of the flap and its bed should be gently cleaned with saline solution. The skin flap should then be carefully replaced into position. The area should be bandaged, if possible, until the veterinarian arrives.

Daily Wound Care for Lacerations
Bandaged Wounds

Wounds that are sutured should be managed as described later for incisions. For unsutured wounds in locations that can be bandaged, the dressing should be changed and the wound inspected daily for the first 3 – 4 days. Depending on how much the wound is oozing, the bandage can then be changed every 1 – 2 days until the wound has healed. If left unbandaged, the granulation bed can dry out or be damaged. This can slow or halt skin cell migration across the wound surface.

The wound should be thoroughly cleaned at each bandage change, taking care to *gently* remove all discharges and crusts from the edges of the wound—this is where the skin cells begin their migration.

Using sterile, non-stick dressings or antiseptic ointment and a gauze pad over the wound makes removing the dressings easier and less traumatic for the wound surface. It is also less painful for the horse. Antiseptic or antibiotic ointment does not prevent or treat wound infection—it just sits on the surface of the wound and too little antibiotic is absorbed to do much good. However, the greasy base helps prevent the dressing from sticking to the wound, and the antibiotic or antiseptic reduces odor in the dressings by controlling bacterial growth.

Some wounds appear to stop healing before the surface is completely covered with skin. This may be due to the pressure of the bandage or the presence of the dressing on the granulation bed's surface. In such cases it is often best to leave the bandage off and treat the wound as an exposed wound.

Exposed Wounds

Because of their location, it is difficult to bandage or otherwise protect some wounds. Unless they were sutured, these wounds should be cleaned twice per day and an antiseptic ointment applied. The ointment keeps the granulation bed from drying out too much. It also makes wound cleaning easier. Fly repellant on or around the wound—depending on the product recommendations—is especially important on exposed wounds during the warmer months.

Hosing effectively cleans large wounds, and the water's massaging action stimulates the granulation bed. However, a fresh wound should not be hosed; it is best to wait 2 – 3 days before beginning hosing. In the meantime, the wound should be cleaned with saline solution or dilute antiseptic. As with bandaged wounds, it is very important to keep the wound's edges clean and free of discharges and crusts. If the wound is oozing serum or pus, a greasy ointment (such as Vaseline™, Desitin®, or lanolin) should be applied below the wound to prevent the discharge from irritating the skin. The ointment also makes cleaning around the wound easier.

Incisions

Incisions are wounds that are created by cutting the skin with a sharp instrument, such as a scalpel blade. Usually, these wounds are not contaminated, the skin edges are neat, and the blood supply is good. Therefore, in most cases they are sutured.

Wound Care for Incisions

The following recommendations apply to incisions as well as lacerations that were sutured. Where possible, the wound should be bandaged to minimize movement and tension on the sutures, prevent fly worry, and keep the horse from chewing at the wound (particularly as it heals and starts to itch). If the incision cannot be covered, fly repellant should be applied around it. The horse's activity should be limited until the sutures are removed.

Many sutured wounds leak a little blood or serum for the first 1 – 2 days. This discharge can be gently wiped away from around the sutures. Even though the wound may not need to be cleaned after this time, it should be inspected every day. Most sutured wounds look good for the first 3 – 4 days. If they break down (open up or pull apart) they usually do so 4 – 6 days after suturing. If at any time the wound begins to swell, ooze serum or pus, or appears to be opening up, the veterinarian should be called.

Skin sutures are usually left in place for 7 – 10 days in horses. More time may be necessary if there is a lot of tension on the wound or the wound has not completely closed. However, it is often difficult to remove the sutures if they are left in for longer than about 2 weeks.

Abrasions

Abrasions are one of the most common skin wounds in horses. Injuries such as scrapes, harness rubs, and rope burns (more an abrasion than a true burn) damage and remove the epidermis. The dermis generally remains intact, although the tiny blood vessels that supply the epidermis may be damaged. Exposure of these epidermal vessels makes the abraded area appear red, and leaked blood creates a fine scab or grainy crust over the wound surface. Abrasions can be painful, but they heal quickly, and without scarring.

Definitions

Epidermis: outer layer of the skin.
Dermis: deep layer of the skin.

Harness Rubs and Saddle Sores

Girth galls and saddle sores are abrasions that can result in mild lameness or reluctance to exercise. Boots, hobbles, or a heart rate monitor can also cause these rubs. They are often overlooked or thought to be unimportant if they are on the body, rather than on the legs. But these wounds can be painful. For example, a girth gall may cause pain every time the horse brings its foreleg forward. This can result in lameness, shortened stride, or reluctance to perform normal activities. In most cases the rub can be confirmed as the cause of lameness simply by removing the tack and watching the horse exercise (either led or longed) without lameness.

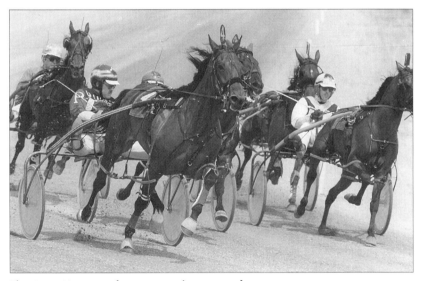

Fig. 13–4. Harness rubs can sometimes cause lameness.

Sometimes the horse's gait may not be normal until the rub has healed. The wound heals quickest if the irritating piece of equipment is not used. However, this is often impossible without interrupting the horse's training program. So, after each exercise session the abraded area should be gently cleaned and an antibacterial ointment applied. Ensuring that the equipment fits the horse properly, and using padding can help to prevent further abrasion.

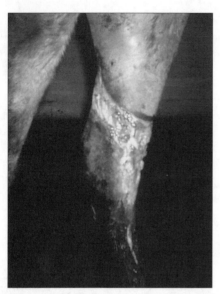

Fig. 13–5. This pressure sore was caused by a rope caught around the horse's leg.

Pressure Sores

Pressure sores are usually caused by a combination of abrasion and pressure. They occur because pressure reduces blood flow to the skin and underlying tissues. If the pressure is severe and prolonged (more than a few hours) cell death results. The dead skin sloughs (lifts away), leaving an ulcerated, crater-like wound. When the injury is caused by trauma, some skin may be lost during the injury. But it may take a few days for the rest of the damaged skin to slough.

Pressure sores can be acute (recent) or chronic (long-standing). Acute pressure sores often develop when a horse is caught in a fence or under a stall partition. The horse in Figure 13–5 was injured when its leg was caught in a lead rope for 4 hours. When the rope was finally removed, a narrow abrasion was found, and the whole lower leg was swollen. The swelling quickly improved, but a few days later a wide strip of skin below the wound began to slough.

Another common example of acute pressure injury is a "bandage bow." Tight bandages can compress the skin and underlying tissues, particularly over the front and back of the cannon. Even if the bandage did not cause a wound, the leg may swell once the bandage is removed. This swelling can give the impression that the flexor tendons have "bowed" *(see Chapter 11)*. Fiberglass casts can also cause pressure sores, especially over bony points such as the front and back of the fetlock. Sometimes the skin damage caused by the bandage or cast is so severe that the hair follicles are destroyed. As a result, the healed area either is permanently bare or has patches of white hairs.

Chronic pressure sores can occur on any part of the horse that is subjected to repeated or prolonged pressure. These sores develop over areas where there is little soft tissue padding between the skin and the bone. One example occurs in horses that are housed on concrete, without enough bedding. They often develop pressure sores on the outside of the hocks and the front of the fetlocks on the forelegs.

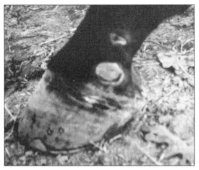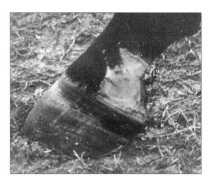

Fig. 13–6. At first (left), the wound did not look very bad. But after a few days (right), it became obvious that the damage was more extensive. The surrounding dead skin has sloughed.

Ill or injured horses that are unable to stand develop pressure sores on the points of the hips and the sides of the elbows. These sores can be very painful to the touch, possibly because the nerve endings in the damaged tissue are chronically inflamed and overly sensitive.

Terminology

Pressure sores in horses that cannot get up are called decubital ulcers.

Wound Care for Pressure Sores

Pressure sores are best treated by relieving the pressure and treating the wound as described earlier for exposed wounds. Acute pressure sores may look worse for several days before they begin to heal, particularly if they result from trauma. The veterinarian may have to trim the sloughing tissue more than once before all of the damaged, devitalized tissue is identified and removed.

When "bandage bows" occur, the swelling can be reduced with a "sweat" or poultice. However, the accompanying bandage must not be fitted tightly, and should not be left on for more than a couple of hours. Cold therapy, NSAIDs, and DMSO can also reduce the swelling and relieve the discomfort. *(See Chapter 5 for more information on these therapies.)*

Pressure sores that develop beneath a bandage or cast can be managed one of two ways. If the veterinarian decides to leave the bandage or cast off, the wound should be treated like an exposed wound. If the veterinarian reapplies the bandage or cast, the bandage will be well padded and snug (but not tight), and applied with even tension so there are no areas of excessive pressure. The cast will be well contoured to the leg. A loose-fitting cast is not only ineffective, but it can cause abrasions and pressure sores. *(Bandaging techniques are discussed in Chapter 4, and casting is discussed in Chapter 6.)*

Pressure sores in a horse that cannot stand are extremely difficult to prevent or treat until the horse is able to get up. Frequently turning the horse from side to side can help. Ensuring that there is always a deep layer of dry bedding beneath the horse can also help. But this is difficult if the horse is moving around a lot or repeatedly struggling to get up.

Puncture Wounds

Punctures are wounds that are much deeper than they are wide. In many cases, the wound at the skin edge is so small that it quickly seals, leaving a contaminated tract or cavity beneath the skin surface. These wounds can cause real problems because the tract or cavity is an ideal environment for bacteria to multiply. Also, the narrow (or sealed) opening in the skin prevents effective drainage from the wound.

Puncture wounds typically are caused by a penetrating object, such as a nail or a piece of wire. However, small, deep lacerations may develop some of the same characteristics that make puncture wounds such a problem. For example, wounds on the top or side of the body may develop a cavity beneath the skin if serum or pus is prevented from draining. This is more likely if the skin wound is small and closes over quickly. The result in these cases, and with true puncture wounds, is a tract or cavity which contains infected material that has no way to escape. Pus can build up and enlarge the space or spread to involve nearby tissues.

Another wound that has some of the characteristics and problems of a puncture wound is the "radiating" wound. With these wounds, the damage beneath the skin is far more extensive than expected from the size of the wound. For example, a kick to the side of the forearm creates a small wound on the skin. However, beneath the skin the force of the kick radiates through the underlying tissues. This causes extensive bruising in the subcutaneous tissue and muscle, and possibly also damage to the underlying bone surface. The skin wound usually closes over quickly, trapping the damaged and contaminated tissue beneath. If the bone surface has been damaged, a piece of bone (a sequestrum) may also be trapped within the wound, and bone infection can develop *(see Chapter 9)*. These horses can be quite lame.

Wound Care for Puncture Wounds
   Treatment of puncture-type wounds involves reopening or enlarging the wound at the skin edge to allow it to drain. *This is a procedure
for the veterinarian to perform.* The wound may also need to be lav-

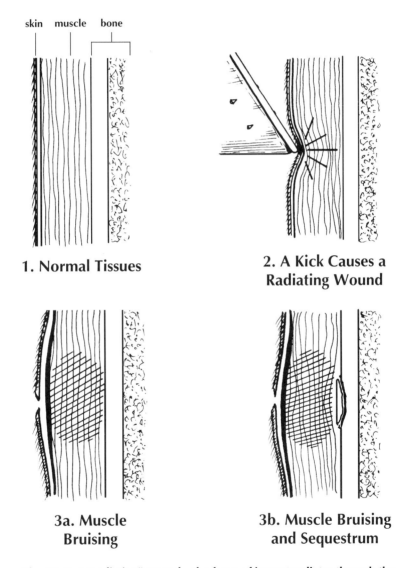

1. Normal Tissues

**2. A Kick Causes a
Radiating Wound**

**3a. Muscle
Bruising**

**3b. Muscle Bruising
and Sequestrum**

Fig. 13–7. A "radiating" wound—the force of impact radiates through the
tissues, causing muscle or bone damage beneath a minor skin wound.

aged (flushed out) at least twice per day with saline solution or dilute antiseptic.

In many cases, massaging upward from below the wound can help move the infected material out of the wound. When this does not work, the veterinarian may make a small hole below the wound into the lower part of the cavity, to allow it to drain. In either case, it is very important that the wound(s) is kept open until the cavity or tract has filled in.

Antibiotics are usually given, although it is up to the veterinarian to decide which antibiotic is most suitable. *Vaccination against tetanus is extremely important* in horses with these wounds because closed cavities or tracts are ideal places for tetanus bacteria to multiply.

Burns

Burns may be caused by excessive heat, such as fire, heat lamps, "firing," etc. However, irritant or caustic chemicals, such as blisters, liniments, and "leg paints," far more often cause burns that result in lameness. In some sensitive horses, even DMSO can cause a mild chemical burn, especially if it is covered with a bandage.

Burns may be partial or full thickness, and are generally defined as first-, second-, or third-degree. First- and second-degree burns involve only the skin's outer layer. Third-degree burns damage the full thickness of the skin, and may extend to the underlying tissues. The first signs of skin damage after a burn are swelling, heat, and pain—typical signs of inflammation. If the burned area is on pink skin, the inflamed skin is also very red. If just the outer layer is burned, there may be no further signs, other than scurfing or flaking after a day or two. However, if a third-degree burn has occurred the signs are more severe, and include blistering, oozing, and sloughing (lifting away) of the skin. Burns are very painful injuries, so horses with second- or third-degree burns on the legs are usually quite lame.

Wound Care for Burns

The burned area should be gently cleaned with saline solution to remove any irritant or caustic substances. The entire wound should then be liberally covered with an antibiotic cream or aloe vera gel. Twice daily cleaning and antibiotic ointment/aloe vera should continue until the burned area has healed. With third-degree burns the veterinarian may need to trim the dead tissue as it sloughs, to allow the underlying wound to heal without complications.

Contusions

Contusions are injuries that do not break the skin surface. But they generally damage the blood vessels within or beneath the skin. Examples include:

* bruises
* hematomas—collections of blood beneath the skin
* seromas—collections of serum beneath the skin

In most cases the lameness is mild, unless the surface of the underlying bone is also damaged.

Wound Care for Contusions

When contusions first occur, ice, cold packs, or cold hosing can minimize the swelling, as can a firm bandage (in suitable areas). It is not a good idea to stick a needle into, or attempt to drain a contusion. The veterinarian may decide to drain the fluid from the swelling at a later date (for a better cosmetic result), but this must be done with strictly sterile technique. Inserting a needle or blade into a hematoma or seroma—sterile cavities containing sterile fluid—can introduce bacteria and cause an abscess to develop. Also, draining a hematoma within 2 – 3 days of injury can cause further bleeding. While the blood is contained beneath the skin it acts like a pressure pad on the damaged vessels. When the swelling is drained, the pressure on the damaged blood vessels is relieved, and bleeding into the cavity can begin again.

Contusions resolve as the body absorbs the fluid. Heat therapy, massage, or other physical therapies (such as magnetic field therapy; *see Chapter 4*) that improve blood flow to the area may speed up the resolution of these swellings. However, these therapies should not

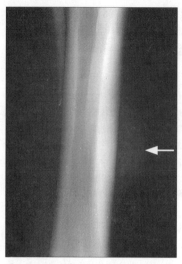

Fig. 13–8. A hematoma on the front of the cannon, which has begun to calcify.

begin until at least 3 days after the injury.

Sometimes contusions over a bony surface, such as the cannon bone, can become calcified and form a permanent, hard swelling. Cold therapy and NSAIDs *(see Chapter 5)*, begun immediately after the injury, can reduce the chance of this blemish developing.

Wounds Involving a Joint

Wounds near joints should always be treated seriously. They should receive immediate veterinary attention, whether or not the joint is obviously damaged.

The joint capsule is the fibrous, outer covering that protects and supports the joint. In most parts of the leg there is very little tissue between the skin and the joint, so wounds over joints can easily damage the joint capsule. When the capsule is damaged, clear, yellow, honey-like joint fluid may leak from the wound, and bacteria

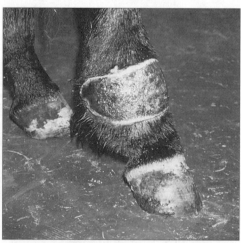

Fig. 13–9. Immediate veterinary attention could have prevented the permanent disability caused by this wound.

and debris may enter the joint space. The result can be septic arthritis, and a permanently disabled horse.

It can be very difficult to determine whether a small wound over a joint is deep enough to have damaged the joint capsule. In many cases the initial lameness is no greater than would be expected for a similar-sized wound on another part of the leg. So, the degree of lameness is not a reliable way to determine the severity of the injury. Because of the serious consequences of joint infection, it is best to call the veterinarian immediately after the wound is discovered.

Initial Care for Wounds Involving a Joint

If joint fluid is leaking from a wound, it is best not to touch the wound, except to carefully remove whatever dirt and debris is possible without contaminating the joint further. Only saline solution should be used to clean these wounds; antiseptic can irritate the joint. The cloth or cotton should not be wiped across the wound because this can deposit dirt or hair into the joint. Also, no attempt should be made to flush the joint because this will almost certainly contaminate it. The wound should be covered with a sterile dressing and a bandage until the veterinarian arrives.

(See Chapter 8 for more information on managing wounds that involve joints.)

Wounds Involving Bone

Injuries that expose or involve bone should receive immediate veterinary attention, whether or not the bone is fractured. The outer surface of the bone is covered by a thin, fibrous membrane called the periosteum, which nourishes and protects the bone surface. If the periosteum is damaged or stripped away during the injury, the outer surface of the bone may become devitalized. A dead piece of bone (a sequestrum) may then act like a foreign object. Bacterial infection of the damaged bone often develops with these wounds. Bone infection, or osteomyelitis, can lead to further bone damage *(see Chapter 9)*. It can also slow wound healing.

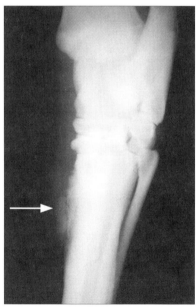

Fig. 13–10. Osteomyelitis on the cannon bone, resulting from a wound just below the hock.

Initial Care for Wounds Involving Bone

These wounds should only be cleaned with saline solution; antiseptic can irritate the bone surface. If the skin cannot be pulled over the bone, a sterile dressing or clean cloth should be saturated with saline solution and placed over the bone to prevent it from drying out. The leg should then be bandaged. If the wound cannot be sutured, the bone should be kept moist with saline-soaked dressings until granulation tissue covers the bone. Injuries this severe should always receive veterinary attention.

Open fractures are injuries in which a piece of bone has penetrated the skin or there is a deep wound directly over a fracture. They are very serious injuries that should be considered emergencies. There may not be a piece of bone visibly protruding from the skin, but any wound over a bone that is known or suspected to be fractured should be viewed with suspicion. The wound should be cleaned with saline solution only if there is a lot of dirt or debris in or around it. Otherwise, it should simply be covered with a sterile dressing or gauze pad. A firm support bandage and splint should be then applied to the limb *(see Chapter 4).* The horse must be kept still until the veterinarian arrives or the horse can be transported to a veterinary hospital. *(See Chapter 9 for information on treating fractures.)*

Note
Whenever a wound is found over an area of extensive swelling in a very lame horse, it is best to assume there is an open fracture until the veterinarian can examine it.

Wounds Involving Muscle

The most common areas in which a wound may involve the underlying muscle are:

- the forearm
- the pectoral area: the front of the chest and between the forelegs
- the side or back of the thigh

These wounds can be several inches long and quite deep; when they gape open they can look awful. Despite their appearance, in most cases the horse is usually only a little stiff, rather than obviously lame. However, the degree of lameness depends on the cause of the injury. For example, if the wound occurred during a trailer wreck, bruising and other tissue trauma cause more pain than if the wound was caused by a wire cut.

Initial Care for Wounds Involving Muscle

Although these injuries can look terrible, they should be managed like a skin laceration (discussed earlier). These wounds do not tend to bleed very much, and the bleeding is usually easy to control with a few minutes of pressure over the worst areas. Many owners and trainers are afraid to clean these wounds, but it is usually safe to gently bathe away any dirt and debris from the wound with saline solution. Done carefully, most horses do not react too much to this procedure. As with skin wounds, the veterinarian will decide whether it is worth suturing the wound. If it can be sutured, the sooner the wound is treated, the better the outcome will be. *(See Chapter 10 for more information on managing wounds that involve muscle.)*

Muscles have a very good blood supply, so unless they are grossly contaminated, these wounds generally heal well. The scar is often smaller than would be expected from the size and depth of the

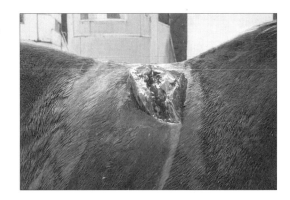

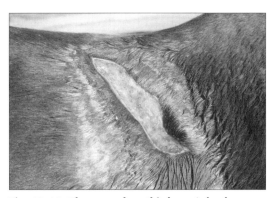

Fig. 13–11. The wound on this horse's back looked bad at first (top), but quickly developed a healthy granulation bed (bottom).

wound. In most cases, the horse can soon return to its normal athletic activities.

Wounds Involving Tendons or Ligaments

Wounds that expose or involve tendons or ligaments can be serious injuries, and need prompt veterinary attention. Any damage to the tendon or ligament fibers weakens the entire structure. If the horse is permitted to move around without adequate support on the injured leg, the tendon or ligament may completely rupture. If one or both of the flexor tendons are severed, excessive strain is placed on the other structures that support the fetlock. The result can be complete breakdown of the suspensory apparatus *(see Chapter 16)*.

Initial Care for Wounds Involving Tendons or Ligaments

When a wound exposes or involves a tendon or ligament, it should only be cleaned with saline solution; antiseptic can be too irritant for these tissues. While waiting for the veterinarian to arrive, a sterile dressing or clean cloth should be saturated with saline solution and placed over the wound. This prevents the tissues from drying out. The leg should then be bandaged.

It is very important that the horse is prevented from moving about if one or both of the flexor tendons are lacerated. A firm support bandage should be applied over the existing wound bandage. The leg should then be splinted so that the horse cannot place the foot flat and bear weight on the leg *(see Chapter 4)*. As an alternative, a wedge of wood can be taped to the underside of the horse's foot so that the heels are raised a few inches and tension on the tendons is relieved.

(See Chapter 11 for more information on managing tendon lacerations.)

DERMATITIS

Dermatitis is inflammation of the skin (dermis and epidermis). It can be caused by several factors, including:

- trauma (e.g. abrasions)
- chemical irritation
- prolonged moisture (e.g. from a damp bandage, or standing in mud)
- bacterial infection
- fungal infection
- certain viruses
- immune-related problems

The skin condition that most often causes lameness in horses is bacterial dermatitis. A couple of less common skin conditions that affect the legs and can cause lameness are also mentioned in this section.

Bacterial Dermatitis ("Scratches")

Definition and Causes

Bacterial dermatitis is skin inflammation caused by bacterial infection. It can occur anywhere on the horse's body. But the most commonly affected area, and the one most likely to cause lameness, is the lower leg. Bacterial dermatitis of the lower leg is the focus of this section. The common name for this condition varies in different parts of the country. One is "scratches"; others are "mud fever" and "greasy heel."

There are several different organisms that can cause this problem. In many cases there is more than one type invading the skin and causing inflammation. The organisms that most frequently cause "scratches" are *Dermatophilus, Staphylococcus*, and *Streptococcus* species. In some cases fungi may also be involved, although they are probably secondary invaders.

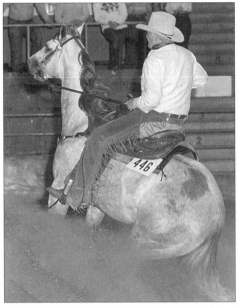

Fig. 13–12. Working on sand can cause abrasions that may lead to "scratches."

None of these organisms can invade normal, healthy skin. There must be a skin lesion—a breakdown of the skin's protective outer layer—for this condition to develop. The skin lesion may only be a minor abrasion, such as can occur when the horse is clipped or regularly worked on sand. The protective barrier is also broken down by constant moisture, such as standing all day in a dirty stall or muddy paddock.

Bacterial dermatitis is more common in horses with white socks or stockings—that is, on unpigmented skin. Presumably, this skin is more easily damaged than pigmented skin. It is also fairly common in draft breeds because when the feathers (the long hairs on the fetlocks and pasterns) get wet, they keep the skin beneath moist. Occasionally, a severe case of thrush can also lead to "scratches."

Signs of Bacterial Dermatitis

No matter what the cause, the skin lesions begin as small, superficial wounds that ooze serum or blood. This dries and forms hard crusts or scabs over the sores. When the crusts are pulled away the hair usually pulls out with it, leaving a raw, weeping sore. This condition is very painful and most horses resent the scabs being lifted.

When the lesions occur on the legs they typically begin at the back of the pastern, and spread around the sides and front of the pastern and up the leg. It is common for the affected leg to be swollen due to cellulitis (discussed later). Lameness often results because movement stretches the damaged skin.

Diagnosis of Bacterial Dermatitis

The diagnosis is usually based on the history, and on the distribution and appearance of the skin lesions. It is impossible to tell just by looking at the leg which organism is causing the infection. The veterinarian may remove some of the scabs and submit them to the laboratory for bacterial identification, or culture and antibiotic sensitivity testing *(see Chapter 2)*. However, in most cases it is not necessary because the treatment is the same, no matter which organisms are present.

Treatment of Bacterial Dermatitis

The organisms themselves may be easy to kill with a number of different antiseptics and antibiotics. However, the condition can be very difficult to resolve, particularly if the horse's environment is not changed. *For the infection to resolve, the horse must be kept in a clean, dry stall or paddock.*

To treat this condition, the scabs must be removed to expose the wounds beneath. There is no point in plastering medication over the top of the crusts—the organisms are in the skin *under* the crusts. The scabs are easier to remove if the skin is soaked with warm water and

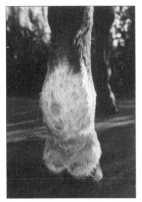 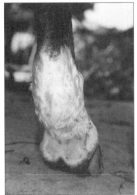 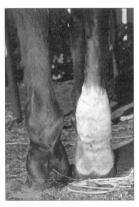

Fig. 13–13. Left: A severe case of bacterial dermatitis, after trimming and cleaning. **Middle:** After a week of treatment, the swelling is reduced and the wounds are healing. **Right:** After 3¹/₂ weeks of treatment, the skin is almost healed.

thoroughly lathered with a medicated shampoo. In some cases it may be necessary to soften the scabs overnight by liberally applying a greasy ointment or Vaseline to the crusts and covering the leg with plastic wrap and a bandage. Softening the scabs makes removing them less painful for the horse and less likely to cause bleeding. It is usually necessary to trim the hair from the affected areas with scissors, especially in horses with long, dense fetlock hair. As with scabs, the medication does no good if it is just applied to the hair.

Once all the scabs are removed, the skin should be gently patted dry with a clean towel or cloth. It should then be allowed to dry out completely before an antibiotic ointment is applied. This process must be repeated once or twice per day until the wounds have completely healed. Ointments that also contain corticosteroids can relieve the inflammation and pain, but they also inhibit the horse's immune response to the infection. The most effective way to relieve the inflammation is by controlling the infection, not by suppressing the inflammation with drugs. In severe cases the veterinarian may prescribe a course of oral or injectable antibiotics to help clear up the infection. However, antibiotics are not a suitable substitute for a clean, dry environment and proper wound care.

Many owners and trainers stop treatment before the wounds have completely healed. This usually leads to persistence or recurrence of the problem because oozing from a wound is all the moisture these organisms need to multiply and re-invade the skin. A vicious cycle develops unless the wounds are completely healed.

Prognosis for Bacterial Dermatitis
The prognosis for full return to athletic activities is excellent once the skin condition is cleared up. However, unless the horse's environment is improved, persistence or recurrence of the infection is likely.

Vesicular Stomatitis
Vesicular stomatitis (VS) is a viral disease of horses and cattle. The virus causes vesicles, or blisters, to form in the mouth. But occasionally lesions also develop on the coronets and cause mild lameness. The blisters may go unnoticed because they are easily ruptured, leaving only small, painful, ulcerated wounds. There is no cure for this disease, but complete recovery occurs within a couple of weeks of infection in all but the most serious cases.

VS is a contagious disease that must be reported to the state veterinary inspector. When VS is diagnosed, the state inspector issues a quarantine order that restricts the movement of livestock into and out of the area.

Immune-Related Skin Disorders
Contact Allergies
Contact allergies are reactions to substances in direct contact with the skin. They can cause dermatitis that may result in mild lameness when it occurs on the legs. Allergies to pasture plants (such as *Paspalum*) are good examples. The skin lesions can look like bacterial dermatitis: painful crusts or scabs. They can be difficult to resolve if the cause of the inflammation is unknown or cannot be removed. In some cases topical (on the skin), oral, or injectable corticosteroids may be necessary to control the condition. However, these drugs do not cure the problem; the dermatitis persists as long as the cause of the allergic reaction is present.

Auto-Immune Diseases
Fortunately, auto-immune diseases, in which the body's immune system attacks its own tissues, are rare in horses. Pemphigus foliaceus is the most common auto-immune skin disorder in horses. Skin lesions can occur anywhere on the body, although they are more often seen on the ears, face, and coronets. When erosions and crusts occur on the coronets, lameness can result. To make this diag-

nosis, special tests must be performed on a skin biopsy sample. Treatment involves oral or injectable corticosteroids *(see Chapter 5)*. Other immunosuppressive drugs may also be used in some cases. Treatment must continue for the rest of the horse's life.

LIMB EDEMA

Edema is diffuse swelling caused by an accumulation of fluid within the tissues. It develops when there is overload or obstruction of the lymphatic vessels. These are the tiny, thin-walled vessels that pick up any extra tissue fluid (called lymph) that has leaked out of the capillaries. The lymphatic vessels return this fluid to the bloodstream.

When the lymphatic vessels in the legs are overloaded or obstructed, tissue fluid builds up. This stretches the skin, which can make movement painful. There are several causes of limb edema; they vary in severity and in their potential to cause lameness. Limb edema may be caused by:

- "stocking up"
- cellulitis
- vasculitis
- ulcerative lymphangitis ("big leg")
- heart or kidney problems

Bruising can also cause diffuse swelling; however, this is not edema. It is leakage of blood from damaged vessels into the tissues. In most cases in which bruising is so extensive that it can be mistaken for edema, there is a history of a traumatic incident or there are marks on the skin that indicate the horse has sustained trauma to that area.

"Stocking Up"

The lymphatic vessels in the horse's legs are tiny and do not have any valves to prevent backflow. The flow of fluid up the leg (against gravity) depends on movement of the tissues around the lymphatic vessels. Inactivity, such as standing around in a stall, can result in the buildup of tissue fluid in the lower legs. This causes a mild swelling called "stocking up."

"Stocking up" does not cause lameness. It merely causes mild edema that begins at the coronet and works slowly up the leg, usually stopping just above the fetlock. In most cases only the hindlegs

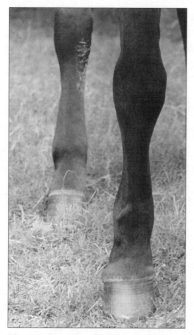

Fig. 13–14. "Stocking up" causes mild swelling in the lower legs.

are affected, although it can occur in all four legs. In either case the swelling is bilateral: the same in both the left and right legs. The skin over the swollen area is of normal temperature or slightly cooler than normal. Although the swollen area may remain pitted when pressed with the thumb—the hallmark of edema from any cause—it is not painful. The swelling quickly and completely resolves with activity. It can usually be prevented by keeping the lower legs bandaged while the horse is in the stall.

Cellulitis

Cellulitis is inflammation of the superficial tissues beneath the skin. It is usually caused by bacterial infection. In nearly all cases cellulitis occurs secondary to either a skin wound (which may only be very small and superficial) or infection of the deeper tissues. For example, cellulitis is commonly found around an abscess or an infected bone, joint, or tendon sheath.

The most consistent sign of cellulitis in a limb is diffuse swelling. This swelling is caused by inflammatory edema—accumulation of tissue fluid as a result of inflammation *(see Chapter 5)*. The amount of fluid that leaks out of the blood vessels in the inflamed area overloads the lymphatic vessels, causing edema. This swelling is hot and painful, and the horse is lame, which differentiates it from "stocking up." Also, "stocking up" causes symmetrical swelling in both hindlegs or all four legs, whereas cellulitis is almost always confined to just one leg.

At first, the swelling begins around the focus of infection (wound, infected joint, etc.). But then it moves down the leg, and may also spread further up the leg. So for the first day or two the location of the swelling can help to pinpoint the site of infection.

When the cause of the infection is not immediately apparent, the degree of lameness can be a fairly accurate way to determine the severity of the primary problem. For example, when cellulitis is the result of a superficial wound, the horse may only be mildly lame (grade 1 – 2 of 5). But when cellulitis develops as a result of septic arthritis *(see Chapter 8)*, the horse is very lame (grade 4 – 5 of 5). A thorough history and physical examination, and possibly other tests are necessary to identify the cause of the infection when it is not obvious.

Treatment

Treatment of cellulitis must begin with managing the primary problem. When cellulitis is secondary to a skin wound, treatment includes:

* proper wound care
* cold hosing
* a "sweat" or poultice, where appropriate
* NSAIDs
* gentle exercise

These measures are usually successful in resolving the swelling within a couple of days. In some cases the veterinarian may also treat the horse with antibiotics.

Managing abscesses and bone, joint, and tendon sheath infections are covered in the relevant chapters.

Vasculitis

Vasculitis is inflammation of the blood vessels. The result is leakage of fluid from the vessels; in severe cases whole blood (fluid and red blood cells) leaks from the vessels. Leakage of fluid results in edema because the lymphatic vessels cannot return this excess of fluid to the general circulation fast enough. Vasculitis in any form is uncommon in horses. Some causes of vasculitis that can affect the limbs are discussed below.

Equine Viral Arteritis (EVA)

Equine Viral Arteritis (EVA) causes vasculitis in several organ systems. Typically, it results in edema in all four limbs, although the swelling is usually worse in the hindlimbs. It can also cause swelling beneath the chest and abdomen, and a watery discharge from the nostrils and eyes. It may cause abortion in pregnant mares.

EVA is an infectious disease, so several or all of the horses at the facility may be affected. In most cases the lameness is mild, although the fever and lethargy that are typical of the disease make the horse reluctant to move around.

<table>
<tr><td>

More Information

The hygiene and isolation procedures outlined in Chapter 4 can limit the spread of this disease within and between facilities.

</td><td>

There is no specific treatment for this infection. Most horses recover fully in 1 – 2 weeks with just supportive care (NSAIDs, oral or IV fluids if necessary, and good nursing care). EVA is important because the virus rapidly spreads from horse to horse in nasal secretions and other discharges.

</td></tr>
</table>

Purpura

Purpura hemorrhagica is a form of vasculitis in which the vessel walls are damaged by immune complexes: antibodies bound to foreign particles, such as bacteria. In most cases this condition develops within a few weeks of an upper respiratory tract infection. Strangles is the classic cause of purpura. (Strangles is a bacterial disease caused by *Streptococcus equi,* in which abscesses form in the glands under the jaw.) However, purpura can occur after infection with other bacteria and possibly also certain viruses.

The signs of purpura include edema of all four legs and the underside of the chest and abdomen. In male horses the sheath may also be swollen. There may be fever and depression, although this is not always the case. In severe cases there may also be small spots of hemorrhage in the mucous membranes—gums, lining of the mouth, inside of the nostrils and eyelids, etc. When the condition is this severe, the limb edema may be so great that patches of skin begin to slough and bloody serum oozes from the wounds. In these horses, walking is obviously painful. When the edema is only mild, the horse may simply walk with a stiff, stilted gait.

Treatment usually includes:

- corticosteroids to inhibit the immune complexes and further blood vessel damage
- antibiotics to help prevent secondary infection
- good nursing care

Firm bandages that begin at the coronet and are applied up the leg can help squeeze fluid out of the lower legs and make the horse more comfortable. Hydrotherapy, massage, and gentle exercise can also reduce the limb edema. *(These therapies are discussed in Chapter 4.)*

The prognosis for full recovery and return to athletic activities is usually quite good, although it may take several weeks for the horse to recover fully after a severe case of purpura. Laminitis may complicate the situation, particularly if corticosteroids were given.

Ehrlichia equi Infection

Ehrlichia equi is a bacteria-like organism in the same group as the organism that causes Potomac Horse Fever *(Ehrlichia risticii).* It is a tick-transmitted disease that can also affect people. This condition was first seen in California, but there is evidence that it is also present on the East coast of the U.S.

The first signs are vague: fever and loss of appetite. After a couple of days the legs begin to swell, and small red spots of hemorrhage develop in the mucous membranes. Some horses are jaundiced, which causes the mucous membranes and the white of the eye to become yellowed. The horse is reluctant to move and may seem incoordinated when made to walk. Unlike Potomac Horse Fever, abortion, diarrhea, and laminitis generally do not occur with this disease.

Treatment consists of antibiotics and supportive care. Other problems, such as secondary bacterial infection, are uncommon, so the prognosis for complete recovery is very good.

Ulcerative Lymphangitis ("Big Leg")

Lymphangitis is inflammation of the lymphatic vessels, usually as a result of bacterial invasion. In most cases the bacteria enter the lymphatic vessels through a wound on the lower leg. This condition is more likely when the normal lymphatic flow is slowed by inactivity ("stocking up") or obstructed by injury further up the leg.

The inflammation that results from bacterial infection further obstructs lymphatic flow and causes fluid to leak from the inflamed tissues. This process may also obstruct the veins, which causes further fluid leakage into the tissues. As a result, the leg becomes hugely swollen, which is why the common name is "big leg." If the immune system cannot control the infection, abscesses break out in several places over the swollen leg. When the condition gets to this stage it is called ulcerative lymphangitis. Fortunately, this is uncommon.

In most cases the hot, painful swelling involves a single hindleg, although occasionally both hindlegs or a foreleg may be affected. Lameness is usually moderate to severe, depending on the stage and severity of the disease.

Treatment of Ulcerative Lymphangitis

Ulcerative lymphangitis can be extremely difficult to resolve. By the time abscesses develop, the infection is well established. Often the invading bacteria is *Staphylococcus aureus,* or "golden staph." This organism is notoriously difficult to kill because it has become resistant to most antibiotics. Other bacteria can also cause this condition, so the veterinarian will sample the discharge from the wounds and submit it to the laboratory for bacterial culture and antibiotic sensitivity testing *(see Chapter 2).* This test is important to identify which organism is causing the infection and which antibiotic will be most effective.

Oral or intravenous antibiotics, poulticing, and physical therapy (such as hydrotherapy and magnetic field therapy) help resolve the infection. NSAIDs are commonly given to reduce the inflammation and pain, although they are not very effective unless the antibiotics can control the infection. Corticosteroids should not be used to treat this condition because they inhibit the body's normal immune response. The horses that develop ulcerative lymphangitis likely have some degree of immune system compromise which allows the bacteria to invade and spread unchallenged. Corticosteroids would further impair the horse's ability to resolve the infection. *(These therapies and medications are discussed in Section II: Principles of Therapy.)*

Prognosis for Ulcerative Lymphangitis

Often the horse must be treated for several weeks before its condition improves. But despite diligent therapy, the prognosis for return to athletic usefulness is poor. Even if the infection can be resolved, the swelling often remains because the lymphatic vessels, and sometimes even the nearby veins are permanently obstructed. Such severe swelling puts tension on the skin, which can make movement of the joints painful. Therefore, chronic lameness and a large, unsightly leg are the common results of this condition.

14

DEVELOPMENTAL
ORTHOPEDIC
DISORDERS

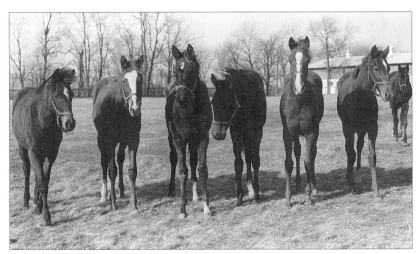

Fig. 14–1.

his chapter covers a variety of musculoskeletal conditions that may either be present at birth or develop as the foal grows. These conditions, collectively called Developmental Orthopedic Disorders (DODs), include:

- angular limb deformities ("crooked legs")
- flexural limb deformities (lax or "contracted" tendons)
- physitis
- osteochondrosis
- osteochondroma

Developmental disorders are very important problems in foals that are destined for athletic or show careers. Some of these conditions, particularly angular and flexural limb deformities, can result in permanent conformational faults. For example, "offset knees," "splay feet," or "pigeon toes" in an adult horse may be the result of an angular limb deformity that was not appropriately treated in the foal.

Throughout this book, conformational faults are listed as potential causes of a wide variety of problems in athletic horses. But conformational faults are not the only result of untreated DODs. Osteochondrosis is one of the factors that can lead to degenerative joint disease, which is a chronic problem that plagues many athletic horses *(see Chapter 8)*. Thus, preventing, or at least recognizing and treating developmental disorders in the foal is extremely important if the adult horse is to have a successful athletic or show career.

Figure 14–2 is a time line that shows the average age when the first signs of the DODs usually appear. This time line highlights the importance of frequently observing all foals, both normal and abnormal, from birth to maturity.

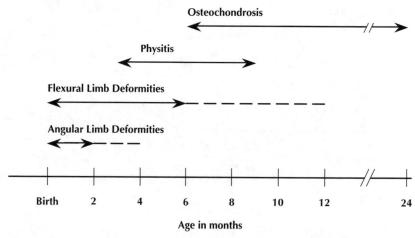

Fig. 14–2. The average age when the first signs of various DODs are noticed.

NORMAL BONE DEVELOPMENT

In fetuses and young animals most of the bones develop and grow in length by replacing the specialized cartilage in their physes and epiphyses with bone. The physis, or "growth plate," is a band of growth cartilage near the end of the bone. It is responsible for lengthwise bone growth. The epiphysis is the area between the physis and the joint surface. In very young animals it is composed of growth cartilage, with a core of new bone, called the epiphyseal growth center. As new bone is produced it radiates out from this center until the entire epiphysis is bone, except for a thin layer of articular cartilage at the joint surface. This process is called ossification.

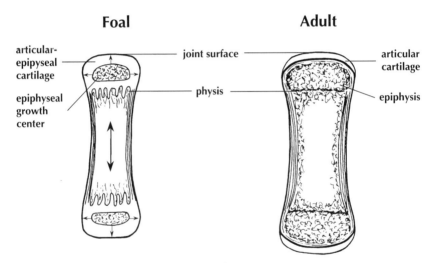

Fig. 14–3. Normal development of a longbone.

Other bones, such as the block-shaped "cuboidal" bones in the knee and hock, also develop from a core of new bone, surrounded by growth cartilage—an area called a secondary ossification center. New bone radiates out from this site until the entire structure is composed of bone, with a thin layer of articular cartilage on the joint surfaces.

FACTORS COMMON TO MOST DODS

Each DOD involves a different part of the musculoskeletal system. For example, physitis primarily involves the physes, whereas osteochondrosis mostly affects the epiphyses. The primary defect with angular limb deformities involves bone growth. But the major problem with flexural limb deformities is slower soft tissue growth.

Despite these differences, DODs share several contributing factors, including:

- rapid growth and large body size
- inappropriate level of activity—either too much or too little
- nutritional imbalance or excess

More specific causes are discussed in later sections on the individual conditions.

Some DODs also have a hereditary component. But for the most part they are the result of management problems. The pregnant mare's diet and health appear to be the most important factors in DODs that are present at birth. When these conditions develop after birth, the critical factors are the foal's diet and level of activity.

Growth Rate and Body Size

DODs are more common in large, rapidly growing foals. This probably explains the higher incidence of these disorders in Thoroughbreds, Standardbreds, Quarter Horses, and Warmbloods. When the foal is growing rapidly, its body weight may increase too quickly for the developing bones and joints to adapt. These structures are easily overloaded during their growth period.

Some developmental problems (especially osteochondrosis) are more common in certain breeds, and even in certain family lines. This has led scientists to speculate that there may be a hereditary component to some DODs. However, this theory has not been proven. More likely, DODs occur more often in these breeds or families because they are genetically programmed for rapid growth and large body size, rather than having a specific defect of bone development.

Exercise

Exercise is crucial for the normal development of the musculoskeletal system, particularly bones, tendons, and ligaments. These structures must be regularly loaded—but not overloaded—if they are to grow normally and be suited to the job they will do when mature. However, too much exercise can be as bad as too little, especially in very young foals.

Normal foals should be allowed to self-regulate their exercise. This is easily done by turning out the mare and foal in a large paddock, either full time or for a minimum of 2 – 3 hours every day. Young foals (in the first few weeks of life) do not need, and cannot tolerate as much exercise as older foals. It is usually best to separate the mares with young foals from the rest of the group.

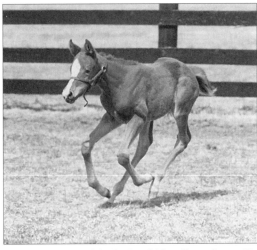

Fig. 14–4. Normal foals should be allowed to self-regulate their exercise.

Foals that are showing signs of DOD also need regular exercise, but it must be controlled. Specific recommendations are given in later sections on the individual DODs.

Diet

Dietary factors have received a lot of attention in recent years. The three main areas of research and management recommendations have targeted carbohydrate excess, calcium-phosphorus imbalance, and copper deficiency.

Carbohydrate Excess

Diets that are high in grain or grain products (meals, pellets, sweet feed, etc.) often provide more carbohydrate than is needed, even for a growing horse. Foals, weanlings, and yearlings that are fed high carbohydrate diets commonly develop DODs, regardless of the amount of protein or calcium in the ration. There may be at least two reasons for this. First, foals on a high carbohydrate diet grow rapidly. They quickly increase their body size and weight, often too fast for their bones and soft tissues to adapt. Second, high carbohydrate diets may suppress thyroid function, which is an important regulator of bone development.

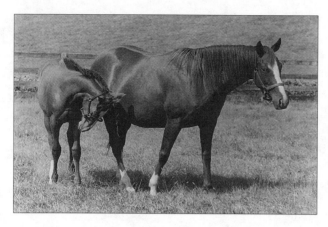

Fig. 14-5. DODs are more common in foals that are nursing from mares fed a high carbohydrate diet.

DODs are also more common in foals that are nursing from mares producing large volumes of milk. These mares usually are fed—or rather, overfed—a ration that is very high in carbohydrates.

Calcium-Phosphorus Imbalance

Low calcium, high phosphorus diets have long been known to increase the potential for DODs, especially osteochondrosis and physitis. Calcium is essential for normal bone production. A diet that is low in calcium and/or high in phosphorus can affect bone production and quality. The typical ration that consists of grain or grain products, grass hay, and no vitamin or mineral supplements does not supply the calcium needs of a pregnant or nursing mare, or a growing horse.

> **More Information**
>
> Figure 9–33 in Chapter 9 shows the calcium and phosphorus content of common hays and grains.
>
> Figure 9–34 gives the calcium and phosphorus requirements for pregnant or nursing mares, and growing horses.

On the other hand, high calcium, low phosphorus diets, such as those based on alfalfa hay, may also cause DODs. Both calcium and phosphorus must be present in the recommended amounts, and in the ideal ratio, for bones to develop normally. Imbalances in either direction can cause abnormal bone development. Incidentally, good quality alfalfa is relatively high in carbohydrates, which could also contribute to abnormal bone development if too much is fed.

The amount and ratio of calcium and phosphorus appear to be important both in the pregnant mare's diet and the foal's diet. Dietary analysis can determine whether the ration meets their calcium and phosphorus needs. It is no use measuring the blood concentration of calcium or phosphorus because the body maintains these minerals within a very narrow range. However, measuring the urinary fractional excretion (FE; *see Chapter 2*) of phosphorus can help identify dietary imbalances of calcium and phosphorus.

Copper Deficiency

Copper is essential for normal bone development. Studies have shown that foals fed a diet that is deficient in copper are much more likely to develop osteochondrosis than foals that receive the recommended amount. In fact, adding copper to the foal's diet can reduce the incidence of osteochondrosis.

The potential for some DODs to develop apparently begins before the foal is born. There is evidence that the mare's copper intake plays an important role. There is very little copper in mare's milk, no matter how much copper is fed to her after the foal is born. The newborn foal must rely on the copper its body stored before birth to meet its needs until it begins to eat enough solid food. In rapidly growing foals, this limited store of copper may be quickly depleted.

The incidence of some DODs, particularly osteochondrosis, can be

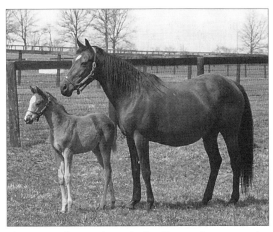

Fig. 14–6. The newborn foal relies on the copper its body stored before birth to meet its needs until it begins to eat solid food.

substantially reduced by adding copper to the pregnant mare's diet, especially in the third trimester. Supplementing pregnant mares with copper is much more effective in reducing the incidence of osteochondrosis than supplementing foals. The National Research Council recommends that growing horses, and pregnant or nursing mares receive 10 mg of copper per kilogram of feed (or 4.5 mg per pound of feed). The maximum tolerated level is 800 mg/kg of feed, so copper appears quite safe to feed in greater than recommended quantities. *(Recommendations for copper supplementation are in the next section.)*

There is little value in measuring the copper concentration in the mare's or foal's blood. Copper is stored in the liver, so unless a liver biopsy is performed—which is *not* recommended—it is impossible to accurately determine whether the foal has adequate copper stores. It is better to analyze the ration (hay, grain, supplements, and pasture) to ensure that the mare and foal receive enough copper.

High levels of calcium and phosphorus in the ration can impair copper absorption from the intestine. So, oversupplementing calcium and phosphorus may cause relative copper deficiency.

GENERAL MANAGEMENT & PREVENTION

Because some DODs may begin before the foal is born, a few general comments about managing these conditions and reducing their incidence on a breeding farm are in order. Specific treatment recommendations are discussed in later sections on the individual DODs.

Careful attention to nutrition and exercise are the keys to minimizing the incidence and impact of these problems. Equally important are frequent observation of every foal from birth to maturity, and prompt and appropriate management of feet and leg problems. With many of these conditions it is too late to correct the fault once the horse is an adult.

When more than one foal is affected, or more than one type of DOD is found on a farm, it should be treated as a herd problem. If only one foal in a group has a problem in just one leg, trauma, infection, or some other isolated event was probably the cause. However, if more than one foal has a DOD, it is a signal that there is a management problem which could affect every foal on the farm.

Professional nutritional advice from a veterinarian or equine nutritionist can minimize the incidence of DODs. The problem may be a dietary imbalance or a deficiency, but in many cases it is nutritional excess. For example, a mare that is overfed and producing a lot of milk is more likely to produce a foal with a DOD. Foals born to such mares should be watched very closely in the first few months of life. DODs can be difficult to manage in this situation because it is hard to control the nursing foal's nutritional intake. Reducing the amount of carbohydrate in the mare's ration may help decrease her milk production. However, this should not be done to the extent that the mare becomes thin or her milk production drops too much.

Specific Preventive Measures

DODs usually are far more easily prevented than treated. Effective prevention must begin with the pregnant mare. Mares should be kept on a good (but not excessive) level of nutrition throughout pregnancy. They should be maintained in good condition, and not allowed to get too fat or too thin. The levels and ratio of calcium and phosphorus in the diet should be carefully regulated. Copper should be supplemented if necessary, so that up to four times the maintenance copper requirement is provided. Higher levels of copper can be fed with safety, but more is not necessarily better.

The preventive measures should not stop once the foal is born. Foals and young horses should be raised on a balanced ration that:

- avoids carbohydrate excess and merely meets the animal's maintenance needs
- ensures steady growth (as much as nature allows)
- avoids deficiencies or excesses of calcium and phosphorus
- contains slightly increased levels of copper (feeding up to seven times the recommended requirement appears to be safe)

For detailed information on feeding all types of horses, read *Feeding to Win II*, published by Equine Research, Inc.

Foals and young horses must also receive daily exercise. Pasture turnout is usually the best option. If the foal must be kept in a stall or small paddock, it should be allowed to exercise freely in a larger area for a couple of hours every day.

ANGULAR LIMB DEFORMITIES
Definitions

Angular limb deformities (ALDs) are deviations of one or more of the foal's legs when viewed from the front or rear. These foals are often called "crooked" foals. Normally, it should be possible to draw a straight line from the point of the foal's shoulder through the center of the leg and foot. In foals with ALDs, the leg deviates from this vertical line.

Valgus is deviation of the leg to the outside below the affected joint. Valgus deformity of the knees results in a foal with "knock-knees." *Varus* is deviation of the leg to the inside below the affected joint. A foal with a varus deformity of the knees appears "bow-legged." Valgus in one leg and varus in the other results in a "wind-swept" foal.

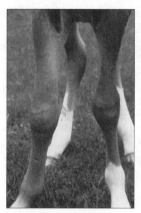 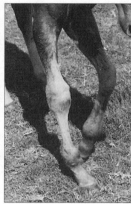 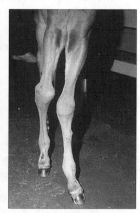

Fig. 14–7. Left: Carpal valgus—"knock-kneed" foal. Middle: Carpal varus—"bow-legged" foal. Right: Carpal valgus and carpal varus—"windswept" foal.

Mild angular deviations at the knees or hocks are very common in newborn foals. In many cases they disappear without specific treatment in the first few weeks of life. However, treatment is necessary to correct the problem if:

1. The deviation is severe.
2. The deviation initially is mild, but worsens.
3. The deviation develops in a foal that was normal at birth.

Causes of ALDs

ALDs can result from one of several abnormalities:

- uneven bone growth at a physis—the most common abnormality
- uneven bone development at an epiphysis
- incomplete development and collapse of the cuboidal bones in the knee or hock
- bowing of the cannon bone

(The first three abnormalities are illustrated in Figure 14–15.)

Bones grow in length as the specialized cartilage in the physes produces new bone *(see Figure 14–3)*. If bone growth on one side of the physis is slowed or stopped, yet the other side continues to lengthen normally, the bone, and the limb, becomes deviated. Sometimes uneven bone growth at the physis also causes the bone to rotate.

Occasionally, ALDs are caused by uneven bone development at the epiphysis. In newborn foals the deviation may be due to incomplete development and collapse of the block-shaped cuboidal bones in the knee or hock. Deviation caused by bowing of the cannon bone is very uncommon at any age.

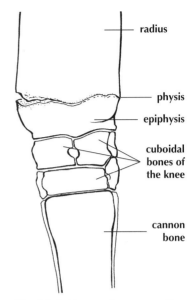

Fig. 14–8. Uneven bone growth at the physis has caused an ALD.

Most of the bone production in the physes of the lower legs occurs either before birth or in the first 6 months of life, so ALD is generally a condition that affects young foals. An ALD can be congenital—present at birth. Or, it can be developmental—develops days, weeks, or even months after birth.

Congenital ALDs

The actual cause(s) of ALD in newborn foals is not known. However, these abnormalities are probably due to a combination of maternal and foal factors. Suggested maternal factors include:

- nutritional imbalances in the diet (discussed earlier)
- severe illness, such as influenza, during pregnancy
- toxic plants, such as locoweed and Sudan grass, eaten during pregnancy

Possible foal factors include:

- abnormal position within the uterus, especially lack of space for a large foal
- prematurity or immaturity

Prematurity or immaturity can result in incomplete ossification of the cuboidal bones in the foal's knee or hock. This can lead to compression of the bones and partial collapse on one side of the joint when the foal stands. Low thyroid function has been suggested as a possible cause. Premature or immature foals often have tendon and ligament laxity (looseness or slackness) and generalized muscle weakness, both of which result in joint laxity. Laxity or collapse of the joint causes immediate deviation of the leg at the affected joint. This abnormal position can cause uneven loading of the physes and epiphyses, leading to further limb deviation if not corrected.

Developmental ALDs

The most common causes of developmental ALDs include:
- pain or injury elsewhere in the leg, not involving the physes
- excessive exercise
- direct damage to a physis
- severe physitis
- conformational faults

Any condition that causes pain in the foal's foot or leg may result in an ALD, whether or not the condition involves a physis. The foal adopts an abnormal position to protect the painful area. For example, the foal may hold the leg out to the side, or walk on the inside of the foot. If this position is maintained for longer than about a week, bone growth in the physes of that limb may be uneven.

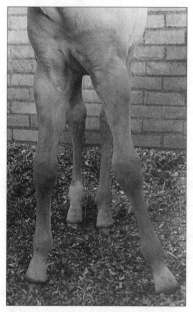

Fig. 14–9. ALDs may develop in an injured leg because the foal holds the leg in an abnormal position.

A deviation may instead develop in the normal, weight-bearing leg as a result of excessive and uneven loading of the physes. For the same reason, too much exercise, even without any pain or injury can cause or worsen an ALD.

A direct blow or a fracture that begins in, or extends into a physis may severely damage the physeal cartilage. This may lead to early closure on one side of the physis, which stops bone development.

Osteomyelitis (bone infection) that involves a physis is uncommon, but it can
also cause early closure and ALD. Severe
physitis may also contribute to the development of ALDs in some foals.

Conformational faults, such as "offset"
or "bench" knees, can result in uneven
loading of the physes, and ALD. On the
other hand, an ALD can *cause* the con-

> **More Information**
>
> Bone problems, includ-
> ing physeal fractures
> and osteomyelitis in
> young foals, are
> covered in Chapter 9.

formational fault. For example, angular
deviation at the fetlock can result in a "splay-footed" or "pigeon-
toed" horse. ALDs can develop in mature horses, but only after a
fracture or collapsed joint heals at an abnormal angle.

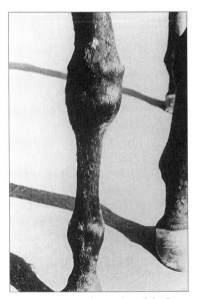

Fig. 14–10. Conformational faults,
such as "offset" knees, can cause
or be caused by an ALD.

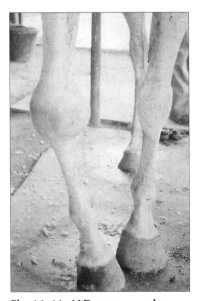

Fig. 14–11. ALDs can occur in mature horses after an injured joint
heals at an abnormal angle.

Signs of ALDs

The signs of ALD are obvious: crooked legs. When looking at a normal foal from the front, it should be possible to draw an imaginary
straight line from the point of the shoulder through the forearm,
knee, cannon, fetlock, pastern, and foot. In foals with ALDs, the part

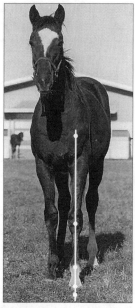

Fig. 14–12. A normal foal.

of the leg below the affected physis or joint deviates from this vertical line. The foot is either outside the line (valgus) or inside the line (varus).

It may help to imagine or stick a dot on the front of the foal's leg, on the point of the shoulder, knee, fetlock, coronet, and toe. By mentally joining the dots, it is easier to identify the site and degree of deviation, and any rotation. Taking a photograph of the foal every couple of weeks is a good way to record and measure changes over time.

Congenital ALDs often are bilateral. That is, the ALD involves a deviation in at least one physis in both forelegs (or both hindlegs). In contrast, developmental ALDs usually only involve one physis in one leg.

The most common ALDs are knee (carpal) or hock (tarsal) valgus—deviation of the lower leg to the outside. The cannon bone and pastern are aligned, but the entire lower leg deviates below the knee or hock. Fetlock varus—deviation of the pastern and foot to the inside—is also fairly common. The upper leg and cannon are aligned, but the pastern and foot deviate. (ALDs of the fetlock and the knee or hock can occur in the same leg.)

Sometimes part or all of the leg also is rotated. When rotation primarily involves the pastern bones, the foal is "pigeon-toed" or "splay-footed." Not only does the foot deviate from the vertical line, the toe also points either in or out. At first, this is

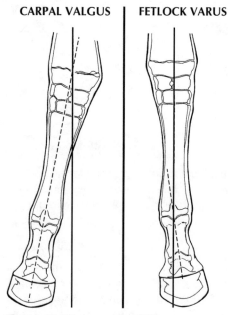

CARPAL VALGUS | FETLOCK VARUS

Fig. 14–13. Two common ALDs.

just the way the foal stands. But over time the pastern bones adapt to the abnormal forces on them, and the rotational deviation can become permanent. When the rotation occurs in the bones of the upper leg, the knee and cannon are rotated as well as the pastern and foot. In these cases the rotation is almost always to the outside.

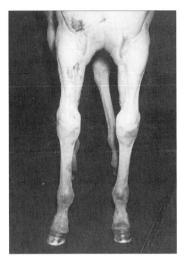 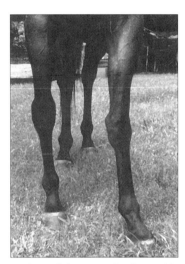

Fig. 14–14. Left: Fetlock valgus with rotation. Right: Carpal valgus with rotation.

Foals with ALDs are seldom obviously lame, although their gait is abnormal. (They may be lame if a painful condition caused the ALD.) If the foal is lame and the physis is swollen, this may indicate physitis or a more serious problem, such as a fracture or infection of the physis.

Diagnosis of ALDs

Diagnosing an ALD is straightforward, and is based on the signs and the foal's age. But to treat the condition properly it is necessary to know exactly where the deviation originates. If the deviation is due to joint laxity or collapse of the cuboidal bones, it should be possible to manually straighten the foal's leg. If, however, the deviation is due to uneven bone growth at the physis or epiphysis, the leg cannot be completely straightened manually.

Radiographs are usually necessary to:

• confirm the exact site of deviation
• determine whether the cuboidal bones are ossifying normally

• identify abnormalities in the shape of the epiphysis or cuboidal bones
• identify differences in the width of the physis between the inside and outside of the leg

To determine the exact site of deviation, a line is drawn on the radiograph, through the center of the bones above and below the affected joint. The point where the lines intersect is the site of the deviation. In most cases it is the physis. Occasionally the epiphysis or the cuboidal bones are where the abnormality occurs.

In ALDs involving the knee, the physis at the lower end of the radius (just above the knee) is the only active physis in this area after birth. In contrast, the fetlock has two physes that may cause a problem: one at the lower end of the cannon bone, and one at the upper end of the first pastern bone.

With any congenital condition, it is important for the veterinarian to examine the foal for other congenital abnormalities, such as "parrot mouth," cleft palate, heart abnormalities, and other leg deformities. In foals that develop an ALD after birth, the cause (for example, injury or infection) should also be investigated and corrected.

Physis   **Epiphysis**   **Cuboidal Bones**

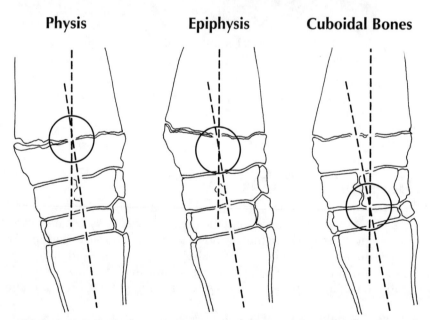

Fig. 14–15. A line is drawn through the center of the bones above and below the affected joint (in this case, the knee). The point where the lines intersect is the site of the deviation.

Treatment of ALDs

There are several treatment options available, ranging from conservative (restricted exercise, hoof trimming, etc.) to surgical. The choice of treatment depends on:

- the type and location of the deviation—physis, epiphysis, or cuboidal bones
- the severity of the deviation
- the age of the foal

In general, the younger the foal, the more quickly the leg responds, and the more likely the deviation will be completely corrected and need no further treatment. In older foals, correction is slower and may be incomplete.

Figure 14–16 summarizes the general treatment guidelines for

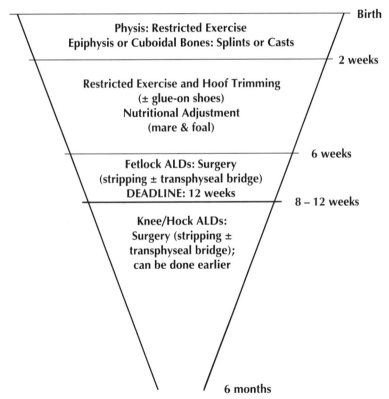

Fig. 14–16. The choice of treatment depends on the type and location of the deviation, and the age of the foal.

ALDs, based on the foal's age and the primary area involved. As the figure illustrates, timing is very important in the successful management of ALDs. *The timeframe narrows quickly as the foal grows.*

Deviation at the Physis
Conservative Management
Many cases of congenital and early developmental ALDs respond well to restricted exercise—provided the problem is identified and treated in the first couple of weeks of life. In other cases hoof trimming and special shoes may be recommended.

Restricted Exercise
The "crooked" foal and its mother should be separated from the other mares and foals, and confined to a stall or small paddock. This allows the owner or breeder to control the foal's activity level. The mare and foal should be turned out on their own for only 1 – 3 hours per day. The more severe the deviation, the more the foal's activity should be restricted.

Hoof Trimming and Other Options

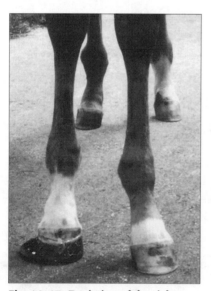

Fig. 14–17. Deviation of the right foreleg was corrected with a glue-on shoe. Unfortunately, deviation then developed in the left foreleg.

In foals older than about 2 weeks, many veterinarians and farriers recommend hoof trimming, with or without plastic glue-on shoes that have side extensions ("wings"). The hoof is usually trimmed by lowering the wall on the "short side" of the leg. For example, the inside of the foot is trimmed if the lower leg deviates to the inside. When glue-on shoes are used, the wing is usually placed on the "long side." For example, the wing is placed on the outside of the foot if the leg deviates to the inside.

Caution must be used when trimming the foal's feet. The height of the hoof wall should not be altered too much. It is usually best just to restore and maintain normal latero-medial hoof balance. Because the bones of young foals are active and responsive, excessive trimming of the hoof wall may encourage abnormal bone growth. Trimming the feet in young foals is best done "little and often"—a little every 2 weeks. Even so, trimming one side of the hoof wall in a young foal affects the pastern and fetlock, but probably has little influence on the knee.

Definition
Latero-medial balance: the height and angle of the hoof wall are identical on both sides of the foot *(see Chapter 7).*

When glue-on shoes are used in foals they should be removed every 10 – 20 days. Some farriers and veterinarians prefer to leave the shoes off for another 2 – 3 weeks before reapplying them. If the deviation has improved, the shoes may no longer be necessary.

Splints and fiberglass casts *(see Chapters 4 and 6)* are not the best options in foals with ALDs originating at a physis. The physis does not respond very well to these devices, and splints and casts can cause pressure sores. Flexor laxity (discussed later) can also occur with these devices.

Surgery

In severe cases that were not corrected with conservative management, surgery is necessary to alter bone growth at the affected physis. The response to surgery and the chances of a successful outcome are greatest if the surgery is performed before the foal is 2 months old. This is when bone growth can be manipulated to the greatest degree. It also allows time for the surgery to be repeated if the condition is not completely corrected on the first attempt. (After about 2 weeks of age, foals tolerate general anesthesia well, although the veterinarian should ensure that the foal is healthy beforehand.)

Bone growth in the fetlock physes is limited after about 3 months of age. It is essentially stopped by about 6 months of age. So, surgical manipulation of the fetlock physes will usually be unsuccessful after 2 – 3 months of age.

Bone growth in the physis just above the knee or hock begins to slow down after about 9 months. By about 2 years of age, it has essentially stopped. Although there is a longer period when the growth at this physis can be manipulated, the surgery is best performed in the first few months of life—the sooner the better. Once the ALD is corrected, the foal will likely need no further treatment. However, if the surgery is delayed, permanent changes may develop in the lower joints as a consequence of the abnormal limb position and uneven loading. So, surgery performed on an older foal may not be completely successful in straightening the limb.

Periosteal Elevation ("Stripping")

The most common surgical procedure used to correct deviation at a physis is periosteal elevation, or "stripping." This is the simplest and most effective surgical procedure, if done early. The aim is to accelerate bone growth on the "short side" of the bone. It involves anesthetizing the foal, making a small incision over the physis on the "short side," and cutting through the periosteum (the bone's fibrous covering) just above the physis in an inverted "T." The edges of the periosteum are then lifted. In most young foals this procedure straightens the leg in 4 – 6 weeks. Overcorrection—deviation in the opposite direction—generally does not occur with this procedure. In severe cases the surgery may need to be repeated in 6 – 8 weeks, provided there is still significant growth potential in the physis.

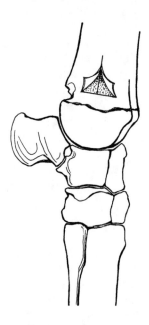

Fig. 14–18. Periosteal "stripping" involves making a small, inverted T-shaped incision through the periosteum just above the physis. The edges of the periosteum are then lifted.

Most veterinarians prefer to use absorbable ("dissolving") sutures beneath the skin to close the incision. These sutures cannot be seen and do not need to be removed. The veterinarian may prescribe antibiotics; NSAIDs, when used, are given for only 1 – 2 days. In all cases the foal's tetanus status must be reviewed *(see Chapter 5)*.

The surgery site is bandaged for 3 – 5 days, and the mare and foal are confined to a stall or small paddock. Exercise should be limited to 20 – 30 minutes of turnout twice per day for about a week. After that time, it is usually safe to turn the mare and foal out for longer periods. The long-term cosmetic result of this procedure is excellent. In most foals the leg is straight and there is little or no scarring.

Transphyseal Bridging

Before periosteal elevation was developed, transphyseal bridging was a common surgical procedure in foals. Now it is used almost exclusively in older foals, when there is limited growth potential in the physis and a rapid result is needed. Young foals with very severe ALDs may also need transphyseal bridging. The aim is to restrict bone growth on the "long side" of the bone, allowing the other side of the physis to catch up. In most cases it is combined with periosteal elevation, which is performed on the opposite side of the physis.

Transphyseal bridging involves

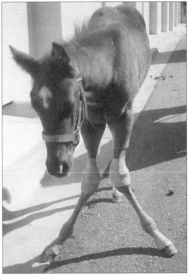

Fig. 14–19. Severe ALDs may require "stripping" and bridging.

spanning the physis on the "long side" with a surgical implant. The surgeon may use a surgical staple, two bone screws and some orthopedic wire, or a small bone plate. These implants restrict growth in the physis on that side, so they must be removed once the deviation is corrected; otherwise, overcorrection can occur.

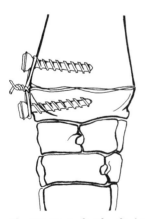
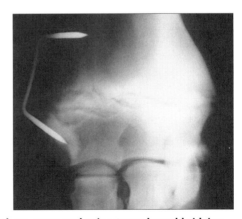

Fig. 14–20. Left: The deviation has been corrected using transphyseal bridging with bone screws and orthopedic wire. Right: Transphyseal bridging using a surgical staple.

Post-operative care following transphyseal bridging is similar to that described for periosteal elevation. In most cases antibiotics and NSAIDs are given for a few days after surgery. The veterinarian may recommend keeping the mare and foal confined for a week or two longer after bridging. Because it involves implants that must be removed during a second surgery, this procedure may leave permanent thickening and a scar.

Osteotomies

Other, more "invasive" surgical procedures may be necessary to correct severe deviations in older foals when there is little or no growth potential in the physis. These procedures are almost always restricted to correcting fetlock deviations, for two reasons. First, the fetlock physes close so early that the owner or breeder may not have sought veterinary advice soon enough for treatment to completely correct the deviation. *(Some people "wait and see if the foal grows out of it"; however, with fetlock deviations this is not a good approach.)* Second, these surgical procedures are very involved, and can have serious consequences. Catastrophic failure is more likely when osteotomies are performed on the larger bones (above the knee or hock) than on the lower end of the cannon bone.

To correct a deviation after the physis has closed, the surgeon must cut through the bone and realign it correctly. Wedge osteotomy involves removing a wedge of bone from the "long side," aligning the bone, and repairing it with a bone plate. Step osteotomy is another approach. It involves

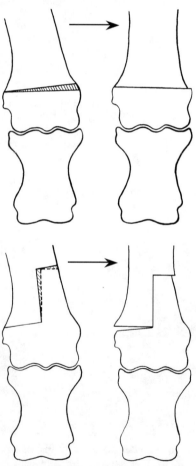

Fig. 14–21. Top: A wedge osteotomy. Bottom: A step osteotomy.

making a horizontal cut halfway through the bone on one side of the leg, making a similar cut on the other side of the leg a few inches above the first cut, and vertically sawing the bone in two between these two cuts. The two halves of the bone are then aligned and re-paired with bone plates and screws.

Since both of these procedures involve sawing the bone in two, the same precautions, post-operative care, and potential complications associated with fracture repair also apply *(see Chapters 6 and 9)*. These are radical procedures—they should only be undertaken after careful consideration of the potential complications and guarded prognosis for future athletic performance. With frequent observation of young foals, and prompt and appropriate treatment of ALDs, osteotomies should never be necessary.

Rotation

When conservative management is unsuccessful, further rotation may be prevented or limited with transphyseal bridging. The implant is placed at an angle across the physis so that both lengthwise growth and further rotation are restricted. In some cases it may be possible to partially de-rotate the bone with this procedure, but only in young foals. As with typical deviations at a physis, the sooner the surgery is performed, the better the outcome will be.

Deviation in the Bones of the Knee or Hock

The decision whether to treat foals with malformation of an epi-physis, or with incomplete development and collapse of the cuboidal bones is based on the severity of the changes, and on the foal's general condition. Severe underdevelopment, deformity, or collapse of these bones in a premature or immature foal carries a poor prognosis for normal development and future athletic function. (Also, these foals often have other problems.) For these reasons, the veterinarian may recommend euthanasia.

Less severe problems with the epiphysis or cuboidal bones are usually treated by placing a splint or fiberglass cast on the leg. The splint or cast should extend from the bottom of the cannon to the top

> **Note**
>
> Splints can quickly cause pressure sores. They should not be left on for more than about 8 hours *(see Chapter 4)*.
>
> A cast should not be left on a young foal for more than 10 – 14 days. Otherwise, growth will be restricted *(see Chapter 6)*.

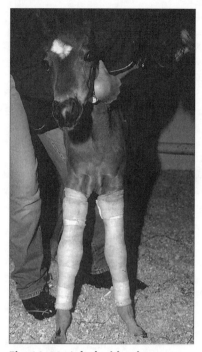

Fig. 14–22. A foal with tube casts on both forelegs.

of the forearm or thigh. It should not encase the fetlock or foot, so the foal can stand and bear weight normally. This type of cast is called a "sleeve" or "tube" cast.

Splints and casts can cause pressure sores if they are not monitored closely and replaced frequently. Flexor laxity should not develop as long as the foal is permitted to use the fetlock and foot normally. The leg should remain splinted or cast until radiographs indicate that the bones are ossifying and developing normally. In most cases these devices are necessary for only 2 – 3 weeks.

If the foal simply has very lax joints, and the bones are normal on radiographs, controlled exercise usually corrects the problem. Exercise should be limited to short periods in a small paddock, twice per day. However, the foal should be closely monitored for worsening of the deviation. Splinting or casting the foal may help prevent stretching of the ligaments on the "long side" of the joint. But it may also worsen the tendon and ligament laxity, so it is not recommended in most cases.

Trimming the hooves and applying special shoes usually does not work in foals with abnormal epiphyses or cuboidal bones.

Bowing

Bowing of the cannon bone may be improved or corrected with periosteal elevation. The incision in the periosteum extends down the length of the bone, from the physis at the top to the one at the bottom. As with other deviations, the sooner the surgery is performed, the better the chances of a good outcome.

Rickets is a bone disorder caused by dietary deficiency of either phosphorus or vitamin D *(see Chapter 9)*. It can cause the longbones to bow. So, close attention to the diet is very important in foals with bowed cannon bones.

Other Management Recommendations

Some amount of exercise is important because it encourages the normal loading and development of the bones. However, unrestricted activity can worsen the ALD in many cases. Also, the footing beneath the stall bedding and in the turnout area should be secure. Slippery surfaces, such as concrete, mud, or wet rubber mats, can encourage further deviation.

Nutritional imbalances (in particular, overfeeding carbohydrates) in both the mare's and the foal's diets can lead to various DODs, including ALDs. To moderate the foal's bone growth, the dietary changes discussed at the beginning of the chapter should be made.

It is very important to frequently re-evaluate the foal—changes for better or for worse can occur in only 1 – 2 weeks. Even after the problem is corrected, the foal should be evaluated at least every week until it is 12 months old.

Prognosis for ALDs

The prognosis for complete correction and future athletic performance is excellent for deviations that involve a physis, as long as the foal is treated early and responds well. Severe ALDs in older foals, and foals that also have rotation may not be completely corrected, even with surgery. These problems can result in permanent conformational faults that predispose to a variety of "stress and strain" injuries once the horse begins training.

The prognosis for a successful athletic career is guarded in foals with abnormal epiphyses, incomplete development of the cuboidal bones, or bowing of the cannon bone. The more "invasive" surgical procedures (osteotomies) also reduce the likelihood of an athletic career.

Prevention of ALDs

It is very difficult to prevent congenital ALDs. Paying careful attention to the pregnant mare's diet and health may control some of the possible causes. Although other factors may not be controllable, prompt treatment and frequent reassessment greatly improve the success rate and minimize the impact on the foal's athletic future.

In many cases developmental ALDs can be prevented (or at least minimized) through close attention to, and prompt and appropriate treatment of any lame foal. Close scrutiny of the foal's legs every week is an important management strategy for preventing this and other DODs.

FLEXURAL LIMB DEFORMITIES

Flexural limb deformities are abnormalities in the position or angle of the lower leg when viewed from the side of the foal. The deformity may be flexor laxity, which is slackness or lengthening. Or, it may be flexor contracture, which is tightening or shortening. These abnormalities involve the flexor unit of the leg.

Structure of the Flexor Unit

The flexor unit consists of a flexor muscle and a flexor tendon. The flexor muscle begins at the back of the forearm or thigh and fuses with its flexor tendon just above the knee or hock. The flexor tendon then continues down the back of the leg. The superficial digital flexor tendon, or SDFT, attaches onto the sides of the pastern. The deep digital flexor tendon, or DDFT, attaches onto the bottom of the pedal bone.

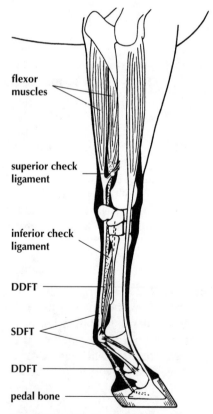

flexor muscles

superior check ligament

inferior check ligament

DDFT

SDFT

DDFT

pedal bone

Fig. 14–23. The flexor units of the foreleg.

The flexor unit may also include a check ligament, which prevents the muscle-tendon unit from being over-stretched. In the foreleg the check ligament for the SDFT is called the superior check ligament. This short ligament begins on the back of the radius and attaches onto the superficial flexor muscle-tendon junction, just above the knee. The inferior check ligament serves the deep flexor unit. It begins at the back of the knee and fuses with the DDFT about halfway down the cannon.

In the hindleg, there is no superior check ligament, and only a small and poorly developed inferior check ligament. Some horses may not even have an inferior check ligament in the hindleg. *(See Chapter 11 for more information on the flexor tendons and their check ligaments.)*

Flexor Laxity

Flexor laxity is slackness or looseness of the flexor unit. It is the one DOD that is not caused by rapid growth and large body size, or an inappropriate level of activity. It is included in the DOD group because it occurs in young foals.

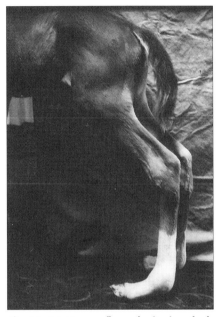

Flexor laxity allows the fetlock to drop and the toe to tip up. In severe cases, the fetlock touches the ground. It is more common in newborn foals that are premature, immature, or ill—conditions that cause generalized muscle weakness. Older foals and adult horses that have worn a cast for more than a couple of weeks may

Fig. 14–24. Severe flexor laxity in a foal.

also develop flexor laxity because the flexor muscles lose tone, bulk, and strength with disuse.

Frequent light exercise is usually sufficient treatment for this condition. Exercise should consist of 20 – 30 minutes of voluntary activity in a small paddock at least twice per day. Most cases resolve or greatly improve in 2 – 4 days. Casts, splints, and heavy bandages should be avoided because they prevent flexor muscle activity, which promotes further flexor laxity. However, a light bandage can help prevent overstretching of the tendons, ligaments, and joint capsules. It also prevents abrasions at the back of the fetlock, pastern, and heels. Abrasions can also be avoided by keeping the foal in a well-bedded stall and exercising it in a small, grassy paddock.

Flexor Contracture

Definition

Flexor contracture is commonly called "contracted tendons."

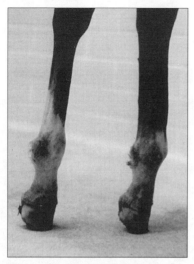

Fig. 14–25. Flexor contracture.

However, tendons do not contract—they simply transmit muscle contraction to the bone they are attached to, which flexes or extends the joint(s).

Flexor contracture is a problem involving the flexor units. In some cases other soft tissues, such as the suspensory ligament, are also involved. Basically, the muscles, tendons, and ligaments fail to lengthen at the same rate as the bones, or a flexor muscle persistently contracts. Either way, the flexor unit becomes shorter than the bones, which causes persistent flexion of the affected joints.

Causes of Flexor Contracture

There are three types of flexor contracture, depending on which joint is primarily affected:

1. Flexor contracture of the fetlock is caused by a problem involving the SDFT and/or its flexor muscle and check ligament. In some cases, the DDFT-muscle-check ligament unit is also involved.
2. Flexor contracture of the coffin joint is caused by abnormalities in the DDFT-muscle-check ligament unit.
3. Flexor contracture of the knee in newborn foals is caused by constriction of the supporting tissues (carpal fascia and palmar carpal ligament) at the back of the knee. This has nothing to do with the flexor units.

(This information is summarized in Figure 14–32.)
Flexor contracture can be congenital—present at birth. Or, it can be acquired—develops after birth.

Congenital

The causes of congenital flexor contracture are not clearly understood. They are probably similar to those listed for congenital angular limb deformities (ALDs; discussed earlier).

Acquired

Flexor contracture may develop as a result of:

- improper nutrition—particularly overfeeding
- confinement or lack of exercise
- rapid growth and large body size
- pain or injury that reduces weight-bearing in the affected leg
- combination of any or all of these factors

Dietary imbalances or excesses, lack of regular exercise, and the genetic potential for rapid growth and large body size are the factors that most often cause this DOD. Rapid bone growth without exercise can lead to failure of the muscles, tendons, and ligaments to lengthen at the same rate as the bones.

Painful foot or leg conditions can make the foal or young horse take some of the weight off the leg by contracting the flexor muscles, which flexes the joints of the lower leg. If this position is maintained for several days, flexor contracture may develop. Trauma, wounds, and hoof infections are examples of painful conditions that can lead to flexor contracture in normal foals. However, other DODs (in particular, physitis and osteochondrosis) can cause pain, and hence flexor contracture in an already "developmentally challenged" animal.

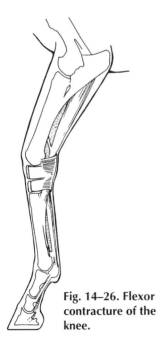

Fig. 14–26. Flexor contracture of the knee.

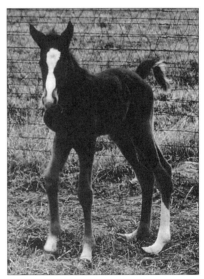

Fig. 14–27. A foal with congenital contracture of the right knee. It also has flexor laxity in both hindlegs.

Occasionally, acquired flexor contracture of the knee is seen in mature performance horses. When it occurs, it is usually a result of injury to the SDFT or inferior check ligament *(both discussed in Chapter 11)*. The fibrous tissue that repairs the damage shrinks as it matures, causing relative shortening of the tendon or check ligament.

Signs of Flexor Contracture

Congenital

Congenital flexor contracture usually involves one or both knees. Occasionally the fetlocks are the joints primarily affected. Flexor contracture of the knee causes the knee to buckle forward. In moderate to severe cases it is impossible to manually straighten the leg. The foal is usually not lame, although its gait is abnormal because it cannot extend the affected joints.

Acquired

There are two types of acquired flexor contracture:

1. **Flexor contracture of the fetlock joint** causes the pastern to appear upright. In moderate to severe cases the fetlock knuckles forward, particularly when weight is taken off the leg. In this condition the foot is placed flat on the ground, in the normal position. This abnormality more often develops in yearlings and 2-year-olds.
2. **Flexor contracture of the coffin joint** causes elevation of the heel, so the foal stands on its toe; the fetlock angle is normal. In mild or early cases the heel is raised and does not contact the ground. But in chronic cases the heel grows very long and eventually reaches the ground. This is called a "club foot"—a box-shaped foot in which the heel is very long and the wall at the toe is nearly vertical. This abnormality more often develops in foals and weanlings.

(These signs are summarized in Figure 14–32 at the end of the section.)
Acquired flexor contracture can affect just one leg or both legs, depending on the cause. It occurs more often in the forelegs, although it can develop in the hindlegs. The degree of gait abnormality or lameness varies, depending on the severity of the signs and on the primary condition that led to the deformity.

Diagnosis of Flexor Contracture

The diagnosis is based on the signs. In young horses with acquired

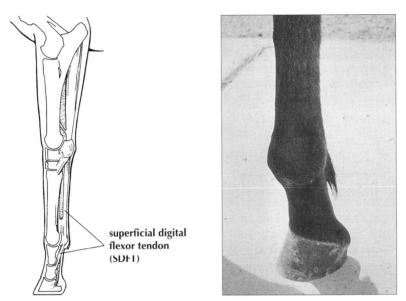

Fig. 14–28. Flexor contracture of the fetlock joint. Left: The shortened SDFT unit makes the normal fetlock angle impossible. Right: A more extreme case where the SDFT unit makes the fetlock knuckle forward.

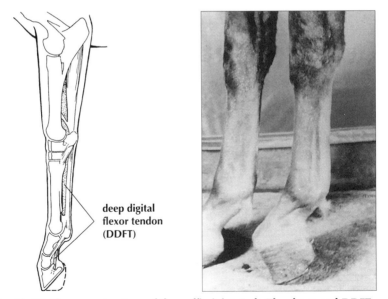

Fig. 14–29. Flexor contracture of the coffin joint. Left: The shortened DDFT unit causes elevation of the heel. Right: A severe case in which a "club foot" is developing.

flexor contracture it is important to identify any predisposing causes, especially painful conditions that prevent the foal from using the affected leg normally. It is also important to define which joint and which structures are involved. This information has considerable bearing on the treatment options.

Treatment of Flexor Contracture
Congenital

Mild cases of flexor contracture in newborn foals usually improve with light exercise, as recommended for angular limb deformities. Physical therapy, in the form of repeated flexion and extension, several times per day can also benefit these foals *(see Chapter 4)*.

Intravenous oxytetracycline (an antibiotic) can be very effective in correcting congenital flexor contracture in young foals, although how it does this is not precisely known. In most cases only a single injection is needed. Oxytetracycline appears to be of most benefit in the first few days of life. It generally is far less effective in older foals. If this treatment is to be used, it should be given within 1 – 2 days of birth. Oxytetracycline should only be administered by a veterinarian because it can cause kidney and red blood cell damage.

If the contracture is severe, or if it does not improve with these treatments, some veterinarians apply PVC splints to the foal's legs *(see Chapter 4)*. Applying splints to correct flexor contracture of the knees is simple, but it is difficult to splint the fetlock joint at the normal angle. A fiberglass cast is a better option for fetlock contracture because it can be molded to the correct shape of the leg.

> **Caution**
>
> If both forelegs (or hindlegs) are splinted, the foal may need help getting up to nurse.

The splints must be placed over a well-padded bandage, and changed frequently because pressure sores quickly develop. Foals often resent splint placement because forced extension of the contracted joints is painful.

In very severe cases that do not respond to these medical options, surgery may be necessary. For contracture of the knee, the connective tissues at the back of the knee are severed. For flexor contracture of the fetlock, the superior check ligament and perhaps also the SDFT must be cut. However, such severe abnormalities and "invasive" surgeries limit the chances of the foal developing normally and having a successful athletic career.

Acquired

Conservative Management

Conservative management of mild to moderate acquired flexor contracture includes:

- correcting the primary problem, if any
- changing the diet, especially reducing the amount of carbohydrate
- allowing daily light exercise, if the primary problem permits
- lowering the heels and applying a shoe with a toe extension or toe wedge for coffin joint contracture

Casts and splints are of little use for these conditions in older foals and young horses. Rather than trying to force the joint into a more normal position, the aims of conservative management are: 1) to slow bone growth in rapidly growing horses, giving the soft tissues a chance to catch up, and 2) to encourage loading and lengthening of the tendons and ligaments involved. These goals can often be achieved just by modifying the diet and providing daily exercise. If NSAIDs are given to enable the foal to exercise more freely with little discomfort, they should be used with caution and only under veterinary advice *(see Chapter 5)*.

Applying a shoe with a metal toe extension *(see Chapter 7)* can help prevent further coffin joint contracture. In mild cases it may also exert enough tension on the DDFT unit to correct the condition. Applying a glue-on shoe with a toe wedge can have a similar effect. The toe wedge raises the foal's toe ¼ – ½ inch (6 – 12 mm), encouraging weight-bearing on the heels.

Surgery

If there is no response to conservative management after a couple of weeks, or if the condition is severe, surgery is usually recommended. The conservative management recommendations outlined above should also be followed for foals and young horses that undergo surgery.

Flexor Contracture of the Fetlock Joint. The surgical procedure for acquired fetlock contracture depends on which tendon is primarily involved. If the SDFT is more

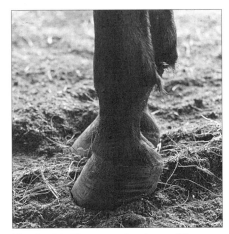

Fig. 14–30. Flexor contracture of the fetlock joint.

taut than the DDFT both when the horse is standing on the leg and when the leg is raised, surgery involves cutting the superior check ligament. If the DDFT is more taut, both the superior and inferior check ligaments are cut. *(These procedures are discussed in Chapter 11.)*

Daily light exercise is essential for a successful outcome after these surgical procedures, and it should be started within a couple of days of surgery. The check ligament rejoins in the 3 months or so following surgery. It is very important that the normal fetlock angle is achieved and maintained during this time so that when the ligament heals it is longer than before surgery.

In severe cases that do not respond to cutting the superior check ligament, the SDFT may need to be cut. Over time, the suspensory ligament may have become involved in the fetlock contracture, and it may also need to be cut if the horse does not respond to the other surgeries. However, cutting the SDFT and suspensory ligament are extreme measures that may allow dislocation of the pastern joint or breakdown of the fetlock. They should only be considered as a last resort—a salvage procedure for an animal with breeding potential. An athletic career is out of the question after such radical surgery.

Flexor Contracture of the Coffin Joint ("Club Foot"). In horses

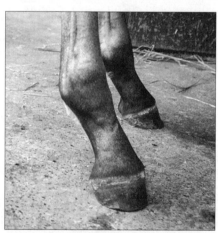

with contracture of the coffin joint, the inferior check ligament is cut a few inches below the knee. This allows the foal to place the foot normally, if the surgery is going to be successful. Surgery should be combined with exercise, hoof trimming, and, in moderate to severe cases, a shoe with a toe extension.

Severe cases of coffin joint contracture may require cutting the DDFT, either at the back of the pastern or midway along the cannon. However, even this fairly radical procedure may not be successful in long-standing cases. Fibrosis (thickening with fibrous tissue) of the joint capsule and surrounding ligaments may cause the coffin joint to be permanently fixed in the abnormal position. Also, changes in the shape of the hoof wall, and even the pedal bone, may only be partially reversible.

Fig. 14–31. Flexor contracture of the coffin joint.

Joint	Age Group	Structure(s)	Signs	Treatment Options
KNEE	newborn foal	fascia and ligaments at the back of the knee	bent knees (usually bilateral)	• exercise • physical therapy • oxytetracycline • ± splints or casts
	mature performance horse	SDFT or inferior check ligament fibrosis	bent knee (one leg only)	• cut superior or inferior check ligament
FETLOCK	yearlings, 2-year-olds (can also occur in newborn foals)	SDFT-muscle-check ligament unit (may also involve DDFT-muscle-check ligament unit)	upright pastern fetlock knuckled forward foot placed flat (normal foot position)	• correct primary problem • modify diet • daily exercise (mild cases) • if severe, cut superior check ligament (also cut inferior check ligament if DDFT involved)
COFFIN	foals and weanlings	DDFT-muscle-check ligament unit	upright or "club foot" normal fetlock angle	• modify diet • daily exercise • lower heels • shoe with toe extension • cut inferior check ligament

Fig. 14–32. Different types of flexor contracture.

(± = may or may not be recommended)

Flexor Contracture of the Knee. Surgical management of flexor contracture in a mature performance horse depends on which structure was damaged. If the fibrosis is in the SDFT, cutting the superior check ligament may improve or correct the knee angle. When the inferior check ligament is the structure causing the problem, it can be cut. Ultrasound examination at the time of injury is the best way to accurately assess the site and degree of damage *(see Chapter 11)*.

Prognosis for Flexor Contracture

Mild to moderate flexor contracture generally has a very good prognosis for complete correction and future athletic function, provided it is treated promptly. More severe or long-standing cases often have a less promising future. This is especially so if the SDFT, DDFT, or suspensory ligament has been cut.

Prevention of Flexor Contracture

Preventing flexural limb deformities involves controlling or eliminating the factors that contribute to them. Overfeeding, insufficient exercise, and painful leg problems are the most common, and most readily managed factors.

Frequent observation and appropriate management of all young horses from birth to maturity is very important in preventing these problems, or at least minimizing their impact.

PHYSITIS
Definition

Terminology
Physeal dysplasia (abnormal growth) is a more precise term for this condition.
"Epiphysitis" is a common, but incorrect term; it is the physis that is affected, not the epiphysis.

Physitis is a very common condition in rapidly growing horses. It causes painful swelling of the physes, or growth plates, just above the knees, hocks, or fetlocks. Although the word "physitis" means inflammation of the physis, the inflammation is secondary to other changes.

Causes

Exactly what causes the abnormality in the physeal cartilage is not known, although it is certain that nutritional factors play a key role. Physitis is most common in large, rapidly growing foals. These foals typically are fed more carbohydrate than they need. This may affect bone development in two ways. First, high carbohydrate diets suppress thyroid hormone production, which, among other things, limits nutrient supply to the cartilage cells. Second, the increase in body weight is often too rapid for the developing bones to accommodate.

There may be a limit to the amount of new bone the physes can produce per day. When the demands on the growth cartilage exceed its ability to produce new bone, problems develop. Instead of maturing into new bone, the cartilage becomes thickened and irregular. This abnormal cartilage is vulnerable, and is easily damaged by trauma or overloading. Crushing of the cartilage and microscopic fractures in the new bone cause inflammation and pain. Some large foals become lame with little or no activity, but in other foals the physes become painful and swollen after excessive or forced exercise.

Physitis at the fetlock usually occurs in foals between 3 and 6 months old. Physitis at the knee usually occurs in foals between 6 and 9 months old; it is occasionally also seen in yearlings. These are the average times when bone growth at these physes begins to slow down (that is, the physes begin to "close"). It is probable that physitis occurs at these times because the loading capacity of the vulnerable cartilage and new bone has finally been exceeded by the young horse's increasing body weight and activity level.

Signs

In most cases there is obvious swelling of the affected physes. This swelling is firm, warm, and painful. Typically, one side of the physis is more swollen than the other. The condition is usually bilateral—it occurs at the same site in both legs, most often the forelegs. In some cases it develops in all four legs. Foals and young horses with physitis may be stiff-gaited or obviously lame. Some are so sore that they are reluctant to move at all.

Note: The physes of normal

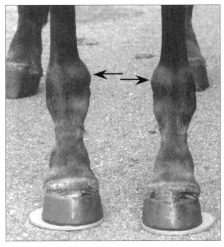

Fig. 14–33. Physitis causes swellings at the physes [arrows]. (This foal is being treated for ALDs.)

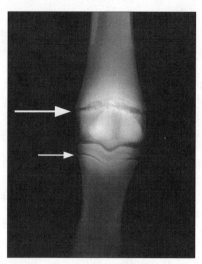

Fig. 14–34. A radiograph of a young foal's fetlock. The lower physis (small arrow) is normal. The upper physis (large arrow) is abnormal.

foals are prominent during the first 6 months. However, they are symmetrical, and are not painful.

Diagnosis of Physitis

The history (age, diet, growth rate, and level of activity) and the signs are generally all that are required to make the diagnosis. If the foal or young horse is very lame, radiographs should be taken to check for more serious problems, such as a fracture or infection in the physis. (Infection is more common in newborn foals; *see Chapter 9*).

Treatment of Physitis

Treatment involves limiting the young horse's activity to daily short periods of voluntary exercise: turn it out into a small paddock, and allow it as little or as much exercise as it wants. Complete restriction may result in flexural limb deformities, so some form of light exercise should be encouraged each day.

The diet should be examined and any imbalances corrected. In particular, the amount of carbohydrate (grain and grain products) should be reduced to a maintenance level. (For more information on feeding horses of any age, read *Feeding to Win II,* published by Equine Research, Inc.)

More Information
Foals are especially vulnerable to the side effects of NSAIDs. (See Chapter 5 for more information on the positive and negative effects of these drugs.)

If the foal is very uncomfortable, small doses of an NSAID can be given for a day or two. But care should be taken to follow the veterinarian's advice closely when giving these drugs to foals. Also, relieving the foal's pain may encourage it to exercise more, which could cause more damage to the physeal cartilage. If the foal is in so much pain that it needs pain-relieving drugs, the veterinarian may need to re-examine it to be certain that a more serious problem has not developed.

Prognosis and Prevention of Physitis

Unless fractures or infection are part of the overall problem, the prognosis for normal development and future athletic function is good with proper management. Severe physitis may result in an angular limb deformity, but this is not common.

Prevention of physitis involves following the management strategies discussed at the beginning of the chapter. Overfeeding carbohydrates should especially be avoided.

OSTEOCHONDROSIS
Definition

Osteochondrosis is a defect of ossification, the process by which new bone is produced from growth cartilage. Normally, specialized cartilage in the physes, epiphyses, and secondary ossification centers matures into bone as the foal grows *(see Figure 14–3)*. The cartilage in the epiphyses is completely replaced with bone, except for a thin layer of cartilage at the joint surface. The bone directly beneath this cartilage is called subchondral bone— literally, "bone beneath the cartilage."

Osteochondrosis involves delayed ossification of the growth cartilage in the epiphyses. Part of the subchondral bone fails to form, leaving thickened, abnormal cartilage at that site. With normal weight-bearing and activity, the joint cartilage can collapse into the underlying bone defect.

Reminder
Physis: area of growth cartilage near the ends of the bones; "growth plate."
Epiphysis: end of the bone, between the physis and the joint surface.
Secondary Ossification Center: core of new bone surrounded by growth cartilage. This is how the bones in the knee and hock develop.

Some osteochondrosis-like lesions may not involve delayed ossification, but instead are caused by physical insult to normal growth cartilage and developing bone (discussed later). But for simplicity, the term osteochondrosis is used throughout this book for all typical lesions involving the joint cartilage and underlying bone in young horses.

Causes of Osteochondrosis

Osteochondrosis can occur in any breed, but it is very common in Thoroughbreds, Quarter Horses, Standardbreds, and Warmbloods. It can occur in virtually any bone, although the bones of the stifle, hock, fetlock, and shoulder are more often affected. Some veterinarians believe that cervical vertebral malformation, or "wobbler" syndrome, in horses less than about 2 years old is caused by osteochondrosis in the cervical vertebrae. *(This neurologic condition is discussed in Chapter 12.)*

The development of growth cartilage is affected by nutrition, especially the availability of certain minerals. It is also affected by physical activity, hormones, toxins, and infection.

Nutritional Factors

Excess carbohydrate in the diet—whether milk in a nursing foal, or grain or lush pasture in a growing horse—can affect bone development in two ways. First, it can increase the body weight too rapidly for the developing bones and joints to adapt. As a result, the growth cartilage and new bone may be overloaded and damaged even during normal activity. Second, excess dietary carbohydrate impairs the production of thyroid hormones, substances that are needed for normal growth. When thyroid hormone production is low, less nutrients are supplied to the cartilage cells.

Dietary calcium and phosphorus are essential for normal bone production; these minerals give bones their strength. Both calcium and phosphorus must be fed in the recommended amounts, and in the correct ratio. An excess or deficiency of one or both can interfere with new bone production, as well as the overall strength of the bone.

Copper is also essential for bone development. Severe copper deficiency leads to fragile cartilage and new bone that is easily damaged during normal loading. Microscopically, tiny fractures are seen in the developing bone. This occurs at multiple sites—that is, in several joints—even when copper is only moderately deficient.

When nutritional factors play a part, osteochondrosis lesions are often found in several joints. This is because bone development is affected throughout the body. Osteochondrosis this extensive is now fairly uncommon because veterinarians and breeders have understood the impact of these nutritional elements for some time.

(Nutritional factors and recommendations are discussed in more detail at the beginning of the chapter.)

Excessive Load

Osteochondrosis lesions are found in fairly predictable locations *(see Figure 14–42)*. At these sites the joint cartilage and subchondral bone bears a lot of weight during activity. Growth cartilage is vulnerable to injury during its development. This fact has led some scientists to believe that excessive load on the developing cartilage and bone is an important contributor to osteochondrosis.

Overloading and Blood Supply

Unlike mature joint cartilage, growth cartilage in the epiphysis is supplied with blood through tiny canals in the cartilage. Trauma to the joint, such as a kick or a fall, may directly damage the cartilage or developing bone. Or, it may crush some of the cartilage canals and interrupt the blood supply to part of the growth cartilage. As a result, the cartilage at that site dies, and fails to develop into new bone.

The cartilage canals may also be crushed during unrestricted or enforced activity, especially in large, overfed, rapidly growing foals. In these foals the body weight often increases too quickly, overloading the developing bone and cartilage. In newborn foals, pasture turnout can result in too much activity, particularly if the mare gallops around a lot.

The growth cartilage in the epiphyses develops into bone in the first few months of life. Studies have shown microscopic evidence of osteochondrosis-type lesions in foals as young as 1 month old. The cartilage canals that nourish the growth cartilage disappear by about 7 months of age. So when physical damage to these canals is a factor, it must occur early in life.

According to one study, by about 7 months of age any bone and/or cartilage lesions are chronic, and new lesions are unlikely to develop. But not all lesions cause obvious signs or are visible on radiographs at that time. Some lesions disappear as the cartilage and subchondral bone heal, but others remain and either stay the same or worsen. Of those that persist, some lesions cause obvious signs, others do not.

Activity may play an important role in determining whether a lesion will become obvious. For example, pasture turnout after a period of confinement, and breaking and training are common activities that could overload the defective cartilage and bone. Being ridden further increases the load on the bones and joint surfaces, particularly if the work surface is hard.

Other Contributing Factors

Heredity

Certain osteochondrosis lesions appear to have a hereditary component. These lesions include 1) bone-and-cartilage fragments on the lower end of the tibia, in the tibiotarsal joint of the hock, and 2) bone-and-cartilage fragments off the top of the first pastern bone, in the back of the fetlock joint. Other osteochondrosis lesions in common locations may also prove to have a hereditary component as more research is done.

However, "heredity" may not necessarily mean a specific defect of bone development. Osteochondrosis is more common in breeds that are genetically programmed and selected for rapid growth and large body size. These characteristics alone could lead to osteochondrosis lesions, especially when combined with breaking and training well before the horse is mature. Heredity could also be responsible for certain conformational faults and congenital deformities.

Conformation and Congenital Deformities

Conformational faults and congenital deformities can contribute to osteochondrosis by overloading part or all of a joint surface. For example, a cow-hocked, toed-out stance places uneven stresses on the hocks and hind fetlocks. Angular and flexural limb deformities also encourage overloading.

Gender

Osteochondrosis is more common in males than females, probably because most male horses are a little larger and heavier than females of the same age. This could contribute to the load on the joint surfaces and developing bone.

Infection

Infectious diseases, such as *Rhodococcus equi,* strangles, and bacterial or rotavirus diarrhea, can affect bone development in at least two ways. First, they cause illness and lack of appetite, which can quickly lead to weight loss and interrupted growth. Once the foal recovers and begins to eat normally, it has a growth spurt to compensate. In some cases the increase in body weight is too rapid for the developing bone; as a result, it may be overloaded during normal activity. Second, if the infection is severe, it can reduce blood flow to the cartilage canals by causing tiny blood clots or clots of bacteria and white blood cells. This can result in defective or interrupted bone development at that site.

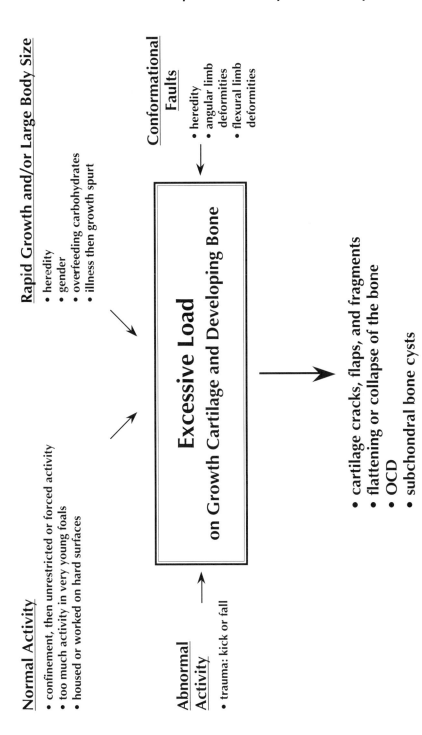

Normal Activity
- confinement, then unrestricted or forced activity
- too much activity in very young foals
- housed or worked on hard surfaces

Abnormal Activity
- trauma: kick or fall

Rapid Growth and/or Large Body Size
- heredity
- gender
- overfeeding carbohydrates
- illness then growth spurt

Conformational Faults
- heredity
- angular limb deformities
- flexural limb deformities

Excessive Load on Growth Cartilage and Developing Bone

- cartilage cracks, flaps, and fragments
- flattening or collapse of the bone
- OCD
- subchondral bone cysts

Fig. 14–35. Summary of how osteochondrosis-like lesions can develop in otherwise normal growth cartilage.

Zinc Toxicity

Foals on a pasture or prepared diet that contains excess zinc have an increased potential for osteochondrosis. High levels of dietary zinc can reduce copper absorption from the intestine. So, even though the ration appears to *contain* enough copper, the foal does not *absorb* enough of it. In severe cases, osteochondrosis lesions and fractures in the new bone develop at several sites throughout the body.

Corticosteroids

Corticosteroids, or "cortisone," are potent anti-inflammatory drugs *(see Chapter 5)*. But their use in foals should be restricted because they can interrupt normal cartilage and bone development.

Manifestations of Osteochondrosis

The type of osteochondrosis lesion depends to some extent on the underlying cause—delayed ossification, or physical damage to otherwise normal growth cartilage.

When ossification is delayed, the thickened, abnormal joint cartilage is easily damaged, leading to cartilage defects. A less common manifestation is collapse of the cuboidal bones in the knee or hock. This causes angular limb deformity in young foals (discussed earlier).

Physical damage to growth cartilage can result in several possible defects:

- cartilage erosions, cracks, flaps, or fragments in the joint
- flattened or collapsed subchondral bone
- fracture through the subchondral bone, causing OCD
- subchondral bone cysts

Cartilage Lesions

The thickened or degenerating joint cartilage is more fragile than healthy cartilage. It is easily damaged during activity, sometimes to the extent that the cartilage lesion exposes the subchondral bone. In some cases the crack creates a cartilage flap, which can break off and float freely in the joint. These pieces of cartilage are often called "joint mice." (Some people refer to bone chips as "joint mice." However, a mouse is small and quiet, and it can cause damage without being seen. Therefore, this term is more appropriate for cartilage fragments—which do not show up on radiographs—than for bone chips, which usually are visible radiographically.)

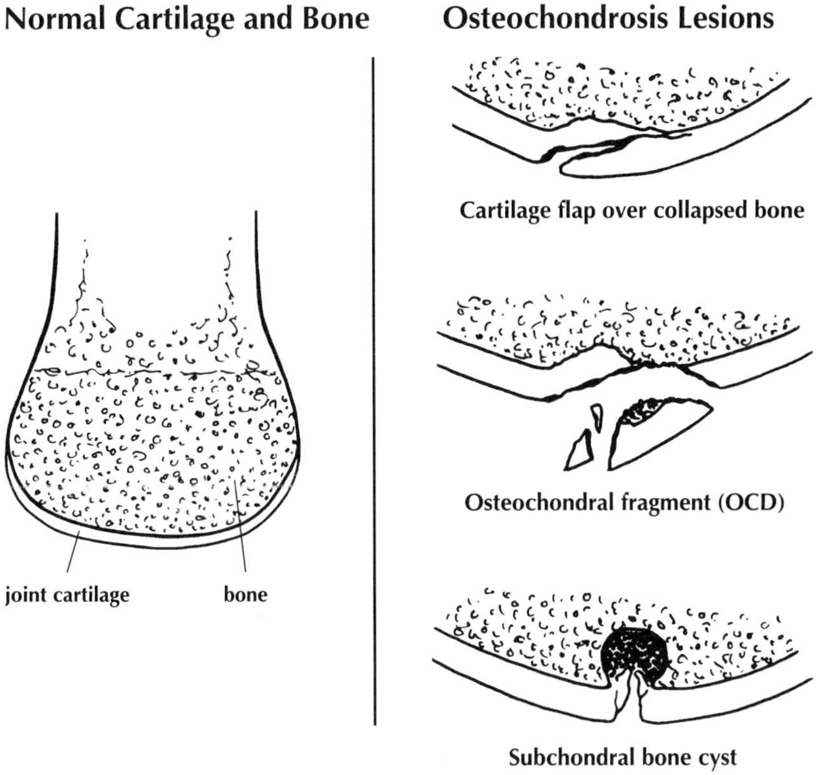

Normal Cartilage and Bone

Osteochondrosis Lesions

Cartilage flap over collapsed bone

Osteochondral fragment (OCD)

joint cartilage   bone

Subchondral bone cyst

Fig. 14–36. Manifestations of osteochondrosis.

Cartilage lesions alone can cause obvious signs of joint disease. But because they cannot be seen on radiographs, they are difficult to diagnose without looking into the joint with an arthroscope *(see Chapter 6)*. As a consequence, cartilage abnormalities probably are missed in many horses. It is likely that these lesions occur much more often than is reported. If so, osteochondrosis is an important cause of degenerative joint disease in young, athletic horses *(see Chapter 8)*.

Flattened or Collapsed Subchondral Bone

Sometimes the only radiographic evidence of osteochondrosis is flattening or other irregularity of the subchondral bone at one of the common sites. Cartilage lesions may also be present over the defective bone, although they cannot be seen on radiographs.

OCD Lesions

The classic type of osteochondrosis lesion is an osteochondral (bone-and-cartilage) fragment. These lesions are called osteochondritis dissecans, or OCD: a "dissected" piece of bone and cartilage. The fragment may remain attached to the underlying bone, or it may break off and float freely in the joint. These lesions usually are visible on routine radiographs, although they may be hidden behind superimposed bone edges on some views. They occur in fairly predictable sites in the commonly affected joints.

Subchondral Bone Cyst

Subchondral bone cysts are circular or oval-shaped cavities in the bone, just beneath the joint surface. In most cases a small hole in the overlying cartilage connects the inside of the cyst with the joint space.

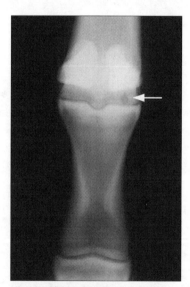

There are at least three possible explanations for why these bone cysts develop. First, it may be failure of normal ossification in a small part of the growth cartilage, resulting in a plug of thickened cartilage within the bone. The retained cartilage dies and leaves a cavity.

Second, trauma to, or overloading of the growth cartilage may damage the cartilage canals, compromising the blood flow to the developing bone. As a result, the cells in that location may die, leaving an area of degenerating bone and cartilage. Subchondral bone cysts typically are found in the part of the joint that sustains the greatest load. Whether or not bone development is abnormal, overloading of the growth cartilage likely plays a key role.

Fig. 14–37. Subchondral bone cyst in the fetlock.

Third, any joint cartilage defect that exposes and damages the underlying bone can lead to a subchondral bone cyst. This can even occur in a mature joint. According to this theory, subchondral bone cysts may just be the result of severe degenerative joint disease, a deep crack or cartilage flap, or even an OCD lesion. That is, they are not necessarily caused by a defect of cartilage and bone development.

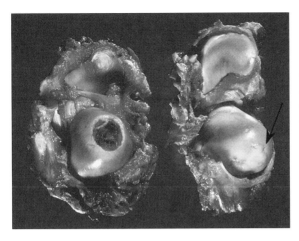

Fig. 14–38. Left: Severe cartilage erosion exposes the subchondral bone. Right: The dimple [arrow] in the opposite joint indicates where a bone cyst exists under the thickened cartilage.

Subchondral bone cysts are less common than OCD, but when they occur, they can be more of a problem.

Signs of Osteochondrosis

The most consistent sign of osteochondrosis is joint effusion—accumulation of fluid within the joint. This may be difficult to detect in some joints, like the stifle and shoulder. Mild to moderate lameness (grade 1 – 3 of 5) is common, although some horses do not show a gait abnormality until they are worked hard. Even then, the only sign may be a reluctance to "stretch out" or perform certain maneuvers. Often the first clue is lameness immediately after a farrier has trimmed the feet. By holding up the leg, the farrier is, in effect, performing a flexion test on the joint *(see Chapter 2)*. Whether or not the horse (or foal) is lame, a positive flexion test is a typical sign of osteochondrosis.

The shoulder is a little different from other commonly affected

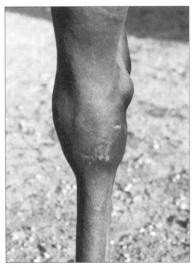

Fig. 14–39. The most consistent sign of osteochondrosis is joint effusion.

joints. Effusion generally is not detectable. But most horses with shoulder osteochondrosis are consistently at least grade 2 of 5 lame.

In many cases, the horse has osteochondrosis in the same joint on the opposite leg (bilaterally), although one joint usually is more obviously affected than the other. When the condition is caused by severe nutritional imbalances, the horse may have osteochondrosis in several sites. So, it is important that the physical examination of the entire horse is thorough.

Diagnosis of Osteochondrosis

The most important parts of the history in horses suspected of having osteochondrosis are:

- age and size
- breed
- level of activity or stage of training

The process of bone development is most vulnerable in the first few months of the horse's life, when bone growth is at its greatest. But often there are no signs of osteochondrosis until the overweight yearling is exercised or the 2-year-old horse goes into training. That is, the signs appear when the cartilage and bone surfaces are loaded.

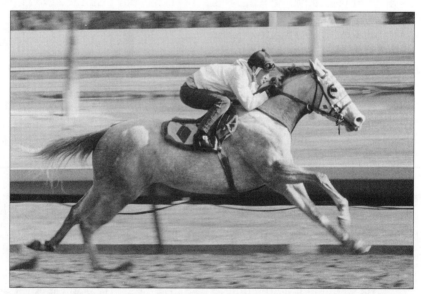

Fig. 14–40. There may be no signs of osteochondrosis until the 2-year-old horse goes into training and the defective cartilage and bone surfaces are "loaded."

Although osteochondrosis may be considered to be a "young horse disease," some horses may not show obvious signs for years. It usually takes a traumatic incident, such as a fall, or a sudden increase in the workload for osteochondrosis to show up in a mature horse.

It is difficult to diagnose osteochondrosis from the signs because they are not very specific. They are similar to those of other non-infectious joint diseases, such as synovitis or DJD *(see Chapter 8).* In fact, these horses actually have synovitis because of the changes within the joint. Horses with osteochondrosis are more prone to develop DJD in affected joints because the cartilage surfaces are abnormal. There is an even greater chance of developing DJD if there is a loose OCD fragment in the joint. For these reasons, it is important to determine whether osteochondrosis is part of the problem in young horses showing signs of non-infectious joint disease.

Radiographs

A series of good quality radiographs is necessary for an accurate diagnosis. Radiographs that are detailed enough to identify bone defects in the joints above the knee or hock can be very difficult to obtain with a portable x-ray machine. They may need to be taken at an equine hospital or referral center where a larger x-ray machine is available.

The fact that osteochondrosis lesions occur at fairly predictable locations can make diagnosis easier. Cartilage defects are not visible on plain radiographs, but in many cases osteo-

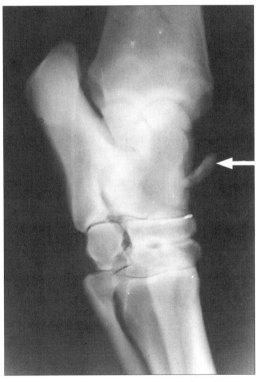

Fig. 14–41. The classic type of osteochondrosis: the OCD fragment. This is a fairly common site in the hock.

More Information

Nuclear scintigraphy is of little value in diagnosing osteochondrosis because these lesions often do not show up as "hot spots." Also, because their physes are normally active, "bone scans" of horses less than 4 years old can be very difficult to interpret *(see Chapter 2)*.

chondrosis may be suspected because the underlying bone at one of the typical locations is irregular. The same joint on the opposite leg should also be radiographed because osteochondrosis is often bilateral. It is common for one joint to be "silent"—showing no outward signs—and yet have radiographic evidence of osteochondrosis.

Radiography is also important for identifying secondary changes within the joint. The presence of degenerative changes may influence how the veterinarian manages the condition, and also the long-term prognosis.

JOINT	LESION TYPE & LOCATION
Stifle	Cartilage or OCD lesions on the femur, in the femoropatellar joint Bone cyst in the lower end of the femur (medial condyle)
Hock	OCD lesions on the lower end of the tibia: • central ridge • medial maleolus OCD lesions on the front of the talus
Fetlock	OCD lesions on the top of P1, at the back of the joint Cartilage lesions and flattening at the back of the cannon bone, opposite the sesamoid bones (?)
Shoulder	OCD lesions or flattening at the top of the humerus (humeral head)
Pastern	Bone cyst at the top of P1

P1 = first pastern bone   (?) = may not be an osteochondrosis lesion

Fig. 14–42. Common sites of osteochondrosis in horses. *Note: These bones and joints are described and illustrated in later chapters.*

Treatment of Osteochondrosis

Conservative Management

Modifying the horse's diet as discussed at the start of the chapter is an important part of managing osteochondrosis. It involves:

- reducing the amount of carbohydrate (grain and grain products)
- ensuring that the ration contains adequate amounts and an ideal ratio of calcium and phosphorus
- adding copper, if necessary

These recommendations are more important in foals and young horses (less than 12 months old) than in older horses because there is more opportunity to influence bone development in young animals.

Rest from training is also important in managing osteochondrosis, even if the horse is not lame. Cartilage damage usually occurs when the joint surfaces are loaded, and it takes at least 3 months for the damaged cartilage to be repaired. Pasture rest is far better than stall confinement, unless the horse or foal is very active in the pasture. Some amount of exercise is essential for the normal development of bones, tendons, ligaments, and muscles. So if the horse or foal must be confined to a stall or small paddock, it should be lightly exercised or turned out into a larger area for a few hours every day.

NSAIDs may reduce the pain and inflammation if the horse is lame, or if joint effusion is severe. However, NSAIDs should be used with caution in foals. Corticosteroids should be avoided in horses and foals with osteochondrosis because these drugs can slow cartilage repair. They can also interrupt normal bone development if overused. Some veterinarians recommend joint medications (hyaluronic acid or GAGs) to promote cartilage repair and limit further cartilage damage. Because more than one joint may be affected, intravenous or intramuscular formulations of these joint medications may be helpful. *(Medications are discussed in Chapter 5.)*

Surgery

OCD fragments that appear to be hanging off or floating free within the joint should be removed using arthroscopy *(see Chapter 6)*. Even if the piece is lodged in a pouch of the joint capsule and is apparently not affecting a joint surface, arthroscopy is warranted in a valuable animal. It is common for the cartilage damage to be more severe than would be expected from the size of the fragment seen on radiographs. Also, smaller, unsuspected fragments of bone and/or cartilage are frequently found during surgery. Arthroscopy also provides the surgeon with an excellent view of most, if not all of the joint's cartilage surfaces. This information helps determine the best way to manage the horse after surgery, and it helps establish an accurate prognosis.

Bone fragments that appear on radiographs to be in their normal position and attached to the underlying bone usually reattach in time. Most veterinarians recommend that the pieces be left alone and the condition managed with paddock or pasture rest, rather than with surgery.

Subchondral bone cysts generally need surgery for the best result. This involves removing the defective cartilage and bone from the cyst. The surgeon may then drill several small holes into the surrounding healthy bone to stimulate it to fill in the defect. This procedure can usually be done with arthroscopy. As an alternative, the surgeon drills through the cyst from the side of the bone and fills the cavity with a bone graft.

In many cases the veterinarian recommends joint medications, either hyaluronic acid or GAGs, after surgery or when the horse begins training.

Prognosis for Osteochondrosis

The joint cartilage of young foals is capable of complete repair. In contrast, joint cartilage in older foals and adult horses has slow and limited repair capabilities. Exactly when this "golden period" of complete repair ends is not known, but it probably occurs before 6 months old. So, young foals with osteochondrosis lesions can have a very good prognosis for future athletic function.

In older foals and adult horses the prognosis for athletic usefulness depends on the location and type of lesion, and the number of joints involved. If only one lesion is found in a single joint (whether one or both legs are affected), the prognosis is generally good with appropriate treatment. Shoulder osteochondrosis is an exception—it always has a guarded prognosis.

The final outcome also depends on the length of time between the lesion's occurrence and treatment. Very few osteochondrosis lesions are diagnosed before the cycle of injury, repair, and reinjury has been repeated. The potential for persistent joint effusion and DJD increases with the delay between injury and treatment.

Various studies have attempted to compare the outcome of conservative versus surgical management in racehorses. Some of these studies have found no difference in race times or earnings between the two treatment strategies. Other studies have shown a definite advantage to surgical treatment.

Prevention of Osteochondrosis

When there is a high incidence of orthopedic problems in foals and growing horses on a farm, and lesions are found in several sites, it is a reliable sign that there is a management problem.

A balanced, mineral-supplemented diet significantly reduces the incidence of osteochondrosis, but it does not eliminate it. Occasional cases will continue to appear, even on well-managed farms. This is because there are several possible contributing factors, one of which (trauma) is virtually impossible to prevent in young horses. Also, osteochondrosis lesions with a hereditary component cannot always be prevented by better nutrition or management.

More information on preventing DODs, both in the individual foal and in a herd, is given at the beginning of this chapter.

OSTEOCHONDROMA

Osteochondromas are rare in horses. The lesion is a bone spur with a cartilage cap, which grows out from the side of the bone, just above the physis. This condition appears to mostly affect young adult horses, although occasional cases have been seen in foals. Exactly why osteochondromas develop is not known, although some scientists believe that they are benign bone tumors. In the few cases that have been reported in horses, the osteochondroma was found at the bottom of the radius (just above the knee) or the tibia (just above the hock).

The signs are nonspecific: mild to moderate lameness (grade 1 – 3 of 5) and soft tissue swelling. There generally are no other signs, and it is often impossible to see or feel the bone spur. The lameness and swelling may worsen with exercise, and decrease or disappear with rest. The diagnosis is made when radiographs reveal the bone spur. In most cases, treatment, which involves surgically removing the bone spur, permanently resolves the lameness.

SECTION

IV

TREATMENT OF SPECIFIC CONDITIONS

This section addresses specific conditions in anatomical order. It begins with the foot and works up the foreleg, then the hindleg, and finishes with the back.

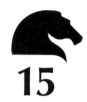

15

THE FOOT

The foot is a very complex structure. The bones and soft tissues are close together, and are therefore subject to the same forces. The foot sustains massive weight-bearing and ground impact forces during exercise. So foot conditions are among the most common causes of lameness in athletic horses. Some of these conditions are mild and easily cured. Others are performance-limiting, career-halting, or even life-threatening.

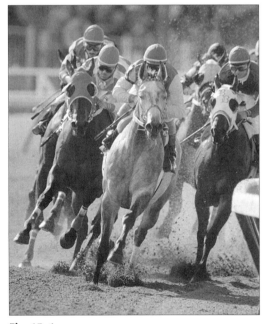

Fig. 15–1.

NAVICULAR SYNDROME

Definition

Navicular syndrome is a complex of inflammatory or degenerative conditions that affect the navicular bone and its supporting structures. (Podotrochleitis is an older term for this condition.) Despite a variety of causes, and the involvement of different structures and processes, the signs are almost always the same.

Preview
The structures of the foot are described and illustrated in Chapter 7. The current chapter covers the following conditions: • navicular bone problems • laminitis • pedal bone problems • puncture wounds • bruises and abscesses • hoof wall problems • other conditions

Navicular Structures

The navicular bone is a small, boat-shaped bone that sits behind the coffin joint. It lies between the deep digital flexor tendon (DDFT) and the back of the second pastern bone and pedal bone. Its role is that of a fulcrum, or point of support, for the flexor tendon as it runs over the back of the coffin joint.

The navicular bone is supported by ligaments above, below, and at each side. The front and back surfaces of the navicular bone are cov-

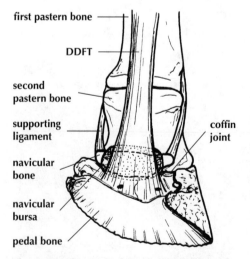
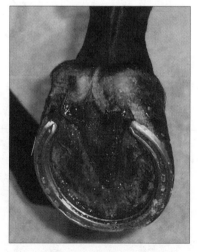

Fig. 15–2. The navicular structures. These structures are located at the back of the foot and pastern.

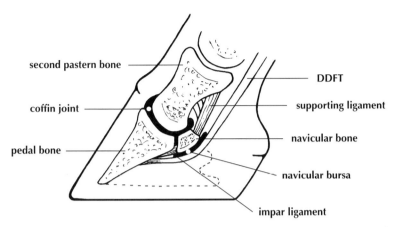

second pastern bone

coffin joint

pedal bone

DDFT

supporting ligament

navicular bone

navicular bursa

impar ligament

Fig. 15–3. The navicular structures from the side. The dotted line indicates the wing of the pedal bone.

ered with cartilage. One side faces, and forms the back of the coffin joint. The other side—the flexor surface—faces the deep flexor tendon. Between the flexor surface and the deep flexor tendon is a small sac: the navicular bursa. It protects the navicular bone and flexor tendon from abrasion as the tendon glides over the bone.

Causes

There is no single known cause of navicular syndrome. The more that scientists investigate the processes involved, the more complex this condition appears. There is no consensus on what starts the process, or which factors are most important in its progression. Several theories about the causes of navicular syndrome are combined in this section.

The navicular bone supports the deep flexor tendon as it runs over the back of the coffin joint and attaches onto the bottom of the pedal bone. In the process, the tendon puts pressure on the navicular bone. As the horse bears weight on the leg the coffin and pastern joints extend, and the navicular bone is squeezed between the deep flexor tendon and the back of the second pastern bone. At the same time, tension is placed on the ligaments that support the navicular bone. Thus, there are two major forces that the navicular structures must withstand: compression and tension. Over time, these forces can cause a variety of navicular bone abnormalities. Figure 15–5 summarizes this process.

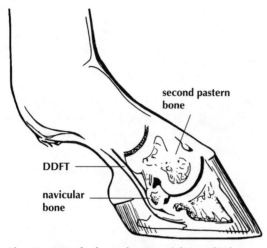

second pastern bone

DDFT

navicular bone

Fig. 15–4. As the horse bears weight on the leg, the navicular bone is squeezed between the flexor tendon and the back of the second pastern bone.

Compression of the Navicular Bone

Repeated compression of a cartilage surface can result in cartilage degeneration *(see Chapter 8)*. The cartilage becomes flattened and less resistant to compression; in severe cases it also becomes eroded. These cartilage changes are very common on the navicular bones of horses with navicular syndrome. They occur most often along the flexor surface.

Sometimes the cartilage erosion is so extensive that the bone underneath is exposed. When this happens the navicular bursa and deep flexor tendon can be damaged by the roughened navicular bone surface. Occasionally, adhesions (fibrous bands) form between the tendon and the navicular bone. Inflammation of the navicular bursa (navicular bursitis) can occur even without severe cartilage damage. This is probably due to compression and friction between the navicular bone and deep flexor tendon.

Chronic compression of the navicular bone can also result in an abnormal increase in bone density directly beneath the cartilage surfaces, especially on the flexor surface. This abnormality can be seen on a skyline radiograph. To obtain this view, the x-ray beam is directed at an angle down the back of the foot to highlight the flexor surface of the navicular bone. Although this increase in bone density is designed to strengthen the bone, it tends to make it more brittle and less "giving," which makes it more prone to fracture. Nevertheless, navicular fractures are uncommon.

Tension on the Supporting Ligaments

The navicular bone is surrounded by supporting ligaments. Some scientists believe that the whole degenerative process starts with excessive tension on these ligaments, which causes strain and in-

Weight-bearing

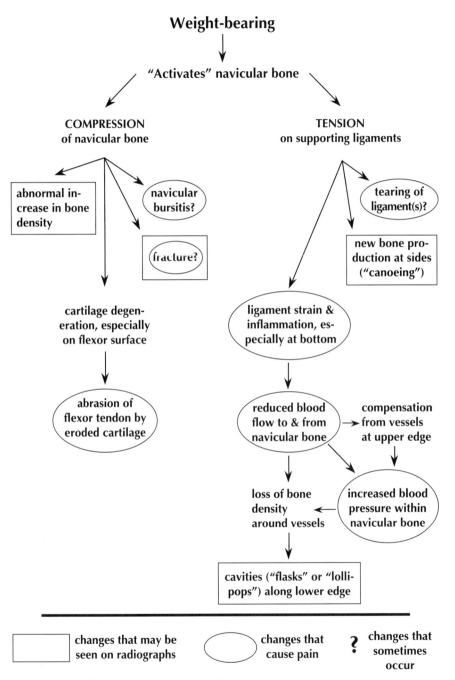

Fig. 15–5. Development of navicular syndrome.

flammation. The blood vessels to and from the navicular bone run through the ligaments that anchor it at the top and bottom. In normal horses, most of the blood supply comes from below the bone, through vessels in the thin ligament that attaches the lower edge of the navicular bone to the back of the pedal bone. This structure is called the impar ligament. The arteries run upward to the bone, which means that blood flow *to* the navicular bone must go against gravity. Blood flow *from* the navicular bone travels downward, through veins in the impar ligament.

Strain and inflammation of the impar ligament can obstruct these blood vessels and reduce blood flow to and from the navicular bone.

Fig. 15–6. Radiographic changes seen with advanced navicular syndrome.

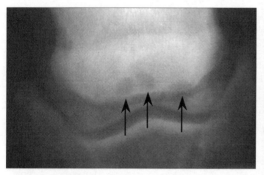 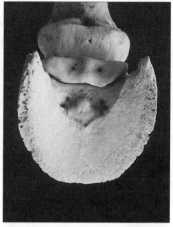

A. Above: The loss of bone density is most obvious along the lower edge of the bone. Right: The flexor surface of the navicular bone.

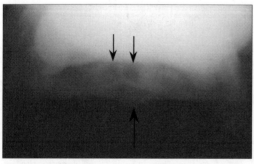 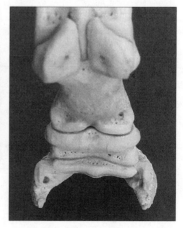

B. Above: Skyline view, showing the cavities in the center of the bone [small arrows] and erosion at the flexor surface [large arrow]. Right: The angle used to take this radiograph.

Over time, the damaged ligament may become thickened with fibrous tissue, which could permanently reduce blood flow. Veins are more easily compressed than arteries, so blood flow *from* the navicular bone is reduced to a greater degree than blood flow *to* the bone. This causes pressure to build up within the navicular bone. The body compensates for the reduced blood supply by increasing blood flow through the arteries that run into the navicular bone from above. This can add to the increased pressure within the bone.

The navicular bone's response to reduced blood supply and increased pressure is to absorb some of the mineral from its center. This remodeling process is most apparent along the lower edge of the bone. Widening of the channels through which the vessels run is seen on radiographs as cavities in the bone. These cavities are sometimes called "lollipops" or "flasks" because of their shape.

Another common abnormality that is seen on radiographs is new bone production (exostoses; *see Chapter 9*) on either side of the bone. Excessive tension on the supporting ligaments at each side of the bone places tension on the bone surface. This results in new bone production at the stress points. Exostoses often make the navicular bone look canoe-shaped on radiographs, which is why this

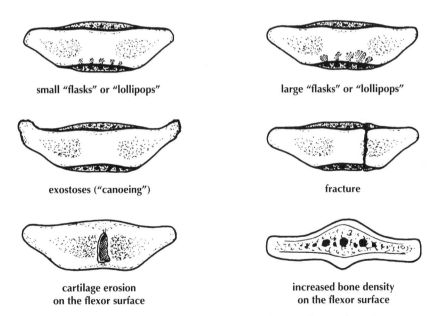

small "flasks" or "lollipops" large "flasks" or "lollipops"

exostoses ("canoeing") fracture

cartilage erosion on the flexor surface increased bone density on the flexor surface

Fig. 15–7. Changes associated with navicular syndrome. The top four drawings are viewed from the front of the bone. The bottom left is viewed from the back, and the bottom right is viewed from above (like a skyline radiograph).

abnormality is called "canoeing." Excessive tension can also tear the ligaments, although this problem cannot be detected on radiographs.

Sources of Pain

Lameness in these horses may come from a variety of sources involving both bone and soft tissues. Strain and inflammation of the supporting ligaments causes pain, whether or not the ligaments are torn. Most of the nerves that supply the navicular bone travel through the impar ligament. So stretching and inflammation of the ligament stimulates these nerves. Reduced blood flow to any tissue causes pain, as does increased blood pressure within a solid structure (in this case, the navicular bone). Damage to the navicular bursa and deep flexor tendon can contribute to the pain and lameness, as can cartilage erosions that are extensive enough to expose the bone beneath.

In many horses with navicular syndrome the lameness is inconsistent. It tends to shift from one leg to the other; it may be worse on some days and absent on others. This can be explained by the fact that the condition involves mechanical factors and blood flow changes, both of which are dynamic (changing) processes. So, the pain varies with the forces sustained by the navicular bone, and the body's response to those forces.

Terminology

Because the navicular bone may not be the only structure causing lameness, some veterinarians and farriers use the term, "caudal heel syndrome," for problems that cause pain in the back part (caudal area) of the foot.

Navicular syndrome, sheared heels, and hoof wall defects at the quarters or heels are the most common causes of heel pain in horses.

Contributing Factors

Foot Shape

Abnormal foot conformation plays a major role in navicular syndrome, although the condition is also seen in horses with normally-shaped feet. There is no single foot shape that exclusively contributes to the condition. However, it is more commonly seen in two types of horses: 1) those with long toes and low heels, which is typical of many Thoroughbreds, and 2) those with narrow, upright feet, which is typical of many Quarter Horses. But navicular syndrome is by no means confined to these two breeds of horses.

The long toe–low heel foot shape encourages overextension of the coffin joint during exercise. It even causes increased pressure on the navicular bone while the horse is standing. Horses with tall, narrow heels have a different problem. This foot shape increases concussion in the heel area, directly beneath the navicular bone. Plus, the heels, frog, and digital cushion absorb less of the concussion than in a normal foot. These concussive forces are transmitted to the deeper structures of the foot, including the navicular bone and its supporting ligaments. Hoof wall pain at the heels is another important contributor to the lameness with either foot shape.

Although improper trimming and shoeing, and long shoeing intervals can contribute to, or worsen these foot shapes, for the most part they are inherited. The farrier can change the foot shape to some degree, but it is generally a basic fault of the horse's conformation that leads to these abnormalities. *(See Chapter 7 for more information on abnormal foot shape.)*

Recently, scientists reported that in young Warmbloods the shape of the navicular bone (which is probably also determined by heredity) may influence which horses will develop the worst signs of navicular syndrome. The practical significance of this information, and whether it holds true for other breeds, remains to be seen. But it strengthens the belief that many different factors are involved in the development of this condition.

Activity

Steep hill work, galloping, and jumping may also contribute to navicular syndrome. These activities place a lot of tension on the deep flexor tendon, and cause overextension of the coffin and pastern joints. Frequent exercise on hard or irregular surfaces may also affect the navicular bone and its supporting structures by increasing the concussive forces on the feet. This holds true for all horses, regardless of foot shape.

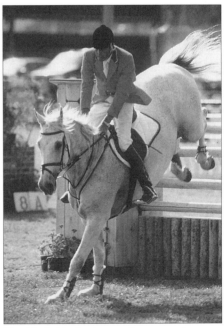

Fig. 15–8. Navicular syndrome can be aggravated by jumping.

It has been suggested that navicular syndrome is a condition of the standing horse, rather than being related to the type and intensity of the horse's activity. The navicular bone is compressed whenever the horse bears weight on the foot. The compressive forces increase with the speed of motion. However, they are intermittent—while the foot is in the air (midstride) there is little pressure on the navicular bone.

In contrast, a horse that is standing around for most of the day is putting constant pressure on its navicular bones. Blood flow to the navicular bones may also be compromised. This is because blood flow in the lower legs is sluggish while the horse is standing still. Tension on the supporting ligaments may further reduce navicular blood flow. Thus, inactivity, such as stall confinement, may contribute to navicular syndrome. On the other hand, frequent low-grade activity, such as is provided by pasture turnout, may help slow or prevent it.

The horse's body weight in relation to its foot size may be another contributing factor. The heavier the horse, the more load is placed on its feet. In a large horse, the smaller the feet, the greater the relative load on the navicular structures. This might help explain why navicular syndrome is not often seen in ponies and Arabians, but it is common in Thoroughbreds, Quarter Horses, and Warmbloods.

Signs of Navicular Syndrome

Navicular syndrome typically causes mild lameness (grade 1 – 2 of 5). The lameness can usually be made more obvious (often one grade worse) by working the horse in a circle or on a hard surface. The condition is almost always confined to the forelimbs. It is often bilateral,

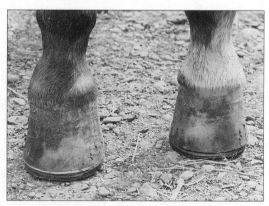

although it is usually worse in one foot on any given day. Many horses with heel pain try to protect the heels by landing toe-first, rather than placing the foot flat. As a result, they take short, "mincing" steps. This gait abnormality can easily be confused with a shoulder problem *(see Chapter 1).*

Fig. 15–9. The more painful foot has become narrow and upright.

Over several months, mismatched feet may develop because of uneven weight-bearing between the two feet. Mismatching means that the feet are noticeably different in size, shape, and angle *(see Chapter 7)*. Typically, the more painful foot becomes narrow and upright. However, mismatching is also seen in other chronic foot conditions, so it is not diagnostic for navicular syndrome.

Diagnosis of Navicular Syndrome

The history, especially the age, breed, and use of the horse, is important in forming a diagnosis. The condition may have been progressing for some time before the horse shows any signs of pain. So, in most cases it is seen in mature performance horses. The foot shape is also an important characteristic when determining whether a horse is a candidate for navicular syndrome.

The signs of navicular syndrome can be vague and inconsistent. They can often be confusing because the lameness may seem to shift from one limb to the other, and fluctuate in severity. Some days the horse may not seem lame at all.

Because the navicular bone is deep within the foot, horses with navicular syndrome do not always respond to hoof tester pressure. They may, however, show a positive response to a fetlock flexion test. This is because flexing the fetlock also flexes the pastern and coffin joints, which affects the navicular area. A toe extension test, where the horse is made to stand with its toe raised for a minute before being trotted off, can also worsen the lameness. This test overextends the coffin joint, which increases compression on the navicular bone and tension on its supporting structures.

A definite diagnosis cannot be made unless a nerve block

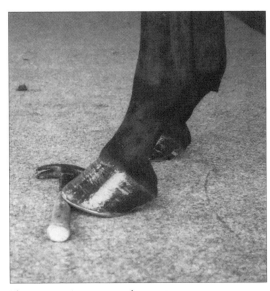

Fig. 15–10. A toe extension test.

localizes the lameness to the back of the foot, and radiographs show obvious changes in the navicular bone. However, this diagnostic approach is not foolproof.

Nerve Blocks

Blocking the Palmar Digital nerves at the back of the pastern temporarily blocks sensation in the structures at the back of the foot. They include the navicular bone and its supporting structures, the back half of the pedal bone, and the sensitive tissues of the frog, hoof wall, and sole. This is called a PD nerve block *(see Chapter 2)*.

In most horses with navicular syndrome a PD nerve block resolves the lameness in that leg. Occasionally, the lameness is just improved, and a higher block is needed to completely resolve it. This may mean that a problem in the pastern or front of the foot is contributing to the lameness. But it could also mean that the nerve supply to the navicular area is a little more complex than normal in that horse. This latter point is important when deciding whether a palmar digital neurectomy ("nerving"; discussed later) would be useful.

Often the horse becomes lame in the opposite foreleg once the "lame" leg is blocked. This indicates that the lameness is bilateral, although one foot was more painful than the other.

Radiographic Changes

The severity of the radiographic changes in the navicular bone are not always consistent with the degree of lameness. Some horses are quite lame, but have only minor radiographic changes. Others are hardly lame, but have obvious, even severe changes. This can be a

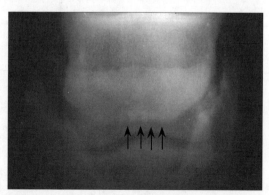

dilemma for the veterinarian, particularly during a prepurchase examination *(see Chapter 3)*. If the feet of a dozen normal horses over 8 years old were radiographed, more than half would probably have some radiographic changes in their navicular bones. In these horses the

Fig. 15–11. Small cavities along the lower edge of the navicular bone.

changes are not causing lameness at the time, and in fact, may never cause lameness. But the changes do indicate that the navicular bones have been responding to the forces on them.

Coffin Joint Block

Some veterinarians block the coffin joint before performing a PD nerve block. The navicular bone forms the back of the coffin joint, and part of the joint capsule lies against the navicular bone's supporting ligaments above and below the joint. Injecting local anesthetic into the coffin joint blocks sensation in the navicular bone and most of its supporting structures. It improves the lameness in many horses with navicular syndrome.

However, it also improve the lameness in horses with coffin joint arthritis and some pedal bone fractures. Another drawback is that extreme care must be taken to prevent infection when performing a joint block *(see Chapter 2)*. Nevertheless, a coffin joint block is warranted when the nerve block and radiographs are inconclusive. If the horse is still lame after a coffin joint block, it is unlikely that it has navicular syndrome.

Nuclear Scintigraphy

Nuclear scintigraphy is sometimes useful if there is any doubt that navicular syndrome is causing the lameness. If there is a "hot spot" over the navicular area, there is a good chance that the navicular bone is the source of lameness and the radiographic changes are significant.

Treatment of Navicular Syndrome

A variety of therapies have been used to treat navicular syndrome. Given that the cause is not precisely known, and probably involves several factors, it is no wonder that no single treatment is universally successful.

The degenerative changes in the navicular bone are often well advanced by the time the horse shows consistent signs and a diagnosis is made. These changes are largely irreversible. So, management is aimed at slowing the progression of the condition and relieving pain in an effort to keep the horse working.

Shoeing

Supportive shoeing is the most important and effective long-term management strategy for horses with navicular syndrome. The farrier must aim to restore and maintain hoof balance and a normal hoof wall angle. Also, the heels must be supported as much as possible. These principles are especially important in horses with low or underrun heels. Some horses can also benefit from shoes that alter breakover, such as a rolled toe or square toe shoe. In horses with narrow, upright feet, the heels may need to be lowered, and a shoe applied that encourages the heels to spread. *(See Chapter 7 for more information on shoeing options.)*

What is necessary in one foot may not be necessary or effective in the other foot, particularly if the feet are mismatched. No matter which type of shoe is used, ensuring that the shoeing interval remains constant is very important in managing navicular syndrome.

After the shoeing changes are made, it often helps to restrict the horse to daily light exercise for 1 – 2 weeks before beginning the modified training schedule. This gives the horse time to adjust to its new shoes, and allows any resulting inflammation to subside.

Training

Reducing the intensity of the training schedule is important, although the horse should still be exercised daily. Other methods of promoting and maintaining fitness could be incorporated into the horse's exercise program. Slow, distance work and swimming are examples of appropriate activities.

It is often best to eliminate, or at least minimize the factors that cause or worsen navicular problems, such as:

- steep hills
- galloping
- jumping
- working on hard or irregular surfaces
- working on deep, shifting surfaces, e.g., sand

Drugs
Vasodilators

Several drugs have been tried in an effort to improve blood flow in the small vessels in the foot. These drugs are called vasodilators. Although mechanical factors affecting the navicular bone and its soft tissues probably start the whole process, they lead to blood flow changes. So drugs that reduce blood pressure and improve blood flow within the navicular bone have some justification.

Isoxsuprine is one such drug that is often recommended for navicular syndrome. There is no conclusive evidence that isoxsuprine is effective in improving blood flow within the navicular bone, but it does seem to help some horses. It usually takes at least 3 weeks of continuous use before an improvement is seen. The lameness may be improved for several weeks after the drug is stopped. But most horses revert back to their former degree of lameness once the drug is no longer given regularly.

Pentoxifylline is another drug that may temporarily improve blood flow within the navicular bone. This drug makes the red blood cells more deformable, so they can squeeze through small spaces without becoming lodged or damaged. In theory, this effect should improve blood flow in small or narrowed blood vessels. Pentoxifylline can make some horses with navicular syndrome more comfortable. However, as with isoxsuprine, the effects only last for as long as the horse is on the medication.

Anti-Inflammatory Drugs

NSAIDs temporarily improve or resolve the lameness in most horses. However, once they are stopped, the lameness usually returns within a few days. High doses given for several days can cause stomach ulcers and kidney damage. But low-dose programs (using the lowest effective dose once per day) may safely allow the horse to continue in training relatively pain-free.

Some veterinarians have tried injecting corticosteroids or other joint medications (HA or GAGs) into the navicular bursa. However, navicular bursitis is only part of the problem. This approach is seldom successful in the long term.

None of these drugs are very effective in halting or slowing the progression of navicular syndrome. They merely treat the primary symptom: pain. But when used with shoeing and training modifications, they can greatly improve or resolve the lameness. When planning a long-term medication program for an athletic horse, the specific competition rules regarding drug administration must also be taken into consideration. *(Medications are discussed in Chapter 5.)*

Surgery

Palmar Digital Neurectomy

Neurectomy ("nerving") involves severing the Palmar Digital (PD) nerves on each side of the deep flexor tendon at the back of the pastern. This eliminates feeling in the back of the foot. In horses that remain lame despite shoeing and training changes and medication neurectomy is an option—but only if a PD nerve block resolves the lameness. However, it is a surgical procedure with several potential

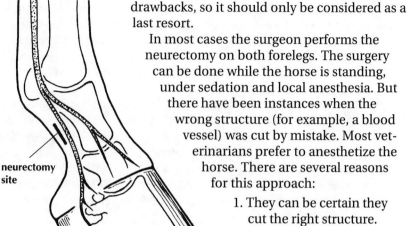

neurectomy site

Fig. 15–12. The nerve supply to the foot.

drawbacks, so it should only be considered as a last resort.

In most cases the surgeon performs the neurectomy on both forelegs. The surgery can be done while the horse is standing, under sedation and local anesthesia. But there have been instances when the wrong structure (for example, a blood vessel) was cut by mistake. Most veterinarians prefer to anesthetize the horse. There are several reasons for this approach:

1. They can be certain they cut the right structure.
2. They can explore the area and make sure they cut any extra nerve branches that are found.
3. They can "cap," freeze, or laser the end of the nerve to reduce the potential for neuroma formation and delay regrowth of the nerve.

Some of the potential complications or inevitable results of neurectomy include:

Wound breakdown—As with any wound at the pastern, skin movement causes tension on, and sometimes breakdown of the sutures. Also, wound infection is possible with any surgical procedure near the foot.

Persistent lameness—The lameness may persist if small nerve branches remain intact. Or, it may persist if due to another, unrelated condition elsewhere in the foot or leg. *(For this reason, it is very important to establish that the lameness can be resolved with a PD nerve block before this surgery is considered.)* Temporary lameness for 2 – 6 weeks after surgery is common, and is usually due to tension on the healing tissues at the surgical site.

Neuroma formation—A neuroma is a small swelling of nerve fibers at the cut end of a nerve. People with neuromas describe them as being very painful. In neurectomized horses neuroma formation can cause pain and lameness weeks or months after surgery. Neuromas can be surgically removed, but they can also re-form.

Undetected injuries at the back of the foot—Because the horse has no feeling in the area, injuries at the back of the foot may go undetected for a long time. Some of the more serious injuries include navicular or pedal bone fractures, and infected puncture wounds. Thus, the horse's feet should be carefully cleaned out and inspected every day.

Regrowth of the nerve and return of the lameness—Although nerves regenerate slowly, in most horses sensation does eventually return, even if the nerve was "capped." It may take months or a couple of years, but neurectomy is generally not a permanent "cure." Repeating the surgery months or years later is more difficult because of the fibrous (scar) tissue at the site.

Reduction in market value—The market value, and even the salability of a horse may be substantially reduced if it is known that the horse has been neurectomized. In some sports neurectomy may make the horse ineligible for competition.

Areas of Controversy

Neurectomy is a somewhat controversial topic. Although its purpose is to relieve the horse's pain, some people feel that it is mutilation to perform this surgery simply so the horse can continue to work. Others feel that it may save the horse's life, or at least ensure that it is well cared for and valued, by allowing it to perform pain-free.

Another area of controversy relates to whether neurectomy may make the horse more likely to stumble and fall. Some people think that neurectomy interferes with the horse's perception of where its foot is placed, causing it to misstep. However, only the back of the foot is desensitized by neurectomy; the front of the foot still retains feeling. Further, many horses with chronic heel pain take shorter strides and tend to stumble. Therefore, neurectomy may actually reduce stumbling by relieving pain at the back of the foot.

In many cases the decision whether to "nerve" the horse comes down to the owner's opinion of the procedure. Liability issues may also be relevant with horses involved in public riding programs. If a rider is hurt because a "nerved" horse tripped and fell, it could cause a serious and confusing legal situation. This dilemma may also arise when a person sells a "nerved" horse without informing the buyer that the surgery has been performed.

Navicular Suspensory Desmotomy

Because the navicular bone's supporting ligaments are involved in the condition, some surgeons have tried severing the ligaments that attach to the sides of the bone. These ligaments can be cut just above the heel bulbs. This procedure, called a navicular suspensory desmotomy, can help some horses by making the navicular bone a little more mobile. This decreases the tension on the other supporting ligaments. However, it reduces lameness in only about 50% of horses.

Post-Operative Care

After either procedure, the wounds should be kept bandaged until the sutures are removed, usually 10 – 14 days after surgery. During that time the horse should be confined in a clean, dry stall, and only hand-walked, if advised by the veterinarian. The bandages should be changed as often as necessary to ensure that the wounds remain clean and dry. Most surgeons prescribe antibiotics and NSAIDs for 3 – 5 days after surgery. The horse's tetanus status should be checked before surgery *(see Chapter 5)*.

As long as the wounds have completely healed, the horse can be gradually returned to regular exercise 3 – 4 weeks after surgery. The shoeing and training recommendations discussed earlier should also be followed in these horses.

Prognosis for Navicular Syndrome

The prognosis for long-term athletic usefulness is guarded in most cases. Navicular syndrome is an all-too-common reason that horses are unable to continue to compete at their former level, or are retired from competition altogether. It eventually becomes necessary to find less strenuous activities for the horse. However, if the horse responds to the shoeing and training modifications, it may remain usable for some time.

NAVICULAR BONE FRACTURES
Causes

The navicular bone is well protected within the foot, both by the hoof wall and the surrounding internal structures. Nevertheless, it can be fractured. Because of the protected location, navicular bone fractures most likely are caused by compression between the back of the second pastern bone and the deep flexor tendon *(see Figure 15–4)*. Navicular bone fractures are quite uncommon, so it would be reasonable to assume that normal navicular bones are very difficult to fracture. In most cases of navicular fracture, there is evidence that the horse has navicular syndrome. Chronic overloading probably weakens the bone, making it more likely to fracture.

Signs

In most cases, the navicular fracture occurs in a forelimb. It can occur in a hindlimb, but this is very unusual. There are no outward signs of a fracture, such as swelling and heat. The lameness is usually moderate (grade 3 of 5), and is consistent.

Diagnosis

The lameness may be partially improved by a Palmar Digital (PD) nerve block. However, often the veterinarian must block the Palmar nerves at the back of the fetlock or block the coffin joint to completely resolve the lameness. The diagnosis can only be confirmed with radiographs. Identifying the fracture line can be difficult, so it is important that the foot is thoroughly cleaned and the frog sulci are carefully packed before the radiographs are taken. Dirt on the hoof, gas lines from the sulci, and improper positioning of the foot, plate, or x-ray beam can each result in misdiagnosis. The fracture may be

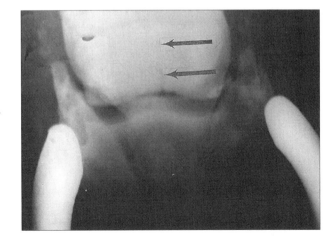

Fig. 15–13. A navicular bone fracture.

missed, or dirt or a gas line may be mistaken for a fracture. In some cases the fracture may not be visible for several days after injury. The diagnosis is made after radiographs are repeated. *(See Chapter 2 for more information on nerve blocks and radiographs.)*

Treatment of Navicular Bone Fractures

Because of the navicular bone's location, surgical repair is very difficult, if not impossible. Also, the potential for infection is great. No matter how well the hoof is scrubbed and disinfected, it is always contaminated. For these reasons, surgical repair of navicular bone fractures is usually not attempted.

Treatment involves confining the horse to a stall and/or small paddock for 4 – 6 months. Some veterinarians recommend a shoe that prevents the hoof wall from expanding, such as a bar shoe with quarter clips or a raised rim. Others prefer an egg bar shoe because it provides stability and support to the back of the foot. Raising the horse's heels with a wedge pad or a shoe with built-up heels can also help by relieving some of the tension on the navicular bone from the deep flexor tendon. *(See Chapter 7 for more information on shoeing options.)*

Navicular fractures generally heal with a fibrous union, rather than a bony callus. So the fracture line usually persists on repeat radiographs. The only way to determine when the horse is ready to return to work is by exercising the horse, watching for lameness or shortened stride. If lameness persists, the horse should be rested for longer.

Prognosis for Navicular Bone Fractures

Persistent or recurrent lameness is fairly common in horses with healed navicular fractures. Therefore, the prognosis for return to full athletic function is usually not very good. Chronic lameness may be caused by one or more of the following problems:

- instability of the fracture, allowing slight movement across the fracture line
- inflammation of the navicular bursa (navicular bursitis)
- adhesions (fibrous bands) between the navicular bone and the deep flexor tendon
- coffin joint arthritis (discussed later)

When rest, shoeing, and time do not resolve the lameness, the veterinarian may suggest a Palmar Digital neurectomy—provided the lameness can be substantially improved by a PD nerve block. *(Neurectomy is covered in the earlier section on Navicular Syndrome.)*

LAMINITIS
Definition

Laminitis, or "founder," is a common and very serious foot condition. Laminitis literally means "inflammation of the laminae." But despite the name, laminitis is not caused by inflammation. The condition begins with reduced blood flow to the sensitive laminae of the hoof wall. This results in cell death and breakdown of the bond between the hoof wall and the pedal bone. Inflammation is just one of the consequences of these much more serious events.

The sensitive laminae are tiny, finger-like projections in the laminar corium. These projections interlock with matching, tiny corrugations, called insensitive laminae, on the inside of the hoof wall. The laminar corium is attached to the surface of the pedal bone. The connection between these two layers keeps the hoof wall and pedal bone tightly adhered along the entire front and side surfaces of the bone. The laminar corium is well supplied with blood vessels and nerves, which makes this hoof wall–pedal bone bond a "living connection." The bond can break down if its blood supply is compromised.

Laminitis may take a few different forms. But basically, the condition can be separated into two broad categories: acute and chronic. Acute laminitis is the active stage of the disease, within the first 72 hours of lameness. Chronic laminitis relates to the persistent

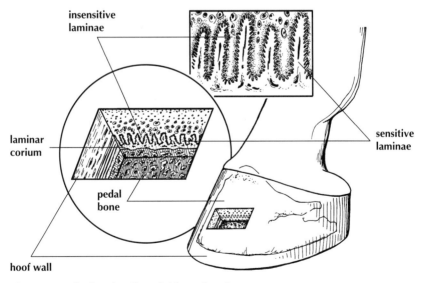

Fig. 15–14. The hoof wall–pedal bone bond.

changes in hoof wall structure and blood supply that result from an episode of acute laminitis. This section deals with acute laminitis. Chronic laminitis is discussed at the end of the section.

Causes of Laminitis

The basic cause of laminitis is thought to be reduced blood supply to the laminae, which results in breakdown of the hoof wall–pedal bone bond. Reduced blood supply may be caused by several specific factors, including endotoxemia, corticosteroids, and extreme load. Understanding the basic process is necessary to appreciate how these specific factors contribute to laminitis.

Basic Process of Laminitis

The disease process appears to begin with constriction of the blood vessels in the foot, and shunting of blood away from the sensitive laminae of the hoof wall. As a result, the cells of the sensitive laminae die, and the bond between the hoof wall and the pedal bone breaks down.

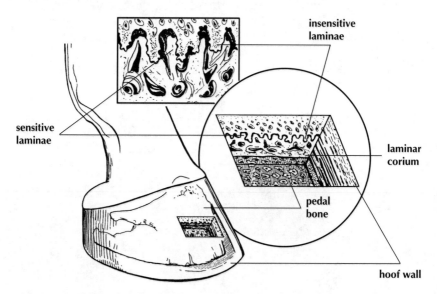

Fig. 15–15. The hoof wall–pedal bone bond is broken. Compare with Figure 15–14 of normal laminae.

Recent research suggests that the blood flow changes may not be the first events in this destructive process. There is a microscopic layer called the basement membrane between the cells of the sensitive and insensitive laminae. This membrane is an essential part of the hoof wall–pedal bone bond. Some scientists speculate that laminitis begins when the basement membrane is damaged by enzymes or inflammatory substances from the bloodstream. According to this theory, blood flow changes occur as a result of this damage. But the opposite may instead be true: reduced blood flow may damage the basement membrane. Research into this process is continuing.

With the bond between them disrupted, the pedal bone can be pulled away from the hoof wall by the deep flexor tendon, which attaches onto the bottom of the bone. The pull of the deep flexor tendon causes the front of the pedal bone to rotate downward. At the same time, the hoof wall can be torn away from the pedal bone by the vertical forces at the ground surface. These forces lever the hoof wall upward, particularly when the horse walks.

In large or heavy horses, the horse's weight may force the pedal bone downward, causing it to drop or "sink" within the hoof. Rotation and sinking are both very serious. Not only do they cause tearing of the sensitive laminae, which is very painful, they can cause irreparable damage to the hoof wall.

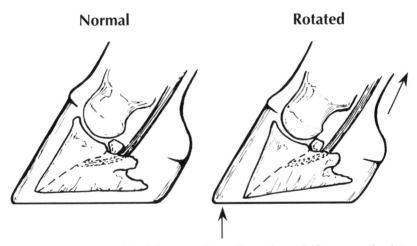

Normal **Rotated**

Fig. 15–16. The deep digital flexor tendon pulls on the pedal bone, causing it to rotate. Ground forces push up on the hoof wall, causing further separation.

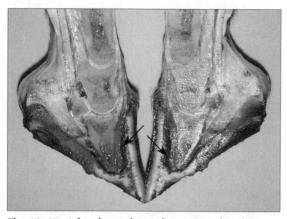

Fig. 15–17. A hoof, cut down the center, showing pedal bone rotation. Note the bruising between the hoof wall and the tip of the pedal bone (arrows).

To add insult to injury, pedal bone rotation can tear the blood vessels that supply the sensitive laminae at the front of the hoof wall. These vessels come from the back of the foot, run under the pedal bone, and track through its tip before emerging at the front and side surfaces of the bone. They then run up the inside of the hoof wall to supply the sensitive laminae with blood. When the pedal bone rotates, it tears away the vessels that run through its lower edge. As a result, the sensitive laminae of the wall are left without an adequate blood supply. This is one of the major changes that contribute to chronic laminitis.

Also, the tip of the rotated pedal bone can put pressure on the

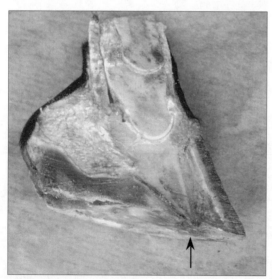

Fig. 15–18. The tip of the pedal bone can penetrate the sole in severe cases.

sole and cause bruising or dropping of the sole. In severe cases, the pedal bone may even penetrate the sole. This latter situation commonly necessitates euthanasia for humane reasons. The resulting pain is severe and unrelenting, and infection and degeneration of the exposed pedal bone is impossible to prevent and extremely difficult to manage.

Contributing Factors

The factors that can cause reduced blood flow to the foot, and therefore acute laminitis include:

- certain bacterial toxins—endotoxemia
- carbohydrate overload
- severe dehydration or shock
- corticosteroids
- pituitary gland dysfunction in old horses
- extreme load
- repeated concussion ("road founder")

Endotoxemia

Certain bacteria can cause more harm when they die than when they are alive. When these bacteria die, their cell walls break down, releasing molecules called endotoxin. If large amounts of endotoxin are absorbed into the bloodstream, it causes a dramatic drop in blood pressure and blood flow to the tissues. The feet are particularly sensitive to the effects of endotoxin, so laminitis is a common consequence when endotoxin enters the bloodstream.

The conditions that can result in endotoxemia—excess of endotoxin in the bloodstream—and hence laminitis include:

- colic that involves interruption of the blood supply to any part of the bowel, e.g. twisted bowel
- colitis, which is inflammation of the large intestine, resulting in profuse, watery diarrhea
- Potomac Horse Fever, which causes colitis
- pleuropneumonia, which is bacterial infection of the chest cavity and lungs
- endometritis, which is infection of the uterus—mares that do not expel the placenta within a couple of hours of foaling are especially vulnerable

The endotoxin-causing bacteria are normally found in large numbers in the bowel. Usually, the bowel can limit endotoxin absorption into the bloodstream. However, when the bowel wall is damaged by severe inflammation or interruption of its blood supply, endotoxin can flood into the bloodstream.

Extra Information

Endotoxin-causing bacteria are "gram negative" bacteria. They include *E. coli* and *Salmonella*. These bacteria are commonly found in the horse's bowel.

Carbohydrate Overload

Overeating carbohydrates, such as grain, grain-based pellets, "sweet feed," and lush pasture, can result in endotoxemia and laminitis. This is because carbohydrate overload creates an acidic environment in the bowel. The endotoxin-causing bacteria are very sensitive to acidity, and are killed in large numbers. The normally adequate protective mechanisms in the bowel are overwhelmed. So even though the bowel wall is not damaged, endotoxin enters the bloodstream.

Severe Dehydration and Shock

Severe dehydration results in a reduction in blood volume, blood pressure, and hence blood flow to the tissues, particularly the extremities (including the feet). Shock, which is circulatory collapse, also results in a dramatic drop in blood pressure and blood flow. As well as directly affecting blood flow in the feet, a severe reduction in blood pressure can also reduce blood flow to the bowel wall. This allows endotoxin to enter the bloodstream. Thus, any condition that causes the blood pressure to drop dramatically could cause laminitis by reducing blood flow both to the feet and the bowel.

Corticosteroids

Corticosteroids, or "cortisone," can make the horse more prone to laminitis because these drugs make the blood vessels in the feet more sensitive to the effects of adrenaline. Adrenaline is a natural substance that is produced by the adrenal glands, near the kidneys. It causes blood vessel constriction, which is essential for maintaining normal blood pressure and blood flow in the body. In high doses, corticosteroids can make adrenaline-induced blood vessel constriction either so profound or prolonged that laminitis develops. *(See Chapter 5 for more information on corticosteroids.)*

Pituitary Gland Dysfunction

Old horses commonly develop a benign tumor (adenoma) of the pituitary gland, which is located at the base of the brain. The pituitary gland normally produces hormones that direct the function of several other glands. Among other things, pituitary gland dysfunction causes the adrenal glands to produce too much cortisol, the body's natural "cortisone." Laminitis occurs in these horses for the same reason as it does with corticosteroid use.

Horses with pituitary adenoma typically have very long, shaggy or wavy haircoats that are not shed in the summer. These horses tend to drink and urinate more than normal. Despite good appetites and diets, they often are in poor body condition. Also, they are prone to infections, such as colds, skin conditions, foot abscesses, eye infections, tooth infections, etc.

Extreme Load

Horses are designed to distribute their body weight over each of the four feet. When one limb

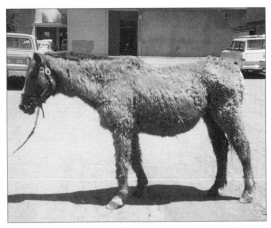

Fig. 15–19. Pituitary adenoma causes a very long, shaggy or wavy haircoat, and poor body condition.

cannot bear weight due to severe injury, the opposite limb must take more weight. For example, if the horse is unable to bear weight on its left forelimb, the right forelimb must take more of the load. If the horse will not bear weight on one limb, the load on the opposite foot cannot be relieved unless the horse lies down—which many are reluctant to do.

The blood supply to the front of the pedal bone and hoof wall comes from blood vessels that run underneath the pedal bone, through the tip, and up the front of the bone. Constant overloading of the foot can compress these vessels, restricting blood flow to the sensitive laminae of the hoof wall. Therefore, laminitis in the weight-bearing foot is a very common consequence of a severe, nonweight-bearing lameness.

"Road founder" may also be due to compression of the blood vessels at the bottom of the pedal bone. However, this rather poorly-defined condition more likely is associated with pedal osteitis and severe sole bruising (both discussed later) than with the process of laminitis.

Signs of Acute Laminitis

Laminitis can affect just one foot, as is typically the case when severe lameness causes laminitis in the weight-bearing foot. Or, it can affect both forefeet, or all four feet. It mostly affects the forefeet, probably because the forefeet bear more of the horse's body weight than the hindfeet. When all four feet are affected, the forefeet are

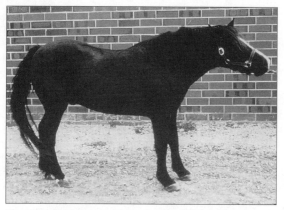

Fig. 15–20. Horses with severe laminitis adopt a typical stance and are reluctant to move.

usually more severely affected, or at least more painful, than the hindfeet.

It can take up to 40 hours from the start of blood flow restriction to when the signs of foot pain are first noticed. The signs are usually mild at first, with the horse merely shifting its weight from one foot to the other. In some cases this is all the discomfort the horse shows. However, in a severe bout of acute laminitis, the signs progress rapidly—over a couple of hours—to a stilted, shuffling gait. The horse then becomes so sore it is reluctant to move. It either stands with its forefeet in front of it and its hindfeet underneath it, or it lies down and refuses to get up. When the pain becomes this severe, the horse's heart rate may be elevated, and the horse may be sweaty and distressed. These signs can be mistaken for colic, or even tetanus when the horse stands "parked out." Occasionally, it may appear as if the horse has a hindlimb problem because it is reluctant to move and has its hindlegs drawn underneath it.

Many people check the hoof wall for warmth, assuming that if the hoof wall is cool, there is no problem. In the early stages of the condition, when blood flow to the hoof wall is restricted, the hoof wall may feel cool. But later, when secondary inflammation develops in the surviving tissues, the hoof wall may feel warmer. The air temperature can also affect the temperature of the hoof wall. Thus, the hoof wall temperature can be deceptive, and should not be relied upon.

More Information

The location and normal feel of the digital arteries are described in Chapter 4, under *Routine Foot Care*.

Digital Pulses

A more reliable indicator is an increase in the pulse pressure in the digital arteries. Laminitis causes a strong, even bounding pulse in the arteries of the affected feet. The increase in pulse pressure can often be detected even before the horse shows obvious signs of foot pain. This is because it is a reflection of the changes in blood flow that are occurring in the feet.

The pulse pressure in the digital arteries increases, despite the fact that blood flow to the sensitive laminae of the hoof wall is reduced. This may sound contradictory, but it makes sense when the blood vessel network in the foot is viewed as a highway that runs through a town. When the highway on the far side of town is partially blocked, outbound traffic builds up in the town, and quickly results in a traffic jam. The same thing happens with the blood flow in the feet. Obstruction of outflow in the veins causes blockage in the capillaries and an increase in pulse pressure in the arteries that supply the feet.

However, an increase in the pulse pressure in these arteries occurs with many foot problems. It is not diagnostic for laminitis.

Diagnosis of Acute Laminitis

The diagnosis can usually be made based on the history and the signs. For example, the history may include recent illness or infection, colic, grain overload, or access to lush pasture. If the horse has had laminitis in the past (which is quite common), there may be "founder rings" on the feet. These rings are horizontal ridges in the hoof wall *(see Chapter 7)*. Other causes of discomfort and elevated heart rate, such as colic, should be ruled out with a thorough physical examination.

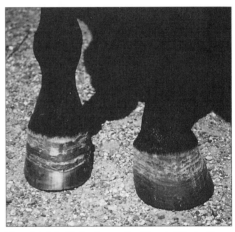

Fig. 15–21. If the horse had laminitis in the past, it may have founder rings.

In mild cases, or when just one or two feet are involved, the veterinarian must examine the feet for other causes of foot pain, such as severe bruising and foot abscesses. Pain in response to hoof testers over much of the sole, especially from the tip of the frog forward, is a strong sign of acute laminitis. In contrast, a sole bruise or abscess usually causes severe pain in a small area.

When laminitis is suspected, the veterinarian usually recommends radiographing the feet. The most telling view is the lateral view, in which the beam is directed across the foot *(see Chapter 2)*. It is on this view that rotation or sinking of the pedal bone is seen. Rotation is more common than sinking, and is easier to identify on radiographs. The front of the pedal bone normally is parallel with the hoof wall at the front of the foot. If these surfaces are not parallel, rotation has occurred. In contrast, when the pedal bone sinks, it usually remains more or less parallel with the hoof wall. Sinking can be difficult to detect unless an earlier radiograph is available that indicates the initial position of the pedal bone.

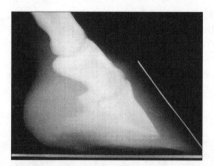 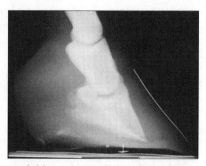

Fig. 15–22. On the left, a normal foot. The pedal bone is parallel with the front of the hoof wall (indicated by the white line). On the right, a laminitic foot. The pedal bone is rotated (the tack indicates the tip of the frog).

These changes in the pedal bone's position do not always happen immediately, and they may continue to slowly worsen over several days. However, it is important that the veterinarian takes a lateral radiograph of both forefeet (or all four feet if the signs warrant) as soon as laminitis is suspected. This gives the veterinarian a "baseline" radiograph of each foot for comparison with later radiographs. Some horses may already have some pedal bone displacement from previous episodes of laminitis. Establishing the initial position of the pedal bone is important for determining the degree of displacement during the current episode. This information is necessary for deciding how to manage the problem, immediately and long-term. It also helps the veterinarian establish an accurate prognosis.

Treatment of Acute Laminitis

There is no universally effective treatment for laminitis. By the time signs are seen, degeneration of the sensitive laminae has already occurred. Therefore, immediate treatment must aim to:

- prevent or limit pedal bone rotation
- relieve the horse's pain
- improve blood flow in the feet
- treat the underlying cause

(Long-term management of a horse with laminitis, once the acute stage has passed, is discussed in the later section on Chronic Laminitis.)

Limiting Pedal Bone Rotation

Limiting pedal bone rotation should be a priority when treating any horse with acute laminitis, whether or not radiographs indicate rotation has begun. There are several options available, the choice depending on the severity, stage, and cause of the condition.

> **More Information**
>
> **The trimming and shoeing options mentioned in this section are discussed and illustrated in Chapter 7.**

Frog Support

Frog support is often recommended in horses with severe lameness. This term does not mean the frog is being supported. It means that the frog is being used to support the rest of the foot. Frog support can prevent or minimize the effects of laminitis in the weight-bearing foot.

Vinyl Lily Pads and metal shoes, such as the heart bar or tongue bar shoe, use the frog for support and help the foot resist large shifts in the position of the pedal bone. Most veterinarians favor Lily Pads (or a suitable alternative) for the first 2 – 3 days because the pads can be quickly and painlessly applied and removed.

Wedges and Trimming

Raising the heels several inches with wooden or plastic wedges can decrease tension on the deep flexor tendon, and reduce the pull on the pedal bone. The wedges can be taped or glued to the feet. (Nailing on a shoe often causes severe pain in a horse with acute laminitis, and may jar the wall enough to separate more of the compromised laminae. Also, the horse is forced to bear more weight on the opposite foot while the shoe is being fitted.) If the wedges are just taped on, they are easy to remove if they make the pain worse, which sometimes happens.

If pedal bone rotation has already occurred, wedges may cause the horse more pain because they tip the weight forward onto the front of the foot. This places more pressure on the already compromised

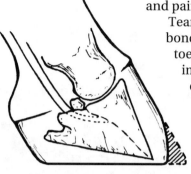

Fig. 15–23. Squaring the toe reduces the lever effect of the ground forces.

and painful hoof wall and pedal bone. Tearing of the hoof wall–pedal bone bond can worsen unless the wall at the toe is trimmed off. Squaring the toe is important to reduce the lever effect of the ground forces on the front of the hoof wall.

Reverse Shoes

Reverse shoes can also limit further breakdown of the hoof wall–pedal bone bond by decreasing the lever effect on the wall at the toe *(see Figure 15–29)*. These shoes relieve the front of the hoof wall from weight-bearing. This eliminates one of the forces that encourage pedal bone rotation: upward pressure on the ground surface of the hoof wall. Without this pressure the intact laminae stand a better chance of maintaining their integrity and resisting further pedal bone rotation. However, the horse may be in too much pain to tolerate the farrier nailing on the shoes. Nerve blocks may be necessary before the shoes can be fitted.

> ## Note
>
> Allowing bedding or manure to pack into the bottom of the feet will worsen the horse's pain. The feet should be picked out at least twice per day, if possible.
>
> If the horse is too sore to allow its feet to be picked up, even for a couple of seconds, removing the wet bedding and manure from the stall at least twice per day may be all that can be done.

Deep Bedding

Horses with laminitis seem to be more comfortable, and may be less likely to rotate their pedal bones, if they are kept on deep sand or shavings. They often burrow their toes into the bedding so that they are standing downhill. This may reduce pain in the foot by decreasing the pull of the deep flexor tendon on the pedal bone. Piling up the bedding this way may also increase frog support, which provides some resistance to pedal bone rotation.

Restricting Exercise

The horse should not be exercised if acute laminitis is suspected. It should be confined to a well-bedded stall or small, sand-filled pen, and moved as little as possible. Activity can cause further tearing of the hoof wall–pedal bone bond, and pedal bone rotation.

Contrary to common belief (and the veterinary advice of a few years ago), exercise does little to improve the blood supply to the feet in horses with acute laminitis. In fact, it probably does considerably more harm than good.

Surgery

In some very severe cases that have not responded to the above measures, the veterinarian may consider surgically cutting the deep flexor tendon. The tendon is cut either at the back of the pastern or midway up the cannon. This extreme procedure can be life-saving because it prevents the pedal bone from rotating further, and perforating the sole. Some horses eventually return to some level of usefulness after this procedure. However, in most cases the severe damage in the feet, coupled with the damaged deep flexor tendon, means the end of the horse's athletic life. This should be considered a salvage procedure.

"Sinkers"

Sinking of the pedal bone often cannot be prevented. Attempting to prevent downward displacement of the pedal bone by putting pressure on the frog is ineffective. Trying to support the pedal bone by applying pressure to the sole, whether with a shoe, a pad, packing, cast material, or bedding, causes severe pain and sole bruising. The only ways to help these horses when they will not lie down are to keep them on deep, dry bedding, provide pain relief, and treat the underlying cause.

Relieving Pain
Medications

NSAIDs are the drugs most often used to manage pain in horses with acute laminitis. These drugs prevent production of the inflammatory substances that cause pain. The inflammatory substances also cause blood vessel constriction, leakage of fluid from the blood vessels, and blood clots (which further reduce blood flow to the tissues). Thus, NSAIDs can reduce the harmful effects of inflammation and improve blood flow in the sensitive tissues of the foot.

NSAIDs can be given orally or intravenously, and should be continued for as long as the horse shows signs of pain. All NSAIDs have the potential to cause stomach ulcers and kidney damage if given at high doses for several days. So, the dose rate should be reduced to the lowest effective level within 3 – 4 days.

Some veterinarians also use DMSO as an anti-inflammatory treatment. It can be painted on the coronary band or given intravenously. DMSO is a potent scavenger of free radicals—harmful substances that are released by damaged cells. So, DMSO may have some added value in the treatment of acute laminitis. It has very few unwanted effects in horses, and is safe to use in horses that are already receiving NSAIDs.

Corticosteroids should not be given to horses suspected of having laminitis. Although they are very effective anti-inflammatory drugs, and may help prevent further cell damage, they can actually cause laminitis. Moreover, they suppress the body's immune response. Horses recovering from acute laminitis often develop foot abscesses. Corticosteroids increase the potential for these infectious problems to occur.

(Anti-inflammatory medications are discussed in more detail in Chapter 5.)

Poultices

Clay-based poultices can provide relief in some horses. Mud has long been known to be of benefit in horses with laminitis, whether because it is cool, it draws fluid from the hoof, or both. If a mud hole is not available, a clay poultice may be a way to achieve the same benefits.

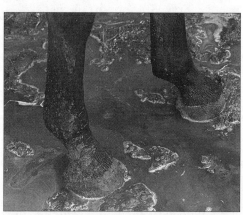

Fig. 15–24. Mud has long been known to be of benefit in horses with laminitis.

Nerve Blocks

Nerve blocks *(see Chapter 2)* can temporarily resolve the pain, and allow the farrier to nail on a shoe. However, it is extremely important that while the feet are blocked, the horse is not permitted to move around more than is absolutely necessary. Otherwise, further rotation and tearing of the hoof wall can result.

Improving Blood Flow
Medications

Various drugs have been used to improve blood flow in the feet. The most commonly used drugs are isoxsuprine and acepromazine. Isoxsuprine is discussed earlier as a treatment for navicular syndrome. Acepromazine, or "ace," is a sedative. It seems to be the more effective of the two drugs. Low doses of acepromazine can be given orally or by intramuscular injection two to three times per day. This dosage maintains dilation of the blood vessels (vasodilation) in the feet. Studies have shown it to be effective in improving blood flow in these vessels. However, the first signs of pain lag behind the start of blood flow restriction by up to 40 hours. So, ace is usually started too late to prevent large-scale destruction of the sensitive tissues of the hoof wall. For this reason, most veterinarians prescribe it for only a couple of days.

> ## Caution
>
> One thing that is guaranteed to increase the horse's pain is removing the shoes and leaving the horse unshod. Without shoes, the sole can contact the ground. This worsens the horse's pain, especially if the pedal bone has already begun to rotate.
>
> If laminitis is suspected, the horse's shoes should be left on until the veterinarian has examined the horse.

Recent research has found that the glyceryl trinitrate (GTN or "nitroglycerine") patches used in people with heart problems can improve blood flow in the feet of horses with acute laminitis. The patches were placed on the skin at the back of the pastern, directly over the digital arteries. Within a few hours, blood flow to the hoof wall was measurably increased. The horses and ponies studied showed a remarkable and speedy recovery, despite being severely lame before the patches were applied. More research is necessary, but this product appears to hold a lot of promise in limiting the destructive effects of acute laminitis.

Other Measures

In theory, placing the horse's feet in warm water should dilate the blood vessels in the feet and improve blood flow. However, in most cases it increases the pain. It may even worsen the problem by increasing the rate of cell activity and the demand for more oxygen and nutrients. When this demand cannot be met by the compromised blood supply, the cells begin to deteriorate. This worsens the inflammation and tissue destruction. If given a choice, horses with laminitis will stand in cool water. This does little to alter blood flow in the feet, unless the water is ice-cold, but it relieves the horse's discomfort.

Prognosis for Acute Laminitis

Except for horses with mild laminitis, the prognosis for future athletic usefulness is guarded, particularly if pedal bone rotation has occurred. Some horses recover from an episode of laminitis with few, if any long-term problems. However, in many horses the hoof wall is damaged to the extent that chronic foot problems result. Repeated episodes of acute laminitis are also fairly common in these horses.

Prevention of Acute Laminitis

The following measures may help to prevent laminitis in some situations:

1. Get prompt veterinary attention for horses with colic, other serious illness, and severe dehydration.
2. Pay careful attention to the horse's diet. Avoid overfeeding carbohydrates, and restrict access to lush pasture in heavy or overweight horses.
3. Never give corticosteroids without or against veterinary advice.
4. Provide frog support for the weight-bearing foot in every horse with a severe, nonweight-bearing lameness.
5. Ensure that horses prone to laminitis are exercised daily.

Idle horses, whether overweight or in normal body condition, seem to be more likely to develop laminitis than horses that are exercised regularly. Therefore, regular exercise may reduce both the potential for, and the severity of laminitis.

Chronic Laminitis

Chronic laminitis is a complex of foot problems that are the direct or indirect results of an episode of acute laminitis. The abnormalities that can cause persistent or recurrent problems include:

• pressure on the sole from a rotated or sunken pedal bone
• breakdown of the hoof wall–pedal bone bond
• permanent changes in the blood supply to the hoof wall

These changes are all related to pedal bone rotation. When the pedal bone rotates it tears the blood vessels that supply the laminae, compromising the hoof wall–pedal bone bond. Also, rotation causes the top of the pedal bone to tip forward. This compresses the blood vessels in the coronary corium between the top of the pedal bone and the inside of the hoof wall. Good blood supply to the coronary corium is essential for normal hoof wall growth, so rotation compromises new horn production at the front of the foot.

As a result of these abnormalities, the horse is more prone to:

- sole bruises
- subsolar abscesses
- flaring and separation of the wall at the toe
- infection beneath the separated wall
- hoof wall cracks
- degeneration of the tip of the pedal bone due to pressure and infection
- chronic lameness due to overloading of the heels (in an attempt to relieve pressure at the toe)
- slowed hoof wall growth at the front of the foot; the hoof wall grows more rapidly at the heels, resulting in a slipper or "duck bill" shaped foot

(These conditions are discussed in later sections, or Chapter 7.)

Chronic laminitis can take several forms, based on the degree of debility:

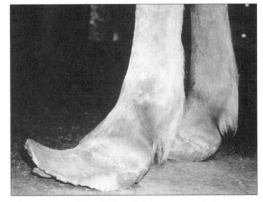

Fig. 15–25. Chronic laminitis can result in a "duck bill" shaped foot.

Progressive—The lameness continues to worsen. This may indicate further pedal bone rotation or imminent penetration of the sole. Or it may simply indicate sole bruising or abscess formation. These conditions can cause severe pain, although the last two are nowhere near as serious as the first two.

Static—The lameness and foot problems are not changing to any measurable degree, despite treatment.

Compensated—The horse can function in some capacity, despite the changes in its feet. For this to be possible, there must be no worsening of the changes, and the pain must be minimal or controllable.

Unstable—The lameness changes from one day, or one week to the next. Sometimes the horse shows little or no discomfort, but becomes lame after only a little exercise, or for no apparent reason. Repeat bouts of acute laminitis are common in these horses.

Certain types of horses are more prone to chronic laminitis and repeat bouts of acute laminitis:

- any horse recovering from a severe episode of acute laminitis
- overweight, "cresty" horses and ponies
- old horses with dysfunctional pituitary glands
- certain families

Overweight or heavy, "cresty" horses and ponies are more prone to laminitis when they are overfed and underexercised. Even if they are turned out on pasture, they may be overeating carbohydrates if the pasture is lush, particularly if they are not exercised regularly. In these animals laminitis is a management problem.

Management of Chronic Laminitis

Chronic laminitis can be difficult to manage. In most cases, the following management recommendations must continue indefinitely. Also, the owner or trainer must constantly be alert for a repeat bout of acute laminitis, or the other foot problems to which laminitic horses are more prone.

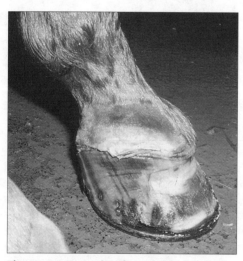

Fig. 15–26. Removing the separated wall is very important.

Shoeing

Regular attention from an experienced farrier is the most important part of managing a horse with chronic laminitis. The aims of trimming and shoeing are to:

- remove all separated wall, no matter how extensive, to prevent infection and further separation
- restore a more normal hoof wall–pedal bone angle
- support the foot, and prevent or minimize pressure on the sole

Remove the Separated Wall

Once the bond between the hoof wall and the pedal bone is broken, the hoof wall can become physically separated from the laminar corium that overlies the pedal bone. This separation typically begins along the ground surface at the front of the hoof wall, and is caused by upward leverage of the wall when the horse walks. Air fills the defect, so the separated area is seen on radiographs as a black gas line within the gray shadow of the hoof wall. Sometimes it is possible to detect these separated areas by tapping on the hoof wall. There is a noticeable difference in pitch of the sound over the air pocket.

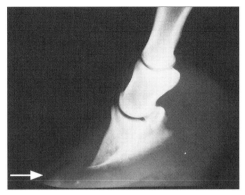

Fig. 15–27. Separation at the front of the hoof wall in a pony with pedal bone rotation.

Removing the separated wall is necessary to prevent or treat infection beneath. This procedure is called hoof wall resection. It also prevents further separation of the wall caused by leverage. Although the result is often unsightly, hoof wall resection is very important.

Restore the Hoof Wall–Pedal Bone Angle

Removing the separated wall also helps restore a normal relationship between the hoof wall and the pedal bone. As new hoof wall grows down from the coronary band, it attaches onto the surface of the pedal bone in the previous area of separation. Provided the laminar corium is not permanently damaged, a healthy hoof wall–pedal bone bond may re-form. However, this is not possible if the hoof wall is continually levered away from the pedal bone.

Lowering the heels and squaring off the remaining hoof wall at the toe further reduces the lever effect on the front of the hoof wall. It also helps to restore a more normal pedal bone orientation within the hoof. The amount of wall that

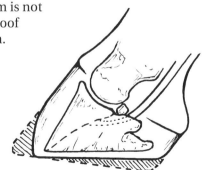

Fig. 15–28. Trimming for chronic laminitis: lowering the heels and squaring the toe.

is trimmed off the heels and toe depends on the degree of pedal bone rotation. Radiographs can be a big help to the farrier in deciding how much wall to remove.

There is a new technique for encouraging hoof wall growth at the front of the foot in horses with chronic laminitis. It involves removing a narrow strip of wall just below the coronary band, around the front and sides of the foot. This is not painful because only insensitive tissue is removed. The aim is to relieve pressure on the coronary blood vessels caused by pedal bone rotation. In some horses this procedure improves hoof wall growth at the toe, promoting a more normal foot shape over time.

Support the Foot

There is no one, universally effective shoeing method that works on every laminitic horse. Some horses benefit just from regular

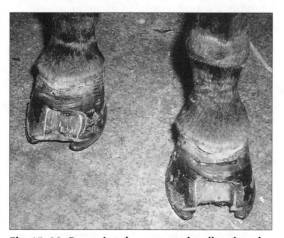

shoes, while others need the added support of a heart bar or tongue bar shoe, which uses the frog for support. Still others do better with reverse shoes, which relieve the toe of all weight-bearing and leverage. Reverse shoes also provide extra support at the heels.

Each of these shoes protects the sole by raising the foot off the ground.

Fig. 15–29. Removing the separated wall and applying reverse shoes relieves leverage at the toe.

However, horses with "dropped soles," in which the rotated pedal bone has caused the sole to bulge down, may require the additional height provided by a rim pad. In severe cases the farrier may need to build up the wall with acrylic resin for extra height. *(See Chapter 7 for more information on shoeing options.)*

It is important to realize that what works at first in one horse may become less effective, or even useless over time. It may be necessary for the veterinarian and farrier to experiment with the type of shoeing (and even the shoeing interval), as the horse's comfort demands.

Diet

Because carbohydrate excess can play a part in the development of acute laminitis, and chronic laminitis is fairly common in overweight horses, careful attention to the horse's diet is essential. Even horses turned out on pasture can develop laminitis if the pasture is lush. Horses in this situation should be watched closely, or confined and allowed only restricted access (a few hours per day) to the pasture during its peak growth period. In most areas pasture growth is at its peak in the spring. However, the pasture may go through other periods of rapid growth after rain in the summer or fall. It is a good idea to feel the digital pulses in these horses at least once per day when the pasture is growing rapidly. Their body weight or condition should also be monitored weekly.

Dietary supplements that improve the quality of the new hoof wall can help horses with chronic laminitis, although the benefits may not be obvious for several months *(see Chapter 4)*. Occasionally, low thyroid hormone production can result in an overweight, lethargic horse. A thyroid hormone supplement may help control the horse's weight. However, these products should not be given unless the veterinarian has confirmed, or has a strong suspicion that the horse has low thyroid activity.

Because of permanent changes in the blood supply within the foot, horses with chronic laminitis are at greater risk of repeated bouts of acute laminitis. Virginiamycin is an antibiotic that has been used experimentally to prevent the rapid multiplication of endotoxin-causing bacteria in the horse's bowel. When added to the feed, it has been shown to prevent laminitis in horses fed grain. This drug may be a good preventive in working horses that have recovered from a bout of laminitis. However, it is not yet commercially available.

Exercise

As long as the horse is comfortable, a little daily exercise can be beneficial: it improves blood flow to the coronary band, which aids hoof wall growth. However, the horse should not be exercised until the farrier has removed all of the separated wall and applied a shoe that adequately supports the entire foot. Allowing exercise before the horse is reshod can be extremely harmful.

Horses with chronic laminitis cannot afford to lose their shoes. Care should be taken to ensure that the work surface or turnout area will not cause the shoes to loosen. In particular, muddy fields and rough, irregular surfaces should be avoided.

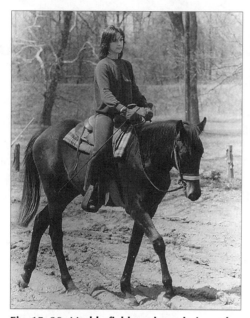

Fig. 15–30. Muddy fields and rough, irregular surfaces should be avoided.

The horse's comfort should be used as a guide to determine the amount and intensity of exercise. If NSAIDs are still necessary, activity should probably be restricted to voluntary exercise in a sand round pen or grassy pasture. However, if the horse is comfortable without NSAIDs, regular work can be introduced and gradually increased. With patience and effective shoeing, the horse may be returned to some form of athletic activity, although it may never regain its former level of performance.

PEDAL OSTEITIS

Pedal osteitis literally means "pedal bone inflammation." It is the term used for inflammatory changes on the bottom, or solar surface,

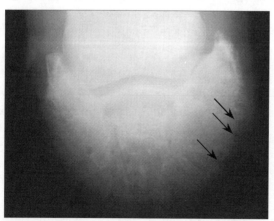

Fig. 15–31. Pedal osteitis results in an irregular border on the outer edges of the pedal bone.

of the pedal bone. This condition is diagnosed when radiographs of the feet show a roughened, irregular border on the outer edges of the pedal bone.

However, these changes may be found in horses that are not lame, or that are lame from another obvious abnormality which does not involve the pedal bone. For example, these changes are commonly seen in horses that have navicular syndrome or ringbone. Therefore, some veterinarians believe that the pedal bone changes are insignificant. Others think of pedal osteitis as an abnormality that does not necessarily cause lameness itself, but is nevertheless a sign of previous or persistent concussion in the feet.

Pedal osteitis is often found in horses with the following problems:

- chronic sole bruising
- laminitis
- chronic subsolar abscesses
- abnormalities of foot shape

Chronic bruising and subsolar abscesses (both discussed later) cause persistent inflammation in the sensitive tissues of the sole. The pedal bone is attached to these tissues, so persistent inflammation can cause a reaction on the surface of the bone.

It has been suggested that pedal osteitis is a form of laminitis. According to this theory, the abnormalities of blood flow and hoof wall–pedal bone attachment involve the sole and the bottom of the pedal bone, rather than the hoof wall and the front of the pedal bone. But it is more likely that it is a *result* of laminitis, especially if pedal bone rotation causes persistent pressure on the sole.

Abnormalities of foot shape, in particular, the long toe–low heel foot shape, and flat, thin soles, can add to the concussive forces on the sole and pedal bone. The result may be inflammation of the bone's surface.

Because pedal osteitis may be present in a horse that is not lame, or is lame for another reason, it is sometimes difficult to be certain whether the pedal bone changes are contributing to the lameness. A positive hoof tester response over the sole can help establish that there is inflammation at the bottom of the foot, but the response may simply be due to sole bruising.

> **More Information**
>
> See Chapter 7 for more information on abnormal foot shape and shoeing options.

Because pedal osteitis is most likely secondary to other problems or chronic concussion, management should aim to resolve the primary problem, and prevent further pressure and concussion on the sole. The sole can be protected from trauma with shoes and pads. Reducing the work intensity and exercising the horse on a softer, more "giving" surface may also be worthwhile. NSAIDs can make the horse more comfortable. However, it is a mistake to use these drugs to manage foot pain if the cause of lameness is not identified.

PEDAL BONE FRACTURES

Pedal bone fractures can occur when the horse forcibly kicks at a stall wall or steps on a rock. But in many cases the cause is unknown. Some pedal bone fractures occur during exercise, particularly in horses working at speed on very hard or irregular surfaces, such as frozen ground or dried clay. Dragging or harrowing an arena or track can create furrows in the solid base beneath the surface material. When these ridges dry out they may become hard enough to cause problems, although the work surface appears even. Standardbred racehorses, endurance horses, fox hunters, and eventers are the horses that more commonly sustain pedal bone fractures during exercise. Like many fractures in athletic horses, the fracture is probably the final result of chronic concussion. *(See Chapter 9 for more information on fractures.)*

Pedal bone fractures can involve the side (wing), center (body), extensor process, or perimeter (solar margin). In most cases, mid-body fractures extend into the coffin joint. Extensor process fractures also involve the joint. Mid-body and wing fractures typically cause moderate to severe lameness (grade 4 – 5 of 5), whereas extensor process and solar margin fractures usually cause low-grade lameness (grade 1 – 2 of 5).

Diagnosing pedal bone fractures can sometimes be difficult. Because the pedal bone is completely encased by the hoof, there are no obvious signs of a fracture, such as swelling and pain during palpa-

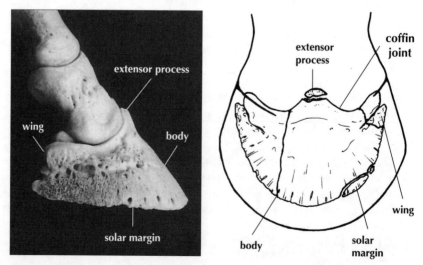

Fig. 15–32. Left: Parts of the pedal bone. Right: Types of pedal bone fractures.

PEDAL BONE FRACTURES

	Wing	Body	Extensor Process	Solar Margin
Involve the Coffin Joint	not usually	usually	yes	no
Degree of Lameness	moderate to severe	moderate to severe	mild	mild

Fig. 15–33.

tion. The digital pulses in that leg may be stronger than normal, but this is found with several other foot problems. Hoof testers may cause a pain response, but usually not in any specific area. In many cases, nerve blocks are necessary to localize the lameness to the foot.

The diagnosis can only be made with radiography. But even with good quality radiographs, the fracture may not be seen for several days. This is because the hoof wall restricts separation of the fracture pieces. Often the diagnosis is only made when radiographs are repeated days later.

Wing Fractures in Foals

An interesting area of debate and research involves apparent wing fractures in foals and weanlings. The wings of the pedal bone in young foals mature from cartilage into bone (ossify) as the foal grows. One theory is that fractures occur in the wing because the developing bone is soft. When the foal turns sharply during exercise, a piece of bone may break off the wing. This is because the deep flexor tendon pulls the pedal bone in one direction and the ground forces push the edge of the bone in the opposite direction.

In fact, these fractures may be osteochondrosis-like lesions, in which the growth cartilage and developing bone are overloaded, creating a fracture through the new bone. Often both forefeet (and occasionally both hindfeet) have similar changes on radiographs, which is typical of osteochondrosis at other sites *(see Chapter 14).*

Another theory is that the supposed fracture line is not a fracture

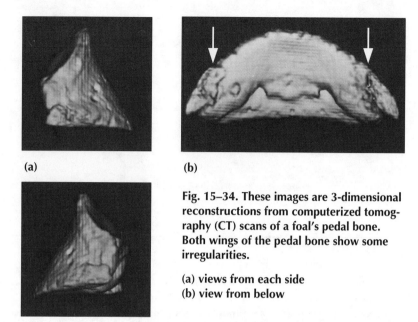

(a)

(b)

Fig. 15–34. These images are 3-dimensional reconstructions from computerized tomography (CT) scans of a foal's pedal bone. Both wings of the pedal bone show some irregularities.

(a) views from each side
(b) view from below

but a thin line of cartilage between the developing wing and the body of the pedal bone. On radiographs the cartilage appears as a black line. Normally, the wing ossifies from the body of the pedal bone outward. But according to this theory, ossification instead begins within the wing cartilage, radiating out from that center to eventually fuse with the body of the pedal bone. This area of ossifying cartilage is called a secondary ossification center.

In any event, many of these foals are not lame. They grow and develop into healthy, mature horses, and the line disappears completely. If the foal is lame, the lameness is only mild and often is traced to some other problem in the foot or elsewhere in the leg. In most cases the lameness resolves with only 4 – 6 weeks of confinement. The line disappears on radiographs by the time the foal is 12 – 15 months old.

Extensor Process Fractures

The extensor process is well protected by the coronary band and hoof wall, so fractures through this area are probably caused by internal forces. The common digital extensor tendon runs down the front of the limb from the forearm or thigh to the foot *(see Chapter 11)*. It attaches onto the extensor process at the top of the pedal bone. Excessive tension on the extensor tendon could tear the extensor process away from the body of the pedal bone. For example, tripping can cause sudden overflexion of the fetlock and knee, placing excessive tension on the extensor tendon. Another instance that may generate extreme tension on the extensor tendon

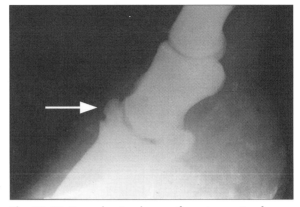

Fig. 15–35. Excessive tension on the extensor tendon can tear the extensor process away from the body of the pedal bone.

is when a horse gets its foot caught and struggles to get free.

It has been suggested that, like wing "fractures" in foals, some supposed extensor process fractures are actually a thin line of cartilage (a secondary ossification center) between the extensor process and the body of the pedal bone. The fact that this line is sometimes an incidental finding in a horse that is not lame strengthens the belief that not all of these lines are fractures.

There is no doubt that fractures of the extensor process really do occur, both in young and mature horses. In fact, the persistence of a cartilage line between the extensor process and the pedal bone may make fracture across this weak point more likely. But unless radiographs show that the extensor process has been pulled upward, or bony changes have developed, it is worth looking for another cause of the lameness.

True extensor process fractures are sometimes managed by surgically removing

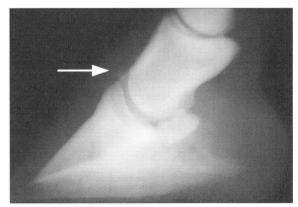

Fig. 15–36. This could be a fracture, but may instead be a secondary ossification center.

More Information

Post-operative care for arthroscopic surgery is described in Chapter 6.

Keeping the surgical wounds bandaged is very important because the risk of infection is greater for any procedure involving the foot.

the bone fragment. If the fragment is small, the surgeon may remove it arthroscopically. Otherwise, it must be removed through a larger incision. Although this procedure frees the end of the extensor tendon, it is attached at several places along its length. It eventually reattaches to the coffin joint capsule or pedal bone, so it is still able to extend the leg.

The back of the extensor process forms part of the coffin joint surface. Degenerative changes may occur in the joint if the fragment is not removed, particularly if it reattaches in an abnormal position. Joint medications may reduce the severity and progression of coffin joint arthritis in these horses *(see Chapter 5)*.

Managing Other Pedal Bone Fractures

Shoeing

The hoof wall normally expands a little as the horse's weight is placed on the foot. When the pedal bone is fractured, hoof wall expansion can create enough movement across the fracture line to slow healing or prevent complete repair. Therefore, most mid-body, wing, and solar margin fractures in adult horses are managed with a shoe that limits hoof wall expansion. A bar shoe with quarter clips or a raised rim are examples of this type of shoe *(see Chapter 7)*. Some veterinarians use fiberglass cast material to encase the hoof and restrict wall expansion.

Surgery

In adult horses, mid-body fractures that involve the coffin joint can sometimes be stabilized with a bone screw. However, pedal bone fractures can be difficult and frustrating to manage surgically for two reasons. First, there is a high risk of infection because the surgery involves making a hole in the hoof wall—a contaminated surface, no matter how thoroughly it is scrubbed and disinfected. Second, it is difficult to place the screw in exactly the right location—the surgeon must drill through the hoof wall "blindly."

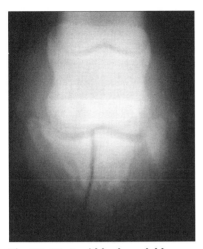

Fig. 15–37. A mid-body pedal bone fracture involving the coffin joint.

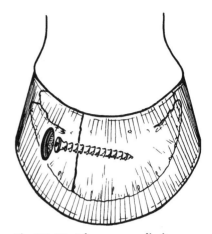

Fig. 15–38. A bone screw limits movement across the fracture line.

Rest

The typical recommendation with most pedal bone fractures in adult horses is 3 – 4 months of confinement in a stall and/or small paddock. This is followed by 4 – 6 months of pasture turnout. The horse's comfort is used as a guide to determine when it can return to training.

Foals and young horses are prone to developmental problems when confined *(see Chapter 14)*. For this reason, it is usually best to place the mare and foal, or young horse in a paddock that is small enough to prevent it from galloping around, yet large enough to allow some amount of activity.

Managing Chronic Lameness

Although the pedal bone has its own ready-made cast (the hoof wall), pedal bone fractures in adult horses sometimes heal with only a fibrous union, rather than a bony callus. The result in many mid-body fractures is that the bone pieces can move a little at the joint surface. Over time, degenerative joint disease develops in the coffin joint, and persistent lameness results. Movement of the pedal bone in these and other types of fractures may also cause tension on the sensitive laminae of the hoof wall. This could add to the lameness.

Chronic lameness in these horses can be very frustrating to manage. Injecting corticosteroids into the coffin joint can improve the lameness for a few weeks or months in some horses with healed mid-body fractures. Egg bar shoes may help other horses by increasing support of the hoof wall, particularly at the heels. Neurectomy ("nerving") only helps in cases where the lameness can be substantially improved or resolved with a Palmar Digital nerve block, which is not very common.

Prognosis for Pedal Bone Fractures

Pedal bone fractures in foals and yearlings have a very good prognosis for complete repair and normal athletic function, if they are diagnosed early and managed properly. In adult horses the prognosis for return to full athletic function is fairly good with fractures that do not involve the coffin joint, and which are managed properly. However, these fractures typically take many months to heal, especially in mature or old horses. Contracted heels in the fractured foot can slow or limit the return to athletic performance in horses treated with restrictive shoes *(see Chapter 7)*.

Chronic lameness is common after pedal bone fractures that involve the coffin joint, even if the fracture was stabilized surgically. But in many cases, surgical repair can substantially speed healing and limit the potential for secondary joint problems.

COFFIN JOINT ARTHRITIS (DJD)

Degenerative joint disease (DJD) is a chronic condition that involves progressive cartilage degeneration. It can be very difficult to diagnose DJD of the coffin joint because it is a small, relatively immobile joint that is encased within the hoof wall. The coffin joint cannot easily be palpated, manipulated, or surgically explored. The diagnosis is most clear when the cause is a condition that damaged the cartilage surface, the joint capsule, or both. If lameness persists after the primary condition is resolved, it is usually safe to assume that DJD has developed. The two most common conditions that typically lead to coffin joint DJD are:

> **More Information**
>
> Arthritis is a common term for DJD. See Chapter 8 for more information on this and other joint problems.

- pedal bone fractures that involve the coffin joint
- deep puncture wounds to the sole or frog that result in infection of the coffin joint

However, it is not necessary for such dramatic conditions to be present for DJD to develop in the coffin joint. Concussion contributes to DJD in other joints, so it probably also contributes to DJD in the coffin joint. Abnormal foot shape, especially narrow, upright feet, can increase the concussive forces on the hoof and internal structures, so coffin joint arthritis may be more likely in these horses.

The coffin joint may not be the only structure affected by concussion. The navicular bone forms the back of the coffin joint, and therefore sustains the same forces or is affected by the same conditions. For example, if the coffin joint suffers repeated concussion to the extent that DJD develops, the navicular bone and its supporting structures may also have been sufficiently stressed to develop degenerative changes. On the other hand, navicular syndrome may lead to inflammation or degenerative changes in the coffin joint.

Thus, coffin joint DJD may not be an isolated condition that can be managed just with joint medications *(see Chapter 5)*. The factors that contributed to the joint changes must be addressed. Because of these complex interactions, and the difficulty in confirming the diagnosis, coffin joint arthritis has a fairly poor prognosis for long-term athletic function.

PUNCTURE WOUNDS

Puncture wounds in the bottom of the foot are fairly common injuries that can be very serious. In most horses the sole is less than ½ inch (12 mm) thick. The weight of the horse as it steps on a nail or a piece of wire can force the object through the sole or frog. The object can directly damage the internal structures of the foot, but more important, it introduces bacteria.

Penetration in the center of the foot could directly damage and infect several important structures, including:

- the pedal bone
- the coffin joint
- the navicular bone and its bursa
- the deep digital flexor tendon (DDFT) and its tendon sheath

Infection of a bone, joint, or tendon sheath can result in severe and persistent lameness, which could halt the horse's athletic career. In

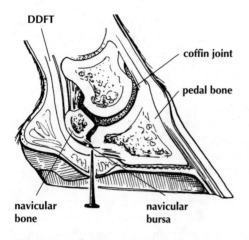

DDFT

coffin joint

pedal bone

navicular bone

navicular bursa

Fig. 15–39. The important structures that can be damaged by a penetrating object.

some cases euthanasia is necessary for humane reasons. *Therefore, penetrating wounds in the center of the foot must always be taken seriously, and should receive immediate veterinary attention.*

Figure 15–40 depicts the bottom of the foot, divided into nine sections. From this angle it is easy to appreciate how a penetrating object in the center of the foot could cause serious damage. In the surrounding eight sections on the diagram, penetration of the sole or frog is less serious. But the closer to the center section the object penetrates, the more likely it is that the pedal bone will be damaged. If the object penetrated the sole with enough force, the pedal bone may be fractured. Or, its surface may be damaged and become infected, leading to osteomyelitis *(see Chapter 9)*.

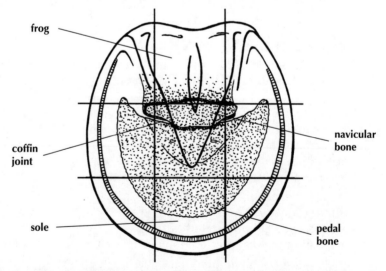

frog

coffin joint

sole

navicular bone

pedal bone

Fig. 15–40. The bottom of the foot, divided into nine sections. Punctures in the center section are more likely to involve important structures.

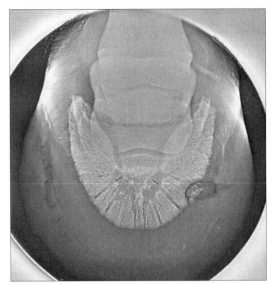

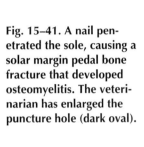

Fig. 15–41. A nail penetrated the sole, causing a solar margin pedal bone fracture that developed osteomyelitis. The veterinarian has enlarged the puncture hole (dark oval).

First Aid Management of Puncture Wounds

Sometimes the object is found in the bottom of the horse's foot. Other times it penetrates the foot then slips out. It often takes a thorough examination to find the puncture hole in those cases. When an object is found in the bottom of the foot, there are two ways to manage the situation until the veterinarian arrives:

1. Remove the object by pulling it out in the direction it appears to have gone in. Use pliers if necessary, but be careful not to break it. Take careful note of exactly where the object was lodged so that the veterinarian knows where to look for the puncture hole. Also make a note of how deeply embedded, and at what angle it was lodged. Save the object for the veterinarian to examine, but do not wipe it clean.

2. Leave the object in place. Tape a block of wood to the bottom of the foot, on either side of the object. This way, if the horse bears weight on the foot, it will not be driven further in.

Some veterinarians prefer the second approach because it gives them an opportunity to see exactly where, at what angle, and how deeply the object penetrated the foot. It also allows them to radiograph the foot with the object in place. This determines, more accurately than any other method, how close to the important structures the object penetrated.

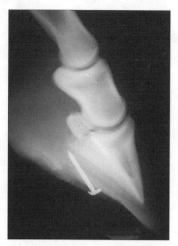

Fig. 15–42. This nail probably missed the important structures.

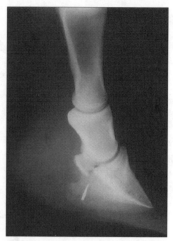

Fig. 15–43. This wire may have penetrated the DDFT.

No matter which approach is used, the foot should be cleaned as thoroughly as possible, taking care not to brush dirt into the hole. An antiseptic-soaked dressing should be placed over the puncture hole, or around the base of the object. The foot should then be bandaged, and the horse confined until the veterinarian arrives, or until the horse can be transported to a veterinary hospital.

Immediate veterinary attention is a *must* for all penetrating wounds in the center of the foot. Many owners and trainers are so relieved by the horse's willingness to bear weight on the foot once the object is removed that they mistakenly believe the problem is solved. But it may be just beginning. The horse may not be very lame until 3 – 4 days afterward. By this time the infection could be so advanced that the chances of a successful outcome are slim. The longer the horse is left without veterinary treatment, the worse the outcome will be. **Note:** Just giving the horse antibiotics after removing the object will not prevent or treat this infection.

Veterinary Treatment of Puncture Wounds

When deciding how to treat the foot, and making an accurate prognosis, the veterinarian considers the following questions:

1. How old is the wound? The longer the time between injury and veterinary attention, the worse the infection, the more costly and lengthy the treatment, and the poorer the prognosis.

2. Where and how deep is the wound? The veterinarian can afford to take a fairly conservative approach if the puncture wound is not very deep, and does not involve the center of the foot. But more extensive treatment is necessary for deep wounds in the center of the foot.

3. Is it a forefoot or hindfoot? The hindfoot supports less of the horse's weight, so puncture wounds in a hindfoot have a slightly better prognosis than puncture wounds in a forefoot.

> **Note**
>
> With any wound, especially one in or near the foot, it is important to make sure that the horse is currently vaccinated against tetanus.
>
> (Preventing tetanus is discussed in Chapter 5.)

Wounds at the Perimeter

Wounds at the perimeter of the sole are usually treated by paring the sole, opening up the puncture hole to its full depth, and removing all damaged and devitalized tissue. This procedure is necessary to treat and prevent infection. If the object contacted the pedal bone, any damaged bone on the surface is also removed. Exploring the sensitive tissues is painful for the horse, so the veterinarian may use a nerve block *(see Chapter 2)* to desensitize the foot.

After being thoroughly cleaned out, the wound is flushed with sterile saline or antiseptic solution (such as iodine), and the foot is bandaged. Depending on the depth of the wound, antibiotics may be given. However, antibiotics are often a waste of time if the puncture hole has not been opened and cleaned out. The horse's tetanus status must also be checked.

The wound should be inspected and flushed daily. The foot must be kept bandaged until the defect in the sole is filled in and is beginning to harden. This process usually takes 2 – 3 weeks. At first, the defect is filled with a blood clot. Healthy, pink granulation tissue replaces the clot in a few days *(see Chapter 13)*. The sole then closes over the defect with new horn, which thickens and hardens (cornifies) as it grows out.

A normal shoe often is all that is needed to protect the sole as it heals. Full sole pads are not recommended. They prevent inspection and treatment of the sole, and they trap moisture between the pad and the sole, which prevents the sole from hardening. However, hospital plates are very good for managing these wounds if the hole in the sole is large *(see Chapter 7)*.

Once the defect hardens and no longer needs treatment, a pad is a good way to protect the sole until it reaches normal thickness. During this time, the horse should be kept in a clean, dry environment.

Wounds in the Center

A fresh puncture wound in the center of the sole or frog that is not very deep can usually be managed much like a wound at the perimeter. However, if the injury is more than a day or two old and the horse is very lame, or if the wound is suspected or known to be deep, treatment must be more extensive.

Determining the Wound's Depth

If the object was removed before the horse was examined, the veterinarian must use contrast material to determine the depth of the tract. This involves injecting contrast material into the puncture hole, then radiographing the foot *(see Chapter 2)*. This technique works best on fresh puncture wounds. The inflammation and soft tissue swelling that result from the injury quickly close the hole, making it difficult for the contrast material to travel all the way up the tract.

The veterinarian may also sample the fluid from the coffin joint or tendon sheath to see if the joint or sheath has become infected. The fluid is submitted to the laboratory for measurement of its white cell count and protein concentration. Bacterial culture and antibiotic sensitivity testing is also performed *(see Chapter 2)*. Occasionally, the veterinarian may inject sterile contrast material into the joint or sheath after sampling the fluid, and before taking radiographs. This procedure is done to see whether the joint or sheath was damaged by the penetrating object. If so, the contrast material leaks into the puncture hole and/or the surrounding tissues.

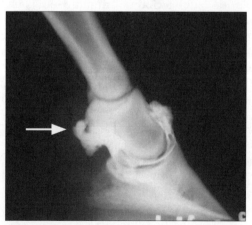

Fig. 15–44. Damage to the coffin joint capsule allowed contrast material to leak from the back of the joint into the surrounding tissues.

Surgery

Whether or not radiographs confirm that important structures are damaged, most veterinarians anesthetize the horse and fully explore the hole. This is essential in horses that have been lame for days before receiving veterinary attention. The procedure is called "street nail surgery." It involves removing a square of sole and/or frog around the puncture hole to expose and remove the damaged tissues. If the tract continues through the deep flexor tendon, part of the tendon must be removed so that infection in the deeper structures can drain freely through the bottom of the foot. The tendon is quite wide at this level, so removing a small section in its center generally does not weaken it that much.

More Information
Bandaging techniques are discussed in Chapter 4.
DMSO, antibiotics, tetanus prevention, and NSAIDs are covered in Chapter 5.

After fully exploring the wound, the veterinarian flushes it with sterile saline solution. A sterile or iodine-soaked dressing is placed over it, and the foot is bandaged. Some veterinarians prefer to use DMSO instead of iodine because of its anti-inflammatory properties. Intravenous antibiotics are given for several days, although without effective drainage, they do little to resolve the infection. The horse's tetanus status must be checked. NSAIDs are important for the horse's comfort, but care should be taken when giving high doses for several days.

Post-Operative Care

The wound must be inspected and flushed at least once per day until the defect has filled with granulation tissue. If the coffin joint or tendon sheath is infected, lavage (flushing) may also be necessary. *(Managing these conditions is discussed in Chapters 8 and 11, respectively.)* Sometimes the granulation tissue that fills the defect restricts drainage from the deeper structures. The veterinarian may have to debride, or trim, some tissue from the wound every couple of days to encourage drainage.

A hospital plate is very useful in these cases. It can improve the horse's comfort and mobility, while protecting the wound and allowing daily inspection and treatment. It is best if the farrier makes and fits the shoe before surgery. This prevents later contamination of the surgical wound. Placing wedge pads beneath the hospital plate can further improve the horse's comfort.

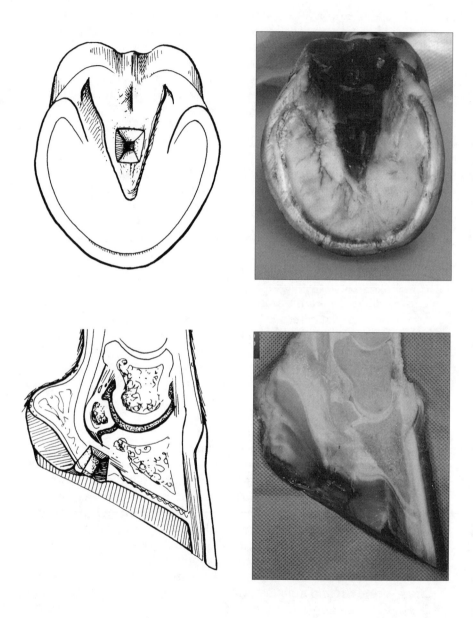

Fig. 15–45. Street nail surgery involves removing a square of sole or frog around the puncture hole.

The opposite, weight-bearing leg needs frog support *(see Chapter 7)* and a support bandage for as long as the horse is very lame. As soon as the horse is able, hand-walking two to three times per day improves drainage from the wound. It also minimizes adhesions (fibrous bands) between the navicular bone and the deep flexor tendon, or the tendon and its sheath.

The deeper layers of the sole and frog (and the tissues beneath them) are sensitive, and surgical exploration in this area is very painful for the horse. So, it is sometimes difficult to tell whether the horse is responding to treatment based solely on the degree of lameness. Most horses are at least grade 3 of 5 lame after street nail surgery, and show little improvement in the first week. If the infection is resolved and the tissues are healing well, the lameness should slowly improve over the next 1 – 3 weeks. Any lameness after this time is probably due to adhesions or coffin joint arthritis (discussed earlier). However, if the horse is still very lame 1 – 2 weeks after the surgery despite proper treatment, it can be assumed that the infection is not under control. The veterinarian must re-evaluate the horse and possibly repeat the surgery; the prognosis must also be revised.

Prognosis for Puncture Wounds

The prognosis for return to full athletic function is good for puncture wounds at the perimeter of the sole, as long as they are treated promptly. It may take a little longer for the lameness to resolve if the surface of the pedal bone was damaged, but in most cases, the horse eventually returns to full use.

When the coffin joint, navicular bone or bursa, or deep flexor tendon and sheath are infected, prompt and aggressive treatment is critical to the horse's athletic future. Even with immediate and appropriate care, the prognosis for return to normal athletic use is guarded. In some cases persistent, severe lameness may necessitate euthanasia for humane reasons. Chronic lameness commonly results from persistent infection, coffin joint arthritis, and adhesions. Laminitis in the opposite, weight-bearing foot is also a common complication, and further worsens the prognosis.

SOLE BRUISES

Like the hoof wall, the sole has an outer, insensitive layer of horn, and an inner, sensitive layer of tissue. The sensitive layer is well supplied with blood vessels and nerves. Excessive pressure on the sole can damage some of these vessels and cause bruising. In severe cases, a pocket of blood (hematoma) may form beneath the sole. Bruising of the sole is commonly called a "stone bruise," regardless of the cause.

Sole bruises are far more often seen in horses with thin soles, especially if the sole is flatter than normal *(see Chapter 7)*. This characteristic is common in Thoroughbreds and draft horses. Bruising is more likely when the horse is worked on hard or irregular surfaces.

Several situations can result in a sole bruise:

- constant, low-grade trauma to any part or all of the sole—most common in flat-footed horses
- a single episode of trauma to a specific part of the sole—the classic "stone bruise"
- repeated or constant pressure in a specific area, such as corns at the heel (discussed later)
- rotation or sinking of the pedal bone during acute laminitis—this causes pressure on the sole from inside the foot

When bruising occurs from constant, low-grade trauma, such as working every day on a hard surface, the horse may have a mild (grade 1 – 2 of 5) intermittent lameness in both forelegs. (The hindfeet can also be bruised, but bruising and lameness are more often seen in the forefeet.) The lameness may shift from one leg to the other. This pattern of vague, shifting lameness can easily be confused with navicular syndrome. However, it is possible to tell the difference using hoof testers. Sole bruising results in a pain response over part or all of the sole. Navicular problems either cause no hoof tester response, or a mild response to pressure across the heels.

When bruising occurs from a single episode of trauma to the sole, such as stepping on a rock, it can cause sudden, moderate to severe lameness (grade 3 – 5 of 5). Sometimes the lameness may be so sudden and severe that the owner or trainer believes the horse has a fractured pedal bone. While it is possible for the horse to fracture its pedal bone this way, the pain and lameness are more likely a result of sole bruising and trauma to the sensitive tissues. Depending on how hard the horse hit the stone, some of the pain may also come from the underside of the pedal bone. This type of injury is more likely to cause a hematoma beneath the sole at the point of impact.

Acute laminitis can result in rotation or sinking of the pedal bone. In some cases the degree of rotation is such that the tip of the pedal bone presses on the sole from above and causes extensive bruising. This can add to the horse's pain and result in persistent lameness.

Typical Sole Bruises
Diagnosis

Diagnosing a sole bruise can be difficult at first. Because of the thickness of the sole, and dark-colored horn in some horses, it is impossible to see red discoloration of the sole until several weeks have passed. It is usually not obvious until the farrier trims the sole in preparation for reshoeing.

There are two conditions that must be ruled out as possible causes of lameness in these horses: a pedal bone fracture and a foot abscess. Hoof testers can often narrow the possibilities to a bruise or an abscess if a specific area of pain is found on the sole. But this approach is by no means foolproof. Radiographs of the foot are usually necessary to definitely eliminate a fracture from the list. But several views and repeat radiographs may be needed before the veterinarian can confidently say there is no fracture. It may also be possible to eliminate fractures and abscesses if, with little or no treatment, the lameness substantially improves in a few days.

The veterinarian or farrier can confirm the diagnosis by making a small exploratory hole in the sole directly over the area of greatest hoof tester pain. If there is a bruise or hematoma, blood oozes from the hole. The sensitive tissues of the sole are well supplied with blood vessels, so deep excavation of a normal sole will cause some bleeding. But fresh blood is bright red, whereas blood that has been pooling beneath the sole is usually dark red-purple.

Note: Although this procedure may seem quick and simple, it should only be performed by a veterinarian or farrier. Removing too much sole can worsen the lameness, prolong the horse's recovery, and expose the pedal bone to damage and infection.

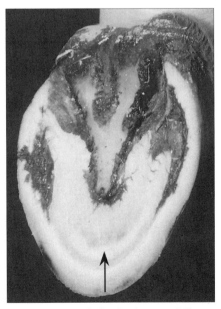

Fig. 15–46. A sole bruise in a partially trimmed foot.

Management of Sole Bruises

Draining the bruise or hematoma usually relieves the pain by relieving the pressure on the sensitive tissues. In most cases the small exploratory hole is enough to allow effective drainage. Provided the hole is small, the defect heals quickly and the horse can usually return to work within a week.

The hole should be covered with an iodine-soaked dressing, and the foot kept bandaged and dry until the defect has filled in. Some veterinarians prefer to use DMSO in place of iodine because DMSO has both antibacterial and anti-inflammatory properties. Checking the horse's tetanus status *(see Chapter 5)* is important whenever the sole has been opened. NSAIDs can relieve the horse's pain. However, they can also mask the persistent or recurrent lameness that indicates the problem is not resolving as it should. Any sole bruise could develop into a subsolar abscess, so bruising should not be taken lightly. It is usually best to give NSAIDs for only 2 – 3 days.

Applying rim or full sole pads *(see Chapter 7)* can help prevent further damage to the sole once it has healed. Packing the bottom of the feet with a clay-based poultice after exercise can also help horses with flat feet or thin soles. Avoiding hard or irregular work surfaces may reduce the incidence and severity of sole bruising.

Corns

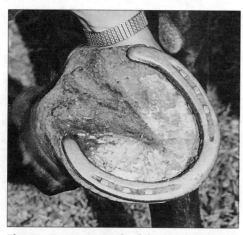

Fig. 15–47. Overgrowth of the hoof wall can allow the shoe to contact the sole between the bar and heel.

Corns in horses are sole bruises caused by the shoe. They are most common at the angle between the bar and the heel. Corns can develop on only one side of just one foot, on both sides of one foot, or in both forefeet. (They can also occur in the hindfeet, but are far more common in the forefeet.) In most cases corns are a sign of improper or overdue shoeing—the shoe should never contact the sole. Applying a shoe that is too small or too short can cause corns, as can pads that are attached to the shoe with rivets (the rivets can press on the sole). However, corns can also develop in a correctly shod horse if it has weak, collapsing heels or underrun heels.

The mild to moderate lameness (grade 1 – 3 of 5) that results may be constant or intermittent. The corn is diagnosed when the foot is examined, and the shoe is seen to be sitting on the sole. Once the shoe is removed and the sole in this area

> **More Information**
>
> Foot abnormalities and shoeing options are discussed in Chapter 7.

is trimmed, reddish discoloration may be seen in white-soled horses. Hoof tester pressure, applied across the heel and bar, often causes a painful response. In many cases the lameness disappears once the shoe is removed.

Corns generally resolve once the foot is trimmed and shod correctly. In horses with weak or underrun heels, shoeing the horse "full," extending the branches of the shoe, or using some other shoe that increases heel support can help prevent corns.

FOOT ABSCESSES

An abscess is an accumulation of pus: a mixture of tissue fluid, white blood cells, cell debris, and bacteria. When bacteria invade a tissue, they create an inflammatory response. Among other things, this response attracts white blood cells into the area and allows fluid to leak from the capillaries *(see Chapter 5)*.

Unlike skin and other soft tissues, the sole and hoof wall cannot expand to accommodate a buildup of fluid beneath their surface. So accumulation of fluid, whether pus or blood from a bruise, beneath the sole or hoof wall causes pain. It also causes an area of separation between the sole or hoof wall and the pedal bone.

The causes and management of abscesses beneath the sole and hoof wall are a little different. Therefore, subsolar abscesses and hoof wall abscesses are discussed separately.

Subsolar Abscesses

Subsolar means "beneath the sole." Subsolar abscesses generally develop as a result of a puncture wound or infection of a sole bruise. The horn of the sole is able to absorb fluid, so bacteria can enter the bruised area through the sole. This is more likely in horses kept in muddy paddocks or dirty stalls. It may also be possible for bacteria to spread to the bruised area via the bloodstream.

Signs of Subsolar Abscesses

Subsolar abscesses usually cause severe lameness (grade 4 – 5 of 5). The infection may have been slowly worsening for several days before it causes obvious signs. In some cases the lameness is so sudden and so severe that the owner or trainer believes that the horse

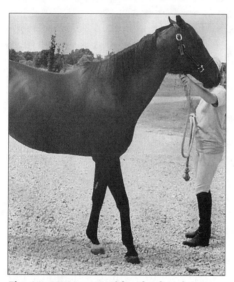

has a fracture. Veterinarians refer to a horse with this intensity of pain as being "fracture-lame." The pain is worse when the horse attempts to put weight on the foot. But the foot is still very painful when no weight is placed on it. So a horse with a subsolar abscess stands with just the toe touching the ground, or with the foot lifted off the ground.

In most cases there are no outward signs of infection, such as swelling or discharge. Occasionally an advanced abscess causes cellulitis, which is bacterial infection of the superficial structures

Fig. 15–48. Horses with subsolar abscesses stand with their weight off the foot.

under the skin *(see Chapter 13).* The result is diffuse swelling that begins at the coronet and spreads upward, sometimes reaching the middle of the cannon. This swelling may be confused with a problem in the fetlock or flexor tendons. However, when a foot abscess is the cause, the swelling is worse at the coronet. With joint and tendon problems the swelling usually is worse at the fetlock.

The affected foot may feel warmer than the other one, and the pulse pressure in the digital arteries is stronger than normal. If the abscess is confined to one side of the foot, it may be possible to detect a difference in pulse pressure be-

More Information

An increase in the pulse pressure occurs with many foot problems that involve inflammation or abnormalities of blood flow. See Chapter 4 for more information.

tween the inside and outside of the leg. The pulse is stronger on the same side as the abscess.

Diagnosis of Subsolar Abscesses

Hoof Tester Response

When faced with a very lame horse, with no apparent abnormalities (other than the stance), most experienced equine veterinarians reach for the foot first, to check for an abscess. Hoof testers produce a dramatic pain response with very little pressure over the abscessed area. A foot abscess can be precisely located with hoof testers if there is little or no pain elsewhere in the foot.

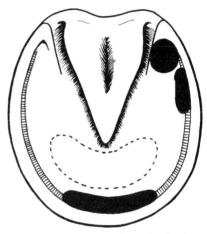

Fig. 15–49. Common sites of subsolar abscess. (The dotted line indicates the common site of sole bruising.)

The other two major causes of severe foot pain are pedal bone fractures and sole bruises. In most cases a fractured pedal bone does not produce as dramatic a pain response to the hoof testers as an abscess. Also, with a fracture the pain may be found over a larger area of the sole, with no specific area worse than the rest.

Sole bruises can also cause a severe pain response to the hoof testers in a specific location. In general, subsolar abscesses tend to develop near the white line. They are most common at the toe, quarter, or heel. Sole bruises are more likely in the center of the sole, from the tip of the frog forward. But these differences are generalizations.

Exploration

In many cases a subsolar abscess can only be distinguished from a sole bruise by finding either pus or blood when the painful area is opened up. It is usually necessary to remove the horse's shoe to examine the sole thoroughly. Many veterinarians and farriers use a nail puller to remove the nails one at a time. This method is slower than the usual way, but it is less painful for the horse. The nail puller is levered against the shoe, not against the hoof wall and sole.

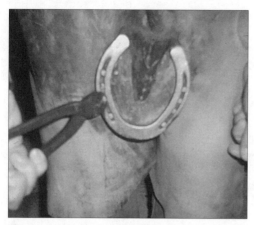

Fig. 15–50. Using a nail puller to remove the nails one at a time is less painful for the horse.

Once the shoe is removed, the sole is thoroughly cleaned with a brush and pared with a hoof knife. The veterinarian or farrier then inspects the sole for punctures or fissures. If a defect in the sole is found or suspected in the area where hoof testers caused the greatest response, the veterinarian or farrier may make a small exploratory hole. If blood oozes from the hole, the diagnosis is a sole bruise. If gray pus drains or spurts from the hole, the diagnosis is a subsolar abscess. Opening up the sole can be very painful for the horse, so some form of restraint or a nerve block *(see Chapter 2)* may be necessary. But once the pressure is relieved, the horse usually stands quietly for the rest of the procedure.

Treatment of Subsolar Abscesses
Drainage

Treatment involves draining the pus from the abscess. The small exploratory hole can be opened a little more to allow effective drainage. It is important that, wherever possible, the veterinarian or farrier limits the size of the hole to about ¼ inch (6 mm). The larger the hole, the longer it takes to close, and the longer the horse is out of work. Also, a large hole in the sole may allow the sensitive tissues to protrude through the opening and be damaged.

Most veterinarians and farriers poultice the foot for a few days to ensure complete drainage. Others simply apply an iodine-soaked dressing beneath a foot bandage. Some veterinarians use DMSO instead of iodine because DMSO is an anti-inflammatory compound, as well as being antibacterial.

Although the horse's relief may be immediate once the abscess is drained, subsolar abscesses take time to completely resolve, so the owner or trainer must be patient. The abscess may have spread quite a way under the sole. It may be necessary for the veterinarian or farrier to make other openings or enlarge the original hole over the next several days. If treatment must continue, or if a large area of the sole has been opened, a hospital plate *(see Chapter 7)* can be very useful. It improves the horse's comfort, keeps the sole clean and protected, and allows the horse to begin light exercise.

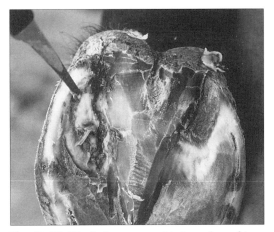

Fig. 15–51. The hole may need to be enlarged to drain the abscess.

Medications

Antibiotics are not usually necessary if the abscess has been drained well; drainage is of far more value. Also, there is some question as to whether antibiotics are able to reach a subsolar abscess because of the poor blood supply to the separated area. But if the horse has swelling in the leg (cellulitis), antibiotics are often a good idea, although they should never be given without or against veterinary advice. In every horse with a foot abscess, the tetanus status should be checked.

NSAIDs can make the horse more comfortable after the abscess is drained. However, they should only be necessary for a couple of days. If the abscess is still active, or has spread to other parts of the sole, NSAIDs may mask the lameness that would indicate the infection is not resolving.

(See Chapter 5 for more information on these medications.)

Chronic Subsolar Abscesses

Occasionally, subsolar abscesses may "smolder" for days or weeks. By the time the abscess is diagnosed, a large part of the sole may have been separated from the sensitive tissue by the buildup of pus. Typically, most of the pus is absorbed by the body, so when the veterinarian or farrier opens the sole, all that is found is a large cavity extending under most of the sole. It is a good idea to remove all of the separated sole and open up any tracts or crevices in the surrounding sole. In most cases, the horse has already begun to produce new horn beneath this area of separation. So all that is necessary after removing the separated sole is to protect the tender, new sole with a bandage and a shoe until it hardens. A pad may keep the sole soft by trapping moisture, and so should not be used until the new sole is hard.

Hoof Wall Abscesses ("Gravel")

Abscesses beneath the hoof wall are the most common type of foot abscess. Hoof wall abscesses begin when dirt and bacteria invade the sensitive tissues beneath the hoof wall through an area of separation at the white line. As dirt, manure, and even gravel (hence the name) pack into the defect, infection develops. It spreads up the wall between the sensitive and insensitive tissue, forming a tract that advances toward the coronary band, along the path of least resistance.

Separation of the sensitive tissues and pressure from the buildup of pus beneath the wall cause moderate to severe lameness (grade 3 – 5 of 5). When an abscess develops at the quarter or heel, the horse may stand with its toe pointed and no weight on the heel. There may be no outward signs of infection at first, although hoof wall abscesses occasionally cause swelling in the lower leg (cellulitis; discussed in the earlier section on *Subsolar Abscess*).

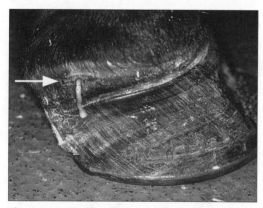

Fig. 15–52. Hoof wall abscesses often break out at the coronary band.

Hoof wall abscesses often break out at the coronary band, causing a slit just below the hairline that oozes pus for a day or so. This wound, which is more common at the quarter or heel, can be confused with an interference mark. In many cases the lameness improves or disappears once the abscess has drained. But if the abscess has not broken out, the diagnosis is made only after hoof testers locate a specific area of pain over the wall.

Infected shoe nail holes are often blamed for causing hoof wall infections if the nail was placed close to, or into the sensitive tissues of the wall. Although it is possible for these nail holes to become infected, the pain and lameness are usually due to inflammation, not infection. Typically, the lameness is resolved by removing the nail and treating the horse with a few days of poulticing, NSAIDs, and rest.

Treatment
Drainage

Treating a hoof wall abscess involves draining the pus from the infected wall. If the abscess has already broken out at the coronet, a poultice may be all that is necessary to completely resolve the problem. However, it is always a good idea for the veterinarian or farrier to remove the shoe and inspect the ground surface of the foot directly below the coronary wound. There will most likely be an area of separation that needs to be opened up and cleaned out. Occasionally, it may be necessary to open up the entire tract beneath the hoof wall to prevent reinfection.

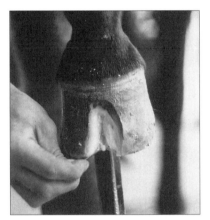 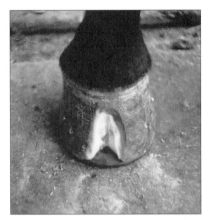

Fig. 15–53. Sometimes the entire tract must be opened up. Although the result may be unsightly, it is necessary to completely resolve the abscess.

If the abscess has not yet drained from the coronary band, it is necessary to open it by making a notch in the wall at the ground surface, over the area of greatest hoof tester response. All tracts beneath the wall should then be explored so that the area is exposed and drained.

Most veterinarians farriers poultice the foot for a few days after opening the infected wall. If the abscess has drained completely and the sole has not been damaged by infection or wall removal, the lameness should improve quickly over the next few days. The shoe can be replaced and the horse returned to work, usually within a week. Any further exploration or resection of the wall can be done with the shoe on, with minimal pain and interference to the horse.

Other Recommendations

It is important to take care of the foot while the shoe is off. The foot should be kept poulticed or bandaged to prevent the wall from chipping, and the horse should be kept in a clean, dry stall or small paddock. If the horse is still lame in 3 – 4 days the veterinarian should be called to re-examine the foot.

Antibiotics are usually not necessary for hoof wall abscesses, provided the abscess is adequately drained. NSAIDs can make the horse more comfortable, although they should only be necessary for a day or two. The horse's tetanus status must also be addressed. *(These therapies are discussed in Chapter 5.)*

Abscesses at the Bar

The bar is located between the heel and the frog. An abscess that forms at the bar may act more like a subsolar abscess than a hoof wall abscess *(see Figure 15–51)*. The abscess should be drained through as small a hole as possible. In most cases it is best to drain it through a small notch in the bar, instead of through the sole or wall. A bar shoe can protect and support the area while it heals *(see Chapter 7)*.

WHITE LINE DISEASE ("SEEDY TOE")

"White line disease" and "seedy toe" are different names for the same condition. White line disease is a better term because seedy toe implies that the condition occurs only at the toe, which is not the case.

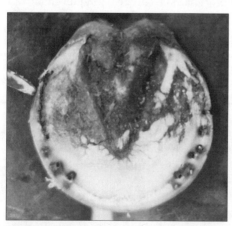

Fig. 15–54. White line disease causes a crevice between the hoof wall and sole.

The basic problem is separation between the hoof wall and sole at the white line. The separated area can spread vertically up the hoof wall, as well as horizontally toward the heel or toe. It may involve any part of the wall from the toe to the heel.

At first, separation of the wall does not cause lameness because it involves only the insensitive tissues. But lameness can occur if the dirt and other material that pack into the crevice results in a hoof wall abscess. Lameness can also occur when the ground forces cause the separated wall to splay out. This can tear the sensitive tissues.

Causes

There are several factors that can contribute to, or cause white line disease:

- hoof wall conformation that causes flaring of the wall; e.g., horses with flat, "pie plate" feet
- irregular shoeing or trimming intervals—this allows the hoof wall to grow long, which encourages flaring or stretching of the wall
- imbalance of hoof moisture, such as environmental conditions that are too wet or too dry, or are alternately too wet then too dry
- laminitis—this causes breakdown of the hoof wall–pedal bone bond (discussed earlier), and separation of the wall at toe
- a hoof wall abscess, which leaves a tract up the inside of the wall
- direct trauma to the hoof wall

Occasionally, the separation begins higher up the hoof, beneath the wall. For example, a hard knock to the hoof wall may cause bleeding in the sensitive tissues beneath the wall. The knock may have been caused by the foot striking a solid jump, a player hitting the hoof with a polo mallet, or some other traumatic incident. The resulting hematoma is like a blood blister beneath a fingernail. It separates the wall at that location. When this defect grows down, the area of separation is seen at the ground surface.

Some farriery publications attribute white line degeneration to fungal infection—a condition they call onychomycosis (literally, "fungal infection of the nail"). Onychomycosis is a term used in human and veterinary medicine for fungal nailbed infections. However, unlike people and dogs, horses do not have a nailbed as such. The hoof grows from the coronary band, not the white line. So fungal infection of the white line in horses is not the same as onychomycosis in people or dogs. Several types of fungi and many species of bacteria can be found in these separated areas of the hoof wall. But these organisms are "opportunistic"—they are taking advantage of the situation. Finding them in the defect does not necessarily mean they caused the problem. (**Note:** This condition is not contagious from horse-to-horse or from horse-to-human. The organisms that invade the separated area are normally found in the horse's environment.)

Treatment of White Line Disease

Treating white line disease involves completely removing the separated wall and opening up any tracts or fissures in the wall above or around the separated area. This procedure is necessary to prevent further separation, and resolve the infection that inevitably develops beneath the wall. The problem cannot be resolved simply by cleaning out the defect; the separated wall must be removed. Resection of the separated wall is not a painful or bloody procedure because the separated part of the hoof wall is insensitive.

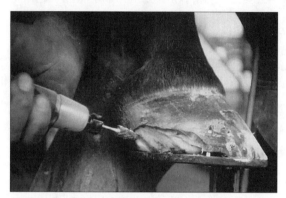

Fig. 15–55. Treating white line disease involves removing all of the separated wall.

If the problem has gone untreated for some time it may be necessary to remove a large area of the wall. The farrier or veterinarian may remove the separated wall in stages so that there is enough wall to hold the shoe nails. Or, the wall can be reconstructed with acrylic resin *(see Chapter 7)*. A shoe that supports the entire foot should be used until the defect grows out. At each subsequent shoeing the farrier may need to explore the wall, searching for new areas of separation or tracts beneath the wall. Unless large areas of the wall have been removed, the horse can usually be exercised normally.

The veterinarian or farrier may recommend topical antifungal medications or disinfectants. However, in most cases the infection resolves without such treatment once the separated wall is removed. Systemic antibiotics are neither necessary nor effective in treating white line disease. Astringents, such as "bluestone" (copper sulfate) and formalin (formaldehyde), are common remedies for white line disease. However, these solutions can overdry the hoof, so they should be used sparingly.

KERATOMA

A keratoma is a non-cancerous tumor involving the tissue that produces the hoof wall and sole. It derives its name from the type of cell involved: the cells that produce keratin. Keratin is the substance that makes up the insensitive layer (horn) of the hoof wall and sole.

Keratomas are extremely uncommon. When they occur, they typically cause the hoof wall or sole to bulge. Once a hoof wall keratoma grows down to the ground surface, it is seen as a whitish mass, pushing out between the white line and the hoof wall. In advanced cases the tumor puts pressure on the pedal bone. Chronic pressure can cause the bone to absorb some of the calcium from that site *(see Chapter 9)*. On radiographs this part of the bone is less dense (less white).

Treatment involves removing the hoof wall or sole overlying the swelling, and removing the entire mass of abnormal tissue. It may be necessary to remove a strip of wall from the ground surface to the coronary band. Although this procedure can be done after a nerve block, it is usually quicker, easier, and less painful if the horse is anesthetized.

After removing the overlying wall or sole and abnormal tissue, the exposed area is covered with an iodine-soaked dressing, and the entire foot is kept bandaged and dry until the exposed tissue hardens. The horse's tetanus status should be checked *(see Chapter 5)*. A shoe that supports the compromised wall should be used until normal hoof wall has grown down to the ground surface *(see Chapter 7)*.

QUARTER CRACKS

Quarter cracks are complete, full thickness hoof wall cracks. They occur anywhere between the quarter and the heel, and extend up into the coronary band. Quarter cracks can appear suddenly, and cause moderate to severe lameness (grade 3 – 4 of 5). Or they can develop slowly, and cause intermittent mild to moderate lameness (grade 1 – 3 of 5).

Note
Causes and management of hoof wall cracks are covered in Chapter 7. Quarter cracks are discussed separately because they typically cause lameness, and require more specific management.

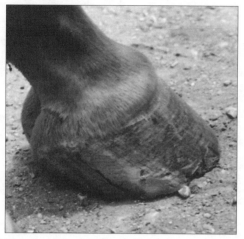

Fig. 15–56. A quarter crack.

Foot conformation is an important contributing factor in the development of quarter cracks. The long toe–low heel foot shape of many Thoroughbreds predisposes to overloading of the heels. At the other extreme, the narrow, upright, long-heel foot shape typically found in Saddlebreds and other "gaited" breeds causes excess concussion on the heels. With either foot shape, the repeated pounding caused by working on hard surfaces can damage the hoof wall at the quarter or heel, particularly if the work surface is irregular. Shoes that are too small or have short branches lessen heel support, so they can also contribute to overloading of the heels and quarters.

Management of Quarter Cracks

Quarter cracks can be very difficult to resolve because the factors that cause them often cannot be totally controlled. Recurrence or persistence of the crack is always a possibility. A concerted team effort by the veterinarian, farrier, and owner or trainer is necessary for the best result.

Management of these cracks has three goals:

- relieve pain
- prevent further wall and coronary band damage
- encourage healthy new horn to grow down in place of the defect

To achieve these goals, the veterinarian and farrier have several options.

Relieving Pain

The pain and lameness occur when the sides of the crack move independently, which pinches or tears the sensitive tissues beneath. This happens because one side of the crack moves more than the other when the horse bears weight on the foot.

Restricting movement across the crack relieves the pain. It can be achieved in a couple of ways. A diagonal or three-quarter bar shoe can be effective because it relieves the damaged heel of all weight-bearing. Alternatively, a narrow strip of wall can be removed along the ground surface behind the crack. This unloads the damaged wall. A full bar shoe is then applied to support the heels. The gap between the wall and the shoe must be

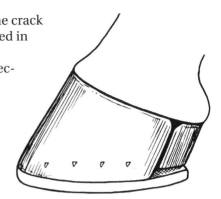

Fig. 15–57. Options for treating a quarter crack.

cleaned out every day with a hoof pick, hack saw blade, or flat-headed screwdriver, to prevent dirt from packing into the defect.

Another approach is to stabilize the crack with an acrylic patch. In most cases the patch is reinforced with wire laces or a small metal plate that bridges the crack. The wall at the ground surface can also be unloaded to minimize stress on the patch.

Preventing Further Damage

Minimizing movement across the crack also prevents further hoof wall or coronary band damage. This is important because scarring of the coronary band can result in a permanent hoof wall defect. There are a couple of other techniques that can be used to prevent further damage. A triangle of wall, with the crack at its center, can be pared out just below the coronary band. Or, the crack can be pared out along its entire length.

Encouraging Normal Wall Growth

Unless the coronary band is permanently damaged, healthy new horn can be encouraged in a number of ways. The techniques mentioned for unloading and supporting the heels can be effective because they prevent the crack from extending into the new horn as it grows down.

But sometimes it is best to remove all of the wall behind the crack. The wall at the heel is removed from the ground surface to the coronary band. This is like wiping the slate clean and starting over. It is painful, so a nerve block or general anesthesia is necessary. The exposed tissue must be protected with a bandage until it hardens, which usually takes 1 – 2 weeks. A bar shoe is needed to support the foot until the new wall has grown down to the ground surface.

LACERATIONS & AVULSIONS

Horses often sustain wounds that lacerate the coronary band or rip up a piece of hoof wall (an avulsion). Getting a foot caught in wire fencing, a cattle guard, or a board wall or partition is a common cause of such injuries. These wounds can be bloody and very painful when they first occur. Nevertheless, it is often remarkable how well they heal with prompt veterinary attention, and diligence on the part of the owner or trainer.

Coronary Band Lacerations

If part of the coronary band is lost or permanently damaged, hoof wall growth from that part will always be defective. The result can be

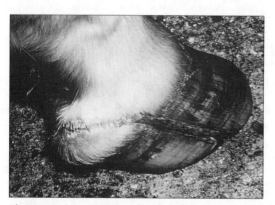

Fig. 15–58. A permanent hoof wall defect result-ing from a coronary band laceration.

a permanently weak-ened wall. For this reason, the veterinar-ian usually makes every effort to suture wounds that involve the coronary band. If the wound is sutured within a few hours of injury, the results are generally very good. The coronary band has an excellent blood supply, so it heals very well with proper care.

First Aid

While waiting for the veterinarian to arrive, the wound should be cleaned and bandaged. It is unwise to cut off a loose piece of skin hanging from the coronet. Doing so can prevent the coronary band from healing without scarring. It can make a real difference to the outcome if the skin flap is cleaned, replaced, and bandaged before the veterinarian arrives.

Management

After treating the wound, the veterinarian either bandages the area or places a bell cast on the foot. A bell cast is a fiberglass cast that completely encases the foot, and extends to the top of the pastern. The cast minimizes movement and tension on the skin. Even if the wound could not be sutured, casting the foot for 2 – 3 weeks can substantially speed healing, as well as improve the cosmetic result. If a cast is not used, the foot should be kept bandaged, changing the bandage as often as necessary (usually every 1 – 2 days). Whether the wound is bandaged or cast, the horse should be confined to a clean, dry stall or small paddock until the wound has completely healed. With any wound, the horse's tetanus status should be checked. *(See Section II: Principles of Therapy for more information on these treatments.)*

After about 2 weeks, the veterinarian inspects the wound and decides whether further bandaging or casting is necessary. By this time, the sutures have done their job. Also, any part of the wound that could not be sutured, or in which the edges pulled apart, has begun to fill in with healthy granulation tissue *(see Chapter 13)*. In many cases the wound can be left uncovered at this point. However, if the wound was deep or extensive, or is not healing well, the veterinarian may keep the area bandaged or apply another cast for a further 2 weeks.

Sometimes a wound that results from the foot being caught in a fence or between two boards actually looks worse over the first 1 – 2 weeks. Most horses struggle to free themselves when the foot is caught; this can tear or destroy the blood vessels in the skin. Even though the wound may not look too bad at first, over the next several days the skin around the wound dies and sloughs (lifts away). As a result, the wound looks larger, and weeps serum or pus. These wounds eventually heal, although they generally take longer than a clean cut, and they leave more of a scar.

Hoof Wall Avulsions

A wound in which part of the hoof wall is torn away is called an avulsion. The veterinarian or farrier must cut off the loose piece of wall as close to the coronet as possible (without cutting the coronary tissue), or at its point of attachment to the wall. It is no use trying to secure the torn piece of wall to the hoof. It will not reattach to the underlying tissue, and infection will inevitably develop underneath. After the damaged wall is removed, the foot should be kept bandaged until the exposed tissue hardens. This usually takes a couple of

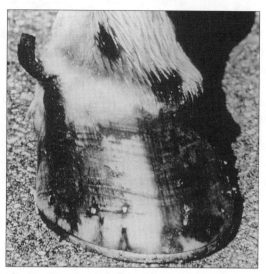

Fig. 15–59. A hoof wall avulsion.

weeks. The horse's tetanus status should also be checked *(see Chapter 5).*

If the avulsion involves the entire length of the wall it takes several months for new wall to grow down to the ground surface. Avulsions at the heel take about 6 months, and those at the toe take about 12 months. During that time a shoe which stabilizes and supports the hoof wall should be used. *(See Chapter 7 for more information on shoeing options.)*

OTHER CONDITIONS
Thrush

Thrush is bacterial infection of the frog. The bacteria that cause the infection are normally found in the horse's environment. They grow very well in wet, unsanitary conditions such as a dirty stall or a muddy paddock. These bacteria prefer a low-oxygen environment, such as is found in the clefts of the frog. Thrush is often seen in horses with narrow or contracted heels because this situation results in a shrunken frog with

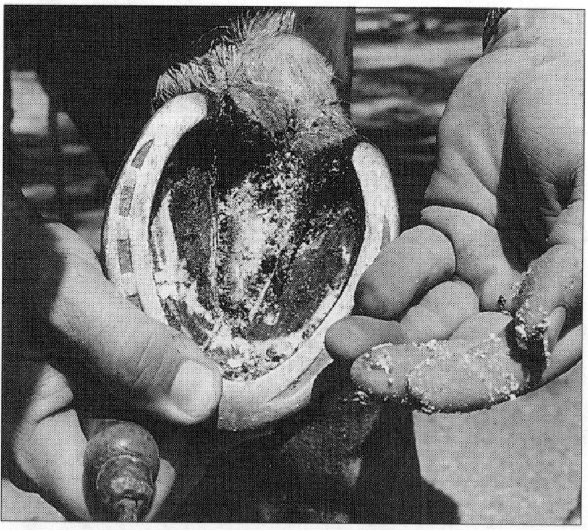

Fig. 15–60. A foot with thrush: the frog's surface is white and crumbly.

deep clefts *(see Chapter 7)*. But thrush can occur in any horse.

The infection is usually identified when the owner or farrier is picking out the horse's feet. The feet have an offensive odor, and the surface of the frog is white and crumbly. Horses with thrush are not necessarily lame. But when the infection invades the sensitive tissues of the frog, it can cause lameness. As a general rule, if the horse reacts when the clefts of the frog are picked out, or if blood is seen, the thrush is severe enough to cause lameness.

When a farrier or veterinarian finds thrush, he or she trims the frog to remove any loose tags of horn and expose the infected areas. Routine treatment recommendations usually include:

- thoroughly picking out the feet
- vigorously cleansing the feet—especially the clefts—with warm water and disinfectant
- painting the frog with an iodine solution or commercial thrush lotion

Medications containing formalin should not be used if the frog is tender when cleaned out. It often helps to pack iodine-soaked cotton balls into the clefts.

The feet should be thoroughly cleaned and painted with thrush medication twice per day, and the horse kept in a clean, dry environment. When an owner finds or suspects thrush, he or she should follow these treatment recommendations, and bring the problem to the farrier's attention at the next visit.

Thrush usually resolves quickly and completely if these steps are taken. However, it may return if the contracted heels are not corrected, and if the horse is not kept in a clean, dry area.

Canker

Canker is another foul-smelling hoof infection that usually involves the frog. But unlike thrush, it often causes chronic lameness. In the past canker was a common problem in draft horses. These days it is very uncommon in any breed, presumably because knowledge and management techniques have improved.

Canker causes the growth of irregular, grayish, granular material from the frog. In severe cases it spreads to the back of the heels.

Canker can be very difficult to resolve. Treatment involves trimming away all abnormal tissue, and diligently treating the underlying area with lotion or ointment that contains antibiotics and corticosteroids. Canker is more commonly seen in horses kept in wet, un-

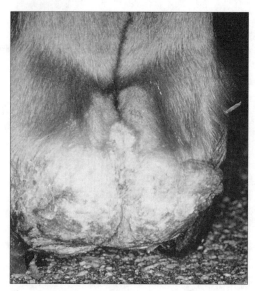

Fig. 15–61. A severe case of canker.

sanitary conditions, so it is essential that the feet are kept clean and dry.

Sheared Heels

Sheared heels develops when one heel is longer than the other on the same foot. It can result from several situations, including:

- uneven weight-bearing due to pain in one heel
- abnormal hoof growth at one heel
- improper trimming, causing uneven heels

Pain in one heel causes the horse to protect that heel by putting less weight on it. As a result, that heel grows longer than the other. In the meantime, the other heel bears more of the horse's weight and sustains more of the ground impact forces during exercise. This alone can cause heel pain and lameness, even before uneven heel height is obvious. Abnormal hoof wall growth at one heel may be due to poor conformation or a coronary band injury.

When the heels are a different height they are not loaded equally. This causes the sensitive tissues of the hoof wall on the longer heel to tear (be sheared) when the horse bears weight on the foot. Tearing or shearing of the soft tissues between the heels can also occur in severe cases. Either situation can result in intermittent or persistent lameness. Because the pain is at the heels, the horse may show gait abnor-

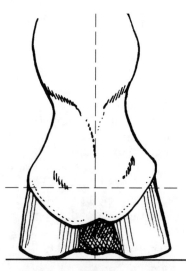

Fig. 15–62. With sheared heels, one heel is longer than the other.

malities similar to a horse with navicular syndrome, although sheared heels often occurs in only one foot.

Treatment involves trimming the heels, and the rest of the foot, evenly. A shoe that supports the heels should then be fitted *(see Chapter 7)*.

Sidebone

On each side of the pedal bone is a large, rounded piece of cartilage called the lateral cartilage. These two cartilages support and protect the soft tissues at the back of the foot. They also support the hoof wall in that area.

Sidebone is a condition in which the lateral cartilages become calcified. These tissues probably calcify because of chronic, repeated concussion, such as frequently exercising on hard surfaces. Although sidebone is seen in horses with normally-shaped feet, it is more com-

lateral cartilage

wing of the pedal bone

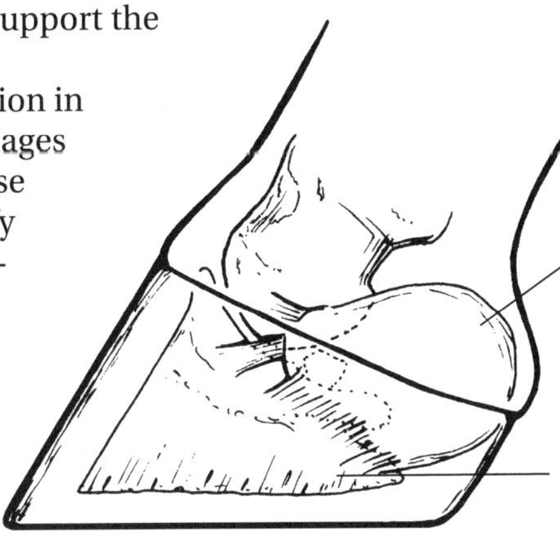

Fig. 15–63. The lateral cartilages support and protect the soft tissues at the back of the foot.

mon in horses with narrow, upright feet. It is also common in horses with unbalanced feet, especially those that toe in or toe out. In most cases, the changes occur in the forefeet. Only one cartilage in just one foot may be calcified. But it is possible to find both cartilages in one foot, one cartilage in each foot, or both cartilages in both feet calcified.

In very severe cases sidebone can be diagnosed with palpation: the normally flexible cartilages just above, and to the outside of the heel bulbs become thickened and hard. However, in most cases sidebone is diagnosed while radiographing the foot for another reason. In other words, sidebone is an incidental finding. It is best seen on the view of the foot that is taken from the front (the dorso-palmar view; *see Chapter 2*).

Mild or early cases of sidebone may be seen as small islands of calcification. Moderate to severe sidebone is seen as calcification of

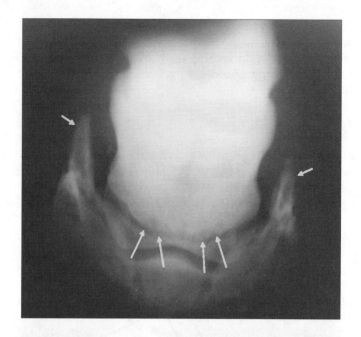

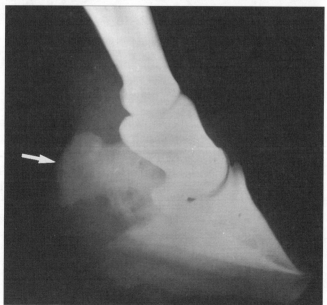

Fig. 15–64. Top: Sidebone is an incidental finding in this horse with navicular syndrome. Bottom: Severe sidebone, visible even on a lateral (side) view.

most or all of the lateral cartilage. In some cases it may appear as if there is line of separation between the calcified cartilage and the pedal bone. This line may be a fracture line, although it could be a line of uncalcified cartilage. This determination is difficult to make.

The importance of sidebone as a cause of lameness is open to question. Sidebone is found in horses that are not lame, or that are lame from another cause. The lateral cartilages are blocked by a Palmar Digital nerve block *(see Chapter 2)*. However, other structures more likely to cause lameness are also desensitized with this block, in particular, the navicular area and the heels. It would be foolhardy to suggest that sidebone is causing the lameness when there are abnormalities in the heel area on examination of the foot or obvious radiographic changes in the navicular bone. Nevertheless, sidebone does indicate that the foot has sustained chronic concussion.

Quittor

Quittor is chronic bacterial infection of the lateral cartilage of the pedal bone. In most cases it involves only one side of one foot. It occurs as a result of one of the following situations:

- a penetrating wound at the heel bulb or side of the foot, involving the lateral cartilage
- spread of infection from a puncture wound or abscess at the quarter or heel (both discussed earlier)

The hallmark of quittor is persistent or intermittent discharge of pus from a wound at the coronet. The wound is found at the quarter or heel—that is, near the infected cartilage. A hoof wall abscess also may erupt at the coronary band in this area and create a wound that drains pus. However, the wound caused by an abscess usually dries up quickly and

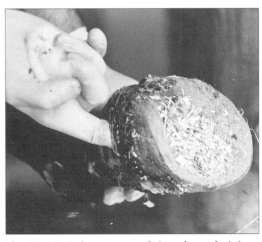

Fig. 15–65. Quittor can result in a deep, draining wound at the coronet.

heals completely. Quittor either continues to ooze, or dries up, only to break out and ooze again. In most cases quittor causes only mild lameness (grade 1 – 2 of 5).

Treatment must include surgical removal of the damaged cartilage, either under nerve block or general anesthesia. Antibiotics alone will not completely resolve the infection—the source of infection (the diseased cartilage) must be removed.

The wound is already contaminated, so the veterinarian may either leave the wound unsutured, or suture it closed but leave in a latex drain tube that allows pus and serum to escape. Post-operative care involves tetanus prevention, antibiotics, NSAIDs, and daily bathing and bandaging of the wound until it has healed *(see Section II: Principles of Therapy)*. However, even with proper surgical treatment, the problem may persist and the veterinarian may need to repeat the surgery.

16

THE PASTERN & FETLOCK

S pecific conditions of the pastern and fetlock are combined in this chapter for two reasons. First, some structures are common to both areas. For example, the first pastern bone forms the lower part of the fetlock joint, and the distal sesamoidean ligaments begin at the fetlock but attach onto the pastern. Second, the forces and factors that damage the pastern also stress the fetlock. So in many cases both areas are strained or injured at the same time.

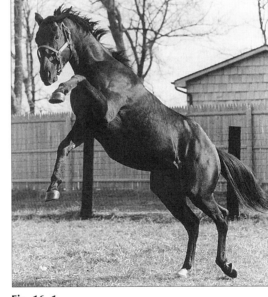

Fig. 16–1.

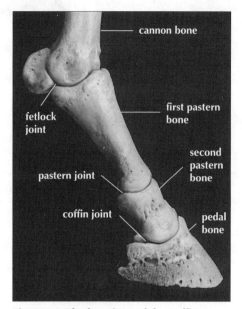

Fig. 16–2. The locations of the coffin, pastern, and fetlock joints.

RINGBONE
Definition

Ringbone is bony proliferation on the pastern bones. Typically, the changes are worse around the pastern joint or coffin joint. In severe and long-standing cases the bony proliferation may extend most or all of the way around the pastern, which is why the condition is called "ringbone."

There are a couple of descriptive terms for ringbone, based on the location of the bony changes. "High" ringbone involves the lower part of the first pastern bone and/or the upper part of the second pastern bone. "Low" ringbone involves the lower part of the second pastern bone and/or the top of the pedal bone. Severe low ringbone may produce an obvious bony swelling at the coronet. This is sometimes called "buttress foot" or "pyramidal disease."

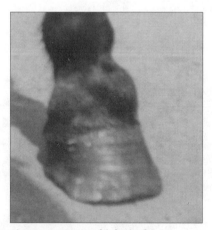

Fig. 16–3. Severe high ringbone.

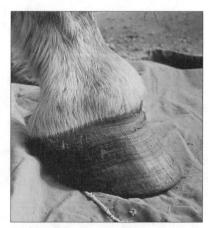

Fig. 16–4. Severe low ringbone.

An important distinction is whether the ringbone is articular or non-articular. Articular ringbone involves a joint and is therefore more likely to cause lameness than non-articular ringbone.

Causes

Ringbone is a process of new bone production on the surfaces of the affected bones. This new bone formation, or exostosis, may be the result of three types of insult:

Definition
Periosteum: the outer covering of a bone. **It is a thin, but very tough membrane that consists of fibrous tissue, blood vessels, nerves, and osteoblasts (bone-forming cells).**

1. Tension on the periosteum from an attached tendon, ligament, or joint capsule. Excessive tension on these structures can strain and inflame the periosteum at the point of attachment, leading to new bone production at the stresspoint.
2. Osteoarthritis of the pastern and/or coffin joint.
3. Direct trauma to the surface of the bone.

The tendons and ligaments that attach onto the pastern bones, and which can result in an exostosis, include:

- the extensor tendon at the front of the pastern
- the superficial digital flexor tendon branches and the collateral ligaments at the sides of the pastern
- the distal sesamoidean ligaments (discussed later) at the back of the pastern

If stretching or tearing of any of these structures results in joint instability, new bone is laid down more quickly and in greater amounts in an effort to stabilize the joint.

In many cases articular ringbone is a form of osteoarthritis—the endstage of severe degenerative joint disease *(see Chapter 8)*. New bone is laid down around the joint in an effort to immobilize the painful joint, and in response to chronic inflammation of the joint capsule. Eventually, the bone bridges the joint, preventing any further movement and pain. However, it may take years for this process to be completed. In the meantime, the inflammation and degenerative changes in and around the joint cause chronic lameness.

Direct trauma to the periosteum caused, for example, by a knock or a laceration, can result in an exostosis at that site. However, unlike

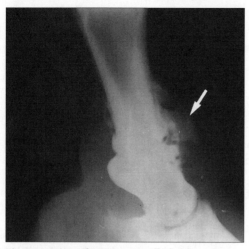

Fig. 16–5. New bone eventually bridges the joint.

ringbone caused by tension on the soft tissues or chronic joint disease, ringbone due to trauma is usually not progressive. That is, the bony changes do not continue to worsen, unless the injury also damaged the supporting soft tissues of the pastern or coffin joint.

Poor pastern or foot conformation and improper shoeing can predispose the horse to ringbone. The following faults are more likely to eventually result in ringbone:

- long, sloping pasterns
- very upright pasterns
- long toe–low heel foot shape
- toed-in ("pigeon-toed") or toed-out ("splay-footed") stance
- unbalanced feet

(Foot conformation is discussed in Chapter 7.)

These faults cause uneven stresses on the lower joints, abnormal tension on some of the soft tissues, and excessive concussion. Each of these stresses can contribute to inflammation and bony changes in or around the pastern and coffin joints.

Signs and Diagnosis of Ringbone

Ringbone is mostly seen in mature horses, particularly those performing strenuous activities. It is much more common in the forelegs than in the hindlegs. Bony changes often develop in both forelegs, but in most cases they are worse in one leg.

High ringbone eventually results in:

- bony swelling around the pastern
- reduced mobility of the pastern joint
- pain during manipulation (flexion and rotation) of the joint
- mild to moderate lameness (grade 1 – 3 of 5)

Early or mild cases usually show mild lameness (grade 1 – 2 of 5), but little or no swelling around the pastern. However, on close inspection, a small amount of thickening may be seen or felt, especially when compared with the opposite pastern. Also, firm palpation and manipulation of the pastern may cause a mild pain response.

Low ringbone may have no outward signs, other than moderate lameness (grade 2 – 3 of

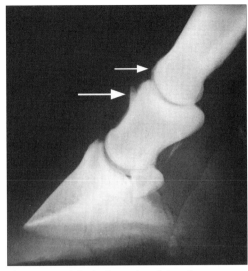

Fig. 16–6. High ringbone involving the pastern joint.

5). Advanced cases may develop a bony swelling at the coronet. Almost all horses with low ringbone are lame because the bony changes are so close to the coffin joint and its supporting structures.

The diagnosis can be confirmed with radiography. This is important in determining whether the ringbone involves a joint. The treatment and the prognosis may depend upon this information.

Treatment of Ringbone

Except for cases caused by direct trauma, ringbone is a progressive, degenerative disease. So, treatment is unlikely to result in a permanent cure. The aims of management are: 1) to slow the progression of the disease by reducing or controlling the mechanical factors that contribute to it, and 2) to relieve the horse's pain.

The farrier must balance the feet as much as possible and apply a shoe that completely supports the heels. When ringbone is advanced, a half-round shoe, which allows the horse to break over at the most comfortable point, can help some horses. *(See Chapter 7 for more information on shoeing options.)*

NSAIDs are important for making the horse more comfortable and reducing inflammation within and around the affected joint(s). In many cases, giving NSAIDs when necessary, or using continual low-dose therapy makes the horse comfortable enough for some type of

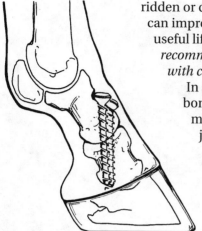

Fig. 16–7. Surgical fusion of the pastern joint.

ridden or driven activity. Daily light exercise can improve the horse's gait and extend its useful life. *(See Chapter 8 for more specific recommendations on managing horses with chronic joint disease.)*

In severe cases of high, articular ringbone, the veterinarian may recommend surgery to fuse the pastern joint. This procedure is called arthrodesis. Under general anesthesia the pastern joint is opened up and the cartilage is stripped away from the joint surfaces. A bone graft is packed into the joint space, and the joint is stabilized with bone screws or a bone plate. A cast is then applied to immobilize the pastern during the first few weeks of healing. *(See Chapter 6 for more information on bone grafts and casts.)*

This invasive procedure may permanently resolve the lameness (after several months of rest) because it eliminates the major source of pain—inflammation and instability of the joint. Articular ringbone is the body's attempt to stabilize a joint, and surgical fusion simply accelerates and completes this process. However, the surgical technique itself can cause extra bony proliferation, so the cosmetic result may not be very good. Arthrodesis of the coffin joint is virtually impossible because the joint is located within the hoof. Also, the functional result of coffin joint fusion is disappointing. Although this joint has a limited range of motion, that small degree of mobility is very important for normal locomotion.

Prognosis for Ringbone

The prognosis for continued athletic usefulness depends on a few different factors, including:

- the location and severity of the bony changes—in particular, how close they are to a joint
- the speed at which the condition is worsening
- the horse's use

A horse that is not exercised intensely (at speed or over high jumps) may remain usable for some time. But a horse that performs

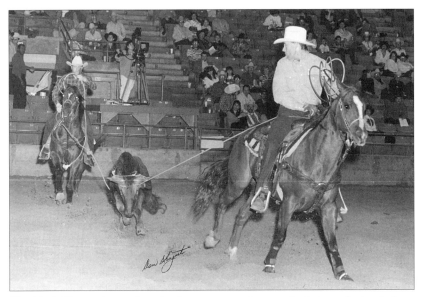

Fig. 16–8. The pasterns of roping horses are under constant stress during training and competition.

strenuous activities, such as a three-day-eventer or calf roping horse, may not be able to train and compete at its former level. These horses are constantly stressing their pastern joints during training and competition.

PASTERN FRACTURES

Fractures of the first pastern bone (P1) or second pastern bone (P2) usually occur during exercise. In most cases a sudden stop or sharp turn causes the fracture, so they are more common in Western performance horses and polo ponies. Pastern fractures can also occur when a horse is turned out after a period of confinement, or breaks away and gets loose. In many cases there is a history of a vague, undiagnosed lameness that was present for days or weeks before the pastern fracture occurred. There most likely was a bone defect, such as a small, incomplete or "stress" fracture, before the fracture occurred. A sharp turn or a wrong step may have created enough stress on the abnormal bone that it fractured.

Pastern fractures can occur in any horse. However, they are more likely in horses wearing shoes with traction devices, such as heel caulks or toe grabs *(see Chapter 7)*. The shoe fixes the foot in place,

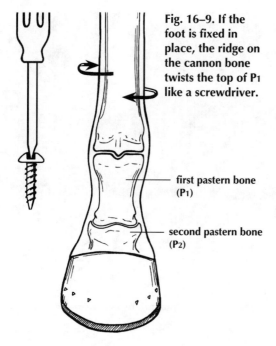

Fig. 16–9. If the foot is fixed in place, the ridge on the cannon bone twists the top of P1 like a screwdriver.

first pastern bone (P1)

second pastern bone (P2)

but as the horse turns, the limb rotates above it; these twisting forces are concentrated at the pastern. Fractures of P1 are sometimes called "screwdriver" injuries. The bottom of the cannon bone has a central ridge that fits into a groove on the top of P1, like a flat-headed screwdriver fits into a screw head. When the horse turns with the foot fixed, the ridge on the cannon bone twists the top of P1. (**Note:** This injury can also occur in horses with regular shoes. Traction devices make it more likely, but they are not the sole cause.)

Pastern fractures in either P1 or P2 can be:

- sagittal—a vertical fracture running down the center of the bone
- comminuted—multiple fracture lines creating several fracture fragments
- avulsion—a piece of bone pulled off by an attached tendon or ligament
- chip fractures within a joint (discussed later)

Sagittal, comminuted, and chip fractures involve at least one joint surface. Depending on the type of fracture and the bone involved, the fetlock, pastern, or coffin joint may be affected.

The treatment and prognosis depend on several factors, but as a general guide the following principles apply:

- displaced fractures are more serious than non-displaced fractures
- P1 fractures are more serious than similar P2 fractures
- fractures that involve two joints are more serious than fractures involving only one joint
- fractures that involve the fetlock joint are more serious than those involving the pastern or coffin joints

Sagittal Fractures

Sagittal fractures of P1 typically start in the shallow groove on the joint surface at the top of the bone. The fracture line then runs vertically down the center of the bone. It may stop halfway down the bone, or it may continue to the lower joint surface. Sometimes the fracture line runs at an angle and comes out at the side of the bone. Sagittal fractures of P2 are very uncommon.

More Information

Types of fractures and treatment options are discussed in Chapter 9.

This section contains specific recommendations for managing pastern fractures.

Signs and Diagnosis

Sagittal fractures can be difficult to diagnose just from the history and signs. Although the horse may develop a sudden, severe lameness (grade 4 – 5 of 5) during exercise, there may be very little swelling around the pastern at first. Sagittal P1 fractures begin in the fetlock joint. The effusion (accumulation of joint fluid) that develops makes it easy to mistakenly focus on the fetlock as the site of pain, rather than on the pastern. However, careful palpation of the pastern usually reveals pain at the front of P1. Compressing the sides of the pastern also causes pain because it exerts pressure across the fracture line. Flexion of the fetlock causes pain, too, although this is true of several joint problems that do not primarily involve the pastern bone. Unless P1 is completely broken in two, crepitus (crunching of bone-on-bone) is not heard or felt.

The diagnosis must be confirmed with radiographs. If the fracture extends to the lower joint surface or out the side of the bone, any weight placed on the leg will have separated the fracture line a millimeter or so. But if the fracture is incomplete there may only be a very thin fracture line. The fracture may not be obvious for several days, so the veterinarian may need to

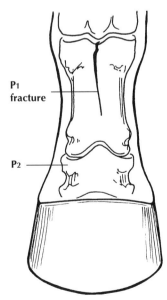

Fig. 16–10. An incomplete sagittal fracture of P1.

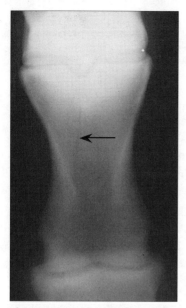

Fig. 16–11. An incomplete sagittal fracture of P₁.

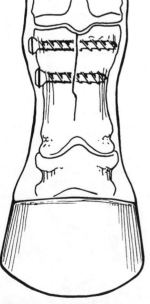

Fig. 16–12. Lag screw repair of a P₁ fracture.

take repeat radiographs before a diagnosis can be made.

When the signs and radiographs are inconclusive, other tests, such as nerve blocks and nuclear scintigraphy, may be necessary to localize the site of lameness *(see Chapter 2)*. However, most veterinarians are cautious about using nerve blocks in a horse suspected of having a fracture. If nuclear scintigraphy is not an option, the veterinarian may simply recommend confining the horse and repeating the radiographs.

Treatment of Sagittal Fractures

Sagittal fractures generally are best repaired with lag screws *(see Chapter 6)*, even if the fracture is incomplete. Any weight-bearing on the leg can cause the fracture to extend and become complete and displaced. Also, because the fracture involves at least one joint surface (typically, the fetlock), it is very important that the fracture line is compressed and the joint surface correctly aligned. Otherwise, degenerative joint disease and chronic lameness will result *(see Chapter 8)*.

Effective compression of the fracture and alignment of the joint surface cannot be achieved with just a bandage or cast. Moreover, a cast cannot prevent the fracture from extending, because it does little to counteract the vertical (weight-bearing) forces on the pastern. But the surgeon may apply a fiberglass cast after surgically repairing the fracture. The cast minimizes movement in the fetlock and pastern joints while the bone heals. It is usually left on, and changed as often as necessary, for 3 – 4 weeks. *(Post-operative care following bone screw repair of a fracture is discussed in Chapter 6.)*

Prognosis for Sagittal Fractures

The prognosis for return to athletic function is fairly good if fracture healing progressed well and degenerative changes in the joints are minimal. In most cases the screws are left in place once the fracture has healed.

Comminuted Fractures

Comminuted pastern fractures, whether of P_1 or P_2, can be devastating injuries in which the bone is completely shattered. In most cases the diagnosis is straightforward. There is usually a history of sudden, severe lameness during exercise. Signs include:

- swelling around the pastern
- reluctance to bear any weight on the leg
- pain and crepitus (crunching of bone-on-bone) when the pastern is manipulated

Radiography is used to confirm the diagnosis and determine the severity of the fracture.

Treatment

Some comminuted pastern fractures can be stabilized with screws or a bone plate, although this is not always possible. The extreme twisting forces that fracture the bone can shatter it into several pieces, none of which is large enough to support the joint above or below it. For satisfactory healing, there must be at least one piece of bone that can act as a

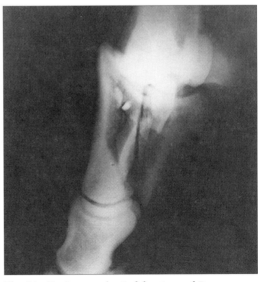

Fig. 16–13. A comminuted fracture of P_1.

support column between the joint above and below it. A bone plate can act as a support, but only if there are bone pieces large enough to hold the bone screws.

To prevent later degenerative joint disease, the surgeon may also surgically fuse the pastern joint (arthrodesis; discussed earlier). As the fracture heals, the joint fuses with new bone, and is no longer a source of persistent pain. However, coffin joint arthrodesis has some practical drawbacks, so it is generally not an option for comminuted P2 fractures. If fetlock arthrodesis is necessary, the horse's athletic career is over; this is just a salvage procedure. (A comminuted fracture that requires pastern arthrodesis may also end the horse's athletic career. But there is some chance that the horse may eventually return to light activities after this procedure.)

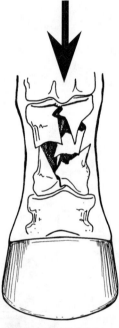

Fig. 16–14. Weight-bearing can cause the fractured pastern bone to collapse.

When surgery is not an option, a fiberglass cast is the only alternative to euthanasia in adult horses with this type of fracture. However, the cast provides little protection against the vertical (weight-bearing) forces on the bone. Even slight weight on the leg causes the bone above the fracture to force the bone fragments apart. As a result, the pastern may collapse. The cast can only prevent gross displacement of the fracture pieces; it cannot prevent collapse of the joints above and below the fractured bone. Therefore, the cast is merely a salvage procedure—a last resort.

Comminuted pastern fractures in foals and small ponies may be managed with an external fixation device *(see Chapter 9)*. Most of the weight on the leg is taken by the device; the pastern is relieved of weight-bearing and the fracture has a chance to heal. Unfortunately, most adult horses are too heavy for this device; the pins bend or break under their weight.

Prognosis for Comminuted Fractures

The prognosis for athletic usefulness is poor with comminuted pastern fractures, even if stability was achieved with bone screws or plates. Chronic lameness is often the result of extensive cartilage damage in the joints above and below the fractured bone. Sometimes the horse is so lame that it must be kept apart from the herd and confined to a small paddock for the rest of its life. These horses cannot cope with being turned out into a pasture. This is an important consideration when deciding between treatment and euthanasia.

Avulsion Fractures

Avulsion fractures at the back of the pastern usually occur when one or more of the distal sesamoidean ligaments tears away, and pulls off a piece of bone. These fragments can be very difficult to surgically remove without causing extensive soft tissue damage. The usual treatment recommendation is several months of paddock rest. *(Distal sesamoidean ligament damage is covered in more detail later in this chapter.)*

CHIP FRACTURES
Definition and Causes

Most bone chips involving the pastern or fetlock occur on the front of P_1, within the fetlock joint. These fractures are thought to be due to direct, but internal trauma. When the fetlock overextends during

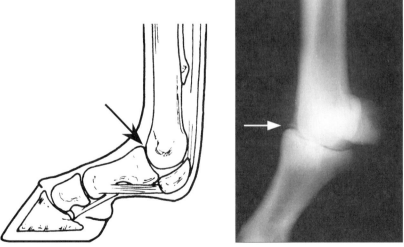

Fig. 16–15. When the fetlock overextends, P_1 hits against the cannon bone, which may cause a chip fracture.

strenuous exercise, the front of P1 hits against the front of the cannon bone. As a result, a small piece of P1 is broken off.

Bone chips occasionally are found in the pastern joint. They are broken off either the bottom of P1 or the top of P2. These fractures may be OCD lesions *(see Chapter 14)*.

Signs and Diagnosis of Chip Fractures

Chip fractures in the fetlock or pastern joint cause signs typical of inflammatory joint disease: joint effusion (accumulation of joint fluid) and mild lameness. Unlike the fetlock joint, effusion in the pastern joint may be difficult to see because the joint capsule is closely attached. The pastern joint has no pouches in which fluid can accumulate. Nerve or joint blocks may be needed to pinpoint the site of lameness *(see Chapter 2)*.

Because these signs are not specific for bone chips, the diagnosis can usually only be made with radiography. Occasionally, ultrasonography can detect bone chips. However, it is usually necessary to confirm their presence and precise location with radiographs.

Treatment of Chip Fractures

In most cases surgical removal of the fragment is recommended. Small chips in the front of the fetlock joint that do not appear to be near the joint surface may be managed conservatively. This involves rest, anti-inflammatory therapy, and joint medications. With larger fragments and those involving a joint surface, degenerative joint disease often results if the fragment remains in the joint. In most cases the bone chip can be removed arthroscopically. The usual recommendation after surgery is 2 – 3 weeks of stall rest followed by about 3 months of paddock rest. *(See Section II: Principles of Therapy for more information on these treatments.)*

Prognosis for Chip Fractures

The prognosis for return to full athletic function is very good if the bone chip is diagnosed and removed soon after injury. But if the chip fracture has been present for some time, degenerative changes may have developed. Also, chip fractures are not the only consequence of repeated fetlock overextension. DJD is very common in the fetlocks of strenuously exercised horses, and is a persistent management challenge.

PALMAR PROCESS FRACTURES
Definition and Cause

The palmar process is a rounded projection at the top of P1, in the back of the fetlock joint. There are two palmar processes in each fetlock joint: one on each side of the joint. Occasionally, a fragment of bone is broken off the palmar process. These fractures are sometimes found in young, adult horses, particularly Thoroughbred and Standardbred racehorses. This has led scientists to speculate that palmar process fractures may actually be osteochondritis dissecans lesions (OCD; *see Chapter 14*). These fractures are often bilateral, meaning they are often found in both forelegs or both hindlegs. This is a common characteristic of OCD lesions in other joints.

> **Terminology**
>
> The hindleg equivalent of this projection is the plantar process. However, for simplicity, the term palmar process is used.

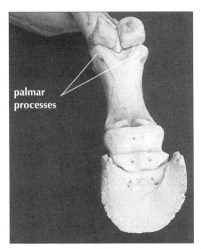 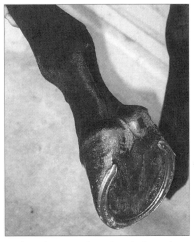

Fig. 16–16. The palmar processes are located at the top of P1, just below the sesamoid bones.

These fractures occur most often in the hindlegs of Standardbreds, usually on the inside (medial side) of the fetlock. There is some evidence that this condition is hereditary, and could be associated with a toe-out stance. This stance may overload the process on the inside of the leg, causing a fracture through the developing bone.

Signs and Diagnosis of Palmar Process Fractures

Also like other OCD lesions, there usually are no obvious signs until the horse's workload is increased. In most cases the lameness is very mild or inconsistent, and the only observation the trainer or rider/driver makes is that the horse is unwilling to stretch out at speed. Although these fractures often are bilateral, the horse may show signs in only one leg.

Because of the fracture's location, the effusion that results usually is very mild. A fetlock flexion test may cause or worsen the lameness; however, this is inconsistent. Desensitizing the fetlock, either with nerve blocks or a joint block *(see Chapter 2)*, temporarily improves the horse's gait, confirming that the fetlock is the site of the problem.

The diagnosis can only be made by radiographing the fetlock. Although some of these fragments are large, they can be difficult to find on routine radiographs. Other structures may be superimposed on the palmar process, hiding the fracture fragment. It usually takes a special, slanted radiographic view of the fetlock to find the fragment.

In most cases only one palmar process is fractured, but occasionally both are fractured. So, it is important for the veterinarian to take a complete series of fetlock radiographs, including the slanted view of each side of the joint. Because this fracture tends to be bilateral, it is also worth taking slanted radiographs of the opposite fetlock.

Treatment and Prognosis for Palmar Process Fractures

Small bone fragments that appear to be physically separated from P1 are often removed with arthroscopic surgery *(see Chapter 6)*. This procedure has excellent short- and long-term results. Large fragments or those that appear to be firmly attached often heal back onto P1 in time. With these fractures the veterinarian may simply recommend several months of paddock rest.

It is important that the veterinarian's recommendations regarding rest are followed. Keeping the horse in training or returning it to training too soon can result in degenerative joint disease. This may lead to chronic lameness.

FETLOCK DJD

This section covers two conditions involving the fetlock. *(The causes, signs, diagnosis, and management of degenerative joint disease [DJD] are discussed in Chapter 8.)*

Osselets

Confusion about the nature of an "osselet" is common because the term means different things to different people. Osselet literally means tiny piece of bone. It is often used to describe bony changes in the front of the fetlock joint. "Green osselet" is soft tissue swelling at the front of the fetlock joint. However, radiographs of green osselets show no bony changes, so the term osselet should not really be used to describe this swelling. Synovitis and capsulitis are more appropriate terms.

There are at least three conditions that can cause bony changes in the front of the fetlock:

- small bone chips within the joint, usually from the front of P1
- new bone production where the joint capsule attaches onto the bone (exostoses)
- calcification of the fibrous pad in the front of the joint: a result of chronic proliferative synovitis

It is important that the veterinarian makes a specific diagnosis in each case. The treatment and prognosis vary with the type of osselet.

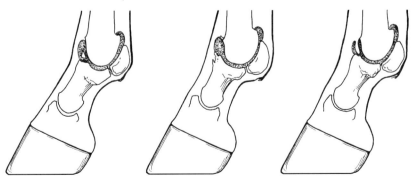

Fig. 16–17. Types of osselets. Left: Chip fracture off the front of P₁. Middle: Exostoses where the joint capsule attaches. Right: Calcification of the fibrous pad.

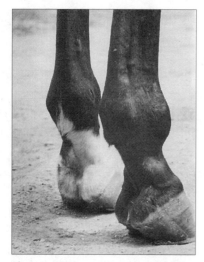

Fig. 16–18. Exostoses cause thickening over the front of the fetlock.

Bone chips and chronic proliferative synovitis are often best treated with arthroscopic surgery. They each have a fairly good prognosis if managed properly. However, exostoses involving the joint capsule cannot be treated surgically, and must be managed as osteoarthritis *(see Chapter 8).*

Flattening of the Bottom of the Cannon Bone

When viewed from the side, the bottom of the cannon bone is rounded. Occasionally, it appears on radiographs to be flattened at the back of the joint, opposite the sesamoid bones. Some veterinarians believe this flattening is a degenerative change, or possibly another manifestation of osteochondrosis *(see Chapter 14)*. However, others are reluctant to give this finding much significance. It may simply be due to slight angling of the leg, x-ray plate, or x-ray beam.

If flattening of the bottom of the cannon bone is the only abnormality found on radiographs, other causes of lameness should probably be investigated.

SESAMOIDITIS
Definition

Sesamoiditis is inflammation and subsequent bony reaction of the sesamoid bones at the back of the fetlock. These triangular bones are supported by several ligaments:

Terminology
In many anatomy texts, the sesamoid bones are called the proximal sesamoid bones.

• suspensory ligament branches
• distal sesamoidean ligaments
• collateral sesamoidean ligaments
• intersesamoidean ligament

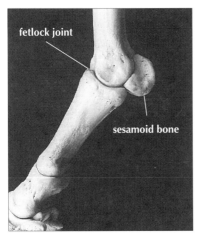
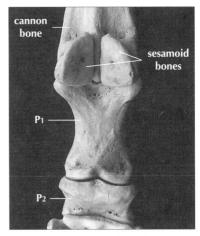

Fig. 16–19. The sesamoid bones are located at the back of the fetlock.

The superficial and deep digital flexor tendons run over the back of the sesamoid bones, and the annular ligament (discussed later) surrounds all of these structures. These tendons and ligaments form the suspensory, or "stay" apparatus of the fetlock joint.

Causes

The sesamoid bones ensure that the flexor tendons glide smoothly over the back of the fetlock joint. In this way, they act like a fulcrum, similar to the purpose served by the navicular bone.

When the fetlock overextends during strenuous exercise, the sesamoid bones are squeezed between the cannon and first pastern bone, and the overlying soft tissue structures. At the same time, the supporting ligaments exert tension on the top, sides, and bottom of the sesamoids. The result

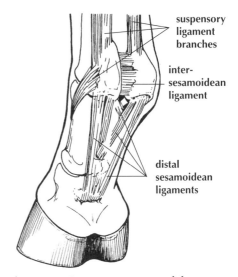

Fig. 16–20. Support structures of the sesamoid bones. (The collateral sesamoidean ligament is hidden beneath the suspensory ligament branch at the side of the fetlock.)

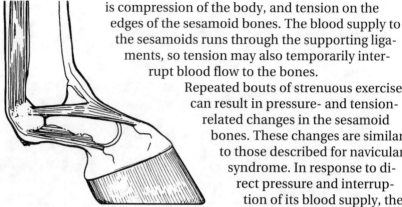

is compression of the body, and tension on the edges of the sesamoid bones. The blood supply to the sesamoids runs through the supporting ligaments, so tension may also temporarily interrupt blood flow to the bones.

Repeated bouts of strenuous exercise can result in pressure- and tension-related changes in the sesamoid bones. These changes are similar to those described for navicular syndrome. In response to direct pressure and interruption of its blood supply, the bone absorbs some of its mineral. This causes a loss of bone density. In severe cases this change is seen on radiographs as thin, dark lines in the sesamoids. The lines represent areas where bone density is reduced, around the blood vessels in the bone. In some cases the loss of bone density may be severe enough to make the sesamoid bones prone to fracture (discussed later).

Fig. 16–21. Fetlock overextension causes compression of the body of the sesamoid bones and tension on their edges.

The other common change seen on radiographs is new bone formation on the bone surfaces (exostoses; *see Chapter 9*). This occurs at the sites of tension, especially where the suspensory branches and distal sesamoidean ligaments attach.

Contributing Factors

Sesamoiditis is most common in young racehorses that have been pushed "too fast, too soon." These horses have not been given enough time to increase the density and strength of their bones in response to intense exercise *(see Chapter 9)*. It takes regular, very short bouts of speed work to cause a significant increase in bone density. In a young, untrained horse, gallops longer than 1 furlong (about 30 strides) can overload the bones. When this pattern is repeated, it can result in sesamoiditis, or other bone problems.

Poor conformation, in particular, long, sloping pasterns, and the long toe–low heel foot shape, can also predispose a horse to developing sesamoiditis. These faults encourage fetlock overextension during strenuous exercise. Improper trimming and shoeing can also encourage fetlock overextension, especially if the heels are not well supported by the shoes. *(See Chapter 7 for more information on hoof conformation and shoeing.)*

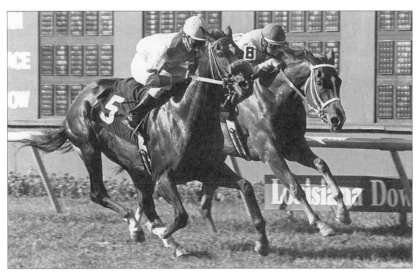

Fig. 16–22. Sesamoiditis is most common in young racehorses.

Signs of Sesamoiditis

Sesamoiditis usually occurs in the forelegs, and is often bilateral. That is, both sesamoid bones in both forelegs are involved. One side is usually more severely affected in horses that work on a circular track.

Horses with mild or early sesamoiditis may show few outward signs, other than vague or mild lameness (grade 1 – 2 of 5). On closer inspection, the back of the fetlock may be a little warmer than normal, and thumb pressure over the sesamoid bones causes mild pain. These horses may resent fetlock flexion, and the lameness may be worsened by flexion.

Severe or long-standing cases often have swollen sesamoid bones or soft tissue swelling around the back of the fetlock. Lameness in these horses is usually moderate (grade 2 – 3 of 5), and light thumb pressure over the sesamoid bones causes

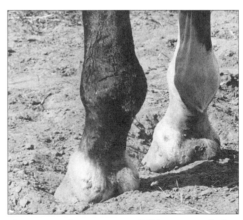

Fig. 16–23. Severe sesamoiditis causes obvious swelling around the sesamoid bones.

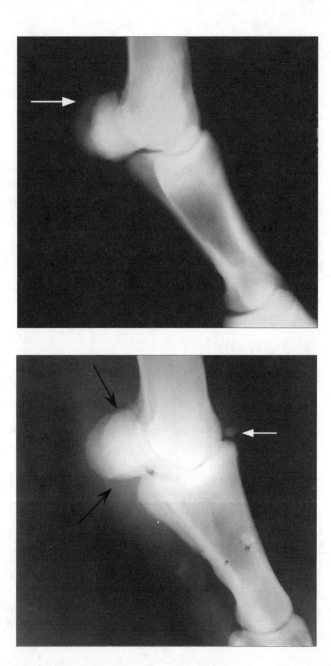

Fig. 16–24. Top: Loss of bone density in the sesamoids, resulting in thin, dark lines. Bottom: Bony changes at the top and bottom of the sesamoids [black arrows]. (Also note the bone chip at the front of the fetlock [white arrow].)

pain. Careful palpation may also reveal pain in the suspensory ligament branches or distal sesamoidean ligaments. It is fairly common
for the supporting ligaments, and even the flexor tendons, to be
strained in a horse with moderate to severe sesamoiditis. Therefore,
the soft tissues at the back of the cannon and fetlock should be palpated in each horse with sesamoiditis.

Diagnosis of Sesamoiditis

It is important to confirm the diagnosis and rule out other more
serious problems, such as a sesamoid fracture, by taking radiographs
of the fetlock. In mild or early cases there may be no obvious radiographic abnormalities on the sesamoid bones; this is a good sign. In
more severe cases radiographic changes are usually apparent: thin,
dark lines (areas of decreased density) within the bone, and/or new
bone formation on the edges. These changes may be seen after only
a few weeks of speed work.

If the swelling and pain are moderate to severe, the veterinarian
may ultrasound the supporting structures at the back of the fetlock.
The forces that caused the sesamoid bone changes may also have
strained or torn the soft tissues that support them, particularly the
suspensory ligament branches.

Back View   **Side View**

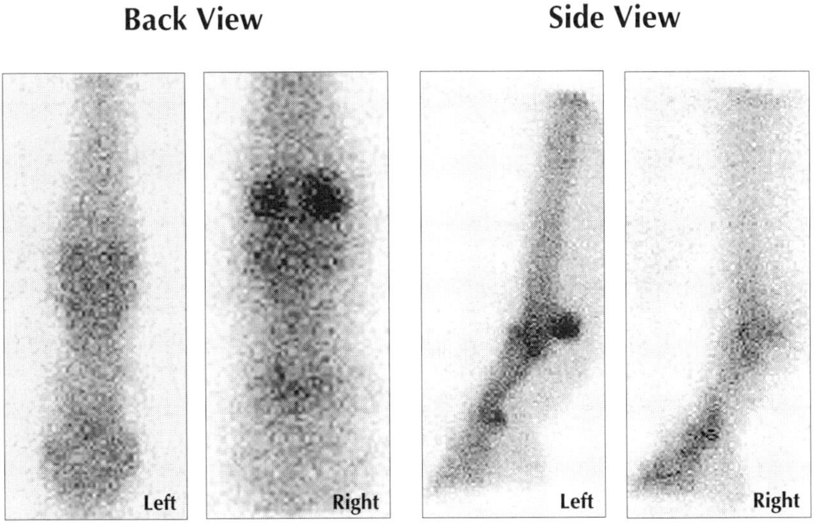

Fig. 16–25. Radiographs did not show any abnormalities, but nuclear scintigraphy showed inflammation in both sesamoids on the right leg.

Interpreting Sesamoid Changes in Mature Horses

Sesamoiditis is very uncommon in mature horses. Once the sesamoid bones have adapted to strenuous exercise, excessive strain or tension is more likely to damage the supporting soft tissues or pull off a piece of bone than cause sesamoiditis. However, dark lines and new bone formation caused by an earlier episode of sesamoiditis may not disappear completely with rest or time. When these changes are seen in a mature, non-racing horse they probably are not significant, especially if the horse is not lame.

Treatment of Sesamoiditis

Initial treatment involves reducing the horse's workload and giving a few days of anti-inflammatory therapy. The horse should be confined to a stall or small paddock. It should be hand-walked or ponied at the walk for at least 20 minutes twice per day until the heat, pain, swelling, and lameness have subsided. This usually takes 2 – 3 weeks in most horses.

More Information
Anti-inflammatory therapy includes:
• NSAIDs
• cold therapy
• DMSO
• "sweats"
(See Chapter 5 for more information.)

Unless there is tendon or ligament damage, or lameness persists, the horse can be returned to regular exercise after this time. There is little to be gained by resting the horse for longer. Bone density will only increase in response to regular exercise. (**Note:** The horse should no longer be receiving NSAIDs when it returns to regular exercise.)

To avoid another bout of sesamoiditis, the recommendations given in Chapter 9 for improving bone quality with training should be followed. Impatience usually results in another episode of sesamoiditis—one that may be more severe and less easy to resolve.

Horses with long, sloping pasterns and those with the long toe–low heel foot shape should be fitted with shoes that completely support the heels. Exercise bandages that limit fetlock overextension *(see Chapter 8)* may be of benefit in all horses, regardless of conformation.

Prognosis for Sesamoiditis

The prognosis for full return to athletic function is excellent in mild or early cases of sesamoiditis that resolve with these recommendations. However, if the horse is again worked up to race speed and distance too quickly, the problem may return. For as long as the horse remains in race training, the inflammatory changes and bone responses could persist and progress. So, it is important to treat the first episode of sesamoiditis properly, and take the steps necessary to prevent its recurrence.

Prevention of Sesamoiditis

Sesamoiditis can be prevented from developing or recurring by taking the following steps:

- ensure that the training program allows the young horse to adequately increase its bone quality
- have a farrier regularly trim and shoe the horse; this is particularly important in horses with the long toe–low heel foot shape
- ensure that the horse is fitted with shoes that completely support the heels
- use bandages that limit fetlock overextension during exercise
- feel the backs of the fetlocks for heat, pain, or swelling before and after each exercise session; reduce the work intensity if any of these signs develop, or if the horse seems uneven or lame

SESAMOID FRACTURES
Definitions and Causes

The sesamoid bones, which are roughly triangular, can fracture at the apex (tip), base, or body (middle). Apex and base fractures usually occur when a supporting structure—either the suspensory ligament branch at the apex or a distal sesamoidean ligament at the base—tears away a piece of bone. This type is called an avulsion fracture.

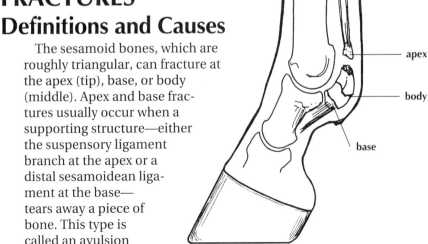

Fig. 16–26. Types of sesamoid bone fractures.

Sesamoid bone fractures generally occur during strenuous exercise. The forces that contribute to sesamoid fractures are the same as those that cause sesamoiditis. These fractures may sometimes be the end result of severe or chronic sesamoiditis, which weakens the bone. Occasionally, the fracture may be incomplete and seen on radiographs as a thin, black line across the bone. It can be hard to tell the difference between these fractures and the lines seen with severe sesamoiditis (compare Figure 16–23, top with Figure 16–27).

No matter where the fracture is located, tension from the ligaments often causes the fracture pieces to be pulled apart. When both sesamoid bones on the same leg are fractured through either the base or the body, the suspensory apparatus of the fetlock can completely break down (discussed later). When this occurs, the fetlock drops and the horse is unable to bear weight on the leg.

Signs and Diagnosis of Sesamoid Fractures

Sesamoid fractures typically cause a sudden, moderate to severe lameness (grade 3 – 5 of 5) during exercise. The degree of the lameness is a general guide to the severity of the injury. In each case radiographs are necessary to confirm the diagnosis and determine the best course of action.

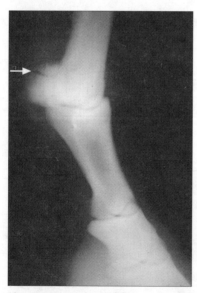

Fig. 16–27. An incomplete sesamoid bone fracture at the apex.

Apex and Base Fractures

With apex or single-sesamoid base fractures there may not be much swelling. But by carefully palpating each sesamoid bone it may be possible to identify a specific area of pain along the upper edge or the bottom of the bone. With apex fractures it is common for there to be thickening or pain in the suspensory ligament branch on the affected side.

Mid-body Fractures

With mid-body fractures the entire fetlock may be swollen, although the worst of the swelling is at the back of the leg, over the sesamoid bones. The sesamoids form the back of the fetlock joint, so mid-body sesamoid fractures can cause joint effusion (accumulation of joint fluid). Palpation of the sesamoid area causes obvious pain, as does fetlock flexion or extension. If both sesamoid bones on the same leg are completely fractured, the swelling may extend above the fetlock at the back of the leg.

Treatment of Sesamoid Fractures

Small Apex and Base Fractures

Small fragments off the apex or base of the sesamoid bone can sometimes be removed surgically. A few of these fragments can be removed with arthroscopy, through the fetlock joint. But others cannot be removed this way. Instead, the surgeon must search for the fragment and cut it free of the attached ligament. This approach can cause more damage to the supporting ligaments, so the veterinarian may recommend several months of paddock rest instead of surgery.

Other Fractures

Larger apex or base fragments and mid-body fractures can sometimes be repaired with bone screws. However, these are frustrating injuries because when weight is on the leg, tension from the supporting ligaments constantly pulls at the fracture pieces. Also, the sesamoids heal slowly and poorly, often with a fibrous union rather than a strong, bony callus.

After surgical repair of a sesamoid fracture, a fiberglass cast is used to immobilize the fetlock and stabilize the repair site during the first few weeks of healing. The cast also takes tension off the ligaments that support the sesamoid bones. When surgical repair is not possible, a cast is usually the only alternative to euthanasia in horses with severe fractures. This is especially true if both sesamoid bones in the same leg are fractured. In these horses the leg must remain in a cast for at least 8 weeks, and the cast changed as often as necessary. *(See Chapter 6 for more information on these procedures.)*

Prognosis for Sesamoid Fractures

The prognoses for sesamoid fractures can be listed from best to worst:

1. apex fractures
2. base fracture involving only one sesamoid bone
3. mid-body fracture involving only one sesamoid bone
4. base or mid-body fractures involving both sesamoid bones in the same leg

The prognosis for return to athletic function is fairly good for small apex or base fractures that are removed without much disruption to the supporting ligaments. But if the fragment cannot be removed, or if extensive ligament damage has already occurred, chronic lameness is a common result.

The prognosis for mid-body fractures is guarded at best. Sesamoid fractures typically heal with just a fibrous union, which is neither as strong nor as stable as a bony callus. The supporting ligaments exert constant tension on the weakened, unstable bone. Furthermore, the sesamoid bones make up the back of the fetlock joint. So even if the fracture repairs well, degenerative joint disease *(see Chapter 8)* and chronic lameness often occur after this fracture.

When both sesamoid bones on the same leg are completely fractured, return to athletic activity is out of the question. The horse may only be comfortable at pasture once this injury has healed.

DISTAL SESAMOIDEAN LIGAMENT DAMAGE
Definition and Causes

The distal sesamoidean ligaments (DSLs) anchor the base of the sesamoid bones to the back of the pastern. This group of short ligaments lies between the back of the first pastern bone and the deep flexor tendon. These ligaments form part of the stay apparatus that supports the fetlock.

Strenuous exercise can strain or tear one or more of the distal sesamoidean ligaments. The result may be just inflammation and pain, or fiber breakage. In severe cases a ligament may be pulled away from its site of attachment on the sesamoid bones or pastern. Occasionally a fragment of bone may pull away with the ligament, causing an avulsion fracture.

Injury to the distal sesamoidean ligaments is a significant cause of chronic lameness in mature performance horses. As with most other exercise-related injuries to the supporting structures of the fetlock, overextension during strenuous exercise places excessive strain on

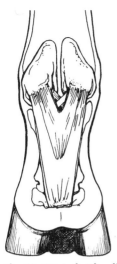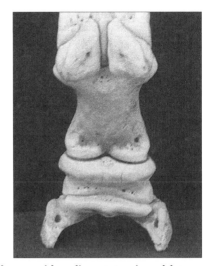

Fig. 16–28. Left: The distal sesamoidean ligaments, viewed from the back of the leg. Right: The same area without the soft tissues.

these ligaments. The same conformational and shoeing factors that contribute to flexor tendon, suspensory ligament, and sesamoid bone injuries also apply to distal sesamoidean ligament injury. *(Flexor tendon and suspensory ligament injuries are discussed in Chapter 11.)*

Signs and Diagnosis

Distal sesamoidean ligament damage causes mild to moderate lameness (grade 2 – 3 of 5), but few other signs. There is little, if any, swelling at the back of the fetlock or pastern unless other structures are also damaged. Deep palpation at the base of the sesamoid bones and back of the pastern usually causes pain. But ultrasonography is the only way to definitely diagnose this condition. Radiography may reveal an avulsion fracture, but it cannot show ligament damage.

Even if none of the ligaments have torn away from the bone, tension and strain may eventually result in new bone production at the site of attachment. The damaged ligament may also become calcified. This may not be seen on radiographs for several weeks after the initial injury.

The bony changes generally do not disappear as the injury heals. When these changes are found on radiographs it is important to correlate them with the signs. If the horse is not lame, the bony changes are unlikely to be significant. (However, they do indicate that there

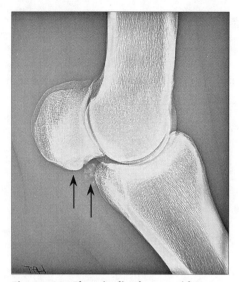

Fig. 16–29. Chronic distal sesamoidean ligament strain can result in bony changes.

has been excessive strain on the ligaments in the past.) If the horse is lame, it is important to rule out other causes of lameness.

Treatment of DSL Damage

Treatment should follow the same guidelines given in Chapter 11 for tendon and ligament injuries. These include rest from regular training, confinement, and a few days of anti-inflammatory therapy. A firm support bandage *(see Chapter 4)* is important in treating distal sesamoidean ligament injury. The bandage should extend from the hoof to the top of the cannon, and have enough padding and bandage material to restrict fetlock flexion. It must act like a cast to minimize movement at the injury site if healing is to proceed quickly. The leg should remain bandaged (and the bandage changed as often as necessary) for at least 3 weeks. During this time the horse should be confined to a stall or small pen.

If the ligament strain is only mild, the horse can then be turned out into a small paddock. Unless the horse is very placid, pasture rest is not ideal. If the horse is too active, healing may be slowed or the damaged ligaments reinjured. A horse with a more serious injury should be kept confined, but can begin daily hand-walking.

This phase of the rest period should continue until repeat ultrasound shows that the ligament has completely healed. In many cases this takes 3 – 4 months, after which the horse can gradually be returned to regular activities. It is important to remember that there are usually no outward signs of injury. The lameness may subside after only a couple of weeks of confinement. But if the horse is returned to regular training before the ligaments have completely healed, reinjury or persistent lameness is likely.

It is usually impossible to surgically remove a bone fragment that was torn away, without causing extensive damage to the ligaments. Therefore, surgery is generally not recommended.

Prognosis for DSL Damage

The prognosis for full return to athletic function is good if the ligament damage is minor and the horse is rested until the injury has completely healed. However, if a ligament was torn, if a bone fragment was pulled away, or if the horse is returned to training too soon, persistent or intermittent lameness may result.

Prevention of DSL Damage

Injuries to the distal sesamoidean ligaments can be prevented by following the same guidelines for preventing tendonitis and suspensory desmitis *(see Chapter 11)*. Ensuring that the shoes completely support the horse's heels is especially important in preventing these injuries and reducing the potential for reinjury.

ANNULAR LIGAMENT CONSTRICTION
Definition and Causes

The annular ligament wraps around the back of the fetlock, encasing the flexor tendons, flexor tendon sheath, and sesamoid bones. It helps support the fetlock and associated soft tissues. But because it is a fibrous, and therefore inelastic tissue, the annular ligament can act like a constricting band under certain circumstances. The conditions that can result in annular ligament constriction are:

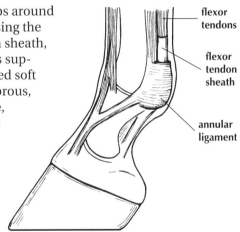

flexor tendons

flexor tendon sheath

annular ligament

Fig. 16–30. The annular ligament wraps around the back of the fetlock.

- annular desmitis—inflammation and thickening of the annular ligament
- flexor tendonitis at the level of the sesamoid bones (a "low bow")
- tenosynovitis of the flexor tendon sheath
- a combination of any of the above conditions

So basically, the circumstances in which annular ligament constriction occurs can be divided into two categories: 1) damage to the annular ligament itself, and 2) damage to the structures beneath a normal annular ligament.

Strain and damage of the annular ligament (annular desmitis) causes thickening of the ligament. The flexor tendon sheath begins above the fetlock and ends just above the navicular bone, within the hoof. It normally has very little fluid in it. But when the annular ligament is thickened, the normal flow of fluid within the sheath is restricted. As a result, fluid builds up in the sheath above the annular ligament. Sometimes the annular ligament is so thickened that it restricts the flexor tendons from gliding smoothly over the back of the sesamoid bones. In very severe cases pressure from the thickened annular ligament can damage the flexor tendons by restricting their blood supply.

Flexor tendonitis in the part of the tendon that is within the tendon sheath can cause an increase in tendon sheath fluid (effusion). This excess of fluid can be restricted from flowing down the tendon sheath by the annular ligament, even if the ligament is normal. Tenosynovitis can also cause tendon sheath effusion, with the same result.

As with most other exercise-related tendon and ligament injuries, the annular ligament is strained by overextension of the fetlock during strenuous exercise. The forces that can strain this ligament may also damage other supporting structures of the fetlock. So it is fairly common to find annular desmitis and flexor tendonitis or tenosynovitis together.

Definitions
Tendonitis: inflammation of a tendon.   **Tenosynovitis:** inflammation of a tendon sheath.   **(See Chapter 11 for more information.)**

Signs of Annular Ligament Constriction

The most consistent feature of annular ligament constriction is a distinctive swelling at the back of the fetlock. The tendon sheath effusion makes the top of the ligament appear as a clearly-defined dent below a large pouch of fluid. In some cases there may also be a smaller pocket of fluid in the tendon sheath at the back of the pastern, over the deep flexor tendon.

Careful palpation of the back of the fetlock is necessary to determine which structures are involved. Thumb pressure directly over the sesamoid bones—particularly in between them—may cause pain if the annular ligament or flexor tendons are inflamed.

The degree of lameness may vary from mild to moderate (grade 1 – 3 of 5), depending on the severity of annular ligament inflammation or flexor tendon damage. In some chronic cases, in which the annular desmitis has settled down and just the tendon sheath effusion remains, the horse may no longer be lame.

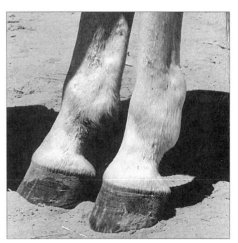

Fig. 16–31. Annular ligament constriction causes a distinctive swelling.

Diagnosis of Annular Ligament Constriction

Ultrasonography is necessary to determine whether the annular ligament, flexor tendons, or tendon sheath is thickened or damaged. The veterinarian can also check for adhesions within the tendon sheath. (Adhesions are fibrous bands. They are a common result of chronic inflammation within the sheath.)

Treatment of Annular Ligament Constriction

Treatment depends, to some extent, on which structure is damaged. If only annular desmitis is present and is fairly acute (recent), treatment should include rest from regular training, confinement, hand-walking, anti-inflammatory therapy, and bandaging, similar to the conservative management of tendonitis. The goal is to resolve the inflammation, and therefore the constriction, as quickly as possible. Most cases of acute annular desmitis settle down in 1 – 2 weeks with these measures, although the tendon sheath effusion may remain.

Annular Desmotomy

If the lameness persists or returns despite treatment, or when a good cosmetic result is desired, surgery to cut the annular ligament and relieve the con-

Definition
Desmotomy: surgically cutting a ligament.

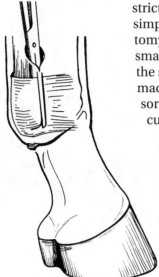

Fig. 16–32. Cutting the annular ligament to relieve the constriction.

striction may be necessary. This relatively simple procedure, called an annular desmotomy, is done under general anesthesia. A small incision is made in the skin at the side of the sesamoid bone. A vertical tunnel is then made in the subcutaneous tissues so that scissors can be inserted and the annular ligament cut through the small skin incision.

If ultrasonography showed a tendon lesion or adhesions within the tendon sheath, the skin incision is extended so the sheath can be opened to expose the tendons. Tendon splitting *(see Chapter 11)* can then be performed if necessary, and any adhesions within the sheath broken down. (Some surgeons prefer to examine the contents of the sheath and break down any adhesions arthroscopically, through the small skin incision.) The sheath and skin are then sutured closed, and the leg is kept bandaged until the skin sutures are removed, usually 7 – 10 days after surgery. Keeping the leg bandaged for a few more weeks can improve the final cosmetic result in many cases.

Most surgeons prescribe antibiotics after surgery. NSAIDs are usually given for a few days to reduce inflammation and discomfort. The horse's tetanus status should be checked before surgery. *(These medications are discussed in Chapter 5.)*

Injecting hyaluronic acid into the sheath, and hand-walking twice daily can help prevent adhesions from re-forming. These treatments may also speed healing. But movement of the skin over the fetlock causes tension on the suture line when the horse walks. So, it is usually best to begin hand-walking only after the wound has healed and the sutures have been removed.

Rehabilitation

Hand-walking should continue for 3 – 4 weeks in cases of annular desmitis—longer if the horse has tendonitis. Horses can function very well without their annular ligaments. So provided the surgical wound has healed well and the horse is not lame, it is usually safe to gradually return the horse to regular training after this time. If there has been flexor tendon damage, the rest period is much longer.

Prognosis for Annular Ligament Constriction

The prognosis for return to full athletic function is quite good, unless there has been severe flexor tendon damage. If just the annular ligament or tendon sheath is involved, and the horse is rested from active training for long enough, there should be no further problems.

"BREAKDOWN" INJURIES

The fetlock is supported in its normal position by the suspensory, or "stay" apparatus, which consists of:

- the flexor tendons
- the sesamoid bones and associated ligaments
- the distal sesamoidean ligaments
- the suspensory ligament

Complete failure of one or more of these structures causes excessive strain on the others, and loss of support to the fetlock. As a result, the fetlock sinks, and in severe cases the horse cannot bear weight on the leg.

Conditions Resulting in "Breakdown"

There are four major conditions that can result in stay apparatus failure, or "breakdown" of the fetlock:

1. Laceration or rupture of the flexor tendons.
2. Fractures through the body or base of both sesamoid bones.
3. Rupture of the distal sesamoidean ligaments.
4. Degeneration or rupture of the suspensory ligament.

Tendon or ligament rupture, and sesamoid bone fractures are catastrophic injuries that occur during strenuous exercise. They are often the final result of chronic strain and overloading of the fetlock's support structures. A recent study indicated that shoes with toe grabs make these "breakdown" injuries up to **16 times** more likely.

When the distal sesamoidean ligaments rupture, they usually pull away from their attachment either at the back of the pastern or the base of the

> ### More Information
>
> Flexor tendon injuries are covered in Chapter 11.
>
> Sesamoid bone fractures were discussed earlier.
>
> Suspensory ligament degeneration is discussed in the next section.

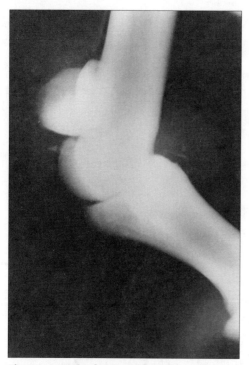

Fig. 16–33. Distal sesamoidean ligament rupture allows the sesamoid bones to be pulled up, and the fetlock to sink.

sesamoid bones. Rupture of these anchoring ligaments allows the suspensory ligament to pull the sesamoids up an inch or two. The same thing happens when both sesamoid bones are fractured through their body or base: the suspensory ligament pulls away the upper part of the sesamoids. In either situation, the fetlock collapses when the horse bears weight on the leg.

In most cases of distal sesamoidean ligament rupture, surgical repair is either impossible or unsuccessful. So treatment involves either casting the leg for at least 8 weeks, as discussed earlier for sesamoid bone fractures, or surgically fusing the fetlock (arthrodesis). But these are only salvage procedures. Return to athletic function is out of the question.

Other Problems

Occasionally, the extreme forces that damage the fetlock's support structures and cause the fetlock to sink may also stretch or tear the digital arteries. These blood vessels run beside the sesamoid bones, on their way down to the pastern and foot. If the digital vessels are severely damaged, the inevitable and devastating result is loss of blood supply and death of the tissues below the fetlock.

Severe blood vessel damage is not obvious just by looking at the leg. It can take days to become noticeable, although the hoof and pastern may feel cold within 24 hours of injury. When the blood supply to the pastern and foot is lost, amputation or euthanasia are the only options.

First-Aid Care for "Breakdown" Injuries

First-aid care of a horse with a "breakdown" injury involves immediately splinting the leg so that the horse cannot place the foot flat and cause the fetlock to sink further. Whatever weight the horse puts on the leg must be taken by the toe and the bottom of the splint.

A thick standard bandage should first be placed on the leg, from the coronet to the top of the cannon. The splint (preferably a narrow board) is then applied at the back of the leg, with the fetlock slightly flexed and the sole flat against the board. The splint should be firmly taped in place so that the horse cannot straighten its fetlock. *(This procedure, and other bandaging and splinting techniques, are discussed and illustrated in Chapter 4.)*

The horse should not be moved, except to walk it to the nearest stall or transport it to a veterinary hospital. NSAIDs should be given to relieve the horse's discomfort, but it is always best to consult the veterinarian first.

Suspensory Ligament Degeneration
Definition and Causes

Degeneration of the suspensory ligament is a fairly uncommon condition. It is the one cause of fetlock "breakdown" that is not usually related to intense exercise. It is associated with chronic degeneration and eventual lengthening of the ligament, rather than sudden, catastrophic rupture.

There are two separate groups of horses that are prone to developing suspensory degeneration: 1) Peruvian Pasos and Paso crosses, and 2) older horses of any breed. The condition is mostly seen in young adult Pasos, about 5 years and older. But it has been reported in Pasos as young as 12 months old. In contrast, when the condition occurs in other breeds, it is usually in horses over 10 years old. Broodmares seem to develop suspensory degeneration more often than male horses.

How or why the degenerative process begins is not known, although heredity may play a role in Peruvian Pasos. Conformation probably contributes in other breeds. Suspensory degeneration is more common in horses with long pasterns and straight hindlegs. It may be more likely in pregnant mares because the weight of the foal places increased load on the legs, particularly the hindlegs. Hormonal changes may also affect the strength of these ligaments in mares.

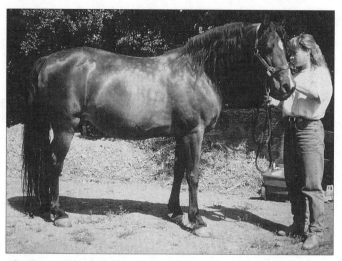

Fig. 16–34. The fetlocks drop and the pasterns become more-or-less horizontal, while the hocks and stifles gradually straighten.

Signs of Suspensory Ligament Degeneration

The result in each case is weakened suspensory ligaments that are easily stretched just by normal weight-bearing at rest. The fetlocks drop and the pasterns become more-or-less horizontal. Ringbone may develop because of the strain this abnormal stance and movement places on the pastern joints. Sudden rupture of the suspensory ligament can also occur in these horses, although it is very uncommon.

This condition generally is bilateral: both forelegs or both hindlegs are affected. Occasionally all four legs have suspensory degeneration. In breeds other than Pasos it occurs more often in the hindlegs. In these cases, the hocks and stifles gradually straighten, losing their normal angle.

There is obvious "sagging" of the fetlocks, which is present at rest and exaggerated when the horse walks. Also, the horse may be reluctant to move around. Movement stretches the suspensory ligaments further, which can cause pain. Often the branches of the suspensory ligament are thickened and painful. During ultrasound examination, fiber degeneration may be seen anywhere along the suspensory ligament, from its origin at the top of the cannon to the branches *(see Chapter 11).*

Management of Suspensory Ligament Degeneration

There is no specific treatment for this condition. Management is aimed at relieving the horse's discomfort and preventing further stretching or rupture of the ligaments. If possible, the horse should be confined to a small paddock; activity in the pasture, even if it is limited, can further stretch the ligaments. Bandages that support the fetlock and prevent overextension may help. NSAIDs can make the horse more comfortable, although they may be counterproductive if they relieve pain to the extent that the horse can exercise freely. More ligament damage will occur if the horse is permitted to run around.

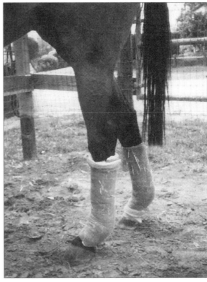

Fig. 16–35. Supportive bandages can limit stretching of the ligaments.

Elongated egg bar shoes *(see Chapter 7)* can help these horses. In fact, they may be a good preventive measure in older horses with long pasterns. However, elongated shoes are not safe on the forefeet. They can easily be caught and pulled loose by the hindfeet.

Prognosis for Suspensory Ligament Degeneration

The prognosis for athletic function is poor once the suspensory ligaments have stretched. The best that can be expected is a horse that is comfortable in a paddock. If the suspensory ligament ruptures, the kindest action may be euthanasia.

17

THE CANNON
&
SPLINT BONES

The cannon is an area of the horse's leg that has long been a focus of attention with horsepeople. Terms like "fine-boned" and "a lot of bone" are still used, and refer to the relative diameter of a horse's cannon bones. Fine-boned horses have narrower cannon bones than horses with a lot of bone.

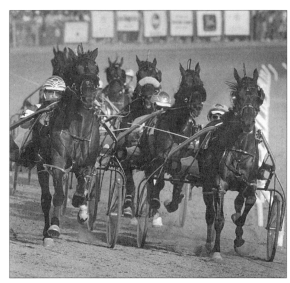

Fig. 17–1.

But fine-boned horses are not necessarily more prone to traumatic or exercise-induced cannon and splint bone injuries.

BUCKED SHINS
Definition

Bucked shins is a condition in which the front of the cannon bone is inflamed and painful. In severe cases, swelling at the front of the cannon gives it a slightly bowed out appearance when viewed from the side. This is where the term, bucked shins, comes from. Another common name for this condition is "shin soreness." (A similar condition in people is called "shin splints.")

Scientists refer to bucked shins as dorsal metacarpal disease. This term means that the front part, or dorsal surface, of the cannon bone on a foreleg—the third metacarpal bone—is abnormal. Dorsal metacarpal disease includes other conditions, in particular incomplete fractures (discussed later).

Cause

Bucked shins is common in young racehorses. It occasionally occurs in other young horses that perform intense exercise. While it is usually seen in 2-year-olds, it is related to the start of fast work, rather than the horse's age. Horses that do not begin training until they are 3 or 4 years old are also at risk of developing bucked shins if they have not been regularly exercised before more intensive training begins.

Bucked shins are almost always confined to the forelegs. More of the horse's (and rider's) weight is taken on the forelegs than the hindlegs. As a result, the weight-bearing and ground impact forces are greatest in the forelegs. These forces are concentrated at the front of the leg. Studies in untrained horses show that the cannon bones in the forelegs bow backward a little when the horse is galloping. This causes compression of the cortex at the front of the leg. The body responds to this stress by laying down new bone under the periosteum to increase the bone's strength and resilience at the stresspoint. This is a normal and appropriate response to regular exercise. In horses that are regularly exercised at speed, more bone is laid down around

Definitions
Periosteum: fibrous membrane covering the bone.
Cortex: dense, outer layer of a bone.
Medullary Cavity: the hollow center of a longbone.
(See Chapter 9 for information on bone structure, improving bone quality, and fractures.)

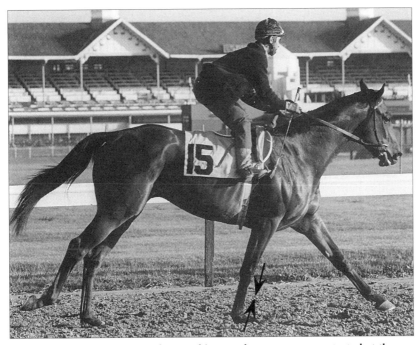

Fig. 17–2. Weight-bearing and ground impact forces are concentrated at the front of the cannon bone (arrows).

the front of the cannon because that is the part that sustains the greatest load. So, when the cannon bone of a trained racehorse is compared with that of an untrained horse, the cortex at the front of the leg is thicker and denser.

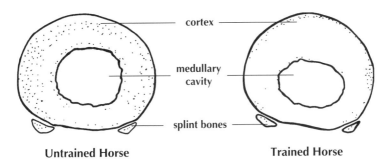

cortex

medullary
cavity

splint bones

Untrained Horse

Trained Horse

Fig. 17–3. The cortex of a trained horse is thicker and denser at the front of the leg than at the sides or back.

It takes regular, very short bouts of speed work for bone density and thickness to be significantly increased. If the horse is worked at speed (three-quarter pace or faster) before the cannon bone has strengthened sufficiently, overloading of the bone can result in:

- inflammation of the periosteum, causing pain and lameness
- areas of new bone production beneath the periosteum, which makes the front of the cannon appear thickened and irregular
- microfractures in the outer part of the bone in severe cases

Microfractures are tiny cracks in the outer few millimeters of the cortex. They are too small to see on routine radiographs. These fractures can weaken the cortex because the body removes some of the mineral deposits before laying down new bone. Occasionally, a microfracture can extend to become an incomplete, or "stress" fracture.

Recent studies have found that the type of work surface and changes in hoof balance and angle have little effect on the load placed on the cannon bones. However, muscle fatigue does increase the load on the bones. So inadequate conditioning probably plays a part in some cases.

Signs of Bucked Shins

Horses with bucked shins usually have a mild to moderate forelimb lameness (grade 1 – 3 of 5), although it may not be obvious at first if both legs are equally sore. In many cases the horse simply appears stiff and reluctant to stride out. Trotting on a hard surface, such as asphalt, worsens the lameness because it increases the concussion on the inflamed bones. In horses that gallop on a circular track, the leading leg is usually more sore than the opposite foreleg. For example, the left foreleg is more

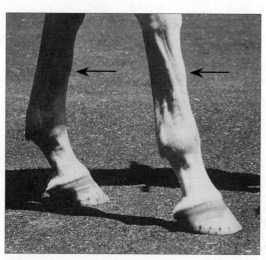

Fig. 17–4. New bone production causes the "bucked" appearance.

sore in horses that work counter-clockwise.

Horses with bucked shins have heat and pain along the fronts of the cannon bones. In moderate to severe cases it takes very little finger pressure to cause a pain response. Horses with microfractures or an incomplete fracture in the bone surface are usually more lame and their cannon bones are more painful during palpation. However, the severity of the signs is not always a reliable way to determine the degree of bone reaction and damage. Some horses with just bucked shins (and no fractures) are very sore.

Once new bone is laid down, the front of the cannon may feel rough and irregular. When new bone is laid down rapidly, it is seldom distributed evenly. Over time, the body remodels this new bone, so the surface of the cannon bone becomes smoother. However, the "bucked" or bowed out appearance may remain.

Diagnosis of Bucked Shins

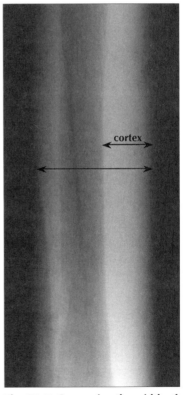

The diagnosis is usually made just on the horse's work history (stage of training, amount and intensity of daily exercise) and signs. If the horse is very sore the veterinarian may radiograph the cannon bones to check for incomplete fractures.

Recent studies have found a way to evaluate the readiness of the cannon bones for intense exercise (galloping). This test can also be used to identify the horses that are most at risk of developing bucked shins. According to these studies, the ability of the cannon bone to resist bending and compression depends on the thickness of the front cortex in relation to the overall width of the bone. The thinner the front cortex, in relation to the bone's width, the less resistant the bone is to loads generated during intense exercise. This relationship

Fig. 17–5. Comparing the width of the cannon bone and front cortex.

is easily assessed by taking a lateral radiograph (from the side) of the cannon bone. The widths of the front cortex and the entire cannon bone are then measured from the radiograph.

Comparing the width of the cortex to the overall width of the bone eliminates the effect of the horse's size. A "fine-boned" horse has narrow cannon bones, but if the front cortex is thick enough in relation to the bone's overall width, the horse is at no more risk of developing bucked shins than a horse with thicker cannon bones. Even a horse with thick cannons will develop bucked shins if it is worked too hard before the cortex has strengthened enough to withstand the load.

Treatment and Prevention of Bucked Shins

Bucked shins is associated with high-speed exercise. So, initial treatment involves reducing the horse's workload and giving a few days of anti-inflammatory therapy. The horse should be confined to a stall and/or small paddock, and hand-walked or ponied at the walk for at least 20 minutes twice per day until the heat, pain, and lameness subside. This usually takes 2 – 3 weeks.

Once the lameness has resolved, and the horse is no longer receiving NSAIDs, the horse should be returned to regular exercise. Prolonged rest does nothing to strengthen the cannon bones—only regular exercise achieves this objective.

Speed work should initially consist of *short* gallops every 7 – 10 days. The rest of the training program should comprise daily exercise of moderate intensity. This "slow" work ensures that the rest of the musculoskeletal system and the cardiovascular system adapt to exercise appropriately. But short bouts of fast work are necessary to stimulate bone to protect itself against the intense stresses it experiences when the horse is galloping. *(It is not necessary to gallop a horse over long distances or too frequently for it to reach peak fitness. Daily exercise of moderate intensity and short gallops once or twice per week are usually enough. This program is discussed further in Chapter 9.)*

If heat, pain, or lameness return at any time during training, the workload should again be reduced until the lame-

---

More Information

Anti-inflammatory therapy includes:

- cold therapy
- NSAIDs
- DMSO
- "sweats"

(See Chapter 5 for information on these treatments.)

ness subsides. Also, the training program should be critically reviewed. Many trainers view bucked shins as inevitable—an occupational hazard of racing. However, *not all racehorses develop bucked shins.* Horses that are conditioned properly seldom develop bucked shins. Also, they lose very few training days due to this or other musculoskeletal problems.

Radiographs may be of value in horses that are still lame after several weeks' rest, or that become lame with just light

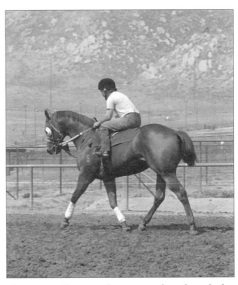

Fig. 17–6. Slow work ensures that the whole horse is conditioned properly.

exercise. Recurrence or persistence of the lameness may be due to an incomplete fracture.

Prognosis for Bucked Shins

The prognosis for return to full athletic function is excellent, provided these management recommendations are followed. However, recurrence or persistence of the problem is common in horses that are brought back to full training too quickly. As long as the horse remains in training, the cannon bones are under stress. Therefore, it is very important that they are given time to adapt to strenuous exercise if delays in training and competition are to be avoided.

INCOMPLETE ("STRESS") FRACTURES

Incomplete, or "stress" fractures involve only one side of the bone—they do not break it completely. Incomplete cannon bone fractures mostly occur in the forelegs of racehorses and other horses performing strenuous athletic activities. There are two distinct types of incomplete cannon bone fractures. Dorsal fractures involve the front (dorsal cortex) of the bone. Palmar fractures involve the back

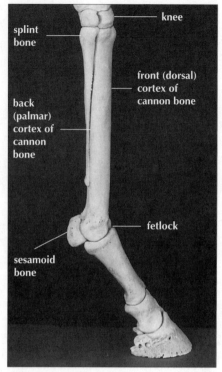

splint bone

knee

front (dorsal) cortex of cannon bone

back (palmar) cortex of cannon bone

fetlock

sesamoid bone

Fig. 17–7. The cannon area without the soft tissues.

(palmar cortex) of the bone.

In either case excessive ground-impact and weight-bearing forces on the cannon bone are the presumed cause. These fractures are the result of repeated overloading of the cannon bone.

Dorsal Stress Fractures

Definition and Causes

Dorsal stress fractures are most common in young Quarter Horse and Thorough-bred racehorses, although they can occur in any young horse that is regularly gal-loped. The fracture typically occurs in the middle of the cannon. It begins at the bone surface and crosses the cortex at an angle. The fracture may or may not extend to the hol-low, medullary cavity in the center of the bone.

Veterinarians sometimes call these fractures incomplete cortical fractures, and group them under the heading, "dorsal metacarpal disease"—a syndrome that also includes bucked shins. In many cases horses that develop these fractures have or recently had bucked shins. Presumably, the same compressive forces that cause bucked shins also cause incomplete fractures in the bone's front cor-tex. Thus, these fractures may be an extension of the bucked shins problem.

In theory, a direct blow to the front of the cannon in other perfor-mance horses could result in an incomplete fracture. For example, the cannon could be struck by a polo mallet or knocked on a jump rail. But in most cases direct trauma simply causes bruising and in-flammation of the bone surface, and possibly a bony swelling. A se-vere, direct blow is more likely to fracture the bone completely, rather than cause an incomplete fracture.

Signs and Diagnosis

The horse may suddenly become moderately lame during or shortly after exercise (grade 3 – 4 of 5). But if the horse also has bucked shins, it may have been mildly lame for a few weeks. There is usually very little swelling at the fracture site, and there are few other signs, except for heat and pain over the front of the cannon. Palpation of the front of the cannon usually causes pain at a very specific location. However, except for the degree of lameness and the fact that it is far more obvious in one leg, these signs could also be taken to indicate a severe case of bucked shins.

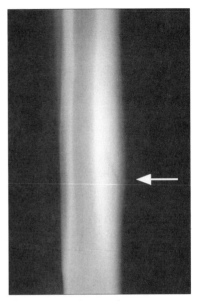

Fig. 17–8. An incomplete cannon bone fracture [arrow] in a horse that also has bucked shins.

The diagnosis must be confirmed with radiographs. Usually, the fracture line is obvious as it runs at an angle across the cortex at the front of the cannon bone. However, it may not be visible for several days after injury. Repeat radiographs or nuclear scintigraphy may be necessary before the veterinarian can make a definite diagnosis.

Treatment

Depending on the size of the fracture, the veterinarian may treat the condition conservatively with 4 – 6 months of small paddock rest. In most cases the fracture line does not extend to the medullary cavity. Nevertheless, there is potential for it to extend and weaken the bone enough that

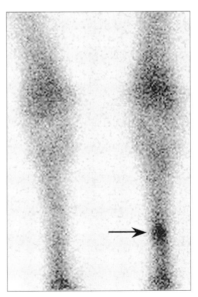

Fig. 17–9. A "bone scan" of a dorsal stress fracture of the cannon bone.

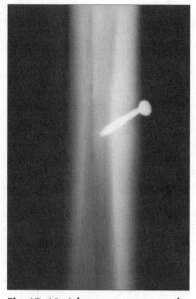

Fig. 17–10. A bone screw across the fracture can add stability.

the entire cannon bone is fractured. For this reason, *training must cease* until the fracture has completely healed.

These fractures, although small, can take several months to resolve. To speed healing, the veterinarian may recommend surgery. The most common technique involves drilling along the fracture line with a surgical drill bit. The surgeon then packs the drill hole with a bone graft to speed up bone production *(see Chapter 6)*. In some cases the surgeon also places a bone screw across the fracture line. Stall rest for 6 – 8 weeks is usually followed by paddock or pasture turnout for at least another 2 months.

Radiographs should be taken before training is resumed. If the fracture line is still visible, the horse should be rested for longer. Once the horse is ready to resume training, the guidelines given earlier for training horses with bucked shins should be followed.

Prognosis for Dorsal Stress Fractures

The prognosis for return to athletic activities after an incomplete cannon bone fracture is very good, provided the fracture heals completely before the horse is returned to regular training. These fractures must be taken seriously. If the horse continues in training or is returned to training too soon, it can shatter its cannon bone—which often results in euthanasia. (Complete cannon bone fractures are discussed later.)

Palmar Stress Fractures

Palmar stress fractures are more common in Standardbred racehorses. The fracture occurs at the back of the cannon bone, just below the knee. In gallopers, the bony reaction or fracture occurs at the front of the cannon bone. Differences in the working gait and speed, as well as the way the horses are trained and shod may account for

the different location of the
bony changes between gallopers and trotters/pacers.

Signs

Other than the lameness,
there are few, if any obvious
signs of a palmar stress fracture. There may be pain when
pressure is applied to the back
of the cannon bone. But the
damaged area is hidden beneath the soft tissues at the
back of the leg: flexor tendons, inferior check ligament,
and suspensory ligament. So
it is very difficult to exert pressure directly over the fracture.

Occasionally, the fracture
extends up the cannon to involve the lower knee joint (the carpometacarpal joint). When this happens
there may be mild effusion in the middle
knee joint (the intercarpal joint). This is
because the joint capsules of these two
joints are connected. However, joint effusion is not a typical feature of palmar
stress fractures.

Unlike dorsal fractures, in which the
lameness may develop suddenly, palmar
fractures usually cause a lameness that is
mild (grade 1 – 2 of 5) and intermittent at

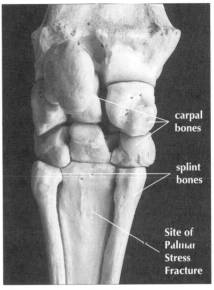

**Fig. 17–11. Location of palmar stress
fractures at the back of the cannon.**

Definition
Effusion: abnormal in-crease in fluid within a joint, causing a soft, fluidy swelling.
(See Chapter 18 for more information on swelling in the knee.)

first. A typical history is of a lameness that worsens as training continues, but disappears with rest. Over time, the lameness becomes
more obvious (grade 2 – 3 of 5) and consistent, particularly if the
horse's workload increases.

Diagnosis

Diagnosing this fracture, or even identifying the site of lameness
can be difficult because it is virtually impossible to specifically block
this area. Also, there may at first be no abnormalities on radiographs.

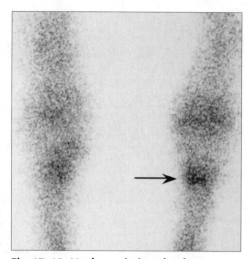

It usually takes several weeks for a fracture line to become apparent.

The best way to diagnose this fracture is with nuclear scintigraphy *(see Chapter 2)*, which shows a distinct "hot spot" on the cannon, just below the knee. Although lameness may be apparent in only one leg, in many cases "hot spots" are seen in both forelegs. There may not be a fracture in both legs, but a stress response in the cannon bone seems to occur in each leg.

Fig. 17–12. Nuclear scintigraphy shows a "hot spot" on the cannon [arrow], just below the knee. A stress response is also present in the other leg.

The history, signs, and diagnostic difficulties are very similar to those found with suspensory origin damage *(see Chapter 11)*. In fact, ultrasound often reveals evidence of suspensory ligament damage in horses with palmar stress fractures. It can be difficult on radiographs to tell the difference between a bone fragment that is torn away by the suspensory ligament (an avulsion fracture) and a palmar stress fracture. However, the distinction is an important one. The suspensory ligament may tear off a piece of bone from the surface of the cannon bone. But palmar fractures occur within the cortex, and therefore weaken the bone.

Treatment of Palmar Stress Fractures

Palmar stress fractures cannot be treated surgically because it is impossible to get to the back of the cannon bone without causing extensive damage to the overlying soft tissues. If the fracture extends up the cannon bone to the carpometacarpal joint, the surgeon can stabilize the top of the cannon with bone screws. Fortunately, this type of fracture is very uncommon.

The usual recommendation for managing palmar stress fractures is 4 – 8 months of paddock rest. If the horse is kept in training, or returned to training too soon, the condition will not resolve. Radiographs or nuclear scintigraphy should be repeated before the horse is returned to training.

Although the training recommendations given in Chapter 9 focus on gallopers, the same principles apply to trotters and pacers. Bone will only increase its strength and resilience in response to regular, very short bouts of vigorous exercise. There is nothing to be gained by increasing the length or frequency of the fast work sessions, particularly in a horse that is recovering from a bone injury. Short bouts of speed work every 7 – 10 days give the best results and minimize the potential for reinjury.

Prognosis for Palmar Stress Fractures

The prognosis for return to full athletic activities is usually quite good, provided the fracture heals completely before regular exercise resumes, and the horse is *slowly* returned to race training.

VERTICAL (CONDYLAR) FRACTURES
Definition and Causes

The lower end of the cannon bone consists of a central ridge and two slightly flared condyles. A condyle is a rounded area of bone at a joint surface. On the cannon bone, there is one condyle on each side of the ridge.

Weight-bearing and ground impact forces during intense exercise can create a vertical fracture that begins at the joint surface, just to one side of the ridge. It runs up the cannon bone, separating one condyle from the rest of the bone. This is called a condylar fracture.

The fracture may be complete or incomplete. Complete fractures usually run at a slight angle up the cannon bone and break out at the side of the bone several inches above the fetlock. Weight-bearing often causes the fracture to displace by a millimeter or so. However, because the horse's weight is

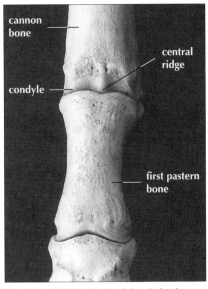

Fig. 17–13. The front of the fetlock.

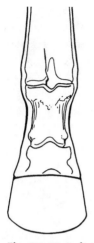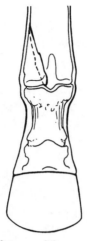

Fig. 17–14. Left: Incomplete condylar fracture. Right: Complete condylar fracture that broke out at the side of the bone. The dotted line is the back of the fracture.

supported by the non-fractured condyle and the central ridge, displacement of these fractures is usually slight. The collateral ligament, which runs down the side of the joint, and the fetlock joint capsule may also help prevent the fractured condyle from displacing very far.

Incomplete fractures do not displace. In some cases the fracture is little more than a crack in the bone at the joint surface; this can be very difficult to see on routine radiographs. Some veterinarians speculate that these fractures begin in an abnormal area of bone. They believe that osteochondrosis may be the basic, underlying bone defect that allows these fractures to develop. *(Osteochondrosis is discussed in Chapter 14.)*

Signs and Diagnosis
Complete Condylar Fractures

Complete condylar fractures cause sudden, moderate to severe lameness (grade 3 – 5 of 5), and moderate swelling around the fetlock. The swelling consists of edema in the superficial tissues and effusion (accumulation of joint fluid) in the fetlock. If the fracture is not displaced, the swelling may only be slight and the lameness moderate. But palpation of the fetlock and cannon causes obvious pain, as does fetlock flexion. Pressing across the cannon bone puts pressure across the fracture line, causing pain. However, crepitus (crunching of bone-on-bone) usually is not heard or felt with this fracture, even when it is displaced. Radiographs are necessary to confirm the diagnosis.

Incomplete Condylar Fractures

Incomplete condylar fractures may not cause obvious lameness until the horse cools down after exercise. Even then, the lameness may only be moderate (grade 2 – 3 of 5). The swelling is usually mild and confined to the fetlock; this can be very misleading. Because the fracture begins in the fetlock joint, effusion makes it easy to mistake an incomplete condylar fracture for synovitis, degenerative joint disease, or other joint problems that do not primarily involve the cannon

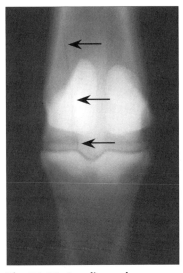

Fig. 17–15. A radiograph confirms the diagnosis of a complete, non-displaced condylar fracture.

bone. However, careful palpation of the bottom of the cannon bone may cause pain, which is not typical of a primary joint problem. Moreover, a joint block may not completely resolve the lameness if there is a condylar fracture.

Radiographs are necessary to confirm the diagnosis. Small, incomplete fractures can be very difficult to detect at first. The radiographs may need to be repeated a few days later; in some cases the fracture may not be obvious for a couple of weeks. Nuclear scintigraphy can help localize the problem to the end of the cannon bone in these cases.

More Information

Joint problems are discussed in Chapter 8.

Diagnostic techniques, including joint blocks and nuclear scintigraphy, are discussed in Chapter 2.

Treatment
Complete Condylar Fractures

Complete condylar fractures are best repaired with bone screws. It is very important that the fracture line is compressed and correctly aligned at the joint surface. Otherwise, degenerative joint disease may result. A cast cannot compress the fracture or align the joint surface enough to guarantee a good result. Still, most surgeons cast

More Information
Bone screw fixation and post-operative care are discussed and illustrated in Chapter 6.

the horse's leg immediately after surgery to protect the repair site from excessive load as the horse gets up after anesthesia. The cast is usually removed within a day or two of surgery and replaced with a bandage.

In most cases the horse is confined for 6 – 8 weeks after surgery, and then rested in a small paddock for another 2 – 4 months. Depending on the surgeon's instructions, the horse may be hand-walked once or twice per day during the confinement period.

The surgeon may recommend that the screws be removed once the fracture has healed. The screws can prevent the normal amount of "give" the cannon bone must have. They may cause chronic, mild lameness, or simply a reduction in athletic performance. However, many horses perform satisfactorily (and race successfully) with screws in their leg. It is not always necessary to take the screws out.

Incomplete Condylar Fractures

Incomplete condylar fractures are usually managed by applying a thick, firm support bandage to the leg from the hoof wall to the base of the knee or hock *(see Chapter 4)*. This type of bandage acts like a cast to restrict movement of the fetlock joint, reducing stress at the fracture site. The bandage should be changed as often as necessary. Depending on how well the fracture is healing, the thick bandage can usually be replaced with a lighter support wrap after 4 – 5 weeks.

In most cases the veterinarian recommends stall confinement for a total of 6 – 8 weeks. When radiographs show that the fracture has healed, the horse can be turned out for another 2 – 3 months of paddock or pasture rest. Even if there is little more than a small crack at the joint surface, most veterinarians recommend these measures because of the potential for the fracture to extend if the horse is exercised. It is not worth risking a complete fracture by continuing to work the horse or turning it out onto pasture immediately after the injury occurs.

Rehabilitation

The return to regular training must be gradual, beginning with the traditional "slow, distance work." Even though the fracture has healed, the horse must be given time to strengthen that area before more strenuous activities begin. Once the horse has had several

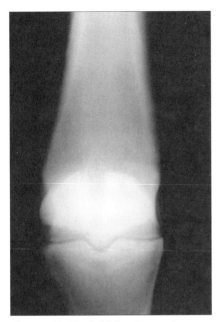

Fig. 17–16. The initial radiograph shows an incomplete condylar fracture behind the left sesamoid bone.

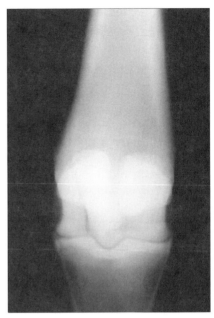

Fig. 17–17. A week later the fracture is complete because the horse was allowed too much activity.

Fig. 17–18. Six weeks later, the fracture has almost healed—there is a white line of mineralization where the dark fracture line used to be. But where the fracture extended into the fetlock joint is still not completely healed [arrow].

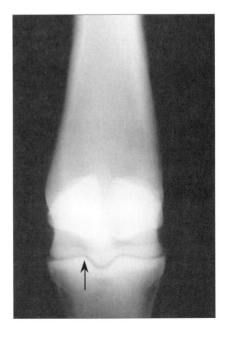

weeks of conditioning work, the guidelines given in Chapter 9 regarding training and bone quality should be followed.

Prognosis for Condylar Fractures

The prognosis for return to full athletic function is usually quite good, even with complete fractures. Of all the different types of long-bone fractures that can occur in horses, condylar fractures have the best outcome. But because the fracture line involves the joint surface, degenerative joint disease is a potential consequence of this type of injury. It is more likely if the surgeon could not perfectly align the bone at the joint surface.

COMPLETE CANNON BONE FRACTURES

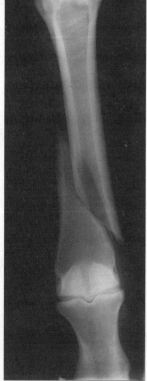

Fig. 17–19. A complete cannon bone fracture.

A complete fracture in the middle of the cannon bone is a devastating injury. These fractures most commonly occur during exercise, although any forceful, direct trauma can completely fracture the bone. Complete cannon bone fractures are usually open fractures. There is very little soft tissue between the bone and the skin in this area, so it is easy for a shard of bone to pierce the skin.

When these fractures occur during exercise, the horse's speed and momentum often keep it going, despite being unable to bear any weight on the fractured leg. Aside from the severe pain, this fracture prevents the horse from bearing weight on the leg because the solid column of bone is disrupted. Any weight on the fracture forces the bone fragments to override (overlap), and causes the cannon bone to collapse.

These fractures occur more often in the forelegs of horses that are not adequately conditioned for strenuous exercise, especially young horses that are "pushed too far, too soon." The fracture may occur when the bone is suddenly and massively overloaded (for example, if the horse stumbles or falls). But in most cases it is the end result of chronic overloading of a bone that has not been given enough time to adapt to the forces placed on it *(see Chapter 9)*. Other evidence of stress in the cannon bone, such as bucked shins or an incomplete dorsal fracture, is common in these horses. A complete fracture occurs when the weakened bone finally gives way.

A "fine boned" horse is at no greater risk of this type of fracture than any other horse. It is the thickness of the cortex (the dense, outer layer of the bone), not the bone's diameter, that determines the strength and resilience of the cannon bone. The thickness of the cortex may be influenced to some extent by genetics, but regular exercise has the most impact on the thickness, and therefore, the strength of the bone. The width of the cannon bone's cortex may be measured from routine radiographs (see the earlier section on *Bucked Shins*).

Management Problems

Euthanasia is often recommended in adult horses with complete cannon bone fractures. It is very difficult to satisfactorily stabilize the fracture, even a simple one. Because of the size and weight of the average adult horse, bone plates and screws often are not strong enough to stabilize and support the fracture. In some cases the bone is shattered into several pieces, which makes surgical repair even more challenging. However, these fractures can sometimes be successfully managed in foals and small ponies.

Despite extreme care and diligent supervision by the surgical staff, the implants may loosen, bend, or break when the horse gets up after anesthesia. Furthermore, because these fractures are often open, bacteria from the skin surface and environment easily invade the dam-

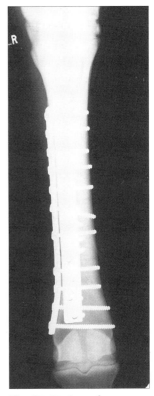

Fig. 17–20. Same bone as Figure 17–19, after surgical repair with two bone plates and over 20 bone screws.

aged bone. This can lead to bone infection (osteomyelitis; *see Chapter 9*). Infection further compromises fracture stability and bone healing.

One other important and common complication of this fracture is laminitis in the opposite, weight-bearing limb *(see Chapter 15)*. Laminitis makes the horse even more uncomfortable. It also causes the horse to shift more weight off the laminitic foot onto the fractured leg, further taxing the implants.

But despite these problems, attempts at surgical repair of complete cannon bone fractures are becoming more successful. As surgical techniques and implants develop, the prognosis will improve. Limb amputation and prosthetic limb technology *(see Chapter 9)* are also advancing, so there may be viable options to euthanasia in some horses.

SPLINTS
Definitions

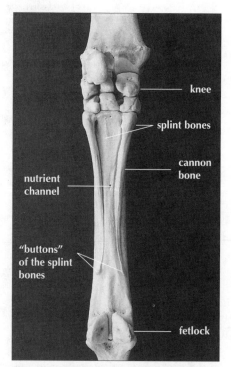

Fig. 17–21. Rear view of the foreleg (tendons and ligaments removed).

A "splint" is a bony swelling on a splint bone or the side of the cannon bone. A "hot splint" is a splint that is inflamed and painful. A "cold splint" is one in which the heat and pain have subsided, and only the bony swelling remains. "Blind splint" is another type of splint (discussed later).

The splint bones are the narrow bones that run down the back of the leg on either side of the cannon bone. They apparently are remnants from when prehistoric horses had five toes on each limb. The cannon bone is the middle (or third) digit and the splint bones are the second and fourth digits. This explains why the cannon bone of the foreleg is called the third metacarpal bone, and the splint bones are called the second and fourth metacarpals. There are no first or fifth metacarpal bones in horses. (In the hindlegs, the cannon and splint bones are called the metatarsal bones.)

Along with the cannon bone, the splint bones form the base of the knee or hock. They are part of the lower knee joint (carpometacarpal joint) and lower hock joint (tarsometatarsal joint). The splint bones narrow as they run down the cannon, and end with a small flare, or "button" of bone a few inches above the fetlock joint.

> **Terminology**
>
> The interosseous ligament between a splint bone and the cannon bone is different from the "interosseus muscle," which is the name for the suspensory ligament in some old texts.

Each splint bone is attached to the cannon bone by a short, dense ligament called the interosseous ligament *(see Figure 17–25).* Although this ligament fixes the splint bone to the cannon bone, a little independent movement of the bones is possible.

Causes

A splint may primarily involve:

- the splint bones
- the cannon bone
- the interosseous ligament ("blind splint")

Direct trauma to the surface of the splint bone or cannon bone can occur with a kick, interference from the opposite foot, or some other injury. It causes inflammation of the periosteum, which is the fibrous outer covering of the bone. As a result, new bone is laid down under the periosteum at that location (exostosis).

However, not all splints

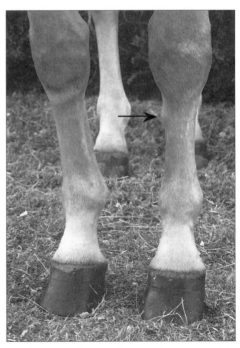

Fig. 17–22. A "cold splint" that was probably caused by trauma.

are caused by direct trauma; concussion is another important cause. The splint bones are free at their lower end; they do not meet another bone at a joint surface. Therefore, they do not sustain the weight-bearing forces that the cannon bone must withstand. But each splint bone is attached to the cannon bone by the interosseous ligament. The concussive ground forces the cannon bone experiences during exercise are transmitted to the splint bones through this ligament. The splint bones narrow a few inches below the knee or hock, and this is the point where most splints develop—presumably, it is a major stresspoint for the splint bones.

Excessive load on a bone results in the production of extra bone to stabilize the stresspoint and make it stronger. It takes several weeks for a bone to significantly increase its density in response to the stresses of exercise *(see Chapter 9)*. Working a young or untrained mature horse at speed before the necessary improvements in bone density have been made can cause splints. Working any horse on a very hard surface increases the concussive forces on the cannon and splint bones. This can also cause splints.

In general, when splints are caused by concussion the swellings are found in the same place on both forelegs (or both hindlegs). That is, the splints are symmetrical. The most common location of these splints is the inside of the forelegs, just below the knees. But when a splint is caused by trauma, the swelling may be present on only one leg. If each leg has a splint the swellings are more likely to be in a slightly different place, and a little further down the leg than those caused by concussion.

"Blind Splints"

Note
Over a period of several years part or all of the interosseous ligament calcifies (is replaced with bone) in many mature horses. However, this does not cause lameness.

The small amount of independent movement allowed by the interosseous ligament can create tension on the periosteum of the splint bone where the ligament attaches. Inflammation and new bone production at this site is called a "blind splint" because it occurs between the cannon and splint bone, rather than as an obvious bony swelling on the outside of the splint bone. "Blind splints" usually cause a lameness that is very difficult to locate.

Signs and Diagnosis of Splints

When splints first form they may cause mild lameness (grade 1 – 2 of 5) and a small, hot, painful, bony swelling on the splint bone or cannon bone. This is a "hot splint." Splints that occur on a splint bone tend to be taller and narrower than those that develop on the cannon bone. Often these initial signs are so subtle and transient, that an owner or trainer may not notice the splint until it has begun to settle down (become a "cold splint"). The splint is found when the horse's legs are examined for another reason. If lameness is present in horses with "cold splints" it can usually be traced to another problem in the leg. In other words, splints do not necessarily cause lameness. In most cases they are only of cosmetic importance.

"Blind splints" can be difficult to definitely diagnose. In most cases the only sign is mild lameness. There usually is no obvious swelling, heat, or pain directly over the affected splint bone. To help diagnose a "blind splint" the veterinarian may inject local anesthetic around the splint bone, aiming to deposit the anesthetic as close as possible to the interosseous ligament. However, it is difficult to block this ligament without also blocking other structures at the back of the cannon, especially the suspensory origin *(see Chapter 11)* and the nerves that supply the lower leg. Accidently blocking these structures can cause confusion or misdiagnosis.

Radiographs of "blind splints" usually show calcification between

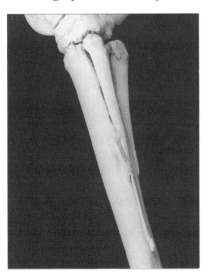 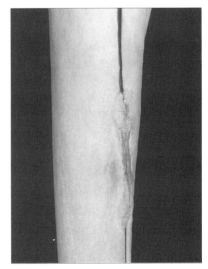

Fig. 17–23. On the left, a "blind splint": new bone production between the cannon and splint bone. On the right, a close-up of the bony proliferation.

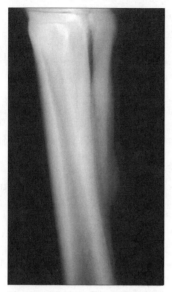

Fig. 17–24. A radiograph of a splint.

the cannon and splint bones. However, if the horse is mature it can be difficult to tell the difference between a "blind splint" and the normal calcification of the interosseous ligament that occurs with age. Nuclear scintigraphy can help; abnormal new bone production causes a "hot spot" over that splint bone.

The veterinarian may also recommend taking a radiograph of a "hot splint," particularly if the swelling and lameness are more severe than usual and persist despite treatment. These signs may be due to a splint bone fracture (discussed later).

Treatment of Splints

Splints resolve when the body remodels the bony swelling by absorbing some of the new bone. The splint flattens out over several weeks, and may disappear completely, provided the cause does not persist. Cannon bone splints usually flatten out and remodel more quickly and completely than those on a splint bone. This is probably because there is a larger area of bone surrounding a splint on the cannon.

Controlled Exercise

No matter what the cause or location, bone remodeling, and therefore resolution of the splint, happens more quickly if the horse's workload is reduced for 1 – 3 weeks. The splint will persist or worsen if the horse remains in training because the splint bone suffers continued concussion. In most cases the horse does not need to be rested from all exercise. Some form of daily, light exercise on a soft, even surface can help stimulate the bone to remodel and resolve the splint. If the final cosmetic appearance is important, it may be best to rest the horse in a stall or small paddock, and only hand-walk it twice per day. Hand-walking prevents the horse from knocking the splint during activity and causing more inflammation.

Medications

A few days of anti-inflammatory therapy, such as cold therapy,

NSAIDs, DMSO, and "sweats" *(see Chapter 5),* is also useful if the splint is hot and painful, or the horse is lame. There are many other medications and therapies that have been tried for resolving splints. Some are more successful than others. But the fact that there are so many implies that none are universally effective. It takes time for the bone to remodel and resolve the swelling. Anti-inflammatory medications may aid this process by reducing inflammation—an important stimulus for new bone production. However, attributing the disappearance of the splint to these medications may be giving them too much credit.

Counter-irritant medications or procedures are aimed at stimulating an inflammatory response in an effort to resolve the bony swelling. However, they often slow the process of bone remodeling and can actually stimulate more new bone. Therefore, counter-irritants are counter-productive.

Surgery

Some veterinarians have attempted surgical removal of large splints. This involves anesthetizing the horse and removing the excess bone with a surgical bone chisel. However, this procedure can stimulate a dramatic bone response, which includes the production of new bone at the surgery site. Surgery improves the appearance of the splint (or resolves it completely) in about one-third of horses. In another third, the splint returns and looks the same. But in the final third of horses the splint becomes larger than it was originally. So the chance of a good cosmetic result with this surgery is only about 30%.

Prognosis for Splints

The prognosis for return to athletic activities is excellent once the inflammation and pain have subsided. With the exception of "blind splints," which may cause pain and lameness until the interosseous ligament is calcified, the lameness caused by a splint usually resolves quickly and completely.

SPLINT BONE FRACTURES
Definition and Causes

A splint bone can be fractured by direct trauma, such as a kick, knock, or blow from a polo mallet. But splint bone fractures also occur spontaneously during exercise; they are not always the result of an obvious traumatic incident. Presumably, the bone fractures because of the same concussive forces that can cause splints. This injury is far more common in racehorses than in other performance horses.

A splint bone can be fractured anywhere along its length. But when the fracture occurs spontaneously it usually does so in the lower half of the bone, most often at the junction between the middle and lower thirds. The interosseous ligament that anchors the splint bone to the cannon bone is much stronger at the top half of the splint bone. Excessive movement of the lower part of the splint bone can cause a fracture in the middle, where the ligament attaches the splint bone more firmly.

It is fairly common for a splint bone fracture to be found in a horse with suspensory ligament strain (suspensory desmitis; *see Chapter 11*). The question is: which occurred first, the fracture or the suspensory ligament problem? The suspensory ligament runs down the back of the cannon, in between the splint bones. It divides into two branches at about the level where the splint bones end. There has been speculation that strain and thickening of one of the suspensory branches may push out the end of the splint bone. This creates greater tension and subsequent fracture further up the bone, where it is more firmly attached to the cannon bone. However, the other possibility is that a fractured splint bone can inflame or damage the suspensory branch which runs so close to it. Unfortunately, science has not yet found a good answer to this question. From a practical standpoint, it is enough to be aware that both conditions often occur together.

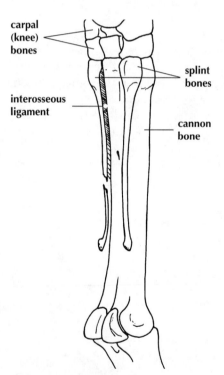

carpal (knee) bones

splint bones

interosseous ligament

cannon bone

Fig. 17–25. The splint bone often fractures in the lower half, where it is less firmly attached by the interosseous ligament.

There are two important questions the veterinarian must address when dealing with splint bone fractures. First, is the fracture open or closed? Second, is the fracture in the upper third or lower two-thirds of the bone?

Open or Closed?

An open fracture is one in which there is a skin wound overlying the fracture. A closed fracture does not involve a skin wound. The bone does not protrude from the skin in open splint bone fractures. However, bacteria from the skin surface and the environment can invade the wound and the damaged bone. These fractures almost always become infected (osteomyelitis; *see Chapter 9*). So, the veterinarian must treat them a little differently than a closed fracture.

Open splint bone fractures generally are caused by direct trauma, such as a kick. They are more likely in pastured horses because when they fight, horses tend to back up and kick one another. These fractures occur more often in the upper half of the bone, and are usually comminuted: more than one fracture line, creating several bone fragments.

Upper Third or Lower Two-Thirds?

The top of each splint bone forms part of the lower knee or hock joint. So, a fracture at the top of the splint bone may be an articular fracture (involving a joint surface). Whether or not the fracture extends into the joint, the splint bones are small but important parts of these joints. Horses need the top parts of their splint bones, but they function very well when the lower part has been surgically removed.

Signs and Diagnosis
Open Splint Bone Fractures

A common scenario with open splint bone fractures is a small wound that appears to heal well, only to swell and ooze pus several days or even a couple of weeks later. At first the wound is little more than a nick on the side of the leg. There is a small amount of swelling and the wound is tender to the touch. The lameness, which usually is mild, is attributed to the wound and the soft tissue trauma around it. So, the owner or trainer simply treats it like any small wound.

This is the problem with these fractures: the delay in proper treatment allows infection in the fracture site to progress and damage the bone further. The skin wound may appear to be healing well, but the swelling and lameness persist or return, and the wound may later break open and ooze pus. When the leg is radiographed, a comminuted splint bone fracture is found; usually, there is also evidence of osteomyelitis. In some cases the surface of the cannon bone directly beneath the fracture is abnormal. Either the cannon bone was damaged at the same time as the splint bone, or the infection spread to involve the cannon bone's surface.

Closed Splint Bone Fractures

Most closed splint bone fractures occur in the lower half of the bone. A typical sign is a small amount of swelling in the middle of the cannon, around the affected splint bone. Careful palpation can locate pain directly over the fracture. When the fracture is "fresh" (within a few days of its occurrence) there may be a more obvious soft tissue swelling over the area. This is a hematoma: an accumulation of leaked blood. If the suspensory ligament is also inflamed, the affected branch is thickened and painful. The lameness associated with this fracture usually is mild (grade 1 – 2 of 5).

The diagnosis must be confirmed, and the precise location of the fracture determined with radiographs. Ultrasonography of the suspensory ligament is also useful. The splint bone fracture can easily be managed. But suspensory ligament injury increases the length of time the horse is out of work, and may worsen the prognosis for future athletic function. *(See Chapter 11 for more information.)*

Treatment
Open Splint Bone Fractures

Open splint bone fractures generally need to be treated surgically. In most cases the infection will not resolve with antibiotics, flushing the wound, or any treatment other than surgical removal of the diseased bone.

When the fracture occurs in the upper third of the bone—particularly if it involves the joint—the splint bone should be stabilized with a bone plate. Instability at this site can prevent fracture healing and result in chronic lameness. (Chronic lameness may also result when the splint bone is fixed to the cannon bone with bone screws. So, a small bone plate with short screws is usually a better method of splint bone repair than regular bone screws.) If removing the infected bone and any small, devitalized bone fragments leaves a large defect, the surgeon may pack the defect with a bone graft. This speeds up bone production and fracture repair *(see Chapter 6)*.

When the splint bone on the outside of the hindleg has a badly comminuted, open fracture near, or involving the joint, removing the entire splint bone can be a viable alternative to surgical repair. Of all the splint bones, the one on the outside of the hindleg contributes the least to joint stability and weight-bearing. This procedure is unsuccessful with the splint bone on the inside of the hindleg or either splint bone on the foreleg. These bones should be repaired with a bone plate.

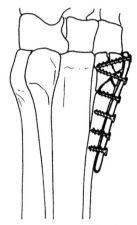

If the fracture occurred in the lower two-thirds of the splint bone, the surgeon may simply remove the part of the splint bone below the fracture. Horses do very well without the lower part of the splint bone, as long as the upper third remains stable.

Fig. 17–26. Repair of a splint bone fracture with a bone plate.

Post-Operative Care

In most cases the skin is sutured closed, and the leg is kept bandaged until the sutures are removed (usually 7 – 10 days after surgery). Antibiotics are given for at least 5 days, and NSAIDs are also given for a few days. The horse's tetanus status should be checked before surgery. *(These therapies are discussed in Section II.)*

Most surgeons recommend keeping the horse confined in a stall or small paddock until radiographs indicate that the fracture has healed. This usually takes 8 – 12 weeks. Another 2 – 3 months of paddock or pasture rest is often recommended after this time. In most cases the bone plate is left in. When part or all of the splint bone is removed, the horse may be able to start light exercise in as little as 4 – 6 weeks after surgery.

Closed Splint Bone Fractures

Closed fractures in the upper third of the bone may require stabilization with a small bone plate. However, they often heal well with just a firm support bandage and 6 – 8 weeks of confinement. The cannon bone acts like a natural splint or support for the fractured splint bone, so conservative management of these fractures can be very successful.

Fractures in the lower two-thirds of the bone are usually treated by surgically removing the fragment of splint bone. In most cases the

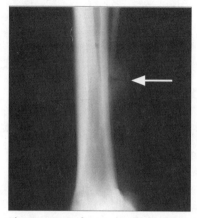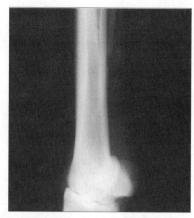

Fig. 17–27. Left: A splint bone fracture that has not healed, despite the bony callus. Right: The same splint bone after surgical removal of the fragment.

functional and cosmetic result is excellent. Unless the horse also has suspensory desmitis, it can usually be returned to regular exercise 4 – 6 weeks post-surgery.

Post-operative care is fairly standard: confinement in a stall or small paddock, bandaging, and a few days of antibiotics and NSAIDs. The horse's tetanus status should be reviewed before surgery. In most cases the leg is kept bandaged until the sutures are removed, usually 7 – 10 days after surgery. To ensure a good cosmetic result the veterinarian may continue to keep the leg bandaged for another 2 – 3 weeks. Daily hand-walking during the convalescent period is useful for horses that are confined to a stall.

Prognosis for Splint Bone Fractures

The prognosis for return to athletic function after an open splint bone fracture is usually fairly good, provided the diseased bone was removed, the infection was resolved, and the fracture was stabilized. Chronic lameness can result from persistent infection or instability of the fracture. If the fracture was articular, degenerative joint disease can also cause chronic lameness.

The prognosis for future athletic usefulness after a closed splint bone fracture is very good for fractures in the upper third, and excellent for fractures in the lower two-thirds of the bone. Provided the fracture was stabilized or the fragment was removed, and the suspensory ligament was undamaged or healed well, these horses have few, if any, long-term problems.

18

THE KNEE

T he knee is a very com-
mon site of injury in
racing Thoroughbreds
and Quarter Horses. Knee
problems are sometimes
seen in other horses that
perform strenuous activities,
particularly jumping. Problems in the knee generally
cause obvious swelling. The
location and severity of the
swelling depend on the
problem. So this chapter is
broadly divided into two sections: conditions that cause
swelling at the front of the
knee, and those that cause
swelling at the back of the
knee.

The knee is a complex
area. Following is a brief discussion of its structures.

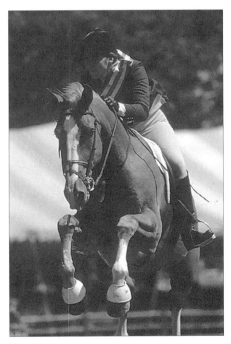

Fig. 18–1.

STRUCTURE & FUNCTION
Bones

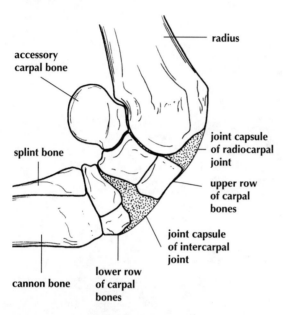

accessory
carpal bone

splint bone

cannon bone

radius

joint capsule
of radiocarpal
joint

upper row
of carpal
bones

joint capsule
of intercarpal
joint

lower row
of carpal
bones

Fig. 18–2. The bones and joints of the knee, seen from the outside.

The knee, or carpus, contains two rows of block-shaped "cuboidal" bones. There are three carpal bones per row. The bones of the upper row are called the radial, intermediate, and ulnar carpal bones. Those of the lower row are called the second, third, and fourth carpal bones (or C2, C3, and C4). These three bones sit directly on top of the cannon and splint bones. At the back of the knee there is an oval-shaped, curved bone called the accessory carpal bone.

Extra Information
Some horses have an extra carpal bone that is about the size of a pebble; a few horses have two. The extra bone is either the first carpal bone on the inside of the leg or the fifth carpal bone on the outside of the leg. They are thought to be remnants from when prehistoric horses had five toes.
These unusual bones could be mistaken for chip fractures because of their small size. However, unlike chip fractures, they are located toward the back of the knee, and they are smooth and round. Their presence, although interesting, does not cause lameness.

Joints

There are three horizontal joints in the knee:

1. **The radiocarpal joint.** This joint lies between the lower end of the radius and the upper row of carpal bones.
2. **The intercarpal joint.** This joint, also called the midcarpal joint, lies between the upper and lower rows of carpal bones.
3. **The carpometacarpal joint.** This joint lies between the lower row of carpal bones and the top of the cannon and splint bones. It is essentially immobile.

There are also several small, vertical, immobile joints in between the carpal bones.

The radiocarpal and intercarpal joints are mobile joints. Most knee problems involve one or both of these joints.

The joint spaces of the radiocarpal and intercarpal joints are separate. So, it is possible to identify the location of the problem with a joint block *(see Chapter 2)* into either the radiocarpal or intercarpal joint.

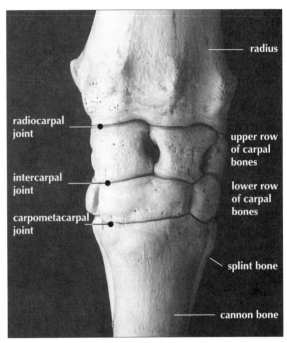

Fig. 18–3. The bones and joints of the knee, seen from the front.

The joint capsules of the radiocarpal and intercarpal joints attach to the front of the carpal bones. With the radiocarpal joint, the top of the joint capsule attaches onto the lower end of the radius. These joint capsules are fairly "roomy" at the front of the joint. This allows the knee to be fully flexed without overstretching the joint capsules. It also means that when there is an accumulation of joint fluid, the joint capsule visibly bulges at the front.

Supporting Structures

There are many small ligaments that support and stabilize the knee. Additional support is provided by the extensor tendons that run over the front of the knee:

1. **The common digital extensor tendon.** This tendon begins as an extensor muscle at the front of the forearm, runs down the front of the leg, and finally attaches onto the top of the pedal bone. Its function is to extend, or straighten the joints of the lower leg (knee, fetlock, pastern, and coffin joint).

2. **The extensor carpi radialis tendon.** This tendon begins as a muscle at the front of the forearm and attaches onto the front of the cannon bone, just below the knee. Its function is to extend the knee.

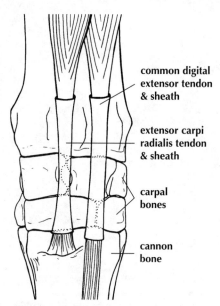

common digital
extensor tendon
& sheath

extensor carpi
radialis tendon
& sheath

carpal
bones

cannon
bone

Fig. 18–4. The extensor tendons at the front of the knee.

Because of their location, these tendons support the front of the knee, particularly when the knee is flexed. They overlie the joint capsules of the radiocarpal and intercarpal joints, so they can create discrete "bubbles" if there is excessive fluid in one of these joints. This fact can help the veterinarian determine the site of the problem.

Joint Mobility

Of all the joints in the horse's body, the knee has the widest range of motion. It is a hinge-type joint, so it is only capable of flexion and extension (closing and opening). In the normal horse the knee can be flexed until the cannon bone and radius are parallel. The back of the foot can touch the back of the elbow without causing any discomfort. The degree of knee flexion a horse allows is an important piece of diagnostic information. If the knee can be fully flexed with little or no discomfort, any problem found in the knee is unlikely to be very serious.

Extra Information

The human equivalent of the horse's knee is the wrist. The wrist has a much more limited range of flexion than the horse's knee, but a greater range of extension. It can also be rotated and bent from side to side.

The human knee, which is equivalent to the horse's stifle, has a range of motion more like the horse's knee. It is only capable of flexion and extension, although it can be fully flexed. The similarities do not end there. As with knee problems in people, knee problems in horses are most commonly seen in young athletes.

SWELLING AT THE FRONT OF THE KNEE

There are several conditions that cause swelling at the front of the knee (also called a "popped knee"). The size of the swelling and the degree of lameness that accompanies it vary with the condition.

Before deciding how to treat the swelling, the veterinarian must determine which structure is involved, and the type and extent of the damage. Some of the questions the veterinarian addresses in the process include:

What is the size, shape, and location of the swelling?

The size, shape, and location of the swelling is a good general guide to which structure is most likely involved. When the problem is located within a joint space, the swelling primarily consists of an accumulation of fluid (effusion) within the joint. This effusion expands the capsule of the affected joint at the front of the knee, so the resulting swelling is quite specific.

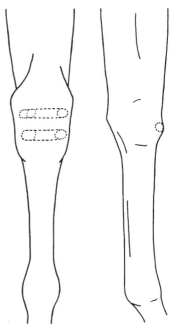

Fig. 18–5. The knee from the front and side, showing the possible location of horizontal swellings and "bubbles."

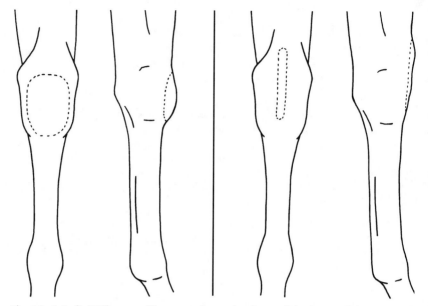

Fig. 18–6. Left: Diffuse swelling over the entire front of the knee. Right: Vertical swelling of the extensor tendon sheath.

When the effusion is great, it pushes out the joint capsule across the entire front of the affected joint, so the swelling is horizontal. But if the effusion is only slight, the extensor tendons that run over the front of the knee may restrict the swelling to a small "bubble" on one side of the joint. The most common place to find such a swelling is toward the inside of the leg, about two-thirds of the way down the knee: that is, over the intercarpal joint.

In contrast, when structures outside the joint capsules are damaged, the swelling is more generalized. Typically, it is a large, fairly even mass that covers most or all of the front of the knee. One exception is when effusion develops in the tendon sheath of one of the extensor tendons. The tendon sheaths are long, narrow cuffs around the tendons, so effusion results in a long, narrow, vertical swelling.

A swelling caused by joint effusion typically disappears when the knee is flexed. This is because flexing the knee puts tension on the joint capsule and prevents it from being expanded by the fluid. On the other hand, fluid accumulation outside the joint is usually still visible or able to be felt when the knee is flexed.

Is the swelling firm or soft?

A firm swelling is likely to be either fibrous tissue or new bone production (an exostosis; *see Chapter 9*) at the site of previous injury. Both of these changes are chronic; they have been developing or present for some time.

A soft swelling may be caused by soft tissue inflammation, a hygroma, or effusion within a joint or tendon sheath. These conditions may be acute or chronic.

Is the swelling painful?

A painful swelling generally indicates that the injury is acute (recent). In most cases, chronic swellings are not painful, unless they are reinjured. The degree of pain is a fairly good guide to the severity of the problem. For example, soft tissue inflammation beneath the skin may only be mildly painful, whereas the swelling caused by a carpal slab fracture is very painful. However, this general trend does not always hold true. A chip fracture may cause a small, non-painful swelling, yet it can have important implications for the horse's athletic future. *(Fractures are discussed later.)*

Once the veterinarian has answered these questions, a diagnosis can sometimes be made and treatment recommended without any diagnostic tests. However, in most instances the veterinarian needs to use radiography and/or ultrasound to identify exactly which structure is involved and determine the severity of the damage *(see Chapter 2)*. The choice of treatment depends on this information, so an accurate diagnosis is very important.

Problems Outside the Joint Capsule

There are three common causes of swelling over the front of the knee that do not directly involve the joints: hygroma, tenosynovitis, and new bone production (exostoses) beneath the extensor tendons. **Note:** Cellulitis occasionally causes generalized swelling over the knee. However, the swelling usually involves the entire knee and part of the cannon or forearm.

> **Definitions**
>
> **Tenosynovitis:** inflammation of a tendon sheath. *See Chapter 11.*
>
> **Cellulitis:** bacterial infection of the superficial tissues. *See Chapter 13.*

Hygroma

Definition

A hygroma is a fluid-filled swelling that develops over a bony surface as a result of trauma. The swelling may be a hematoma or a se-

> ## Definitions
>
> **Hematoma:** collection of blood beneath the skin.
> **Seroma:** collection of serum, the clear yellow, liquid portion of the blood, beneath the skin.

roma beneath the skin. Or it may be excess fluid in a bursa, in this case the supracarpal bursa at the front of the knee.

A bursa is a fluid-filled sac that lies between a tendon and a bone. It protects the tendon from pressure and friction. Like a joint capsule, a bursa has a fibrous, outer layer, and a lining that secretes fluid into the sac. Inflammation of the bursa, whether caused by pressure, friction, or direct trauma, causes an increase of fluid within it. This condition is called bursitis. Fluid accumulation in a bursa is limited by the size of the sac. So, a hygroma that develops due to bursitis is usually not as large as that caused by a hematoma or seroma.

"False Bursa"

Some veterinary texts use the term, "false bursa," for hygromas. This is because a hematoma or seroma can develop some of the same characteristics as a bursa—a fluid-filled, fibrous sac—if the area is repeatedly traumatized. When a tissue is damaged, fibrin, a blood-clotting protein is released into the area to prevent further

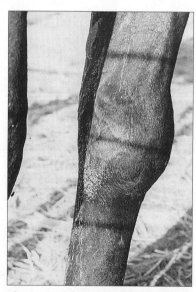

Fig. 18–7. A hygroma over the knee.

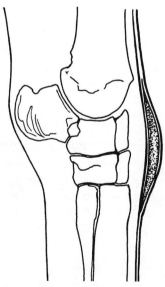

Fig. 18–8. A "false bursa."

blood or serum leakage, and to begin repairing the damage. The body organizes the fibrin within the hematoma/seroma into fibrous tissue. If the area is damaged again the inflammation persists and more serum leaks into the swelling. The end result is a layer of fibrous tissue around a fluidy swelling: a "false bursa."

Causes of Hygromas

A hygroma may form suddenly as the result of a single traumatic incident. For example, a horse that falls onto the front of its knee or hits a jump rail with its knee may develop an acute hygroma. Other hygromas develop more slowly. For example, chronic hygromas often develop in horses that repeatedly paw and knock the stall door or feeder with their knees. Horses that are kept on concrete without enough bedding can also develop chronic hygromas. When horses rest lying down, with their forelegs tucked under their chest, the front of the knee is pressed against the floor. Over time, this can cause inflammation of the bursa and/or soft tissues beneath the skin, and a hygroma.

Signs and Diagnosis of Hygromas

When the hygroma first develops, the soft, fluidy swelling may be warm and mildly painful. In some cases the hygroma is large, covering most or all of the front of the knee. The heat and pain usually subside in a couple of days, although the fluid takes longer to be absorbed. With hematomas or seromas the fluid often gravitates to the lower part of the knee and forms a "baggy" swelling.

Lameness, if present, is usually mild (grade 1 – 2 of 5). Hygromas caused by sudden trauma, such as a fall, are more likely to be painful and cause lameness than those that develop gradually. Other tissue damage is also likely in cases of sudden trauma, and

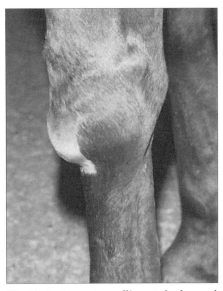

Fig. 18–9. "Baggy" swelling at the base of the knee. The area has been shaved in preparation for drainage.

it may cause a more obvious lameness than just the hygroma alone.

The diagnosis is usually based on the type of swelling and the horse's history. If the lameness is worse than is usual for a hygroma, or does not resolve in a couple of days, the veterinarian may radiograph the knee and ultrasound the swelling. These procedures are needed to see whether any other structures have been damaged. Ultrasound is also the best way to distinguish between bursitis and a hematoma/seroma. This is worthwhile if the swelling is to be drained.

Treatment of Hygromas

In most cases the lameness resolves quickly with a few days of rest, anti-inflammatory therapy (cold therapy, NSAIDs, DMSO, etc.) and daily light exercise, for example, hand-walking. More extensive treatment is usually only necessary for cosmetic reasons. *(See Section II: Principles of Therapy for more information on the therapies mentioned in this section.)*

Drainage

The veterinarian may drain the fluid from the swelling. For a hematoma or seroma this procedure is usually not performed for at least 3 days after an acute injury. When a hematoma first forms, the pressure that builds up within the swelling acts as a bandage to prevent further bleeding from the damaged vessels. Draining the swelling relieves the pressure and allows bleeding to continue. Therefore, if the swelling is to be drained, it is best to wait until a few days after the injury.

> **Caution**
>
> Inserting a needle or a blade into a hygroma could cause infection or damage a joint capsule. This procedure must only be performed by a veterinarian.

After draining the fluid, the veterinarian may inject corticosteroids into the cavity to settle down the inflammation. These drugs also slow the production of fibrous tissue, so they have added benefit for hygromas. But if there is any risk of infection, corticosteroids should not be used. A skin wound over the swelling increases the risk of bacteria invading the hygroma.

Bursitis is often treated with an injection of corticosteroids or hyaluronic acid, sometimes both, into the bursa. Hyaluronic acid relieves inflammation (although not as well as corticosteroids), and it helps prevent fibrous adhesions between the tendon and bursa.

Keeping a firm, well-padded bandage on the knee for 1 – 2 weeks (changing it as often as necessary) can improve the cosmetic result. It can be difficult to maintain a comfortable bandage that does not slip and provides enough pressure over the front of the knee, without causing pressure sores. These problems are less likely if the horse is kept confined while wearing the bandage.

Activity

Daily light exercise or paddock turnout, and passive motion exercises (repeated flexion and extension) are a good alternative to confinement and bandaging in some cases. Activity stimulates blood flow, so provided it is begun at least 3 days after injury, it can speed up absorption of any remaining fluid. It also reduces the potential for adhesions (restrictive fibrous bands) to form between the skin and the joint capsules or tendons. So, this approach can help preserve normal joint mobility and movement. It can also produce a fairly good cosmetic result.

Surgery

Draining the fluid, injecting corticosteroids into the cavity, and keeping the knee bandaged usually resolves, or at least reduces the size of the swelling. However, if the knee is traumatized again, the hygroma may re-form, and a "false bursa" develop. In chronic or persistent cases the veterinarian may surgically remove the fibrous tissue that forms the wall of the sac.

To ensure the best possible cosmetic result following surgery, the veterinarian may recommend that the horse is confined to a stall or small pen. A firm, well-padded bandage is kept on the knee for 1 – 2 weeks, and changed as often as necessary. Antibiotics may be given for a few days following surgery. NSAIDs usually are given to minimize post-operative discomfort and swelling. The horse's tetanus status should be checked before surgery.

No matter how the hygroma is treated, it is important to prevent further trauma. Even after surgical removal of the fibrous tissue, a hygroma can re-form if the horse is permitted to re-traumatize its knee.

Prognosis for Hygromas

The prognosis for athletic function is very good, whether or not the swelling resolves completely. The cosmetic result is more variable. Even with surgical removal of the fibrous tissue, the front of the knee may always be thickened.

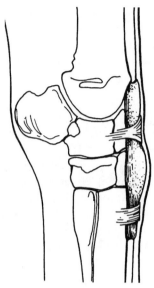

Fig. 18–10. Tenosynovitis in a tendon sheath over the front of the knee causes a distinctive swelling.

Tenosynovitis

Definition and Causes

Tenosynovitis is inflammation of a tendon sheath. In this case it involves the tendon sheath of one of the two extensor tendons that run over the front of the knee. Overstretching or direct trauma to a tendon and/or its sheath causes inflammation, which leads to an accumulation of fluid within the sheath. *(Tenosynovitis is discussed further in Chapter 11.)*

Extensor tenosynovitis is fairly common in jumping horses, particularly if they knock a jump rail with the front of their leg, or trip and fall with their knees flexed. If the horse falls onto its knee while the knee is flexed, the extensor carpi radialis tendon *(see Figure 18–4)* can be torn away from its attachment at the front of the cannon bone. As a result, the tendon sheath may fill with blood. This is a very uncommon injury.

Signs

Tenosynovitis involving an extensor tendon results in a long, narrow, soft swelling that often begins just above the knee. There are some fibrous bands that run across the tendons to hold them in place. These bands cause the swelling to have a slightly irregular outline when seen from the side.

When tenosynovitis first occurs, the swelling may be warm and mildly painful during palpation. In general, if just the tendon sheath is inflamed, the horse usually is not lame. However, if tendon fibers are damaged—which is far less common—mild lameness (grade 1 – 2 of 5) usually is present.

The initial signs of swelling, heat, and pain are more severe if the extensor carpi radialis tendon is partially or completely torn. The horse is still able to straighten the knee and bear weight on the leg because the common digital extensor tendon is intact and functioning normally. However, the lameness is usually moderate to severe (grade 3 – 4 of 5).

If the knock or fall caused a wound that damaged the tendon sheath, persistent inflammation, adhesions, and thickening of the sheath lining may develop. The body controls the infection, but the changes in the sheath cause chronic swelling and low-grade lameness, even after the wound has healed.

Diagnosis

In most cases the veterinarian can make the diagnosis based on the signs. If the horse is lame, ultrasounding the swollen tendon sheath may reveal tendon fiber damage or adhesions. This is important because if the tendon is damaged, the horse must be rested from regular training for longer.

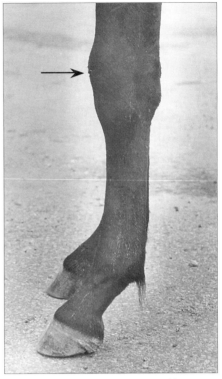

Fig. 18–11. Tenosynovitis caused by trauma to the front of the knee.

Treatment

When the injury first occurs, rest and a few days of anti-inflammatory therapy may relieve the inflammation and resolve the swelling if it is mild. Anti-inflammatory therapy includes cold therapy, NSAIDs, and DMSO *(see Chapter 5).* In most cases the horse can be lightly exercised each day, and can resume regular training in 2 – 3 weeks. Light exercise involves hand-walking or riding/driving at the walk for at least 20 minutes twice per day. It helps resolve the swelling and reduces the potential for adhesions (fibrous bands) to form within the sheath.

Drainage

When the swelling is more pronounced, or a good cosmetic result is

> **More Information**
>
> Treating tenosynovitis with hyaluronic acid and corticosteroids is discussed in Chapter 11.
>
> Applying a comfortable yet effective knee bandage is described in Chapter 4.

important, the veterinarian may need to treat it more aggressively. If done within a couple of days of injury, draining the excess fluid, injecting hyaluronic acid or corticosteroids into the sheath, and keeping a firm bandage over the knee can resolve the swelling.

If the swelling has been present for several days, treatment may not permanently resolve the swelling. By this time the swollen sheath has been stretched, and will continue to fill to its new capacity. But this swelling should not affect the horse's performance once the acute inflammation subsides and any tendon damage heals. It is merely a blemish.

Activity

The presence and degree of tendon fiber damage dictates how long the horse must be rested from regular training. Unless the extensor carpi radialis tendon is completely ruptured, horses with extensor tendon damage benefit from a gradually increasing program of light exercise. Activity not only promotes blood flow to the injured tendon, it prevents adhesions from forming and restricting normal tendon function. The horse can be turned out onto pasture, but better results are usually obtained by hand-walking the horse twice per day for the first 3 – 4 weeks after injury. The duration of each session can be gradually increased over that period. Provided repeat ultrasound examination indicates that the tendon is healing well, ridden/driven exercise can begin after this time, and gradually increase over the next 4 – 6 weeks.

Surgery

When the extensor carpi radialis tendon is ruptured, the veterinarian may recommend surgical repair. The tendon will eventually heal without surgery. However, fibrous thickening over the front of the knee typically remains. Also, adhesions between the torn tendon and the tendon sheath (or even the surrounding tissues) could restrict normal knee flexion. Surgical repair of the tendon can speed healing and improve the chances of a good result. A firm, well-padded bandage, which may include splints to prevent the horse from flexing its knee, and strict stall confinement are necessary for 4 – 6 weeks. Once repeat ultrasound examination indicates that the repair site is healing well, it is usually safe to begin the program of gradually increasing, light exercise.

When a penetrating wound causes chronic lameness, the most effective treatment is surgery. The sheath is opened, the adhesions and thickened lining are removed, and the outer layer of the sheath and the skin are sutured closed. Hand-walking and passive motion exercises for at least one month after surgery usually have very good results.

Prognosis for Tenosynovitis

The prognosis for athletic function is excellent with tenosynovitis of the extensor tendons. Treatment is usually only necessary for cosmetic reasons. Unless extensive tendon damage has also occurred, the heat, pain, and lameness settle down quickly and generally do not return. However, the swelling may remain. The prognosis for return to athletic function after extensor carpi radialis tendon rupture is fair, although recovery may take several months.

Exostoses Beneath the Extensor Tendons

An exostosis is new bone production, usually at a stresspoint *(see Chapter 9)*. In this case it occurs where short ligaments anchor the extensor tendons to the front of the carpal bones and radius. Excessive or repeated strain on these ligaments when the tendons extend the knee causes new bone production beneath the periosteum. It is most often seen along the front of the upper row of carpal bones.

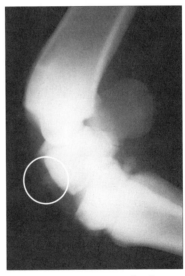

When the exostoses are large or extensive they cause mild thickening over the front of the knee that can be seen and/or felt. Unless the tendon sheath or the extensor tendon itself is inflamed, this condition usually does not cause lameness. It is fairly common in mature performance horses, and is often found when the knees are radiographed during a prepurchase examination. Provided no other

Fig. 18–12. Exostoses at the front of the knee.

abnormalities are present, and the horse does not resent full knee flexion, these exostoses usually are not significant. Although, they do indicate that the structures at the front of the knee have been strained at some time.

Problems Within the Joints

There are several conditions within the knee joints that can cause swelling over the front of the knee. No matter what the underlying problem, the result in each case is effusion—accumulation of joint fluid. So, these conditions may all be similar in appearance, although the degree of effusion and lameness vary.

Despite the variety of potential causes, some people refer to effusion in the knee joints as "carpitis." But carpitis just means inflammation of the carpus, or knee. It is not a very useful term because it is not specific. The conditions that most often cause inflammation and effusion within the knee joints include:

- synovitis and degenerative joint disease (DJD)
- intercarpal ligament damage
- carpal bone fractures

More Information
Synovitis is inflammation of the synovium, which is the joint capsule lining. Synovitis and degenerative joint disease are covered in Chapter 8.

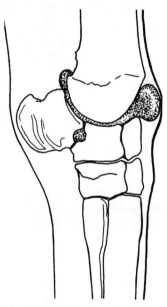

Fig. 18–13. Inflammation in the radiocarpal joint causes a swelling over the front of the knee.

Synovitis and DJD

In most other joints, synovitis and DJD are usually caused by joint capsule strain and repeated cartilage compression during intense exercise. However, in the knee they are just as often the result of a carpal bone fracture, most commonly a chip fracture. That is, they sometimes are secondary to other problems in the joint.

The carpal bones are arranged like children's building blocks. When the horse is bearing weight on the leg, the upper row of carpal bones is stacked on top of the lower row, and the facing surfaces of the bones are touching *(see Figure 18–3)*. These bones have a layer of cartilage on their upper and lower surfaces. When a fracture occurs, cartilage damage is present at the fracture site. But the fracture fragment can also cause cartilage damage on the facing joint surface. Veterinarians sometimes call this other cartilage erosion a "kissing" lesion. It occurs where the two cartilage surfaces meet face to face. Thus, cartilage damage in the knee is often more extensive than would be expected just from the size of the bone lesion seen on radiographs. Cartilage damage is one of the key factors in the development and progression of synovitis and DJD.

Intercarpal Ligament Damage
Definition and Cause

The intercarpal and radiocarpal joints are hinge-type joints. When the knee is flexed these joints open at the front, but remain fixed at the back. This action is possible because the carpal bones are held together at the back of the knee by a tight joint capsule, a dense, fibrous ligament (the palmar carpal ligament), and other small supporting ligaments. The intercarpal joint is also supported by two short, strong ligaments called the intercarpal ligaments. They are located inside, but toward the back of the joint.

As arthroscopic surgery for knee chip removal became more common, surgeons realized that the intercarpal ligaments can be torn in horses that are exercised intensely, particularly racehorses. Presumably, these ligaments are damaged when the knee overextends (bends back slightly) during strenuous exercise.

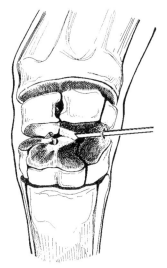

Fig. 18–14. A torn intercarpal ligament, seen during arthroscopic surgery. (The knee is slightly flexed.)

Signs and Diagnosis

The signs of intercarpal ligament damage are not specific, and only indicate that the joint is inflamed. These signs include mild joint effusion, and mild to moderate lameness (grade 2 – 3 of 5) that is made worse by knee flexion. Although these signs point to the knee as the area involved, the veterinarian may need to block the intercarpal joint to pinpoint the exact site of the problem.

There are no abnormalities seen on radiographs, unless there is other damage within the joint, such as a chip fracture. A definite diagnosis of intercarpal ligament damage is only possible with arthroscopy, when the ligaments can actually be seen. Because of the expense of arthroscopic surgery and the potential risk of general anesthesia, many owners are reluctant to submit their horses to this surgery just as a diagnostic procedure. Unfortunately, this often means that intercarpal ligament damage is not diagnosed until one or both of the ligaments are completely torn, and bony damage has occurred.

Treatment of Intercarpal Ligament Damage

Although the surgeon can trim the torn fibers from the damaged ligaments with the arthroscopic instruments, the ligaments cannot be repaired. The only treatment that may resolve the lameness and prevent its return when the horse resumes training is 4 – 6 months of paddock or pasture rest. The horse may have had arthroscopic surgery for bone chip removal, and need only 2 – 3 months of rest for that problem. But it is very important that the horse is rested for longer if the intercarpal ligaments are damaged.

The veterinarian may also recommend a short course of NSAIDs and joint medications to settle down the inflammation within the joint. Though the damage occurs in the back of the joint, harmful inflammatory substances are released from the damaged ligaments into the joint fluid, and distributed to the entire joint. Anti-inflammatory therapy is important to break the vicious cycle of inflammation and cartilage damage that can occur within the joint. *(See the section on Synovitis and DJD in Chapter 8.)*

The potential for reinjury can be reduced by ensuring that the horse is properly conditioned, and its shoes adequately support the heels *(see Chapter 7).*

Prognosis for Intercarpal Ligament Damage

If both ligaments are completely torn, the prognosis for return to strenuous athletic activities is guarded. Chronic or recurrent lameness, due to loss of these stabilizing structures, and DJD are common in such cases. Intercarpal ligament damage is seldom present alone.

Carpal Bone Fractures

There are four types of fracture that can involve the carpal bones:
- chip
- slab
- sagittal
- comminuted

The first three are the most common; and chip fractures are much more common than slab or sagittal fractures. The fourth type, although relatively uncommon, is the most serious.

Definitions

Chip Fractures

Chip fractures are small fragments of bone that typically break off the front edges of the carpal bones. Occasionally, a chip fracture may occur on the lower end of the radius, within the radiocarpal joint.

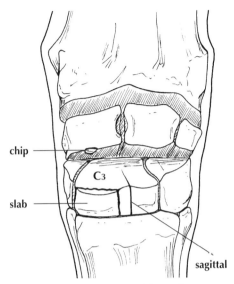

Fig. 18–15. Types of carpal bone fracture.

Slab Fractures

Slab fractures are larger bone fragments that break off the entire front of the bone, like a slab of rock from a cliff face. Sometimes they are little more than a sliver of bone. These fractures damage both the upper and lower joint surfaces of the carpal bone.

Sagittal Fractures

A sagittal fracture is a vertical line that runs from the front surface into the center of the bone. In most cases the fracture does not continue all the way through the bone, although it does involve both the upper and lower joint surfaces. Sagittal fractures almost always occur in the third carpal bone (C3, the largest carpal bone). This bone is located in the middle of the lower row.

Comminuted Fractures

A comminuted fracture is one in which several fracture lines create multiple bone fragments. The carpal bone shatters into several pieces and collapses. This is a very serious injury that cannot satisfactorily be repaired, and means the end of the horse's athletic career.

Comminuted fractures often cause fissures in the bone that look like cracks in a windshield, radiating out from a central defect. These fractures are sometimes called "star" fractures because of their appearance on radiographs.

Causes of Carpal Bone Fractures

In the overwhelming majority of cases carpal bone fractures occur in young racehorses, particularly Thoroughbreds and Quarter Horses. These fractures all occur at the front of the joint. Presumably, they develop when the knee overextends (bends back slightly) during strenuous exercise *(see Figure 18–25).* This action compresses the front edges of the carpal bones. It would be reasonable to assume that landing after a jump causes more stress on the front of the carpal bones than galloping. However, these fractures are far less common in horses that jump than in young racehorses. So, immaturity and the intensity of training probably play important roles in the development of these fractures.

Overextension of the knee is more common in horses that are not well conditioned for strenuous exercise, particularly when muscle fatigue develops. Poor conformation, such as "back at the knee," and the long toe–low heel foot shape encourage overextension during exercise. Improper shoeing, especially inadequate heel support, can also contribute. *(Foot shape and shoeing are discussed in Chapter 7.)*

Signs of Carpal Bone Fractures

With each type of fracture, the signs develop during or shortly after exercise. These signs include:

- lameness
- joint effusion (accumulation of fluid within the joint), which causes a distinct swelling over the front of the knee
- heat
- pain during palpation and flexion of the knee
- positive flexion test—the lameness is worsened by knee flexion

The degree of lameness, swelling, heat, and pain are good indicators of the injury's severity.

Diagnosis of Carpal Bone Fractures

A slab or comminuted fracture may be suspected from the severity of the signs. However, in cases involving a chip or sagittal fracture, the veterinarian may need to perform a joint block to confirm that the knee is the site of the lameness. The signs accompanying these latter two fracture types are often mild and are nonspecific. Also, it is easy to overlook or underestimate the significance of mild joint effusion in the knee. By blocking the intercarpal and radiocarpal joints separately, it is possible to localize the lameness to one specific joint.

CARPAL BONE FRACTURES

FRACTURE	Lameness	Effusion	Pain During Palpation	Response to Flexion
Chip	mild to mod. (grade 1 – 3 of 5)	mild to mod.	mild or absent	mild
Slab	mod. to severe (grade 3 – 4 of 5)	mod. to severe	mod. to severe	severe
Sagittal	moderate (grade 2 – 3 of 5)	mild	mild or absent	mild
Comminuted	severe (grade 4 – 5 of 5)	severe	severe	severe

Fig. 18–16. Typical signs seen with different carpal bone fractures.

Radiographs

When the joint block temporarily improves or resolves the lameness, radiographs are taken. In most instances the veterinarian takes a full series of radiographs because the fracture may be visible on only one of the four routine views. Repeat radiographs at slightly different angles, and special views may be necessary if there are no obvious abnormalities on the routine radiographs. For example, the veterinarian may need to have an assistant flex the knee before repeating the lateral view (from the side). This view can be very useful for highlighting small chip fractures. When the lateral radiograph is taken while the horse is standing on the leg, the chip may be hidden by the superimposed bones.

Sagittal and some slab fractures are also difficult to diagnose on the routine views because of superimposed bones. These fractures often are only visible on a skyline view, in which the knee is flexed and the x-ray beam is directed down the front of the knee. Although these extra views take time, and the

> **More Information**
>
> **Diagnostic techniques, including joint blocks and radiography, are covered in Chapter 2.**

horse may resent having its knee flexed for the radiographs, they are important in making an accurate diagnosis and deciding on the best treatment method.

Sometimes these fractures occur together. For example, the horse may have a sagittal fracture and one or two small chip fractures. Another common injury is a chip fracture in both the intercarpal and radiocarpal joints, or in both knees. For this reason, many veterinarians routinely take radiographs of both knees.

Although these fractures have several features in common, they also have several distinctive differences. Their specific signs, treatment, and prognosis are discussed separately.

Chip Fractures
Signs

Chip fractures usually cause mild to moderate lameness (grade 1 – 3 of 5). The amount of joint effusion is usually also mild. If there is only one bone chip, the effusion is confined to the joint where the chip is located. For example, if the bone chip is broken off the lower edge of one of the carpal bones in the upper row, effusion is seen in the intercarpal joint. Chip fractures only cause effusion in both the intercarpal and radiocarpal joints if there is a bone chip in each joint.

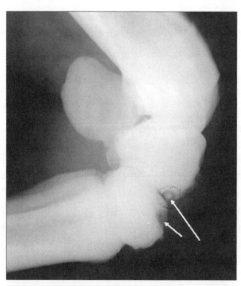

Fig. 18–17. The upper arrow points to a chip fracture. The lower arrow points to other degenerative changes.

Horses with chip fractures may not always show pain when the knee is palpated. But by flexing the knee a little and carefully feeling along the front edges of both rows of carpal bones it is sometimes possible to detect a specific site of pain directly over the chip. However, the chip itself generally cannot be felt. In most cases the horse will not show a pain response until the knee is fully flexed; even then, it may only flinch a little.

Because these signs are not very specific, and often are fairly mild, they can go unnoticed for some time. This is even more likely if the horse has a chip fracture in both knees, which is quite common. The bilateral lameness makes the horse's gait appear more even. Also, when there is swelling in both knees, it is easy to assume that "puffy knees" are normal for that horse.

Treatment

Chip fractures are often best treated by arthroscopic removal of the fragments. Like a pebble in a shoe, as long as the bone fragment remains in the joint, inflammation and lameness may persist. Also, degenerative changes in the joint are more likely and progress more rapidly if the chip is not removed. When chip fractures are removed soon after they occur, cartilage damage is minimal, post-operative recovery is shorter, and the potential for DJD is small.

A major benefit of arthroscopic surgery is that the surgeon can examine the surfaces of virtually the entire joint. This allows a much better understanding of the degree of cartilage damage. Treatment is more likely to be successful when the veterinarian has an accurate idea of the degree of joint damage.

Depending on the size of the chip and the degree of associated cartilage damage, the veterinarian may recommend that the horse is confined to a stall or small paddock for 1 – 4 weeks, followed by 2 – 4 months of paddock or pasture rest. Cartilage defects are slow to heal, usually taking at least 3 months to fill the erosion with new cartilage. The replacement cartilage is not as thick or resilient as normal, healthy cartilage. So, it is important for the horse's athletic future that it is rested for the full time prescribed by the veterinarian. Joint medications *(see Chapter 5)* may be recommended either soon after surgery or once the horse resumes training.

> ### More Information
>
> Post-operative care following arthroscopic surgery is discussed in Chapter 6.

Prognosis

Provided the bone chip is identified and removed soon after it occurs—that is, before extensive cartilage damage develops—the prognosis for return to athletic function is usually very good. However, when the chip has been present for weeks or months, the surgeon often finds large areas of cartilage erosion opposite the fracture site (a "kissing" lesion; discussed earlier). DJD may become a persistent management problem in these horses.

Prevention of Chip Fractures

Carpal bone fractures are most often seen in strenuously exercising horses, particularly young racehorses. While it is impossible to prevent these injuries in every horse, the chance of them occurring is

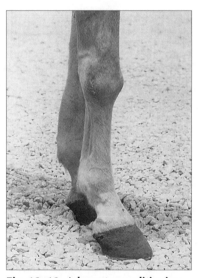

reduced by ensuring that the horse is adequately conditioned for strenuous exercise. Bones must be given time to adapt to the stresses of exercise by increasing their strength and resilience. Strenuous exercise before the body has made these adjustments can result in musculoskeletal injuries, including carpal bone fractures. *(See Chapter 9 for more information on training and bone quality.)*

Ensuring that the horse's feet are regularly trimmed and properly shod is also important in preventing these injuries, particularly in horses with less-than-ideal conformation. Adequate heel support is especially important in galloping horses *(see Chapter 7).*

Fig. 18–18. Adequate conditioning and proper shoeing may have prevented this horse's injuries.

Slab Fractures

Signs

Slab fractures typically cause a sudden, moderate to severe lameness (grade 3 – 4 of 5). Because these fractures involve both joint surfaces, there usually is effusion in both carpal joints if the slab involves a bone in the upper row. But when the slab involves a bone in the lower row, effusion is seen only in the intercarpal joint. This is because the carpometacarpal joint (between the lower row of carpal bones and the cannon bone) is essentially immobile and has a very tight joint capsule. Effusion in this joint is not noticeable.

Some slab fractures cause a large amount of effusion, and the fracture fragment itself can cause the front of the knee to bulge slightly. This can appear as generalized swelling over the front of the knee, which at first glance could be mistaken for a hygroma (discussed earlier). However, the degree of pain and lameness makes it easy to distinguish between a slab fracture and a hygroma.

Light finger pressure over the front of the carpal bones causes a pain response in these horses. The pressure compresses the fracture line by pushing the slab fragment toward the main part of the carpal bone. Horses with slab fractures usually resent any amount of knee flexion because flexing the knee tightens the joint capsules at the front of the knee. This has a similar effect to pressing the slab fragment with the fingertips.

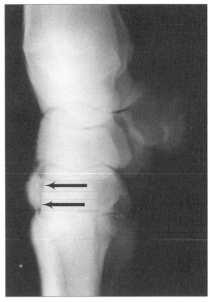

Fig. 18–19. A slab fracture.

Treatment

Provided the bone fragment is thick enough, slab fractures usually are repaired with small bone screws. The fracture would eventually heal without surgery; however, it would probably not heal with the joint surfaces perfectly aligned. Degenerative cartilage changes (DJD) inevitably result on both affected joint surfaces and also on the facing joint surfaces. So, for the horse's athletic future, surgery should be performed within a few days of the injury.

If the fragment is so thin that it could break when drilled, it is usually left alone to heal back onto the main part of the bone. Removing the fragment would damage the joint capsules because they attach onto the front of the carpal bones. In other words, the capsules are attached to the slab. When the slab is thin, very little of the cartilage surface is damaged, so DJD is less of a concern than when a larger slab is left untreated.

Post-operative care is similar to that discussed for chip fractures. The veterinarian usually recommends a longer period of stall confinement and paddock/pasture rest following slab fracture repair, usually at least 6 months. In most cases the bone screw does not need to be removed.

Prognosis and Prevention

If the fracture is diagnosed early and treatment is successful, the prognosis for return to full athletic function is fair. However, cartilage damage is usually more extensive than with chip fractures.

Unless the surgeon was able to perfectly align the fragment at the joint surfaces, DJD is a common sequel in these horses.

Preventing this injury involves following the guidelines discussed earlier for chip fractures.

Sagittal Fractures

Signs

Sagittal fractures usually cause moderate lameness (grade 2 – 3 of 5). The lameness may have been present for several weeks, disappearing with rest and then reappearing when the horse is returned to training. But in most cases the lameness worsens and becomes consistent over time.

These fractures involve both joint surfaces of the third carpal bone. But because this bone is in the lower row, effusion is only seen in the intercarpal joint. In most cases the effusion is mild.

Typically, there is little or no pain during palpation of the knee, and only a mild pain response (if any) when the knee is flexed. Nevertheless, a flexion test often worsens the lameness.

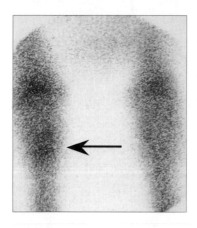
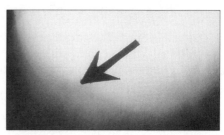

Fig. 18–20. Left: A "bone scan" shows inflammation over the third carpal bone in the horse's right knee. Above: A skyline radiograph revealed a sagittal fracture.

Treatment

Sagittal fractures are incomplete fractures which consist of a fissure that runs into the bone without fracturing it completely. Because of the irregular shape of the third carpal bone and the location of the fracture line, it is very difficult to repair it with bone screws. So, sagittal fractures are usually managed with just an extended rest period. In most cases 4 – 6 weeks of stall or small paddock confinement is followed by at least 6 months of pasture rest.

Although the lameness may resolve after a couple of months, it is important that the horse is rested for the period of time the veterinarian prescribes. Returning the horse to training before the fracture has healed may cause repeated lameness, DJD, and possibly even a disastrous, complete fracture. It is usually best to rest the horse from regular training until repeat radiographs indicate that the fracture has completely healed.

Prognosis and Prevention

Although they do not look as bad as slab fractures, sagittal fractures can be far more frustrating. Chronic lameness is a common result. Therefore, horses with sagittal fractures have a guarded prognosis for return to athletic activities.

Following the guidelines discussed for preventing chip fractures can reduce the potential for this injury to occur.

Comminuted Fractures

Signs

Comminuted fractures cause severe lameness (grade 4 – 5 of 5), and obvious swelling, heat, and pain at the front of the knee. The other, undamaged carpal bones support the joint, so the horse can still bear weight on the leg—as much as the pain allows.

Treatment

Comminuted carpal bone fractures usually cannot be repaired surgically. In most cases the veterinarian places a fiberglass cast or thick support bandage on the leg to prevent the horse from flexing its knee while the fracture heals. The cast or bandage must be applied with great care, monitored closely, and changed as often as needed. These measures are necessary to prevent pressure sores, which often develop over the bony points at the back and inside of the knee. *(See Section II: Principles of Therapy for more information.)*

The horse must be confined to a stall until radiographs indicate

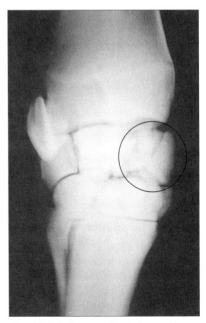

Fig. 18–21. A comminuted carpal bone fracture.

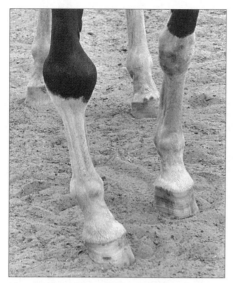

Fig. 18–22. Although the damage was extensive, this horse remained "pasture sound" for several years.

that the fracture is healing well; this usually takes at least 6 weeks. It can then be turned out into a small paddock. While the horse is not bearing much weight on the fractured limb, a frog support *(see Chapter 7)* and a support bandage should be kept on the opposite, weight-bearing limb.

Prognosis for Comminuted Fractures

The degree of joint damage that typically occurs with a comminuted carpal bone fracture generally prevents the horse from returning to athletic activities. However, it may eventually be "pasture sound." In some cases the severity of the injury and the prospect of chronic lameness may prompt euthanasia for humane reasons.

It may be possible to reduce the chances of this injury by following the guidelines for preventing chip fractures.

SWELLING AT THE BACK OF THE KNEE

Swelling at the back of the knee is much less common than at the front of the knee, and there are far fewer conditions that can cause it. The two most common conditions are carpal canal syndrome and accessory carpal bone fracture.

Of Interest

In people the comparable structure is called the carpal tunnel. Problems in this area are referred to as carpal tunnel syndrome.

Carpal Canal Syndrome
Definition and Causes

The carpal canal surrounds the soft tissues at the back of the knee. These tissues include the superficial and deep digital flexor tendons (and their tendon sheath), and the major blood vessels and

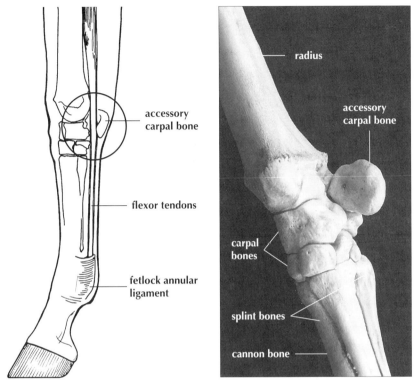

Fig. 18–23. Left: The carpal canal [circled]. The carpal annular ligament has been removed to show the tissues beneath. Right: The back of the knee, viewed at an angle.

nerves that supply the lower leg.

The individual structures that make up the walls of the carpal canal include:

- the back of the carpal bones
- the accessory carpal bone
- the carpal annular ligament

The carpal annular ligament is a broad, dense, fibrous structure that runs around the back of the flexor tendons, from the accessory carpal bone to the carpal bones on the inside of the leg. It is similar in structure and function to the annular ligament at the back of the fetlock.

Carpal canal syndrome can occur under two circumstances. Either the soft tissues inside the canal are damaged, or the structures that make up the walls of the canal are damaged.

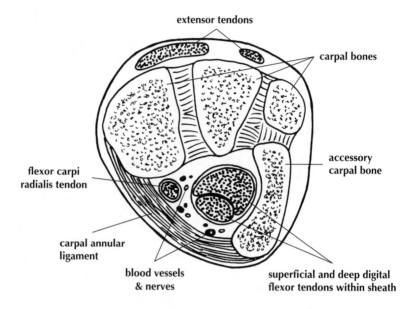

Fig. 18–24. Cross-section of the carpal canal. The front of the knee is at the top.

The carpal annular ligament is a fibrous, inelastic structure. It can act like a constricting band if any of the tissues within the canal are inflamed and swollen. For example, strain of the tendon sheath (tenosynovitis; *see Chapter 11*) or flexor tendons results in an accumulation of fluid within the tendon sheath. The carpal annular ligament prevents the fluid from expanding the canal, so pressure builds up within. As a result the contents of the canal are compressed, which leads to further inflammation and swelling. This vicious cycle of swelling and constriction causes persistent or recurrent pain and lameness—a condition called carpal canal syndrome.

Strain and thickening of the carpal annular ligament, or fracture of the accessory carpal bone can narrow the canal and compress the structures within it. Even if the tendons and their sheath are not damaged at first, compression by the structures that form the canal can result in inflammation, swelling, and further compression of the canal's contents.

Presumably, the initial strain and damage of the flexor tendons, tendon sheath, or carpal annular ligament occurs when the knee overextends during strenuous exercise. This explains why carpal canal syndrome is more common in horses that perform demanding activities, such as galloping, jumping, and polo.

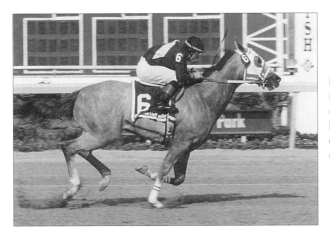

Fig. 18–25. The initial injury occurs when the knee overextends during strenuous exercise.

Signs of Carpal Canal Syndrome

The signs associated with carpal canal syndrome are vague. In most cases the lameness is mild (grade 1 – 2 of 5). The typical pattern is chronic, low-grade lameness that decreases or disappears with rest, but returns when training resumes.

Swelling within the canal is difficult to detect because it is restricted by the fibrous, carpal annular ligament. When the horse's leg is lifted, tension is taken off the flexor tendons. It may then be possible to detect a small amount of swelling around the tendons above or below the canal. To identify this swelling it is usually necessary to compare this area with that of the other leg. The horse may show a mild pain response when the back of the knee is palpated. Most horses with carpal canal syndrome resent full flexion of the knee, and flexion usually worsens the lameness.

Diagnosis of Carpal Canal Syndrome

Because the signs are vague, the diagnosis often depends on three factors:

- detecting pain when the back of the knee is palpated
- finding no bony abnormalities on radiographs that would explain the lameness and pain during knee flexion
- finding excess fluid in a carpal tendon sheath or thickening of the carpal annular ligament during ultrasound examination

Nerve blocks and tissue blocks are usually unrewarding because it is virtually impossible to just block the carpal canal. Blocking the structures within the canal can desensitize the entire lower leg because the canal contains the nerves that supply the lower leg. However, it may be worth performing joint blocks in the intercarpal and radiocarpal joints to eliminate them as possible sites of lameness and pain during knee flexion. *(These diagnostic techniques are discussed in Chapter 2.)*

Treatment of Carpal Canal Syndrome

Treatment involves rest from regular training, and a few days of anti-inflammatory therapy, such as NSAIDs, cold therapy, and DMSO *(see Chapter 5).* The horse can either be rested in a pasture, or confined to a stall or small paddock and hand-walked for at least 20 minutes twice per day. In most cases the inflammation and lameness subside in 1 – 2 weeks, but it is best to suspend training for another 4 – 6 weeks, to be sure the injury has completely healed. It is common for the lameness to disappear with rest and reappear when training resumes. Even though the signs may resolve in only a couple of weeks, it is best to rest the horse for longer.

Under certain circumstances, the veterinarian may recommend surgery to cut the carpal annular ligament and relieve the pressure on the structures within the canal. These circumstances include 1) severe or unresponsive cases, and 2) chronic lameness caused by an accessory carpal bone fracture. The carpal annular ligament eventually heals and re-forms the canal a little wider than before the surgery. Provided adhesions (fibrous bands) do not restrict the normal movement of the tendons within the canal, this surgery can improve or resolve the lameness. NSAIDs and daily hand-walking can reduce the potential for adhesions to restrict tendon function as the ligament heals. In many cases the horse can be gradually returned to regular exercise, beginning 6 – 8 weeks after surgery.

Prognosis for Carpal Canal Syndrome

The prognosis for return to athletic activities is usually fairly good, although lameness will persist or return if the horse is returned to strenuous exercise too quickly.

Accessory Carpal Bone Fractures
Definition and Causes

The accessory carpal bone is the oval-shaped, curved bone that protrudes from the back of the knee on the outside of the leg. Its back edge forms the bony point at the back of the knee. This bone is the point of attachment for some of the flexor muscles of the forearm. It also forms the outside of the carpal canal.

The accessory carpal bone can be fractured by direct, external trauma, such as a knock or a kick, or by internal trauma. A classic instance in which this fracture occurs is when a horse falls onto the front of the knee while it is flexed. The bottom of the radius and the top of the cannon bone can fracture the accessory carpal bone like a nut in a nutcracker.

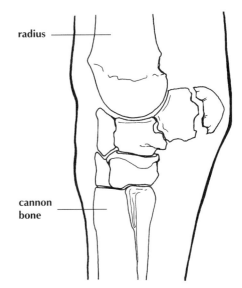

radius

cannon bone

Fig. 18–26. An accessory carpal bone fracture.

Signs and Diagnosis

The lameness that results from this fracture usually is moderate (grade 3 – 4 of 5). The accessory carpal bone does not bear any weight so, unless other bones are also fractured, these horses are not extremely lame. The entire knee may be swollen, although most of the swelling is at the back of the knee, around the accessory carpal bone. Palpation and flexion of the knee causes obvious pain, and in some cases crepitus (crunching of bone-on-bone) may be heard or felt during palpation. The diagnosis is confirmed with radiographs.

Treatment

Some of these fractures can be repaired with a bone screw, but because the bone is curved it is often difficult to adequately stabilize the fracture. Most times the veterinarian simply recommends that the horse is rested in a stall for 6 – 8 weeks. These fractures heal best when a thick support bandage from fetlock to mid-forearm is kept on the leg for at least the first month (and changed as often as necessary during that time; *see Chapter 4*). Once radiographs indicate that the fracture has healed, another 3 – 4 months of pasture rest is usually recommended.

Prognosis for Accessory Carpal Bone Fractures

Accessory carpal bone fractures often heal with a fibrous union rather than a bony callus. Nevertheless, most horses return to full athletic function once the fracture has completely healed. Sometimes these fractures result in carpal canal syndrome if the displaced bone narrows the canal and puts pressure on the structures within.

Other Conditions

There are a few other conditions that can cause swelling at the back of the knee. Specifically, the conditions discussed in this section typically cause swelling just above the knee.

Superior Check Ligament Strain

Definition and Causes

The superior check ligament is a short, fibrous ligament that anchors the superficial digital flexor tendon to the radius, just above the knee. It prevents the tendon and its attached flexor muscle from being overstretched during strenuous exercise. But in the process, the check ligament can be strained or torn. This injury is quite uncommon; it is far more common for the flexor tendon to be damaged. However, the signs of superior check ligament strain are vague, so this condition may be more common than it seems.

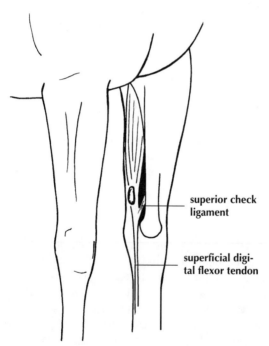

superior check ligament

superficial digital flexor tendon

Fig. 18–27. The location of the superior check ligament.

Signs

The superior check ligament is hidden beneath the muscles at the back and sides of the forearm. So, swelling of the ligament is very difficult, if not impossible to detect. The signs simply include mild lameness (grade 1 – 2 of 5), and mild pain when the check ligament area is palpated. The superior check ligament cannot be felt with the fingertips. But pressure can be applied to it by pressing firmly with the fingertips just in front of the chestnut, on the inside of the forearm. This area is only a couple of inches above the carpal canal, so the symptoms of check ligament strain and carpal canal syndrome are similar.

Diagnosis and Treatment

By ultrasounding the superior check ligament area it may be possible for the veterinarian to confirm that the ligament is thickened or torn. It is also worth ultrasounding the carpal canal to check for abnormalities. Palpating the flexor tendons as they run down the back of the cannon is also important. They could have been strained when the check ligament was damaged.

Treatment involves a few weeks of rest from regular training, and a few days of anti-inflammatory therapy, including NSAIDs, cold therapy, and DMSO *(see Chapter 5)*. As with most other tendon and ligament injuries, daily hand-walking improves the blood supply to the damaged ligament and speeds healing. Pasture rest is a suitable alternative with this injury, unless the horse is very active when turned out. When abnormalities are found during ultrasound examination, it is worth re-ultrasounding the area before deciding when to return the horse to regular exercise.

The recommendations given in Chapter 11 for preventing flexor tendon injuries are wise precautions following superior check ligament strain.

Prognosis

The prognosis for superior check ligament strain is quite good. However, if training resumes before the ligament has completely healed, the lameness will likely persist or return.

Osteochondroma

An osteochondroma is a bone spur that can develop just above the lower physis (growth plate) of the radius. The signs usually do not

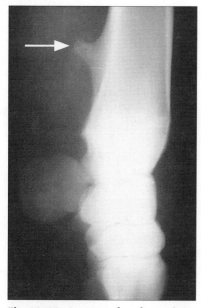

Fig. 18–28. An osteochondroma just above the knee.

appear until the young adult horse begins training. *(Typical signs, diagnosis, and treatment are discussed in Chapter 14.)*

Although osteochondromas are rare, they can cause swelling and pain at the back of the knee. In some cases the bone spur irritates the sheath surrounding the flexor tendons at the back of the knee. Effusion in the sheath causes swelling just above the knee and carpal canal syndrome-like symptoms.

Blood Vessel Tumor

Another very uncommon condition in horses is an aggressive blood vessel tumor (hemangiosarcoma). There have been a few cases in which this tumor has caused lameness and diffuse swelling just above the knee in young, athletic horses. In these cases, the swelling was worst on the inside of the leg. The diagnosis is based on the appearance of the mass on ultrasound, and biopsy of the tissue. There is no specific treatment for this tumor. It is extremely difficult to surgically remove all of the tumor. This is because it usually has invaded the muscle and other soft tissues by the time the signs are noticed and the diagnosis is confirmed. Therefore, euthanasia has been the eventual outcome so far. But anticancer drugs and radiation therapy are being tried for various tumors in horses. They may help control this tumor, if started early. ◄

19

THE UPPER FORELEG

L ameness involving the upper foreleg is relatively uncommon. Although, "shoulder lameness" is a fairly common complaint. This gait abnormality gives the impression that the horse is reluctant to swing its leg forward because its shoulder hurts. But in most cases, the site of lameness is actually in the lower leg, usually the foot *(see Chapter 1)*.

Nevertheless, significant problems do sometimes occur in the upper foreleg. They are discussed in order of anatomic location, from the radius to the shoulder.

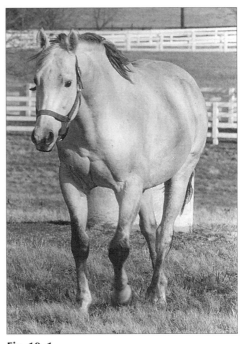

Fig. 19–1.

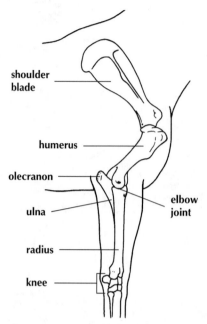

shoulder blade

humerus

olecranon

ulna

elbow joint

radius

knee

Fig. 19–2. Bones of the forearm.

RADIUS

The radius is the main bone in the forearm; it connects the knee and the elbow. The ulna is a smaller, shorter bone that forms part of the elbow joint. It fuses with the radius about half-way down the forearm, so only the radius forms a joint (articulates) with the bones of the knee.

Radial Fractures

Radial fractures are almost always caused by direct trauma, such as a fall or a kick. The fracture may be incomplete, involving only one side of the bone. Or, it may be complete, breaking the bone into two or more pieces.

Incomplete Radial Fractures

Definitions and Causes

There are two types of incomplete radial fracture. The first is a long crack in one side of the bone. The second is a small piece of bone that is broken off the bone's surface. Both are caused by direct trauma, and both may be present together. That is, the traumatic incident may crack the bone and also chip off a small piece of bone at the point of impact. When a piece of bone is broken off the surface, it may lose its blood supply. The fragment then dies and becomes a sequestrum—a devitalized piece of bone that the body treats as foreign material.

Unlike incomplete cannon bone fractures and incomplete tibial fractures, incomplete radial fractures are not usually caused by exercise-induced stress on the bone.

Signs

It is fairly common for a horse with an incomplete radial fracture to have a small wound on the side of the forearm, probably caused

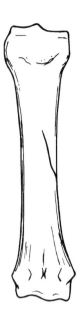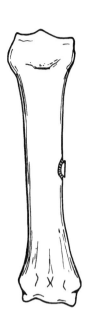

Fig. 19–3. Two types of incomplete fracture. Left: A long crack in the side of the radius. Right: A sequestrum.

by a kick. Because the front and back of the forearm are well covered with muscle, these fractures usually occur on the outside or inside of the leg. The frequent result is a "radiating" wound in which there is severe bruising and bone damage beneath a minor skin wound *(see Chapter 13).*

It is common for a sequestrum and the underlying bone surface to become infected because the skin wound allows bacteria to invade the damaged bone. So, although the wound seems minor, it may fail to heal. Or, it heals only to break open and ooze pus several days or a few weeks later. Lameness in these horses usually is mild to moderate (grade 2 – 3 of 5), and persists even if the wound seems to have healed.

If the traumatic incident cracked the bone without damaging the skin, the only signs (other than lameness) may be a small amount of swelling and pain during palpation of the swollen area. The possibility of an incomplete fracture may not be obvious. These horses often are more lame, and the lameness persists for longer than would be expected just from bruising. This is an important clue that there may be more significant damage.

More Information
Sequestrum formation and bone infection within a wound are discussed in the *Superficial Osteomyelitis* section in Chapter 9.

Diagnosis of Incomplete Radial Fractures

Ultrasonography is sometimes more useful than radiography for identifying a sequestrum in this part of the leg. This is especially true for wounds close to the elbow. The higher up the injury, the more awkward it is to take radiographs of the radius because it is difficult to position the x-ray plate behind the elbow. Nevertheless, the veterinarian should attempt to take at least two views of the radius in case the bone damage is more extensive than just a sequestrum. A crack that is undetected can result in a disastrous, complete fracture if the horse is permitted unrestricted activity.

Treatment of Incomplete Radial Fractures

When a sequestrum is found it should be surgically removed. The problem generally will not resolve as long as it is present. In some cases the veterinarian may perform this procedure under local anesthesia. But if the sequestrum is large or the wound is deep, general anesthesia and thorough exploration of the wound may be necessary. It is important for the veterinarian to carefully examine the radiographs for a more extensive fracture before anesthetizing the horse. If there is a crack in the bone, the radius can fracture completely when the horse gets up from anesthesia. *It is not worth taking this risk.* If there is any doubt, the veterinarian may take more radiographs before deciding on the best way to deal with the sequestrum.

Once the sequestrum and any surrounding damaged bone are removed, the bone and the skin wound usually heal quickly. In most cases the veterinarian prescribes a few days of antibiotics and NSAIDs following surgery. The horse's tetanus status should have been reviewed when the wound was first discovered; if not, it must be done before surgery *(see Chapter 5).*

For a sequestrum, 4 – 6 weeks of stall and/or small paddock rest is usually sufficient before regular training resumes. Daily hand-walking is often advised for horses that are confined to a stall during this period.

With a more extensive incomplete fracture, the horse should be confined in a stall or small pen for 6 – 8 weeks. Ideally, the radiographs should be repeated before the horse is turned out into a larger paddock or pasture for another 2 – 3 months. If the fracture line is still visible, the horse should be confined for longer. After the period of paddock or pasture rest, the horse can resume regular training.

Prognosis for Incomplete Radial Fractures

The prognosis for return to athletic activities is very good with either type of incomplete fracture. Of the two, an extensive incomplete fracture takes longer to heal and has the greater potential to be a major problem. This fracture should be taken very seriously. Failing to confine the horse, or returning it to training too soon can have disastrous consequences. But with appropriate care, the fracture should heal completely and cause the horse no more problems.

<table>
<tr><td>

Definitions

Comminuted: fracture with more than one fracture line and more than one bone fragment. **Open:** fracture that involves a skin wound.

(See Chapter 9 for information on fractures.)
</td></tr>
</table>

Complete Radial Fractures

Complete radial fractures are classic longbone fractures. In many cases the fracture is comminuted, and sometimes it is open. There may not necessarily be a shard of bone protruding from the skin. But if there is a wound overlying a very swollen area in a severely lame horse, an open fracture should be suspected. *(See Chapter 13 for information on first aid for open fractures.)*

Management Problems

Complete radial fractures are dramatic injuries that almost always have a disappointing outcome in adult horses. The radius is a large bone. It is very difficult to stabilize the fracture and adequately support the bone with metal implants, even when two large bone plates are used. A full-limb fiberglass cast or thick support bandage can reduce some of the forces on the surgical repair site. However, on its own a cast or bandage cannot adequately stabilize a complete radial fracture. To stabilize a fracture with a cast or bandage, the joints above and below the fracture must be immobilized. It is not possible to immobilize the elbow joint with a cast or bandage. So, the only chance of success is with surgical repair.

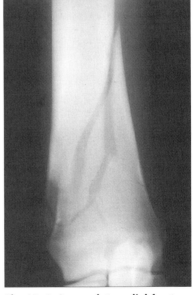

Fig. 19–4. A complete radial fracture that starts just above the knee.

More Information
Bandaging is discussed in Chapter 4.
Bone plates and fiberglass casts are discussed in Chapter 6.

But despite diligent supervision by the surgical staff, the extreme forces across the fracture when the horse gets up from anesthesia can loosen, bend, or break the metal implants. This is because the lower leg acts like a lever that concentrates the weight-bearing forces at the weakest point: the fracture. If it is an open fracture, bone infection (osteomyelitis; *see Chapter 9*) is inevitable and further compromises fracture stability and healing. Laminitis in the opposite, weight-bearing limb is also a common complication of this severe injury. Laminitis causes the horse to shift more weight off the laminitic foot onto the fractured leg, further taxing the implants.

For these reasons, euthanasia is usually recommended in adult horses with a complete radial fracture. The chance of surgical success is better in foals and small ponies because they weigh much less than adult horses. Fracture stability with bone plates may therefore be more effective. However, flexor contracture and angular limb deformities can result from such a severe injury in foals *(see Chapter 14)*.

ELBOW

The elbow is both a general area of the foreleg and a specific joint. The elbow joint consists of three bones: the radius, ulna, and humerus.

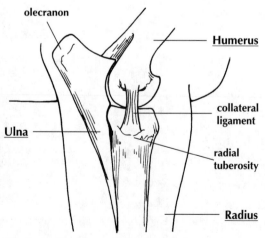

Fig. 19–5. The parts of the elbow joint.

olecranon
Humerus
collateral ligament
Ulna
radial tuberosity
Radius

Fractures
Radial Tuberosity Fracture

On the outside of the elbow is a bony knob called the radial tuberosity. It is like the bony point on the outside of the elbow in people. One of the collateral ligaments of the elbow joint and some of the forearm muscles attach to this knob.

A kick to the side of the elbow can fracture the tuberosity, although this is a very uncommon injury. The collateral ligament is important for joint stability. If the tuberosity is completely broken off, the elbow joint may become unstable, and degenerative joint disease (discussed later) may develop. Thus, surgical repair is usually recommended. In most cases a bone screw is used to reattach the tuberosity onto the radius.

The veterinarian usually recommends a few weeks of confinement, then 4 – 6 months of paddock or pasture rest. Unless the fracture is more extensive and either damages more of the radius or continues into the elbow joint, the prognosis for return to athletic activities is quite good.

Olecranon Fractures

Definition and Causes

The olecranon is the upper part of the ulna, from the bottom of the elbow joint up. It forms the point of the elbow. The triceps are a large, flat group of muscles that begin along the back of the shoulder blade and attach onto the top of the olecranon. When they contract they extend (straighten) the elbow and flex the shoulder.

There is very little soft tissue overlying the olecranon. So, it is easily fractured by direct trauma, such as a kick to the side or back of the elbow. Because the ulna forms the back of the elbow joint, fractures in the lower part of the olecranon may be articular. When a fracture occurs in the upper part, it may miss the joint entirely, creating a non-articular fracture. In foals and yearlings the olecranon may fracture across the physis (growth plate) at the top of the bone. This is called a physeal fracture. *(See Chapter 9 for more information on fracture types.)*

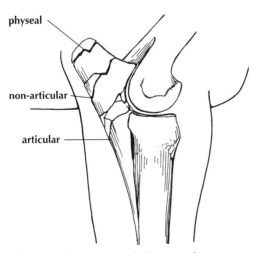

physeal

non-articular

articular

Fig. 19–6. Three types of olecranon facture.

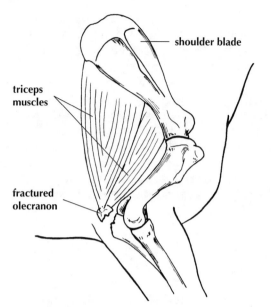

triceps
muscles

shoulder blade

fractured
olecranon

Fig. 19–7. The triceps muscles displace the fractured olecranon.

When a complete fracture occurs in the upper part of the olecranon, the triceps muscles may displace the fracture. Sometimes they pull the top of the olecranon up several millimeters. This makes fracture repair more difficult because there is constant tension on the bone fragment by the triceps muscles. When a complete fracture occurs in the lower part of the olecranon, the joint capsule and supporting ligaments limit fracture displacement.

Signs of Olecranon Fractures

Olecranon fractures may not be immediately obvious, even when the fracture is complete and articular. There usually is generalized swelling around the elbow, and the point of the elbow is no longer distinct. However, this may not be obvious in heavily muscled horses. In other horses the swelling could at first be mistaken for a "capped elbow" (discussed later). However, palpating the fractured olecranon causes pain, as does moving the leg forward and back, which flexes and extends the elbow. Sometimes it is possible to feel movement of the fracture fragment and crepitus (crunching of bone-on-bone) when the elbow is palpated.

The degree of lameness varies a little depending on the location and severity of the fracture. Most horses with an olecranon fracture are at least grade 3 of 5 lame; some cannot bear any weight on the leg at all. Technically, the horse should be able to bear weight on the affected leg because the radius is undamaged. However, if the fracture is displaced, the horse may not be able to fix its elbow in the standing position. This is because when the triceps muscles contract they pull away the fractured piece of olecranon, instead of extending the elbow. As a result, some horses with a complete olecranon fracture have a "dropped" elbow—the elbow joint is lower than normal—and they are unable to bear weight on the leg. This stance can easily be mistaken for radial nerve paralysis (discussed and illustrated later).

Diagnosis of Olecranon Fractures

Radiographs of the elbow usually are necessary to confirm the diagnosis and decide on the best treatment. Two views of the elbow should be taken if possible: one from the side (a lateral view) and one from the front. It can be difficult to get good quality radiographs of the elbow in a conscious horse with an olecranon fracture. To take the lateral view, the horse's leg must be pulled forward. This allows the x-ray beam to be directed through the elbow joint without the interference of the ribs and breastbone. But it can be painful for the horse. Sedating it with a drug that is also an analgesic (pain-killer) makes this procedure less painful for the horse and easier for the veterinarian and assistants.

Treatment of Olecranon Fractures

Most incomplete fractures and non-displaced, complete fractures are treated conservatively. This involves 6 – 8 weeks of confinement in a stall or small pen, followed by 3 – 4 months of paddock or pasture rest. Ideally, repeat radiographs should be taken before the

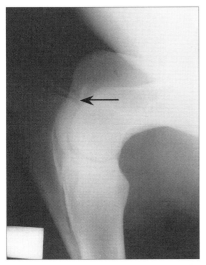 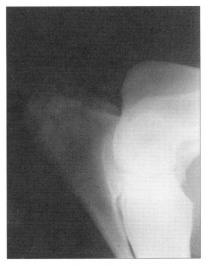

Fig. 19–8. This complete olecranon fracture (left) was allowed to heal on its own, and has done remarkably well (right).

horse is turned out into a paddock or pasture. The precautions discussed in Chapter 9 about long-term NSAID use in horses with fractures are relevant when managing olecranon fractures.

Displaced olecranon fractures are often best repaired with a bone plate, or bone pins and orthopedic wire *(see Chapter 6)*, particularly if the fracture involves the joint. With articular fractures, degenerative joint disease (DJD) commonly develops unless the fracture line is compressed and the joint surface is realigned. Complete fractures through the physis do not involve the joint, but they are also best repaired with a bone plate or bone pins. It is difficult for any type of displaced olecranon fracture to satisfactorily heal while the top of the olecranon is constantly being pulled away by the triceps muscles. So, surgical repair is usually the best method of treatment. The rest periods given above also apply following surgery.

When surgery is not an option, 3 – 4 months of stall confinement can be a reasonable alternative to euthanasia—but only if the horse can bear some weight on the limb. If the horse cannot stand on the fractured limb, laminitis is likely to develop in the opposite limb, which complicates matters. Olecranon fractures have a better outcome than most other complete, articular fractures because the olecranon does not bear weight. *However, DJD and chronic lameness are far more likely when a complete, articular fracture is treated conservatively rather than surgically.*

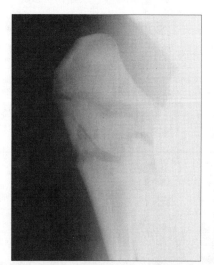 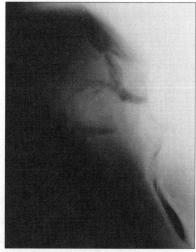

Fig. 19–9. Left: A comminuted olecranon fracture that was not repaired surgically. Right: The fracture has not healed well and this horse almost certainly has degenerative joint disease.

Prognosis for Olecranon Fractures

The prognosis for athletic usefulness is guarded if the fracture involves the elbow joint. DJD often develops unless the joint surface is perfectly realigned, which is not always possible. Incomplete fractures and complete, non-articular fractures have a better outcome, provided they heal completely before the horse is allowed any activity.

Most physeal fractures heal well after surgical repair, and usually cause the foal or young horse no further problems. The physis on the olecranon contributes very little to the growth of the leg. So, interrupted growth and angular limb deformities are unlikely to occur in the fractured limb. They may, however, develop in the opposite limb as a result of excessive load. Also, if the foal cannot bear any weight, flexor contracture may develop in the fractured limb. Thus, surgical repair is very important in foals and young horses with a displaced olecranon fracture.

> **Definitions**
>
> **Angular Limb Deformity:** deviation in the angle of the limb when viewed from the front; "crooked legs."
> **Flexural Limb Deformity:** deviation in the angle of the limb when viewed from the side.
>
> **These conditions are covered in Chapter 14.**

Degenerative Joint Disease

Degenerative joint disease (DJD) in the elbow is almost always secondary to another problem, such as:

- an articular fracture
- joint instability from collateral ligament stretching or rupture
- joint infection (septic arthritis)

The signs of elbow DJD are vague, consisting only of mild to moderate lameness (grade 1 – 3 of 5) and mild pain when the foreleg is pulled forward. Joint effusion (accumulation of fluid) is usually not noticeable because the elbow has a tight joint capsule. Although moving the horse's leg forward, back, and to the side may cause pain, these maneuvers also tax the shoulder joint and muscles. It is virtually impossible to manipulate the elbow without also moving the shoulder. Therefore, these signs are not specific for elbow lameness.

It usually takes an injection of local anesthetic directly into the elbow joint to make the diagnosis (joint block; *see Chapter 2*). If the joint is the source of pain, this procedure temporarily improves or resolves the lameness. Radiographs should then be taken to check for an incomplete fracture or bony changes around the joint. Bony changes are evidence of osteoarthritis, which is the endstage of DJD.

Managing DJD is discussed in Chapter 8. Injecting corticosteroids into the elbow joint can substantially improve the horse's gait in many cases. However, corticosteroids can speed up cartilage degeneration, so their overuse may shorten the horse's athletic career rather than extend it *(see Chapter 5)*.

The long-term prognosis for elbow DJD is guarded in athletic horses. Because the signs are so vague, there may be extensive changes within and around the joint by the time the diagnosis is made. Also, the cause may be impossible to control.

Capped Elbow

A "capped elbow" is a hygroma at the point of the elbow. Hygromas are soft, fluid-filled swellings beneath the skin, over a bony point. They are caused by trauma. There are two basic types of hygroma. The first type involves inflammation of a bursa (bursitis), in this case the small bursa between the olecranon and the short tendons of the triceps muscles. The other type involves a hematoma or seroma. Most capped elbows fall into this category. With repeated trauma, the swelling may develop into a fibrous sac filled with serum. This structure is sometimes called a "false bursa."

Some people call the swelling a "shoe boil," although it is not usually a "boil," or abscess. This term identifies the cause of most of these

Definitions
Hematoma: collection of blood beneath the skin.
Seroma: collection of serum, the clear, yellow, liquid portion of the blood, beneath the skin.
Bursa: small sac of fluid between a bone and a tendon.
(Chapter 18 contains more information on the development and treatment of hygromas.)

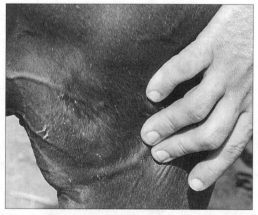

Fig. 19–10. A "capped elbow" may begin with minor skin irritation.

hygromas: the horse's shoe. When the horse is lying down, resting on its chest, the heels of the shoe lie against the point of the elbow. The shoe can cause enough pressure to inflame the skin and underlying tissues. In mild or early cases constant pressure by the shoe causes a

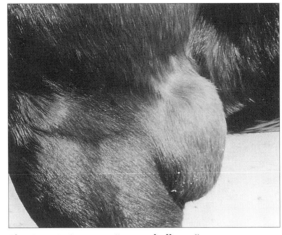

Fig. 19–11. A severe "capped elbow."

patch of thickened, flaky or hairless skin. In more severe or chronic cases a hygroma develops.

"Capped elbows" rarely cause lameness, although if the hygroma develops suddenly, it may be painful for the first few days. Occasionally, the skin is damaged and the hygroma becomes infected. This causes a painful swelling that must be surgically drained like an abscess.

Treatment

In most cases "capped elbows" only require treatment for cosmetic reasons. The best results are obtained by treating it soon after it develops. Unless the hygroma is infected, most veterinarians drain the fluid from the swelling and inject corticosteroids into the cavity. This approach usually resolves an acute hygroma. However, if the swelling has been present for longer than about a month, surgical removal of the fibrous sac may be necessary.

Prevention

Unless repeated trauma to the elbow is prevented, the hygroma can re-form, even after surgery. So, the best long-term treatment is prevention. Commercial "shoe boil" boots are available for this purpose. They consist of a thick, rubberized ring that fits around the pastern and prevents the heels of the shoe from touching the elbow when the horse is lying down. The boot should be left on whenever the horse is in its stall, even during the day.

Making a "Shoe Boil" Boot

An effective boot can be made out of a piece of stirrup leather and some padding. To make a "shoe boil" boot, cut an old stirrup leather to 10 – 14 inches (25 – 35 cm) long and punch a few holes in the new end. Wrap a couple of layers of roll cotton or some other padding material around the strap. Then cover the padding completely with duct tape, leaving the buckle and an inch or two at the other end free. The result is a comfortable, water-resistant strap that can be buckled around the pastern as needed.

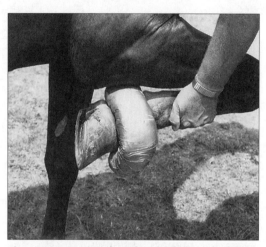

Fig. 19–12. Testing the "shoe boil" boot by lifting the horse's leg and flexing the knee.

The strap does not need to be fitted tightly, although it should be snug enough that it cannot slip down over the horse's foot or up over the fetlock. The padding should be thick enough to prevent the heels from touching the elbow. An easy way to test this is by lifting the horse's leg and flexing the knee.

HUMERUS

The humerus lies between the elbow and the shoulder joint. It is a thick bone that spirals slightly along its length. At its lower end it forms a joint (articulates) with the radius and ulna. At its upper end it articulates with the shoulder blade. Several muscles attach to, or overlie the humerus, so it is not possible to directly palpate much of this bone.

Humeral Fractures

Definition and Causes

The humerus is not often fractured. When it is, the fracture is usually a very serious, complete, comminuted (multiple fragment) fracture in the middle or lower third of the bone. Most humeral fractures are caused by direct trauma to the side of the shoulder, such as a fall or a collision with a solid object. Incomplete fractures can occur in the humerus, although they are very uncommon.

The signs, treatment, and prognosis differ, so complete and incomplete humeral fractures are discussed separately.

Complete Humeral Fractures
Signs and Diagnosis

Because of the muscle mass that surrounds the humerus, the swelling that accompanies a complete fracture may not be very obvious at first. However, palpating the area causes pain, as does moving the leg. The muscles that attach to the humerus usually pull on the fracture pieces and cause them to over-ride (overlap). When this occurs, crepitus may not be heard or felt during palpation. But moving the leg out to the side may cause this grinding noise, as well as extreme pain.

When the humerus is completely fractured, the horse cannot bear weight on the leg. The humerus is one of the supporting bones of the forelimb. When the bone is disrupted, any weight on the leg causes the bone to collapse.

In some cases the horse also shows signs of radial nerve paralysis: "dropped" elbow, inability to straighten the knee and fetlock, etc.

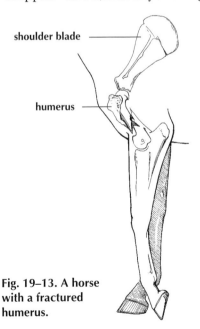

shoulder blade

humerus

Fig. 19–13. A horse
with a fractured
humerus.

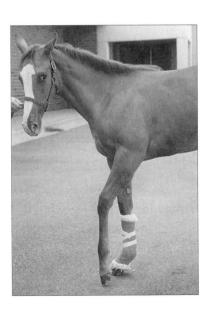

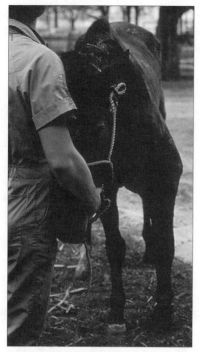

Fig. 19–14. A horse with a severe, displaced humeral fracture.

(discussed later). The radial nerve runs across the back and side of the humerus, on its way to the triceps muscles and the extensor muscles at the front of the forearm. If the nerve is damaged by a bone fragment or compressed by soft tissue swelling, radial nerve paralysis may result.

The diagnosis may be obvious from the signs. But radiographs are useful if an attempt is to be made to surgically repair the fracture. However, radiographs of the humerus are very difficult to obtain without anesthetizing the horse. This is because the leg must be brought as far forward as possible to prevent interference from the ribs and breastbone. This position causes extreme pain, even if the veterinarian gives the horse analgesics (pain-killers).

Treatment of Complete Humeral Factures

In most cases a complete, displaced humeral fracture in an adult horse requires euthanasia for humane reasons. Fracture repair with bone plates or pins *(see Chapter 6)* may be possible for certain humeral fractures in young foals and small ponies. However, these techniques are generally unsuccessful in larger foals and adult horses because of their size and weight. The metal implants often loosen, bend, or break. Furthermore, in any horse, it is difficult to fit a bone plate to the humerus so that it adequately stabilizes the fracture. This is because the bone spirals slightly and its surface is uneven.

In small ponies and horses less than about 12 months old, less complicated fractures may heal without surgery. But the horse must be confined to a stall or small pen for at least 3 months, and then rested in a small paddock for another 3 – 4 months.

Potential Complications

In young horses, flexor contracture is likely because the horse cannot bear weight on the leg. Angular limb deformities are also likely in the opposite leg because of the excessive load. These abnormalities of limb growth are discussed in Chapter 14. A full-limb bandage with PVC splints *(see Chapter 4)* may help prevent flexor contracture. The bandage and splints also make it easier for the foal to swing the leg forward and place it properly if there is radial nerve paralysis. However, it is nearly impossible to prevent angular limb deformities in the opposite leg as long as the foal can bear weight on both forelegs.

Confinement may result in acceptable fracture healing with some simple, non-displaced humeral fractures in adult horses. However, laminitis is common in the weight-bearing limb. Also, there is a risk that the fracture may become displaced and over-ridden when the horse gets up after lying down. Such a fracture has a poor chance of healing. Cross-tying the horse for the first few weeks to keep it from lying down may help to prevent the fracture from displacing. But unfortunately, keeping the horse from lying down increases the potential for laminitis to develop in the opposite limb.

The precautions discussed in Chapter 9 concerning long-term NSAID use in horses and foals with fractures should be considered when treating humeral fractures.

Prognosis for Complete Humeral Factures

The prognosis for future athletic usefulness following repair of a complete humeral fracture is guarded at best. Even if the fracture is relatively uncomplicated and eventually heals well, other musculoskeletal problems often compromise the chance of a successful outcome. For example, development of an angular or flexural limb deformity may limit a foal's athletic potential. Laminitis in the opposite, weight-bearing limb may cause long-term problems (or prompt euthanasia) in an adult horse.

Incomplete Humeral Fractures
Signs and Diagnosis

The signs of an incomplete humeral fracture are vague. The lameness is usually only moderate (grade 2 – 3 of 5), and can be very difficult to localize. Pain during palpation over the humerus helps to pinpoint the source of the lameness. However, this is not specific for a humeral fracture, and it is not always present. Nuclear scintigraphy is the best way to locate the site of lameness in these horses. However, a definite diagnosis can only be made when radiographs reveal a crack in the humerus. Having said that, it can be very difficult to get good radiographs of the humerus because of its location. Also, the

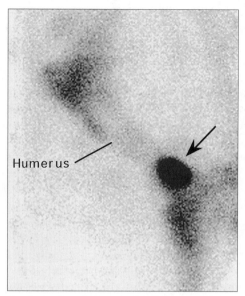

Fig. 19–15. A "bone scan" of an incomplete fracture on the lower end of the humerus, just above the elbow joint.

fracture line may not be obvious because of the bone's irregular surface and overlying muscle.

Treatment and Prognosis for Incomplete Humeral Factures

Incomplete fractures are usually managed with 2 – 3 months of confinement in a stall or small pen, followed by 3 – 4 months of rest in a small paddock. If the crack appears to be extensive, the veterinarian may recommend keeping the horse cross-tied in a stall for the first few weeks. This measure prevents the horse from lying down and completely fracturing the bone when it gets up. It is usually best to keep the horse confined until radiographs and/or nuclear scintigraphy indicate that the fracture has healed. It is not worth allowing the horse unrestricted pasture activity, or returning it to training before this time.

Incomplete fractures generally heal well, allowing the horse to be returned to normal athletic activities. However, the rest period may be several months long.

Radial Nerve Paralysis

The typical stance of radial nerve paralysis is a "dropped" elbow and flexed lower leg. This stance can easily be confused with that of a horse with a complete, displaced olecranon or humeral fracture. In fact, it is not unusual for a humeral fracture to damage the radial nerve and cause temporary or permanent paralysis.

More Information

Radial nerve paralysis is a condition of the nervous system. Its causes, diagnosis, and management are covered in detail in Chapter 12.

Paralysis vs. Olecranon Fracture

There are two important differences between radial nerve paralysis and a complete, displaced olecranon fracture. First, radial nerve paralysis results in an inability to use the extensor muscles at the front of the forearm. The horse cannot extend (straighten) its knee, fetlock, or pastern. In contrast, a horse with an olecranon fracture should still be able to extend these joints, bring the leg forward, and place the foot normally. (However, it may not be able to bear weight on the leg if the top of the olecranon is pulled away by the triceps muscles.) Second, horses with radial nerve paralysis typically lose feeling (skin sensation) over the front and outside of the forearm. This is not the case in horses with an olecranon fracture.

The one feature common to both injuries is the "dropped" elbow; however, the reason for this stance differs. The elbow appears dropped in a horse with radial nerve paralysis because the nerve supply to the triceps muscles is interrupted. As a result the muscles are unable to contract and fix the elbow in the standing position. In contrast, the triceps muscles in a horse with a complete olecranon fracture function normally. However, when they contract they may pull away the top of the olecranon, which allows the rest of the ulna, and the elbow joint, to drop.

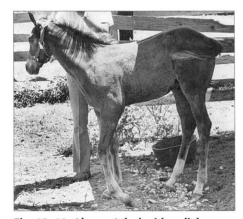 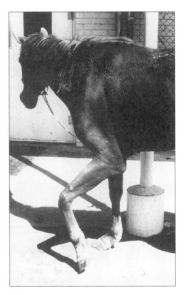

Fig. 19–16. Above: A foal with radial nerve paralysis. Right: A horse with a complete olecranon fracture. While they appear similar, note that the horse is able to bring its leg forward—the foal cannot.

RADIAL NERVE PARALYSIS VS. FRACTURES

	Dropped Elbow	Normal Foot Placement	Skin Sensation	Weight-Bearing
Radial Nerve Paralysis	yes	no	no	no
Olecranon Fracture	maybe	yes	yes	maybe
Humeral Fracture	no	yes	yes	no

Fig. 19–17. Comparing the signs of three upper foreleg conditions. Note: If the radial nerve was also damaged when the humerus was fractured, the horse will show signs of both radial nerve paralysis and humeral fracture.

Paralysis vs. Humeral Fracture

Distinguishing between radial nerve paralysis and a complete humeral fracture usually is straightforward based on the degree of swelling and pain over the humerus. However, radial nerve paralysis caused by a humeral fracture may not be readily apparent because the fracture is the most striking feature, and of most concern. In many cases nerve damage is irrelevant because the fracture alone may prompt euthanasia.

Nevertheless, there are a few signs that differentiate between a humeral fracture alone and a humeral fracture with radial nerve paralysis. When the radial nerve is undamaged, the horse should be able to straighten its knee and lower joints, although it will be very reluctant to do so because of the pain. Some of the extensor muscles of the forearm attach to the lower part of the humerus, and when they contract they pull on the fractured bone. A more useful sign is the position of the elbow; it is in the normal position (that is, not "dropped") if the radial nerve is undamaged. The elbow may in fact be slightly higher or further forward than normal if the fracture pieces over-ride, because this shortens the humerus. Finally, the horse should have normal skin sensation on the front and outside of the forearm if the radial nerve is intact.

Bicipital Bursitis

Definition

The bicipital bursa is a long, narrow sac that lies between the biceps brachii tendon and the top of the humerus at the front of the shoulder joint. Below the joint the biceps brachii muscle continues down and attaches onto the radius at the front of the elbow. Its functions are to flex the elbow and support the shoulder joint in the normal standing position.

Bicipital bursitis is inflammation of the bicipital bursa. When a bursa is inflamed, its lining secretes more fluid and the bursa becomes swollen.

> **Definition**
>
> **Bursa:** a thin sac that lies between a tendon and a bone to ensure that the tendon glides smoothly over the bone's surface.
> **A bursa has a fibrous, outer covering and a thin lining called the synovium, which secretes fluid into the sac.**

Causes

Bicipital bursitis may be due to either direct trauma over the point of the shoulder, or excessive pressure and friction between the bone and the biceps tendon. Bicipital bursitis is fairly uncommon in any type of horse, but it is seen most often in Standardbred racehorses. One factor may be their extreme stride length at race speeds. These horses fully extend their elbows when they are trotting or pacing at speed. When the leg is back and the elbow is extended, there is increased tension on the biceps tendon, and on the bicipital bursa beneath. In pacers, the hobbles may make this problem more likely. The biceps brachii

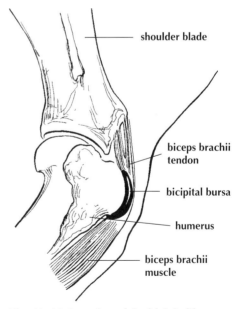

Fig. 19–18. Location of the bicipital bursa at the front of the shoulder.

shoulder blade

biceps brachii tendon

bicipital bursa

humerus

biceps brachii muscle

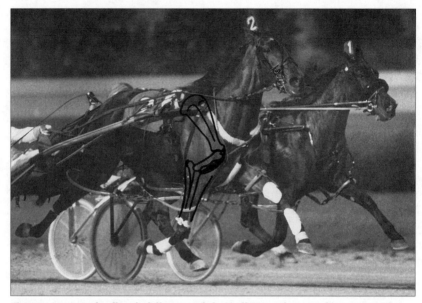

Fig. 19–19. Standardbreds fully extend their elbows when working at speed. This may increase tension on the biceps muscle and tendon (shown in black).

muscle contracts to bring the foreleg forward. But if the hindfoot is not yet lifted, the hobbles prevent the foreleg from being brought forward. As a result, excessive tension is placed on the biceps brachii tendon and the underlying bursa for a brief moment during each stride.

Signs and Diagnosis of Bicipital Bursitis

Bicipital bursitis usually causes mild to moderate lameness (grade 1 – 3 of 5), and few, if any other signs. Often the lameness disappears with rest, but returns when training resumes. In some cases even the lameness is questionable. The only sign may be a reluctance to stride out at high speed, and reduced athletic performance.

Careful palpation around the point of the shoulder may cause a mild pain response. But because the bursa is hidden beneath the biceps tendon and overlying muscles, swelling can rarely be detected with palpation. Lifting the horse's leg and pulling it back may also cause pain. But this is true of other problems in the upper foreleg; it is not specific for bicipital bursitis. It is usually necessary to eliminate other, more likely causes of lameness before focusing on the bicipital bursa.

Injecting local anesthetic directly into the bursa may temporarily resolve the lameness. But it can be difficult to be certain that the needle is in the right location without ultrasound to guide needle placement. Also, if the biceps tendon itself has been strained or torn, injecting local anesthetic into the bursa may not affect the lameness. Therefore, the simplest and best way to diagnose this condition is with ultrasonography *(see Chapter 2)*. When the front of the shoulder is ultrasounded, excess fluid can be seen in the bicipital bursa. Ultrasound is also the only way to detect tendon fiber damage.

Treatment of Bicipital Bursitis

Bicipital bursitis generally is caused by strenuous exercise. So, treatment should include rest from regular training, and a few days of anti-inflammatory therapy (cold therapy, NSAIDs, DMSO, etc.; *see Chapter 5*). Some veterinarians also drain the excess fluid from the bursa; this is easiest to do when guided by ultrasound. After draining the fluid, the veterinarian may inject hyaluronic acid or corticosteroids into the bursa. These medications settle down the inflammation and prevent adhesions (fibrous bands) from forming. However, corticosteroids should not be used if there is tendon damage.

Light exercise can also help reduce adhesions. Such activity includes hand-walking the horse for at least 20 minutes twice per day or turning the horse out onto pasture. Passive motion exercises and other physical therapies, such as laser therapy, therapeutic ultrasound, and magnetic field therapy, can also speed healing *(see Chapter 4)*.

It is usually necessary to suspend regular training for at least 6 weeks to allow the damaged bursa to heal. A longer rest period is needed if there is also tendon fiber damage. Returning the horse to training too soon may cause persistence or recurrence of the lameness. In particular, it is counter-productive to inject the bursa with corticosteroids and continue to work the horse, especially if there is tendon fiber damage. The problem is likely to persist or worsen if it is not given enough time to heal. Repeat ultrasound examination is useful to decide when the horse can return to training.

Prognosis for Bicipital Bursitis

The prognosis for return to strenuous athletic activities usually is good, provided the condition is diagnosed and treated early. However, because the lameness is vague and difficult to localize, the condition usually is chronic before the diagnosis is made. Chronic inflammation and tissue damage is much more difficult to resolve than an acute injury.

SHOULDER

The shoulder is both a general area and a specific joint. Several structures are found in the shoulder area:

- the top of the humerus
- the shoulder joint
- the shoulder blade and its overlying muscles
- the triceps muscles

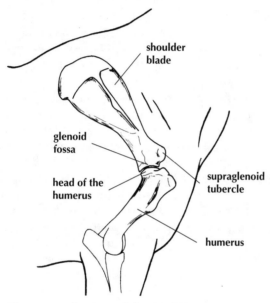

Fig. 19–20. The parts of the shoulder.

Thus, the general term, "shoulder," can cover a large area and various structures. It is important to be specific when describing the location of an injury in this area.

The shoulder joint is a "ball and socket" joint. The "ball" is the rounded head of the humerus, and the "socket" is the shallow cup, or glenoid fossa, on the lower end of the shoulder blade. The joint is supported by the joint capsule and collateral ligaments. It is also stabilized by the tendons of the muscles that lie along the side of the shoulder blade—the supraspinatus and infraspinatus muscles.

The point of the shoulder is a familiar landmark to most horse people. It consists of the supraglenoid tubercle at the lower end of the shoulder blade, and the top of the humerus.

Osteochondrosis (Including OCD)
Definition

Osteochondrosis is an abnormality of developing bone that is fairly common in young horses. It results in defects in the cartilage or underlying bone at the affected joint surface.

The shoulder is one of the classic sites for osteochondrosis, although it is a far less common location than the hock or stifle. In many cases the lesion consists of a bone and cartilage fragment—an osteochondritis dissecans (OCD) lesion. The other common defect is flattening or

> **More Information**
>
> Osteochondrosis is discussed in detail in Chapter 14.

irregularity of the bone at the joint surface. Both types of lesion may be found together in some horses. The typical location for these lesions is on the head of the humerus, toward the back of the joint.

Signs and Diagnosis

Although osteochondrosis is a developmental problem, in most cases the signs of shoulder osteochondrosis are not seen until the horse begins training. In some cases there may be no obvious problems until the workload is increased.

The signs of shoulder osteochondrosis are vague. The lameness may be moderate (grade 2 – 3 of 5), and the horse's stride shortened, particularly in a circle. But there is no visible swelling around the shoulder joint, and palpation usually does not cause pain. The horse may resent the veterinarian bringing the leg forward, back, or to the side, but this is not specific for shoulder osteochondrosis. In fact, it is not specific for any shoulder joint problem; the shoulder muscles and elbow are also affected by these manipulations.

Injecting local anesthetic into the shoulder joint (joint block; *see Chapter 2*) usually improves the lameness, which confirms that the shoulder is the site of lameness. However, this can be a difficult block to perform. Nuclear scintigraphy can be useful for localizing an obscure lameness to the shoulder. But in many horses with shoulder osteochondrosis nuclear scintigraphy reveals no abnormality.

Radiography

Good quality radiographs of the shoulder are necessary to definitely diagnose osteochondrosis. However, the shoulder is a difficult area to radiograph. To get good images, the horse's leg must be pulled as far forward as possible to prevent interference from the ribs and the other shoulder. Many horses resent having their leg pulled forward if their shoulder is painful. Furthermore, in large, heavily muscled horses a powerful x-ray machine is necessary to get good quality radiographs. Some portable machines are not powerful enough to do this, so the horse may need to be transported to a vet-

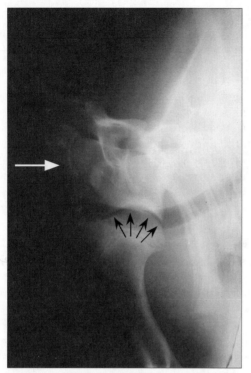

erinary hospital that has a larger x-ray machine. In some cases the veterinarian may need to anesthetize the horse to get good shoulder radiographs.

Osteochondrosis often is bilateral, so both shoulders should be radiographed, even though the horse may be lame in only one leg. Osteochondrosis occasionally affects several other joints in the body. A thorough physical examination should be performed on every horse suspected of having shoulder osteochondrosis. Any joint showing effusion (accumulation of joint fluid) should be radiographed.

Fig. 19–21. Radiograph of a normal shoulder joint in a young horse. The white arrow indicates the supraglenoid tubercle. The black arrows indicate the shoulder joint.

Treatment of Osteochondrosis

If just flattening or irregularity of the bone is seen on radiographs, the veterinarian may recommend resting the horse from regular training for 3 – 4 months. Paddock or pasture rest is better than confinement in a stall or small pen, especially in young horses. If the horse must be confined, it should be hand-walked for at least 20 minutes twice per day.

The veterinarian may also suggest treating the horse with a joint medication, such as hyaluronic acid or Adequan *(see Chapter 5)*. However, if an OCD lesion is found, surgery is often recommended. Of all the locations in the horse's limbs where osteochondrosis typically occurs, OCD lesions in the shoulder have the worst outcome with conservative management (rest and medication). Surgery generally offers the best chance of a satisfactory outcome. In most cases the fragment can be removed arthroscopically *(see Chapter 6)*. This procedure is followed by 2 – 4 weeks of confinement, and then 3 – 6 months of paddock or pasture rest. Joint medications may also be advised following surgery.

Prognosis for Osteochondrosis

The prognosis for return to full athletic function in a horse with shoulder osteochondrosis is guarded, although surgery improves the horse's chance of a successful athletic career. Shoulder osteochondrosis has about the worst prognosis for athletic function of any joint. Chronic, low-grade lameness caused by degenerative joint disease is the common result.

Degenerative Joint Disease

Degenerative joint disease (DJD) in the shoulder is fairly uncommon in horses. It is almost always secondary to another condition, such as:

- osteochondrosis
- a fracture that involves the joint—an articular fracture
- joint instability
- joint infection (septic arthritis)

An articular fracture may involve either the head of the humerus or the cup of the shoulder blade. Instability of the shoulder joint may be due to a joint capsule or collateral ligament tear, or sweeney.

The signs of shoulder DJD are vague. Chronic shoulder joint problems usually do not cause obvious swelling or pain during palpation, although septic arthritis causes both when it is "active." The lameness associated with shoulder DJD is mild to moderate (grade 1 – 3

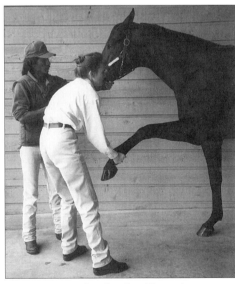

Fig. 19–22. Testing for shoulder pain.

of 5). It can often be worsened by pulling the horse's leg forward and holding it in that position for 30 – 60 seconds before trotting the

horse off. Injecting local anesthetic into the shoulder joint temporarily improves the lameness. But radiographs should be taken to
check for other joint problems, such as osteochondrosis or incomplete fractures, before making a diagnosis of DJD.

Treating DJD in the shoulder should follow the guidelines given in
Chapter 8 for managing chronic joint disease. In many cases the degenerative changes are advanced by the time consistent signs are
seen and the diagnosis is confirmed. As a result, the prognosis for
long-term athletic function is poor, particularly if there are bony
changes within or around the joint.

Shoulder Blade (Scapular) Fractures
Definitions and Causes

The shoulder blade, or scapula, is a broad, flat, oar-shaped bone
that lies at a slight backward angle against the side of the horse's
chest. A narrow ridge of
bone, called the spine
of the scapula, runs
down the outer surface
of the bone. This ridge
can be felt (and in thin
horses, seen) on the
side of the shoulder.
The muscles that help
stabilize the shoulder
joint lie flat against the
scapula on either side of
this ridge.

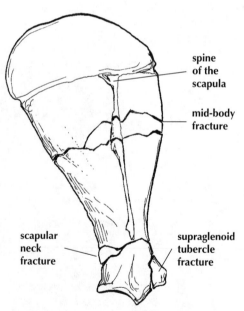

The lower part of the
scapula narrows into a
region called the scapu-
lar neck before it fans
out to form the shoul-
der joint with the head
of the humerus. At the
front of the shoulder
joint, on the lower end
of the scapula, is a bony knob called the supraglenoid tubercle.

Fig. 19–23. Types of scapular fracture.

Scapular fractures are uncommon in horses. In most cases they are
the result of direct trauma, such as a fall or a collision between two
horses. Depending on the site and intensity of the impact, the frac-

ture may be a simple, incomplete fracture—little more than a crack in the bone. Or, it may be a complete, comminuted fracture, in which the bone is broken into several pieces.

Scapular fractures may occur anywhere along the bone's length. Generally they can be divided into three categories:

1. Mid-body fractures, involving the broad, flat surface and vertical spine.
2. Scapular neck fractures, occurring across the narrow "neck" just above the shoulder joint.
3. Supraglenoid fractures, involving the supraglenoid tubercle.

Some fractures of the scapular neck or supraglenoid tubercle are articular, extending into the shoulder joint. Mid-body fractures are not articular, unless they extend across the scapular neck into the joint. The biceps tendon (discussed earlier) attaches onto the supraglenoid tubercle. So, complete supraglenoid fractures may be displaced and the bone fragment pulled forward and down by the biceps brachii muscle.

The signs of scapular fractures vary, depending on their location and severity. Treatment also varies with the location and type of fracture.

Mid-body or Scapular Neck Fractures
Signs and Diagnosis

Simple, incomplete fractures in the body or neck of the scapula may not cause obvious swelling. So, it is sometimes difficult to identify the site of the lameness, which is usually mild to moderate (grade 2 – 3 of 5). Careful palpation may locate a specific site of pain, although it is not possible to directly palpate much of the scapula because of the overlying muscles. Deep pressure is usually necessary to find pain over the fracture site in these horses. Crepitus (crunching of bone-on-bone) is not found with an incomplete fracture.

In most cases pulling the horse's leg forward, back, or to the side causes pain, although this is not a very specific test for bone or joint pain in and around the shoulder. Problems with the humerus or elbow can result in pain during these manipulations. Horses that have exertional rhabdomyolysis (ER or "tying up"; *see Chapter 10*) may also react to these procedures. Pain during palpation over or behind the scapula is fairly common in horses with ER. This is because ER often causes the shoulder muscles (particularly the triceps muscles) to become tense and painful.

Confirming the diagnosis of an incomplete scapular fracture requires radiographs. The horse may need to be taken to a veterinary

Extra Information

A powerful x-ray machine is needed to radiograph the scapula because the x-ray beam must travel through both shoulders and the ribcage. It is not possible to radiograph just one scapula.

hospital that has a powerful x-ray machine, because it is very difficult to get good quality radiographs of the scapula. Sometimes it is even necessary to anesthetize the horse. However, anesthetizing the horse can have disastrous consequences because the horse can completely fracture the scapula when it gets up after anesthesia. Nuclear scintigraphy can help locate the source of lameness, although it is not possible to make a definite diagnosis with scintigraphy.

Complete Fractures

Complete mid-body or scapular neck fractures often collapse and over-ride (overlap) when the horse bears weight on the leg. Thus, these fractures usually cause moderate to severe swelling over the side of the shoulder, obvious pain during palpation, and severe lameness (grade 4 – 5 of 5). Crepitus may sometimes be heard or felt during palpation of the scapula or manipulation of the leg. Making the diagnosis usually is straightforward, although radiographs may be necessary in some cases.

Treatment of Mid-body or Scapular Neck Fractures

Most incomplete and nondisplaced, complete fractures in the body or neck of the scapula are treated conservatively. This consists of 2 – 3 months of stall confinement, followed by 4 – 6 months of pasture rest. The side of the chest and the muscles over the scapula act like a natural splint, so most of these fractures eventually heal. However, care must be taken to keep the horse as quiet as possible. It is usually best not to hand-walk the horse at all for the first 4 weeks or so. The veterinarian may also recommend cross-tying the horse for the first few weeks to prevent it from lying down. This is important because an incomplete fracture may become a complete fracture when the horse gets up.

A few simple, complete fractures in the body of the scapula may be repaired with bone plates, although most mid-body fractures cannot be repaired surgically. Because of the shape of the scapular neck, fractures at this location also cannot be repaired surgically. If the fracture is severe, displaced, and over-ridden, the veterinarian may recommend euthanasia for humane reasons. Over-ridden fractures generally do not heal well.

Scapular fractures typically cause muscle atrophy (wasting) over the side of the shoulder from lack of use. If a scapular neck fracture damages the suprascapular nerve, the resulting loss of nerve supply causes more rapid and severe muscle atrophy (sweeney). The atrophy that accompanies most scapular fractures usually is reversible once the horse can use the leg normally. However, sweeney may result in permanent muscle atrophy if the nerve is severely damaged. Electrical muscle stimulation *(see Chapter 4)* can help reverse the muscle atrophy, but it should not be started until at least 4 weeks after the fracture occurred.

(The issues regarding long-term NSAID use that are discussed in Chapter 9 apply to horses with severe scapular fractures.)

Prognosis for Mid-body or Scapular Neck Fractures

The prognosis for return to athletic function following an incomplete scapular fracture is reasonably good with appropriate care. But the prognosis is guarded to poor with complete mid-body and scapular neck fractures. Because the scapular neck is much narrower than the body of the scapula, fractures at the scapular neck are more likely to displace, and therefore, less likely to heal well. DJD is a common complication of scapular neck fractures that extend into the shoulder joint.

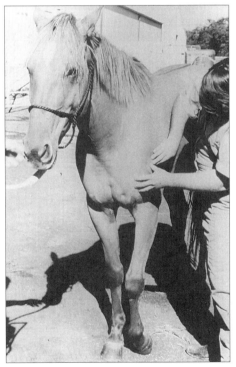

Supraglenoid Fractures
Signs and Diagnosis

Supraglenoid fractures occur at the front of the shoulder joint. If the fracture is complete, it causes swelling over the point of the shoulder. This swelling is painful during palpation, but crepitus usually is not

Fig. 19–24. Careful palpation may locate a specific site of pain.

felt. The horse can still bear weight on the leg because the humerus and the joint surface of the scapula are intact. In most cases the lameness is moderate (grade 3 – 4 of 5), although the horse is very reluctant to swing its leg forward when it moves. To bring the leg forward the horse normally flexes its elbow. The biceps brachii is one of the muscles that flexes the elbow. It is attached to the supraglenoid tubercle by the biceps tendon. When this muscle contracts, tension is placed on the fractured tubercle, which causes severe pain. In some cases the horse stands with the foreleg out in front, a stance which takes tension off the biceps tendon.

A skin abrasion or wound over the point of the shoulder is a clue that there may have been trauma of enough force to fracture the tubercle. However, there do not need to be any marks on the skin for the tubercle to be fractured.

This part of the shoulder can easily be radiographed without anesthetizing the horse. The x-ray plate is held up against the side of the shoulder and the x-ray machine is placed on the other side of the horse. The beam is directed from just in front of the opposite shoulder across the front of the affected shoulder.

Treatment of Supraglenoid Fractures

Supraglenoid tubercle fractures may either be managed conservatively or surgically, depending on the type of fracture. Incomplete fractures and complete fractures involving only a small piece of bone usually are managed conservatively. Complete fractures that involve a large, displaced fragment or that extend into the shoulder joint are usually best treated surgically.

Conservative management is similar to that described for mid-body and scapular neck fractures, although cross-tying is not necessary. The horse should be confined to a stall or small pen for at least 2 months, and then rested in a larger paddock or pasture for at least another 3 months.

Surgical management involves either reattaching the fragment with bone screws or, if the fragment is too small, removing it. If the fracture extends into the shoulder joint, reattachment of the tubercle with bone screws gives the horse the best chance of returning to athletic activities. Post-operative care includes a few days of antibiotics and NSAIDs. The horse's tetanus status should be checked before surgery *(see Chapter 5)*. Confinement for 6 – 8 weeks, followed by 2 – 3 months of paddock rest is the usual recommendation after surgery.

Prognosis for Supraglenoid Fractures

Supraglenoid tubercle fractures that do not involve the joint have a fairly good outcome. Provided the bone fragment was surgically removed or reattached with bone screws, or it healed back onto the scapula with just rest, the horse should eventually return to athletic activities. If the fracture extended into the shoulder joint, DJD may develop. However, the supraglenoid tubercle makes up a very small area of the joint surface, so any degenerative changes within the joint will likely be manageable.

Sweeney

Sweeney is the result of nerve damage at the front of the shoulder blade. Its signs include muscle atrophy along the side of the scapula and instability of the shoulder joint. Sweeney can develop following a scapular neck fracture or as the result of a direct blow to the front of the shoulder.

The suprascapular nerve runs around the front of the scapular neck on its way to the muscles that overlie the scapula: the supraspinatus and infraspinatus muscles. Trauma to the nerve, or compression by a bone fragment or surrounding soft tissue swelling can result in loss of nerve supply to these muscles. Within a couple of weeks, the muscles atrophy because they are no longer stimulated to contract. These muscles are important because they help support the side of the shoulder joint. Loss of muscle function allows the joint to "pop out," or partially dislocate to the side when the horse bears weight on the leg.

> **More Information**
>
> Sweeney is a condition of the nervous system. Its causes, diagnosis, and management are discussed and illustrated in Chapter 12.

20

THE HOCK

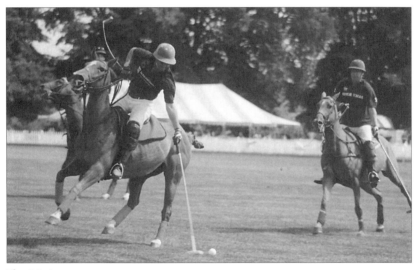

Fig. 20–1.

The hock is the most common site of hindlimb lameness, no matter what the horse's age or athletic activity. Some conditions are of more importance than others. For example, curb and thoroughpin generally are just blemishes, whereas bone spavin can cause chronic, career-halting lameness. Conditions involving the hock joints are discussed first, followed by fractures, problems at the back of the hock, and other conditions.

CONDITIONS OF THE HOCK JOINTS

The hock is a complex area that primarily consists of one large, hinge-type joint, and three narrow, horizontal, relatively immobile joints. There are also some small, vertical, essentially immobile joints between the tarsal bones. The important hock joints are (from top to bottom):

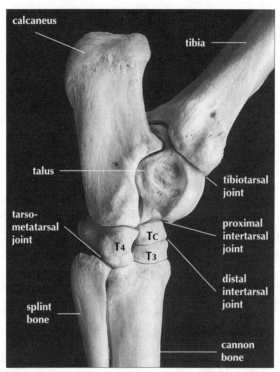

Fig. 20–2. The bones and joints of the hock, viewed from the outside.

• the tibiotarsal joint, between the lower end of the tibia and the talus
• the proximal intertarsal joint, between the talus and the central tarsal bone (Tc)
• the distal intertarsal joint, between the central and third (T3) tarsal bones
• the tarsometatarsal joint, between the third and fourth tarsal bones and the top of the cannon and splint bones

The tibiotarsal joint is the major hock joint, in that it enables the hock to flex. Its joint capsule attaches onto the lower end of the tibia above, and the top of Tc below. It is "roomy" enough to allow the hock to be fully extended (straightened) without putting excess tension on the joint capsule. The capsules of the lower hock joints are much smaller because these joints are essentially immobile.

Of Interest

In people, the equivalent joint to the hock is the ankle. The heel corresponds to the point of the horse's hock (the calcaneus).

Bog Spavin

"Bog spavin" is a non-painful, fluidy swelling at the front and sides of the hock. The swelling is the result of effusion (accumulation of fluid) in the tibiotarsal joint. Because the joint capsule is so "roomy," excess fluid within the joint causes the capsule to pouch out between the tendons and ligaments that run over the hock.

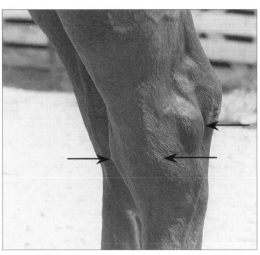

Fig. 20–3. Bog spavin causes fluid-filled swellings around the hock.

This can result in distinct swellings at a few different locations around the hock. The largest pouches occur at the front of the joint, one toward the inside and one toward the outside of the leg. If the effusion is great, smaller pouches may also be seen toward the back of the hock, on either side of the leg.

Causes

Bog spavin is a *symptom*, not a specific disease. The most common causes of joint effusion are synovitis and degenerative joint disease (DJD). Repeated or excessive strain of the joint capsule can result in synovitis and joint effusion. But most cases of bog spavin in horses less than about 3 years old are due to a physical defect within the tibiotarsal joint, such as osteochondrosis (discussed later). In mature horses, bog spavin is more likely due to chronic strain and stretching of the joint capsule.

More Information

Synovitis is inflammation of the synovium, which is the joint capsule lining. Synovitis and degenerative joint disease are covered in Chapter 8.

Not all horses with bog spavin are obviously lame; often lameness is not seen until the horse's workload is increased. Many people consider bog spavin to be unimportant—a blemish. However, the effusion is a clue to the presence of joint disease that could have a significant impact on the horse's athletic future. Therefore, every case of bog spavin should be investigated by a veterinarian, even if the horse is not lame.

Management of Bog Spavin

Most veterinarians radiograph the hocks to check for bony problems within the joint before deciding on the best way to manage the swelling. Draining the excess fluid from the joint is not effective when there is an underlying condition that is not addressed. Within a couple of days the joint will refill if the primary problem is not treated. The longer the effusion is present, the more likely the joint capsule will be stretched, and will then continue to fill to its new capacity. If the cosmetic appearance of the joint is important, this is another good reason to have the veterinarian examine the horse as soon as the effusion is noticed.

More specific management recommendations depend on the underlying problem.

Osteochondrosis (Including OCD)

Definition

Osteochondrosis is an abnormality of developing bone that is fairly common in young horses. It causes defects in the cartilage or underlying bone at the affected joint surfaces.

The hock is the most common site of osteochondrosis in horses. The lesions most often seen are:

- bone-and-cartilage fragments—osteochondritis dissecans (OCD) lesions
- flattening or irregularity of the bone at the joint surface

These lesions occur in fairly predictable locations in the tibiotarsal joint. One frequently affected site is the lower end of the tibia. Another is the ridge on either side of the central groove of the talus (*see Figure 20–12*).

> **More Information**
>
> Osteochondrosis and other Developmental Orthopedic Disorders are discussed in Chapter 14.

Signs

The signs of either type of osteochondrosis lesion include non-painful joint effusion (bog spavin) and mild lameness (grade 1 – 2 of 5). But the lameness may not be seen until the horse's workload is increased or the horse sustains some type of trauma, such as a fall or a kick. Often there are no obvious signs of osteo-chondrosis until the joint is "stressed."

A hock flexion test often causes or worsens the lameness. This test is useful when bog spavin is present but the horse is not lame. If it causes lameness the flexion test indicates that there may be a signifi-cant physical defect in the joint. In some cases the farrier is the first person to notice that hock flexion causes the horse pain. This is be-cause he or she must flex the horse's hocks to trim or shoe the hindfeet. Some horses with hock osteochondrosis resist the farrier, and they may be lame after being trimmed or shod.

Osteochondrosis frequently is bilateral—present in the same joint in both legs. It may also be present in other joints. A thorough physi-cal examination and gait evaluation should be performed to reveal problems in joints other than the hocks.

Diagnosis

The signs are not specific for osteochondrosis; they simply indicate synovitis or DJD. Radio-graphs are necessary to make a definite diagno-sis. A full series of radio-graphs should be taken because the lesion may be visible on only one of the four standard views *(see Chapter 2).* The fact that these lesions typi-cally occur in just a few locations helps the vet-erinarian to find small fragments and subtle changes, such as flatten-ing of the bone. Because osteochondrosis often is bilateral, most veterinar-ians radiograph both hocks, even though the effusion and lameness may be obvious in only one leg.

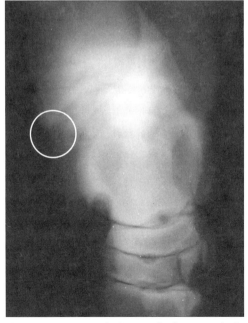

Fig. 20–4. An OCD lesion on the lower end of the tibia.

Treatment of Osteochondrosis

OCD Lesions

When OCD lesions are found on radiographs, the usual recommendation is surgical removal using arthroscopy *(see Chapter 6)*. Sometimes the fragment appears to still be attached to the main part of the bone, and only separated by a thin line. In these cases the veterinarian may simply recommend 3 – 6 months of paddock rest to allow the bone fragment to heal back onto the bone. This approach is successful in many cases. If the fragment appears to be free in the joint, it should be removed to prevent more cartilage damage and persistent joint problems.

Flattening or Other Irregularities

If just flattening or irregularity of the bone surface is seen, most veterinarians recommend paddock or pasture rest for 3 – 6 months. However, cartilage erosions, flaps, or fragments often occur with osteochondrosis. These cartilage lesions do not show up on radiographs. So, if there is just flattening or irregularity of the bone, and the horse has persistent joint effusion and lameness, arthroscopic examination may be worthwhile. It is common to find cartilage fragments in these joints. Removing them is often best if chronic joint problems are to be prevented.

Post-Operative Care

The usual recommendation after surgery is stall confinement for 1 – 4 weeks, depending on the degree of cartilage damage seen during surgery. This is followed by 3 – 4 months of paddock or pasture rest. Cartilage defects take about 3 months to fill in, and the defect is replaced with cartilage that is not as strong or resilient as healthy cartilage. Therefore, it is very important that the horse is rested for the full time prescribed by the veterinarian. Returning the horse to training too soon can result in DJD and chronic lameness. *(See Chapter 6 for more information on post-operative care following arthroscopic surgery.)*

Many veterinarians prescribe joint medications (hyaluronic acid or Adequan; *see Chapter 5*) either during the convalescent period or just before the horse begins training. These products may not significantly speed up cartilage repair or improve the quality of the new cartilage. However, they can settle down inflammation within the joint and provide the cartilage with an environment that is more suited to its repair.

Prognosis and Prevention of Osteochondrosis

If the veterinarian's treatment recommendations are followed and the defects are given time to heal, the prognosis for future athletic usefulness is usually very good. Of all the joints where osteochondrosis develops, the hock has one of the best outcomes with appropriate treatment.

Preventing osteochondrosis must begin with the pregnant mare and continue with the growing foal. Specific recommendations are given in Chapter 14.

Bone Spavin
Definition and Causes

Bone spavin is a type of osteoarthritis—the endstage of degenerative joint disease (DJD) in one or more of the three lower hock joints. It most commonly affects the lower two joints (tarsometatarsal and distal intertarsal); the proximal intertarsal joint is not often involved. These joints are illustrated in Figure 20–2.

Two major factors lead to the development of DJD in the lower hock joints. The first is cartilage compression. The lower tarsal bones have cartilage on their upper and lower surfaces, and they are stacked on top of one another like building blocks. Excessive compression plays a key role by causing cartilage degeneration. Over time, the cartilage surfaces become flattened and eroded, and the joint spaces narrow. Eventually the joints space may fill in with new bone.

The other major factor is uneven loading. When the lower hock joints are unevenly loaded, there is excessive compression of the cartilage and underlying bone on one side. On the other side there is strain on the joint capsules and supporting ligaments. Repeated overloading of a joint surface can cause remodeling and new bone production (exostoses, or bone "spurs") at the edges of the bone. Likewise, excessive and repeated strain on the joint's soft tissues can cause exostoses around the joint.

These bony changes—narrowing of the joint space and bone spurs around the joint—are the hallmark of bone spavin.

More Information

DJD results in:
- **inflammation of the joint capsule and its lining (synovium)**
- **cartilage degeneration**

Osteoarthritis is a severe form of DJD in which bony changes develop in or around the joint.

(These conditions are discussed in Chapter 8.)

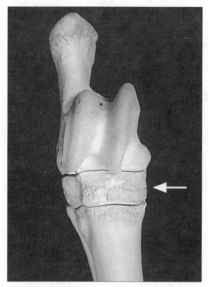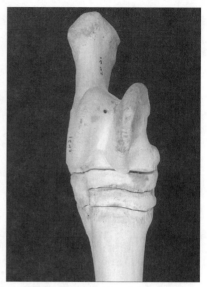

Fig. 20–5. Left: Bone spavin has fused the distal intertarsal joint. Right: Normal hock joints. (Note: The tibia has been removed from each hock.)

Contributing Factors

Bone spavin is a "wear and tear" injury. It is the result of repeated, excessive and/or uneven load on the lower hock joints. Thus, it is commonly seen in mature horses that perform activities that require a lot of hock flexion, such as dressage, or cause jarring, such as jumping. Sudden stops and turns on the hindquarters during roping, reining, and other Western activities can also contribute. In Standardbred racehorses, repeated concussion, pulling a load (jog cart and driver), and gait-modifying shoes may be the most important factors that lead to bone spavin. Poor conformation, particularly "sickle hocks" or "cow hocks," can cause uneven loading of the lower hock joints in any type of horse, as can improper trimming and shoeing.

Occasionally, bone spavin is seen in horses less than about 3 years old; this condition is called "juvenile spavin." Because it sometimes develops before the horse has done much work, some veterinarians believe it may be another manifestation of osteochondrosis. Bony changes typical of advanced bone spavin are sometimes seen in these young horses.

Signs of Bone Spavin

In most cases the initial signs of bone spavin are subtle, consisting

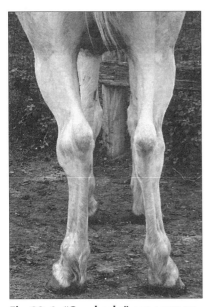

Fig. 20–6. "Cow hocks" can cause uneven loading of the hock joints.

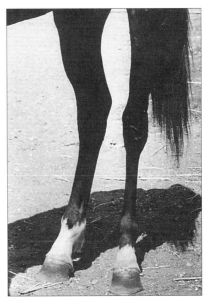

Fig. 20–7. "Sickle hocks" can also lead to bone spavin.

of a vague, intermittent hindlimb lameness that may shift from one leg to the other. The lameness disappears with rest or anti-inflammatory medications, but reappears when training resumes or the drugs are stopped. Over a period of weeks or months, the lameness gradually becomes more consistent and obvious (grade 2 – 3 of 5).

Horses with bone spavin tend to land toe-first, and have a lower and shorter arc of foot flight *(see Chapter 1)*. This gait is an attempt to reduce concussion and hock flexion. It often results in dragging and wearing of the toe on the affected hindlimb.

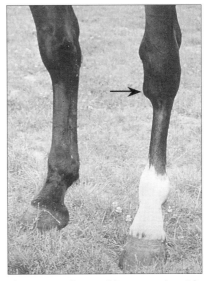

Fig. 20–8. Advanced bone spavin with bony swelling around the lower hock joints.

In most cases bone spavin is bilateral, although one leg is usually more severely affected than the other. In advanced cases there may be bony swelling around the lower hock joints, most often on the inside of the hock. Bone spavin does not cause joint effusion (bog spavin) because it does not directly involve the tibiotarsal joint. If bog spavin is present, there most likely are other problems in the hock.

Diagnosis of Bone Spavin
Flexion Test

In most cases the lameness is worsened by hock flexion, hence the common term, "spavin test," for the hock flexion test. However, it is not possible to flex the hock without also flexing the stifle. So, a positive spavin test does not always mean that the horse has bone spavin. Other changes within or around the hock, or elsewhere in the upper leg may be responsible for the lameness and the positive flexion test.

Some veterinarians modify the spavin test by lifting the leg to a comfortable height and putting firm finger pressure over the lower hock joints on the inside of the leg. This position is held for about a minute, then the horse is trotted off. If there are active bony changes around these joints, this test can worsen the lameness.

Radiographs

When the physical examination, gait evaluation, and flexion tests localize the lameness to the hocks, most veterinarians then radiograph the hocks. Unless the horse has very mild or early bone spavin, the radiographs typically show some new bone production (bone spurs) and narrowing of the joint spaces.

Bone spurs are the more reliable finding. Normal joint spaces can be made to look

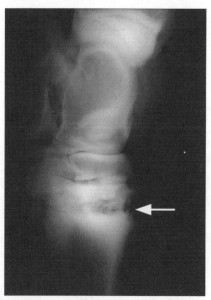

Fig. 20–9. Bone spurs and narrowing of the tarsometatarsal joint space.

narrow if the x-ray beam is at a slight angle, rather than being aimed horizontally through the lower hock joints. Therefore, narrowing of the joint spaces must be interpreted in light of other radiographic findings and the results of the physical examination, gait evaluation, and flexion tests. If it is the only abnormality found on radiographs, other tests may be necessary to confirm the diagnosis.

In advanced cases the joint spaces may be partially or entirely fused (ankylosed), and there may be a callus of bone bridging the joint. These are the horses that have an obvious bony swelling on the side of the hock.

The severity of the bony changes does not always match the degree of pain and lameness. In many cases the horse is obviously lame, but there is only mild bone proliferation around one joint. At the other extreme, some horses in which the affected joints are almost completely fused may no longer be very lame.

Other Tests

Many mild or early cases have no conclusive radiographic changes. In these horses the diagnosis must be confirmed with either a joint block or nuclear scintigraphy. It can be difficult to block the lower hock joints because they are very narrow. Bone spavin narrows the joint space even more, making this joint block a little more difficult. *(See Chapter 2 for more information on these diagnostic techniques.)*

Treatment of Bone Spavin

There is no specific treatment for bone spavin; the changes are irreversible. However, the pain and lameness

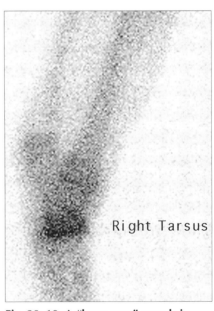

Fig. 20–10. A "bone scan" reveals inflammation in the lower hock joints.

often can be controlled with medication and shoeing, and by modifying the horse's training program. These measures can also slow the condition's progress in some horses. In unresponsive cases, surgery may be recommended.

More Information

Chapter 5 contains more information on medications:

- NSAIDs
- corticosteroids
- HA, GAGs, etc.

Medications

NSAIDs

The veterinarian has a few options for managing bone spavin with drugs. NSAIDs temporarily resolve, or at least improve the lameness in most horses. However, these drugs have two important drawbacks. First, high doses of NSAIDs given for several days can cause stomach ulcers and kidney problems. It is best to reduce the dose to the lowest effective level in the first few days. Second, assuming the NSAIDs allow the horse to train and compete pain-free, these drugs may be prohibited in performing horses. Stopping the drugs for several days before competition may be necessary to comply with specific competition rules. The horse's regular veterinarian is the best person to provide specific dose recommendations and withdrawal times for competition.

Corticosteroids

Injecting long-acting corticosteroids into the lower hock joints usually resolves the lameness for weeks or months, and may be repeated as necessary. Repeated injections of corticosteroids are not recommended in other joints because they can accelerate cartilage degeneration. However, this may have a positive effect in the lower hock joints (discussed later).

Although the drug is injected into the joint space, some of it is absorbed into the bloodstream. It may show up on a pre- or post-competition drug screen. The length of time a drug can be detected in the blood or urine varies among products and horses. Some long-acting corticosteroids can be detected for over 3 weeks after injection. Again, the horse's regular veterinarian is the best person to advise on withdrawal times for these drugs.

Other Drugs

Other joint medications, such as hyaluronic acid and Adequan, may help resolve the pain associated with mild bone spavin. However, these drugs are most useful in acute joint conditions; they are of limited value in horses with moderate to severe bone spavin. Oral products, such as MSM and compounds containing GAGs, can also improve the lameness in some horses with mild or early bone spavin.

Shoeing

Regular shoeing by an experienced farrier is *essential* to managing bone spavin. Various types of shoes have been tried. The ones that are most consistently helpful are those that aid breakover, such as a rolled toe or square toe shoe. Raising the heels with wedge pads can also help some horses by aiding breakover. In addition, most horses benefit from the stability and heel support provided by egg bar shoes. *(Shoeing options are discussed in Chapter 7.)*

Training

Horses with chronic joint disease should be exercised every day *(see Chapter 8)*. In horses with bone spavin, longeing or free-schooling in a round pen is not ideal because it places uneven stresses on the sides of the lower hock joints. Pasture turnout, while good for the horse's overall health and attitude, may not be enough if the horse just stands around or grazes quietly. Ridden or driven exercise is better than longeing, round pen exercise, and pasture turnout.

Reducing the intensity of each training session, while ensuring that the horse remains fit with daily, moderate exercise helps many horses withstand the rigors of training and competition. But bone spavin is a progressive, degenerative disease. Therefore, the horse may not be able to sustain its former level of performance once the lameness becomes consistent. It eventually becomes necessary for the owner or trainer to re-evaluate the horse's athletic future. When the horse can no longer cope with intense training and frequent competition, it is time to find something less strenuous for the horse to do. For example, an upper level event horse may become a schoolmaster for a less experienced rider. Or, a rodeo pick-up horse may be used to "pony" horses at the racetrack. Any type of light exercise is better than inactivity—long-term pasture turnout may spell the end of the horse's useful life.

Surgery

The lameness may eventually resolve once the joints completely fuse with bone. This is because the body has effectively controlled the joint instability and pain. However, this process takes several years, and sometimes these joints never completely fuse.

Surgical treatment of bone spavin is aimed at accelerating the process of joint fusion. It involves destroying some of the cartilage in the lower hock joints with a surgical drill bit. The surgeon may also fill the drill holes with bone grafts for more rapid joint fusion *(see Chapter 6)*. A nonsurgical method of speeding up fusion involves injecting a sterile, caustic agent into the lower hock joints to destroy the cartilage.

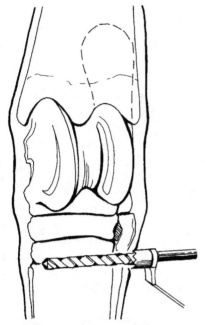

Fig. 20–11. Surgical treatment for bone spavin—fusing the tarsometatarsal joint.

Both procedures worsen the pain until the joints have fused. So, the horse may remain lame for weeks or months after either surgical or chemical fusion.

Exercise can speed joint fusion. In most cases the veterinarian recommends a program of gradually increasing, light exercise, beginning with hand-walking a few days after surgery or injection. NSAIDs usually are recommended to make the horse more comfortable for the first few weeks of exercise.

Prognosis for Bone Spavin

The prognosis for continued athletic function depends on several factors:

- the number of joints involved
- the severity of the bony changes
- the speed at which the condition is worsening
- the horse's use

The long-term prognosis for high-level athletic function is not good in most cases. However, the horse may be useful for light activities, such as pleasure riding, for years.

Dislocation of the Hock

Fortunately, dislocation (luxation) of the hock is rare in horses. It takes extreme force at a very unusual angle to dislocate the hock, either at the tibiotarsal joint or one of the lower hock joints. The supporting ligaments of the hock are strong, and they must be ruptured or badly stretched for the hock to dislocate.

Hock dislocation causes a sudden, nonweight-bearing lameness (grade 5 of 5). The hock may be moderately swollen, but the most dramatic feature is the abnormal angle of the lower leg below the hock. In horses less than about 12 months old it can be difficult to distinguish between hock dislocation and a fracture through the lower physis of the tibia *(see Chapter 21)*. Radiographs usually are necessary to make an accurate diagnosis, and to decide on the best course of action. Radiographs are also valuable in adult horses because the end of the tibia or one of the tarsal bones may be fractured when the hock dislocates.

Treatment and Prognosis

Sometimes surgical repair or reinforcement of the damaged ligaments is possible. However, in many cases all the veterinarian can do is anesthetize the horse, realign the joint, and place a full-limb fiberglass cast or thick support bandage on the leg. If a bandage is used instead of a cast, splints may be added for extra support *(see Chapter 4)*.

The hock must be stabilized with a cast or bandage for at least 6 weeks, and the cast or bandage changed as often as necessary. The horse must be confined to a stall or small pen until the joint is relatively stable. The cast or bandage can then be left off and the horse rested in a small paddock for another 2 – 3 months. Joint stability is only regained when the supporting soft tissues heal with fibrous (scar) tissue. This process takes several weeks, and the fibrous tissue probably does not reach peak strength until at least 3 months after injury. So, the horse should not be permitted any activity before this time.

The prognosis for future athletic activity is poor. Such profound disruption of the joint's supporting structures often results in degenerative joint disease *(see Chapter 8)*. Also, the hock will never be as stable as it was before the injury, so vigorous activity may result in a second dislocation.

TARSAL BONE FRACTURES

Fractures of the hock, or tarsal bones are fairly uncommon. Some specific types of tarsal bone fractures are briefly discussed below.

Slab Fractures

The central and third tarsal bones (Tc and T3) are broad, flat, block-shaped (cuboidal) bones. Although it is an uncommon injury, a tarsal slab fracture can occur during exercise, probably due to

Note
Slab fractures also occur in the cuboidal bones of the knee. This fracture is illustrated in Chapter 18.

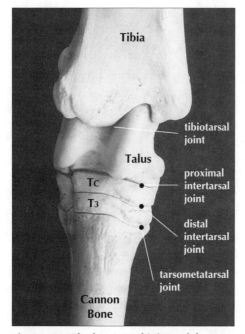

Fig. 20–12. The bones and joints of the hock, viewed from the front.

extreme compressive force from the bones above and below. Compression breaks off a piece of bone from the front of the tarsal bone, like a slab of rock from a cliff face.

Tarsal slab fractures cause sudden, moderate to severe lameness (grade 3 – 4 of 5), and swelling at the front of the hock, just above the cannon. Joint effusion (bog spavin) may develop if Tc is fractured. Radiographs of the hock are necessary to make the diagnosis.

Treatment and Prognosis for Slab Fractures

Tarsal slab fractures usually are surgically repaired with bone screws *(see Chapter 6)*, unless the fragment is very thin. These fractures do eventually heal without surgery. However, the uneven joint surfaces result in degenerative joint disease, which may rapidly progress to bone spavin and cause persistent lameness. But bone spavin can develop even with surgical repair. To avoid this problem, the surgeon may stimulate fusion of the joint above and below the fracture (as described earlier for bone spavin) after repairing it. The affected hock joints then fuse while the fracture heals.

In most cases the surgeon recommends confining the horse to a stall for 4 – 6 weeks, followed by at least 3 months of paddock rest. The prognosis for return to athletic activities is fairly good if the fracture is surgically repaired within a few days of injury. Slab fractures involving a thin bone fragment also have a reasonably good prognosis, after several months of rest.

Maleolus Fractures

The lower end of the tibia has a small bony projection on each side. These bony knobs are called the medial (inside) and lateral (outside) maleolus. The collateral ligaments of the tibiotarsal joint attach onto these structures.

There are a few possible causes of a maleolus fracture. First, because of their fairly exposed location on the side of the hock, direct trauma, such as a kick, can break off a maleolus. Second, the joint surface of the medial maleolus is one of the common sites of hock osteochondrosis

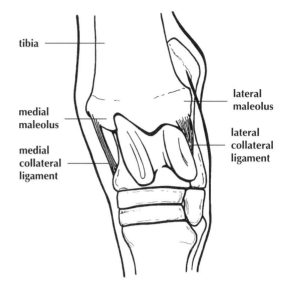

Fig. 20–13. Location of the maleoli and collateral ligaments of the left hock, viewed from the front.

(discussed earlier). It is thought that many of these fractures are actually OCD lesions. The medial maleolus is fractured more often than the lateral maleolus, despite the fact that the inside of the leg is less likely to be traumatized than the outside. Also, maleolus fractures are more common in horses less than about 3 years old. These two facts add weight to the argument that most maleolus fractures are OCD lesions. The third possibility is that the attached collateral ligament tears away a piece of bone, creating an avulsion fracture. But this is probably only possible if there is already a defect in the bone.

No matter what the cause, the bone fragment usually breaks off within the tibiotarsal joint. Therefore, the signs are similar to those seen in horses with osteochondrosis. Lameness is more consistently seen in horses with a maleolus fracture, particularly if trauma is the cause. Radiographs are necessary to confirm the diagnosis and determine the best course of action.

Treatment and Prognosis

If the fractured maleolus is in its normal position, and is therefore still attached to the tibia, most veterinarians recommend conservative management. A few weeks of confinement should be followed by a few months of paddock rest.

If the maleolus appears to be displaced, the veterinarian usually recommends surgical repair or removal, depending on the size and location of the bone fragment. Post-operative care is similar to that described earlier for arthroscopic removal of OCD fragments.

The prognosis for future athletic function is usually very good with appropriate treatment.

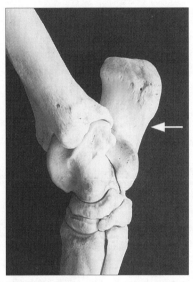

Fig. 20–14. The arrow points to the calcaneus.

Calcaneus Fractures

The calcaneus is the bone that comprises the point of the hock. Calcaneus fractures are uncommon in horses, even though this bone protrudes out the back of the hock. In most cases these fractures are caused by a kick from another horse or kicking at a solid object.

The Achilles tendons (discussed later) attach onto the top of the calcaneus. When the muscles of the Achilles tendons contract, the hock is extended, or straightened. Thus, if the calcaneus is completely fractured, tension from the Achilles tendons can cause the fracture to displace upward and forward.

Treatment and Prognosis

A displaced calcaneus fracture should be surgically repaired with bone screws, pins, or a bone plate for the best result. Additional support with a full-limb fiberglass cast or thick support bandage may also be needed for the first few weeks to counteract the pull of the Achilles tendons. After surgery the usual recommendation is 6 – 8 weeks of confinement in a stall or small pen, then 3 – 4 months of paddock rest. The prognosis for return to athletic function is guarded with most of these fractures.

Calcaneus Fractures in Foals

In foals the calcaneus may be fractured across the physis (growth plate) at the top of the bone. In many cases the Achilles tendons pull off the top of the calcaneus. This injury causes a painful swelling at the point of the hock that can be mistaken for a "capped hock." However, a fracture should be suspected if the foal cannot bear weight on the leg, and palpation of the point of the hock causes severe pain.

This injury is best repaired surgically. A full-limb cast or thick support bandage may also be necessary for the first few weeks to counteract the pull of the Achilles tendons. (**Note:** The cast must be replaced every 10 – 14 days in young, rapidly growing foals; *see Chapter 6.*) The prognosis for future athletic function and a good cosmetic result is usually quite good with appropriate treatment.

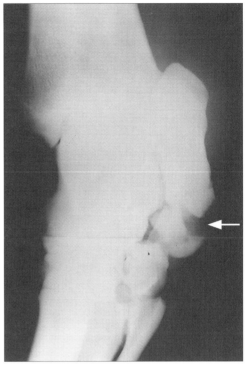

Fig. 20–15. A displaced calcaneus fracture.

Incomplete Fractures

In adult horses a kick to the side or back of the hock more often causes a small piece of bone to break off the surface of the calcaneus. This piece of bone may die and become a sequestrum: an island of devitalized bone that the body treats as "foreign" material *(see Chapter 9)*. Often there is a wound over the sequestrum, which leads to

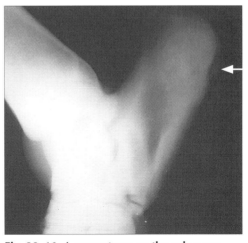

Fig. 20–16. A sequestrum on the calcaneus.

infection of the damaged bone (osteomyelitis). Surgically removing the bone fragment and underlying damaged bone is necessary to resolve the problem. With proper treatment, the prognosis for complete recovery and return to athletic function is very good with this type of calcaneus fracture.

CONDITIONS AT THE BACK OF THE HOCK

Problems at the back of the hock involve the soft tissues that support the joint or attach onto the point of the hock.

Capped Hock

A "capped hock" is a hygroma—a fluid-filled swelling—over the point of the hock. It is caused by trauma. The swelling may be due to inflammation and fluid accumulation in a bursa (bursitis). There are three bursas over the point of the hock:

- a small one between the bone and the Achilles tendons
- a large one between the two tendons
- a small one between the tendons and the skin

It is this last bursa that is most often inflamed.

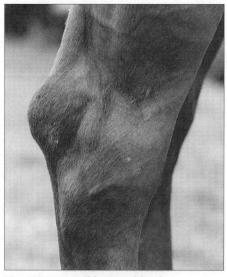

Fig. 20–17. A mild capped hock.

Definitions

Hematoma: collection of blood beneath the skin.
Seroma: collection of serum, the clear yellow, liquid portion of the blood, beneath the skin.
Bursa: small sac of fluid between a bone and a tendon.

(Chapter 18 contains more information on the development and treatment of hygromas.)

In other cases the swelling begins as a hematoma or seroma beneath the skin. With repeated trauma, the swelling may develop into a fibrous sac filled with serum. This structure is sometimes called a "false bursa."

Although it is possible for a single traumatic event to suddenly cause a capped hock, in most cases it is caused by repeated trauma. For example, it is common in horses that repeatedly kick at the stall wall or the back of the trailer.

Capped hocks seldom cause lameness, unless the swelling becomes infected. In most cases treatment is only necessary for cosmetic reasons. It involves anti-inflammatory therapy, including cold, NSAIDs, and DMSO *(see Chapter 5)*. In some cases the veterinarian may also drain the fluid and inject corticosteroids into the cavity. If treated early, the cosmetic result can be quite good.

However, repeated trauma can cause the swelling to persist or return. In these cases it may be necessary to surgically remove the fibrous tissue that forms around the hygroma. But whenever the horse flexes its leg, there is tension on the skin over the point of the hock. This can cause the incision to break down (pull apart) after surgery. To limit hock flexion the veterinarian may place a thick support bandage on the leg from pastern to mid-thigh, until the wound has healed. During this time the horse must be confined to a stall or small pen.

Prevention

Even with surgical removal of the fibrous tissue, the hygroma may re-form if the horse is permitted to re-traumatize the hock. Protecting the hocks with padded boots may help prevent recurrence of the hygroma during transport. Turning the horse out into a paddock or pasture for several hours per day can help prevent boredom-induced kicking. Ensuring that the horse has compatible company while in the stall, or no company if that is what the horse prefers, can also reduce the incidence of stall kicking.

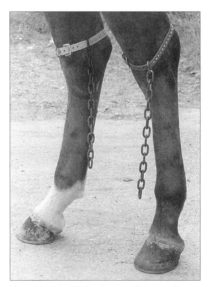

Fig. 20–18. Kick chains distract the horse and may stop it from kicking.

Diversions such as stall toys can help in some cases. Examples include hanging plastic bottles or commercial horse toys. In other horses a "kick chain" may be more effective. This consists of a short piece of lightweight, metal chain that hangs from a leather strap buckled loosely around the leg, just above the hock. The chain hangs down the front of the hock and jangles against the cannon whenever the horse flexes its leg to kick. This can divert the horse's attention enough to stop it from repeatedly kicking the wall.

Achilles Tendon Injuries

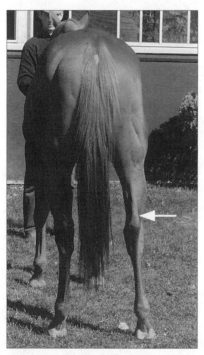

Fig. 20–19. The Achilles tendon.

The Achilles tendon is a human medical term. But it is commonly used to describe the large tendonous structure that runs down the back of the gaskin and attaches onto the point of the hock in horses. This structure consists of two tendons: the gastrocnemius ("gastroc") tendon and the superficial digital flexor tendon (SDFT). Both of these tendons begin as large muscles at the back of the thigh. The "gastroc" tendon ends where it attaches onto the point of the hock *(see Figure 20–20)*. The SDFT continues over the point of the hock and down the back of the cannon before attaching onto the sides of the pastern.

The conditions that can affect the Achilles tendons are discussed below, from more common to least common, which is also from least serious to more serious. However, none of these conditions are very common.

Tendonitis

Tendonitis is inflammation of a tendon; in some cases it includes tendon fiber damage. When the Achilles tendons are inflamed, the most common cause is a "bandage bow": pressure from a tight ban-

---

Extra Information

The Achilles tendons make up part of the "stay apparatus" of the hindlimb. This complex structure consists of:

- the quadriceps muscles above the stifle
- the peroneus tertius tendon at the front of the gaskin
- the Achilles tendons
- the tendons and ligaments of the lower leg

The "stay apparatus" supports the hindlimb in the standing position and allows the horse to rest standing up.

(See Chapter 21 for illustrations of the quadriceps muscles and the peroneus tertius tendon. See Chapter 11 for illustrations of the tendons and ligaments of the lower leg.)

---

dage. It is very difficult to bandage the hock firmly enough that the bandage does its job and stays in place, but not so tightly that it creates a pressure sore. Swelling and skin damage often develop over the Achilles tendons or the point of the hock. *(Bandaging the hock correctly is discussed in Chapter 4.)*

Overstretching of one or both of the Achilles tendons can also cause tendonitis, although it is an uncommon injury. It is most likely the result of sudden, forced flexion of the hock while the muscles of the Achilles tendons are contracting. Examples include a sudden, sliding stop, or slipping backward in the trailer when the driver accelerates too rapidly.

The signs of Achilles tendonitis include mild swelling and pain during palpation of the Achilles tendons, and mild to moderate lameness (grade 2 – 3 of 5). If the injury was caused by a tight bandage, there may also be an area of inflamed skin or a pressure sore along the top of the tendons. The diagnosis can usually be based on the signs. However, the veterinarian may also ultrasound the tendons to check for fiber damage. In most cases fiber damage is seen only when the tendon is overstretched; it is not a typical feature of "bandage bows."

Treatment and Prognosis

Treatment generally involves rest from regular training, and a few days of anti-inflammatory therapy (cold therapy, NSAIDs, DMSO, etc.; *see Chapter 5*). Managing "bandage bows" is discussed in Chapter 13. If ultrasound revealed damaged fibers, tendon splitting may help speed healing.

More Information
Managing tendonitis with tendon splitting and controlled exercise is covered in Chapter 11.

Achilles tendonitis heals best with a program of gradually increasing, light exercise. It should begin with daily hand-walking, then slowly increase in duration and intensity. If no obvious tendon fiber damage is seen on ultrasound, the horse usually can return to regular training in 4 – 6 weeks. If tendon fibers are damaged, light exercise should continue until repeat ultrasound examination indicates that the tendon has completely healed. This may take 3 – 4 months.

The prognosis for full return to athletic activities is usually quite good, provided the horse is rested for long enough.

SDFT Dislocation

An unusual, but serious Achilles tendon injury is dislocation of the SDFT from the point of the hock (the calcaneus). The SDFT runs over the point of the hock and continues down the cannon. At the top of the calcaneus there is a short, strong ligament on each side of the SDFT that anchors it in place and prevents it from slipping off the

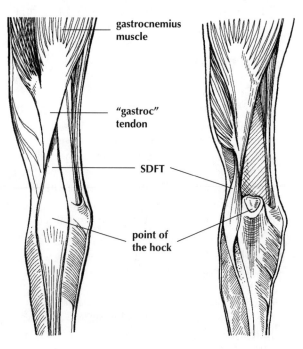

Fig. 20–20. Left: The Achilles tendons in a normal leg, seen from the rear. Right: Dislocation of the SDFT from the point of the hock.

gastrocnemius muscle

"gastroc" tendon

SDFT

point of the hock

bone. When one of these ligaments is torn, the SDFT can slip off to the side of the calcaneus.

This injury usually is caused by direct trauma to the point of the hock. The ligaments may also be torn during the same types of traumatic incident that can cause Achilles tendonitis. At first, the swelling that results may be mistaken for a capped hock. However, the dislocated tendon can be felt or seen to one side (usually the outside) of the calcaneus. It can be manually replaced onto the top of the bone, although it slips off again as soon as the horse takes a step. In some horses the tendon slips on and off the point of the hock with each step. Unlike a capped hock, this condition usually causes moderate lameness (grade 2 – 3 of 5), which is due to pain and mechanical factors *(see Chapter 1)*.

Although the diagnosis is fairly clear based on the signs, most veterinarians radiograph the hock to check for bone damage at the point of impact. Occasionally, the ligament may tear away a bone fragment from its site of attachment, creating an avulsion fracture.

Treatment and Prognosis

The most effective treatment is surgical repair of the torn ligament, and repair or removal of any bone fragments. In some cases it is necessary to reinforce the ligament with surgical mesh, which is a fine-woven nylon netting. But despite reinforcement, tension on the ligament whenever the horse flexes its hock often results in tearing at the repair site. To prevent this, the surgeon places a full-limb fiberglass cast or thick support bandage on the leg for 4 – 6 weeks (changing it as often as necessary; *see Chapters 4 and 6*).

During this time the horse must be confined to a stall or small pen. Once the cast is removed, the horse should remain confined for another 6 – 8 weeks. It takes at least 3 months for the fibrous tissue that repairs torn ligaments to reach peak strength. Activity before this time can result in tearing of the repaired ligament and repeat dislocation of the SDFT.

The repaired ligament is not as strong as an undamaged ligament, so even when surgery is successful, there is the potential for repeat dislocation. Nevertheless, many horses cope well with persistent dislocation of the SDFT. The SDFT still flexes the lower joints, and the undamaged gastrocnemius tendon extends the hock. The horse may eventually return to athletic activities when surgery is not performed, or if it fails. Some may even race again. But the persistent gait abnormality and thickening at the back of the hock spell the end of a horse's show career.

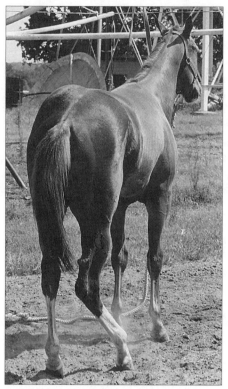

Fig. 20–21. A deep wound above the hock has severed the Achilles tendons.

Tendon Rupture or Laceration

A traumatic incident that causes sudden, forced overflexion of the hock may tear the "gastroc" tendon away from the point of the hock. Fortunately, this is a very uncommon injury. As long as the SDFT is undamaged, the horse can still fix the hock and bear weight on the leg, although walking is painful.

A deep wound over the back of the leg, just above the hock may sever one or both of the Achilles tendons. If both tendons are severed, the hock drops and the horse cannot bear weight on the leg because it is unable to fix its hock in the standing position.

Treatment

These injuries are very serious. Surgical repair is often unrewarding because there is constant tension on the sutures. If surgery is attempted, a full-limb fiberglass cast or a thick support bandage is used to prevent the horse from flexing its hock. This reduces tension on the repair site. If just the "gastroc" tendon is ruptured and the SDFT is still intact, the veterinarian may treat the injury with just a cast or bandage and not attempt surgical repair. It is very difficult to reattach the tendon to the bone.

In either case, the cast or bandage must be kept on the hock for at least 6 weeks, and changed as often as necessary. The horse must then remain confined in a stall or small pen for another 2 – 3 months. Daily hand-walking should not begin until ultrasound examination

More Information

See the section in Chapter 11 on *Flexor Tendon Lacerations & Rupture* for more information on managing this type of injury.

indicates that the tendon is healing well. Activity must be reintroduced very gradually.

Prognosis

The prognosis for return to athletic function is poor. The repaired tendon is not as strong as a normal, healthy tendon, and the load on the Achilles tendons is great. Therefore, the potential for rupture of the repaired tendon generally prevents the horse from returning to strenuous athletic activities. Also, adhesions between the tendon and the surrounding tissues may restrict normal tendon function, resulting in chronic lameness.

Thoroughpin

Thoroughpin is a soft, fluid-filled swelling at the back of the hock. It is located in the groove in front of the Achilles tendons, just above the point of the hock. The swelling, usually about the size of a hen's egg, is the same size and shape on each side of the leg.

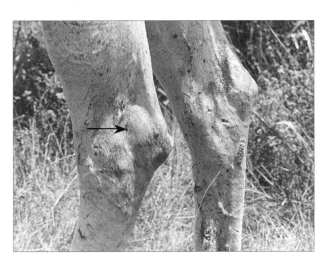

Fig. 20–22. Mild thoroughpin.

This swelling is caused by fluid accumulation (effusion) in the tendon sheath that surrounds the deep digital flexor tendon as it runs over the back of the hock. The fluid accumulates a few inches above the hock because there is a fibrous band that surrounds the deep flexor tendon, preventing the sheath from expanding lower down.

Thoroughpin is usually the result of tendon sheath strain (tenosynovitis; *see Chapter 11*). It may be caused by strain of the deep flexor tendon within the sheath, but this is uncommon. In most cases it does not cause pain or lameness. The swelling may develop suddenly, although in many cases the fluid builds up gradually. If it developed suddenly, there may be mild heat and pain during palpation for the first few days. But these signs usually disappear quickly without treatment.

Treatment is usually only necessary for cosmetic reasons. Draining the fluid and injecting corticosteroids into the sheath may be effective if performed within a few days of the swelling's appearance. However, in most cases the effusion returns. It is impossible to apply pressure to the sheath with a bandage because of its location. Also, a firm bandage over the hock often causes a pressure sore along the Achilles tendons.

The prognosis for continued athletic function is excellent, whether or not the swelling is treated.

Curb

Curb is a small, firm swelling at the back of the leg, a couple of inches below the point of the hock (the calcaneus). The swelling is caused by thickening of the plantar tarsal ligament. This ligament runs down the back of the calcaneus and attaches onto the back of the lower tarsal bones and the top of the cannon and splint bones. Its role is to stabilize the base of the calcaneus and counteract the pull of the Achilles tendons.

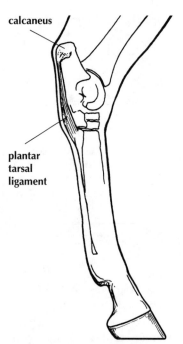

Fig. 20–23. Curb: Thickening of the plantar tarsal ligament.

Inflammation of the plantar tarsal ligament can occur due to trauma, such as kicking at a solid object or being kicked by another horse. However, in horses with poor hock conformation—particularly "sickle hocks"—it is probably due to chronic strain on the ligament. Sudden overflexion of the hock can also strain it, as can sliding stops and cutting cattle.

The horse may be mildly lame (grade 1 – 2 of 5) when the swelling first develops. The lameness usually subsides with rest from regular training, and a few days of anti-inflammatory therapy (cold therapy, NSAIDs, DMSO, etc.; *see Chapter 5*). However, the swelling generally remains. The veterinarian may inject corticosteroids around the ligament. This can improve the cosmetic appearance if it is done when the swelling first occurs. But it is usually ineffective if the curb is more than

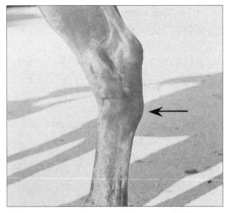

Fig. 20–24. Curbs are often seen in horses with "sickle hocks."

about a week old. Physical therapies, such as laser, therapeutic ultrasound, and magnetic field therapy, may also help if the swelling is acute (recent).

The prognosis for future athletic function is very good. Once the inflammation subsides, most curbs are just blemishes. However, if the curb developed because of poor hock conformation, the horse may be prone to other hock problems, such as bone spavin. In reining and cutting horses, the lameness may persist unless the horse is rested from active training for several weeks.

OTHER CONDITIONS
Extensor Tenosynovitis

Tenosynovitis is inflammation of a tendon sheath. In this case it involves the tendon sheath surrounding the common digital extensor tendon as it runs over the front of the hock, on its way down the leg. Inflammation of the sheath, or the tendon itself, causes fluid

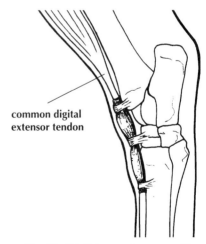

common digital extensor tendon

Fig. 20–25. Extensor tenosynovitis.

accumulation (effusion) within the sheath. This results in a long, narrow, fluidy swelling at the front of the hock and top of the cannon. There are a couple of narrow bands that run across the tendon to keep it in place. These bands can give the swelling a slightly irregular outline.

The tendon sheath probably is strained by a minor accident in which the hock is suddenly extended (straightened). Examples include slipping on a wet surface, or getting a hindleg caught and struggling to break free. But in many cases the owner or trainer is unaware of the incident; the swelling seems to appear spontaneously.

Except for the first few days after injury, the swelling is not hot or painful, and the horse is not lame. So, treatment is only necessary for cosmetic reasons. Treatment follows the same guidelines as those given in Chapter 18 for tenosynovitis at the front of the knee. It involves anti-inflammatory therapy (cold, NSAIDs, DMSO, etc.) and light exercise. The veterinarian may also drain the fluid and inject corticosteroids or hyaluronic acid into the sheath for a better cosmetic result. But keeping an effective bandage on the hock is difficult.

The prognosis for continued athletic function is excellent. However, the swelling often remains.

Cunean Bursitis

Definition
Bursa: a thin sac between a tendon and a bone; it ensures that the tendon glides smoothly over the bone. **A bursa has a fibrous, outer covering and a thin lining called the synovium, which secretes fluid into the sac.**

Bursitis is inflammation of a bursa. In this case it involves the small bursa beneath the cunean tendon. The cunean tendon is a narrow tendon that runs at an angle over the front of the hock and attaches onto the lower row of tarsal bones on the inside of the leg. This tendon and its attached muscle help to flex the hock.

The cunean bursa may be inflamed by pressure or excessive friction from the cunean tendon. Strain and inflammation of the tendon itself can also contribute to the mild lameness. These problems are caused by overextension and/or uneven loading of the hock and its soft tissues. The following factors can place increased tension on the cunean tendon and its bursa:

- poor hock conformation, particularly "cow hocks"
- unbalanced feet
- shoes that alter foot flight or landing, such as one-sided heel extensions *(see Chapter 7)*

Cunean bursitis is almost exclusively seen in Standardbred race-horses, probably because of the stresses their hocks sustain at race speeds and the gait-modifying shoes often used.

Many horses with cunean bursitis also have bone spavin. This could be because the factors that cause cunean bursitis also contribute to the development of bone spavin. It is also possible that the inflammation and bony proliferation around the lower hock

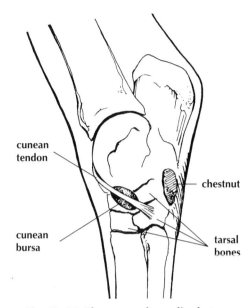

Fig. 20–26. The cunean bursa lies between the cunean tendon and the tarsal bones.

joints which is typical of bone spavin can inflame the cunean bursa, and even the tendon itself.

Signs

On its own, cunean bursitis results in very mild swelling over the cunean bursa, low-grade pain during palpation, and mild lameness (grade 1 – 2 of 5). However, when bone spavin is also present the lameness typically is more obvious (grade 2 – 3 of 5). In these cases bone spavin is the bigger problem for both the horse and the trainer.

Treatment and Prognosis

Cunean bursitis can be treated with rest from regular training, and a few days of anti-inflammatory therapy, including NSAIDs, cold therapy, and DMSO *(see Chapter 5)*. The veterinarian may also inject corticosteroids into the bursa to provide more long-lasting relief. When these measures fail, the cunean tendon can be cut. This procedure is called a cunean tenectomy. It can be done while the horse is standing, under sedation and local anesthetic.

However, bone spavin presents much more of a challenge. Even with the management changes discussed earlier, bone spavin can interrupt the horse's training schedule, and may even end its competitive career. Cunean bursitis is of little importance in these cases.

Stringhalt

The hallmark of stringhalt is exaggerated hock flexion. In most cases the hock is hyperflexed when the horse is walking or turning, but in very severe cases it may also occur while the horse is standing still.

More Information
Stringhalt is a condition of the nervous system. Its causes, diagnosis, and management are covered in Chapter 12.

Although the cause is not fully understood, stringhalt probably has a neurologic basis. That is, the underlying problem is with the nerves that supply the extensor muscles of the hock.

Wounds at the Front of the Hock

Wounds at the front of the hock are common injuries in pastured horses. There is very little tissue between the skin and the joint capsule at the front of the hock, so these wounds can damage the joint capsule and expose the joint to infection. Nevertheless, serious joint infection (septic arthritis; *see Chapter 8*) is quite uncommon with these wounds. More often, the extensor tendon that runs down the front of the hock is damaged. For the most part, horses can walk quite well with a severed extensor tendon *(see Chapter 11)*. So, as long as the wound is properly cared for, this injury eventually heals well, and the horse is able to use the leg normally. The wound may, however, leave an unsightly

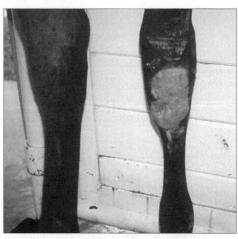

Fig. 20–27. Wounds at the front of the hock usually heal well if managed properly.

scar and some thickening over the front of the hock. *(Wound management is discussed in Chapter 13.)*

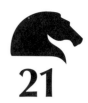

21

THE UPPER HINDLEG

Injuries and other problems involving the upper part of the hindleg are many and varied, but all are relatively uncommon. In this chapter these problems are discussed in order of anatomic location, beginning just above the hock and including the pelvis.

TIBIA

The tibia is the bone that connects the hock and the stifle. It is a large, thick bone that is the sole weight-bearing structure in the gaskin.

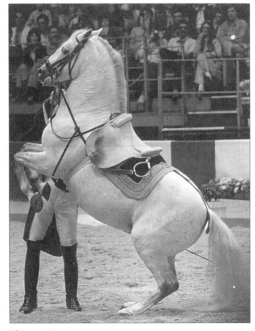

Fig. 21–1.

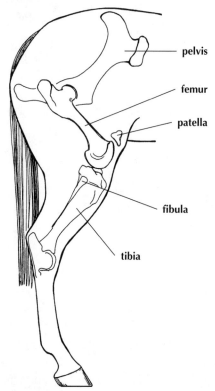

Fig. 21–2. The bones of the upper hindleg.

Definitions

Incomplete fracture: only one side of the bone is cracked.
Complete fracture: the bone is broken into two or more pieces.
Cortex: dense, outer layer of a bone.

(See Chapter 9 for information on bone structure, training and bone quality, and fractures.)

Tibial Fractures

Incomplete and complete tibial fractures can be caused by direct trauma, such as a kick or fall. But the tibia is also prone to incomplete (or "stress") fractures as a result of exercise-induced overloading of the bone.

Incomplete (Stress) Fractures

Definition and Causes

Incomplete tibial fractures usually begin as little more than a short crack in the bone's cortex. Like incomplete cannon bone fractures *(see Chapter 17),* these stress fractures often are the result of overloading during strenuous exercise.

It takes several weeks of training for a bone to increase its density and strength enough to withstand the forces placed on it during strenuous exercise. When young horses are worked "too hard, too soon"—before the bone has had time to adequately increase its strength and resilience—an incomplete fracture can develop. This fracture is most common in young racehorses, especially Thoroughbreds and Quarter Horses.

In older horses, layoffs of more than about 2 months could contribute. This is because bone responds to inactivity by decreasing its density. If a horse is rested for several weeks and then is quickly brought back into full training, the bone may be overloaded.

Most of these fractures occur on the inside of the leg. Because of the tibia's shape and the direction of loading forces on it during weight-bearing, these fractures may extend and spiral up or down the bone if the horse continues in training. Unrestricted pasture activity can also extend the fracture. When this happens, there is a risk that the tibia may fracture completely during activity.

In mature horses this fracture may be caused by a single incident in which unusual twisting forces are placed on the bone. That is, the bone has not necessarily been chronically over-loaded by strenuous exercise. For example, a horse may rear and spin while playing in the pasture or on a hot-walker, and suddenly de-velop an incomplete tibial fracture. However, this is an unusual injury.

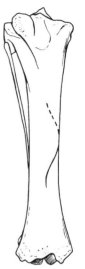

Direct trauma to the tibia may also cause an incomplete fracture. However, a kick or fall that is hard enough to fracture the tibia is more likely to fracture it completely. A less forceful

Fig. 21–3. An in-complete tibial frac-ture. The dotted line indicates the back of the fracture.

kick could cause a "radiating" wound and sequestrum (fragment of dead bone). The causes and management of this injury are similar to those discussed for incomplete radial fractures *(see Chapter 19)*.

Signs

Small stress fractures in the tibia typically cause a mild to moder-ate lameness (grade 2 – 3 of 5) that can be very difficult to locate. In many cases the lameness improves or disappears with only a few days of rest. However, it reappears when the horse is next exercised. Usually, there is no obvious swelling around the fracture site. But with careful palpation it is sometimes possible to detect a specific site of pain on the inside of the leg. Hock flexion may not alter the lameness, although flexing the opposite hindleg may worsen the lameness. This is because the horse must bear more weight on the lame leg for a minute or so while the opposite leg is held up.

If the fracture is more extensive, the lameness is moderate (at least grade 3 of 5) and consistent, and it does not disappear with rest. There may be a little swelling on the inside of the leg, and there is distinct pain during palpation over the tibia. Hock flexion in either leg usually worsens this lameness.

Diagnosis of Incomplete Tibial Fractures

Small stress fractures are a challenge to diagnose. The signs are vague, and physical examination, gait evaluation, and flexion tests may fail to locate the site of lameness. It is not possible to temporarily improve or resolve the lameness with either nerve blocks or joint blocks *(see Chapter 2)*. But these procedures can help rule out other, more likely sites of pain, such as the foot or hock.

Nuclear scintigraphy is the best way to locate the site of lameness in these horses. When the hindlimb is "scanned," a "hot spot" appears in about the middle of the tibia. Radiographs are necessary to confirm the diagnosis. However, the fracture line may not be immediately obvious. Repeat radiographs taken 2 – 3 weeks later may be necessary before a definite diagnosis can be made. But even then, the fracture line may be small and difficult to see because of the ir-

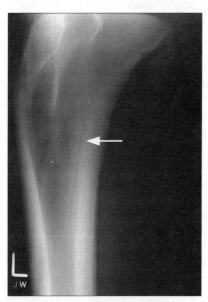

Fig. 21–4. A tibial stress fracture.

regular contour of the bone's surface and the overlying muscles. Sometimes the only abnormality is a small callus on the bone's surface as the fracture heals.

Diagnosing a more extensive incomplete fracture is fairly straightforward. The signs typically indicate pain associated with the tibia, and radiographs usually reveal the thin fracture line. Most of these spiraling tibial fractures begin as a small stress fracture. Because of this potential, the veterinarian may take several different views of the tibia before being satisfied that a small fracture is not more extensive than it seems.

Treatment of Incomplete Tibial Fractures
Conservative Management

Most incomplete tibial fractures are treated conservatively with at least 6 weeks of confinement in a stall or small pen. Horses with small stress fractures can be hand-walked each day during this period, if they are well behaved on the lead. Once repeat radiographs or nuclear scintigraphy show that the fracture has healed, the horse is then rested in a paddock for at least 2 more months before being gradually returned to regular training.

These fractures must be taken very seriously. The tibia can fracture completely if the horse is kept in training or allowed unrestricted activity. Furthermore, there is the potential for the horse to fracture the leg completely when it gets up after lying down. To reduce this risk, the veterinarian may recommend cross-tying the horse for the first few weeks to prevent it from lying down. A complete fracture is most likely in the first 3 weeks. After this time it becomes progressively less of a risk as the incomplete fracture heals. However, many horses do not tolerate cross-tying for this long.

There is no point in putting a cast or thick support bandage on the leg to prevent an incomplete tibial fracture from extending and fracturing completely. In fact, these measures may make a complete fracture more likely by concentrating the levering forces at the top of the cast or bandage—in the upper part of the tibia. (Because of the shape of the horse's leg, the cast or bandage finishes below the stifle.)

Thus, in most cases the owner or trainer must simply accept that there is a small, but real risk that the horse may fracture its tibia completely during the initial confinement period.

The recommendations for returning a horse to training after an incomplete cannon bone fracture also apply to horses with incomplete tibial fractures *(see Chapter 17)*.

Surgery

Sometimes surgery is recommended to stimulate bone healing in small stress fractures. This procedure involves drilling along the fracture line with a surgical drill bit, and filling the drill hole with a bone graft. The bone graft does not provide strength or stability, but it can improve the rate and quality of bone production at the fracture site. Following surgery the horse must be confined in a stall or small pen for at least 4 weeks, and then rested in a small paddock for another 2 – 3 months. The veterinarian may also recommend cross-tying the horse for the first couple of weeks after surgery. This is because the horse is just as likely to completely fracture the leg as a horse that did not have surgery.

When a more extensive incomplete fracture is found, the veterinarian may recommend surgery to prevent a complete fracture. This procedure involves

---

More Information

Surgery, including bone grafts, bone plates, and bone pins, is discussed in Chapter 6.

Post-operative care and rehabilitation are also covered.

stabilizing the bone with two large bone plates. However, there is a risk that the horse may completely fracture its leg when it gets up, despite the metal implants and special care by the surgical staff. This risk, together with the expense of surgery, must be weighed against the possible benefits. The location and extent of the fracture, and individual circumstances must also be factored into this decision. Furthermore, in a horse that is intended for athletic activities, the metal plates must be removed once the fracture has healed. This adds to the expense and the length of time the horse must spend out of training. The many screw holes in the bone are areas of weakness that must fill in before the horse is allowed any exercise more demanding than hand-walking.

Prognosis for Incomplete Tibial Fractures

The prognosis for return to full athletic function is fairly good with small stress fractures, provided they heal completely before the horse returns to training. The prognosis for more extensive fractures is guarded because of the potential for serious complications.

Complete Tibial Fractures

The signs, management, and prognosis for complete tibial fractures depend on the age of the horse and the location of the fracture. In mature horses the tibia usually fractures in the middle of the bone. In foals the tibia may fracture through one of its physes (growth plates).

Fractures in the Middle of the Tibia

Complete fractures in the middle of the tibia are classic longbone fractures. They result in sudden, nonweight-bearing lameness, extensive swelling, severe pain during palpation, and crepitus. Many of these fractures are open, meaning that a piece of bone penetrates the skin. This is because there is very little soft tissue between the skin and the bone on the inside of the leg. Complete fractures usually are caused by direct trauma, although they may be the end result of an incomplete fracture.

The same management problems encountered with complete radial fractures *(see Chapter 19)* also apply to complete

> **Definitions**
>
> **Crepitus**: grinding or crunching sensation heard and/or felt when a fractured bone is palpated or manipulated.
> **Displaced:** the bone fragments are separated.

tibial fractures. These fractures typically have a disappointing outcome in adult horses, so the usual recommendation is euthanasia. The prognosis is a little more favorable in foals and small ponies, although it is still not good. Surgical repair with bone plates or pins may be possible in some of these animals.

Fractures Across a Physis

The tibia has two physes: one at the top of the bone just below the stifle, and one at the bottom just above the hock. Direct trauma can cause a fracture through one of these physes in foals (up to about 12 months old).

Upper Tibial Physis

A fall or a kick to the side of the foal's stifle can fracture the tibia across its upper physis. The result is swelling around the stifle (often worst on the inside of the leg), and severe, nonweight-bearing lameness. Palpating

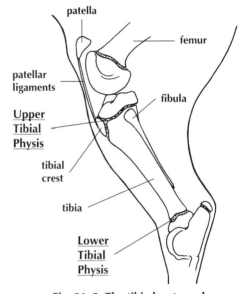

Fig. 21–5. The tibia has two physes.

the stifle or moving the leg causes obvious pain; crepitus may also be heard or felt. Radiographs typically show a fracture straight across the physis or a fracture that starts in the physis on one side of the leg and continues down the tibia for a few inches on the other side.

These fractures should be repaired surgically. Managing them with just stall confinement generally is very disappointing, especially if the fracture is displaced. Displaced fractures in any location do not heal well. Also, bone growth from the damaged physis may be restricted, so angular limb deformities are likely and are very difficult, if not impossible to correct *(see Chapter 14)*. Angular limb deformities can also develop in the opposite, weight-bearing leg because the foal remains very lame for weeks or months. Casting or bandaging the leg is not an option because it is impossible to effectively stabilize a fracture in the top part of the tibia with these methods. In fact, casting or bandaging the leg can make matters worse by concentrating the levering forces at the fracture site.

> **More Information**
>
> Fracture repair and
> post-operative care are
> discussed in Chapter 6.
>
> Long-term use of
> NSAIDs in horses and
> foals with fractures is
> covered in Chapter 9.

Surgical repair involves stabilizing the fracture with a bone plate and bone screws. NSAIDs usually are prescribed for pain relief; however, these drugs must be used with care in foals.

To avoid restricting bone growth in the physis, the bone plate and screws must be removed once the fracture has healed, which usually takes 6 – 8 weeks. During that time, the foal must be kept confined in a stall or small pen. Another 2 – 3 months of confinement in a small paddock is usually recommended before the foal can be turned out onto pasture.

The prognosis for complete fracture healing and normal growth of the tibia is reasonably good, provided surgical repair stabilizes the fracture, and the metal implants are removed once the fracture has healed. The prognosis for future athletic usefulness is also fairly good with proper care.

Tibial Crest "Fracture"

There is a vertical ridge of bone at the front of the tibia, just below the stifle; this is called the tibial crest or tuberosity. It is like the bony ridge just below the knee in people.

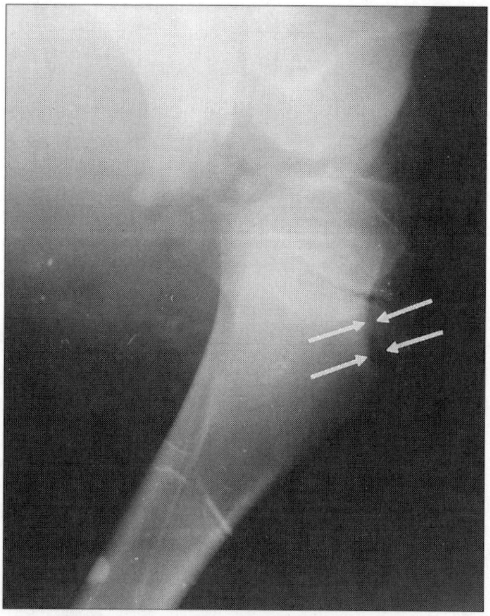

Fig. 21–6. A normal physis can look like a fracture on radiographs.

The physis at the top of the tibia continues down the tibial crest, between the ridge and the rest of the tibia. This physis, which normally looks irregular on radiographs, can be mistaken for a fracture line in foals that have stifle swelling and lameness. Although it is possible for the tibia to fracture along this physis, it is extremely uncommon in horses. If the tibial crest is fractured, the bone is pulled upward by the patellar ligaments that attach to it. So, if there is just a "fracture" line and no displacement of the tibial crest, it probably is not fractured.

If the physis appears to be more irregular than normal in a foal with stifle swelling, pain, and lameness, it is more likely due to inflammation of the physis (physitis; *see Chapter 14*). The lameness usually resolves with 3 – 4 weeks of confinement in a stall or small paddock, and dietary changes.

Lower Tibial Physis

Direct trauma to the hock or the lower part of the foal's gaskin may cause a fracture across the lower tibial physis. The result is sudden, severe lameness and painful swelling around the top of the hock. There may be crepitus if the fracture is displaced. If the lower leg is at an abnormal angle, it can be difficult to tell the difference between a fracture through the lower physis and dislocation of the hock *(see Chapter 20)*.

Radiographs are necessary to confirm the diagnosis and decide on the best treatment method. If the fracture is not displaced, a full-limb cast can be effective. It must be left on (and changed frequently; *see Chapter 6*) for at least 6 weeks. If the fracture is displaced, surgical repair usually is the best option. It gives the foal the best chance of complete fracture repair, normal growth, and future athletic usefulness. Depending on the shape of the fracture, bone screws or a plate may be used to repair it. The surgeon may also place a cast or thick support bandage on the foal's leg to provide extra stability for the first couple of weeks.

The metal implants must be removed once the fracture has healed, to ensure that bone growth from the physis is not restricted. The prognosis for future athletic function is reasonably good, provided the fracture heals well and the bone continues to grow normally.

Peroneus Tertius Rupture

The peroneus tertius is a tendon that starts at the lower end of the femur and attaches onto the front and outside of the hock and the top of the cannon bone. Its functions are to prevent overextension of the hock, and ensure that when the stifle is flexed the hock is also flexed.

The peroneus tertius is protected from direct trauma by the overlying muscles at the front of the gaskin. However, it can be ruptured by sudden, forced overextension of the hock. For example, the peroneus tertius can be damaged when the horse gets a hindfoot caught behind it in a fence or stall partition and struggles violently to get free. A bad fall and slipping on a muddy surface are other incidents that have caused this injury. In many cases, however, it is not known how

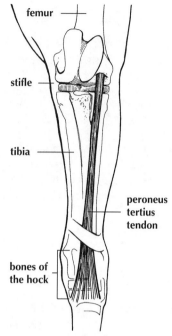

femur

stifle

tibia

peroneus
tertius
tendon

bones of
the hock

Fig. 21–7. The peroneus tertius tendon, viewed from the front of the leg.

the horse damaged the tendon.

The signs of a ruptured peroneus tertius are fairly distinctive. The lameness, which is mild to moderate (grade 2 – 3 of 5), is mostly due to mechanical factors, rather than pain *(see Chapter 1)*. The stifle can now be flexed without also flexing the hock. So, when the horse lifts the leg the hock is flexed very little, and the lower leg dangles as if it is fractured. However, when the foot is placed, the horse can bear full weight on the leg without pain.

When the veterinarian lifts the horse's leg (which flexes the stifle), the hock can be fully extended behind the horse. This is not possible if the peroneus tertius is intact. Extending the hock this way may cause the Achilles tendons to "ripple" because there is no longer any tension on them. There is no obvious swelling at the front of the leg, although palpation along the front of the gaskin may cause a mild pain response.

The tendon usually heals with 6 – 8 weeks of confinement in a stall or small pen. This is followed by 2 – 3 months of gradually increasing, light exercise, beginning with daily hand-walking. The prognosis

Extra Information

The peroneus tertius tendon and the superficial digital flexor muscle–tendon at the back of the gaskin make up the "reciprocal apparatus." These two structures have opposing actions on the stifle and hock. They "tie" these joints together such that the stifle cannot be flexed or extended without also flexing or extending the hock. This is important because, for efficient locomotion, the horse must flex both joints when bringing its hindleg forward.

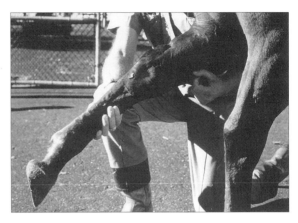

Fig. 21–8. With a ruptured peroneus tertius tendon, the hock can be fully extended while the stifle is flexed.

for full recovery is very good, provided the horse does nothing to aggravate the injury while it is healing.

FIBULA

The fibula is a narrow bone that is attached to the outside of the tibia, just below the stifle. It ends about halfway down the tibia without forming a joint (articulating) with any bone *(see Figure 21–5)*. The fibula is a little like a splint bone, in that it is a small bone that does not bear any weight.

Problems with the fibula are very unusual. They probably only occur along with other, more significant injuries to the tibia or the muscles on the side of the gaskin. Radiographs of the fibula often show a thin, horizontal, dark line about one-third of the way down the bone. This line, which looks like a fracture, is found in many horses that are not lame. It is an area of incomplete bone development and is not significant.

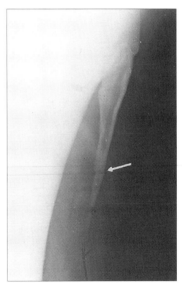

Fig. 21–9. The "fracture" line is just an area of incomplete bone development.

STIFLE
Structure and Function

The stifle is a fairly complex joint. Before discussing the problems that can occur, it is important to understand the location and functions of the structures that make up the stifle.

Bones

The stifle consists of three bones: the tibia, femur, and patella. This joint is similar to the knee in people: the tibia is the shin bone, the femur is the thigh bone, and the patella is the kneecap.

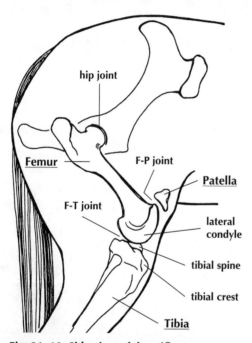

On the upper end of the tibia is a narrow peak of bone called the tibial spine. This structure is important for two reasons. First, it separates the femorotibial joint into two parts: medial and lateral. Second, the tibial spine can be fractured by excessive tension on the cranial cruciate ligament, which attaches to it.

The tibial crest is the bony ridge at the front of the tibia. It is where the patellar ligaments attach.

Fig. 21–10. Side view of the stifle.

The femur is the bone that connects the stifle and the hip joint. At its lower end there are two rounded projections of bone called condyles; there is a large, medial condyle and a slightly smaller lateral condyle. Between the condyles, on the front surface of the bone is a shallow channel called the trochlear groove. The patella slides up and down along this groove.

The patella is a small, pyramid-shaped bone that has cartilage on its underside, the surface that faces the trochlear groove. It also has a hook-shaped extension of fibrous cartilage on its medial (inside) surface. The patella is a sesamoid bone, similar to the sesamoid bones at the back of the fetlock. It is anchored in place by tendons and ligaments, and it helps the stifle maintain its normal, flexed angle.

Joints

The stifle consists of three joints:

- the femoropatellar (F-P) joint, between the femur and the patella at the front of the stifle
- the lateral femorotibial (F-T) joint, between the bottom of the femur and the top of the tibia on the outside of the leg
- the medial femorotibial joint, between the bottom of the femur and the top of the tibia on the inside of the leg

Each of these joints has its own joint capsule. In about two-thirds of horses the F-P joint connects with the medial F-T joint through a small hole. In a few horses the F-P joint and the lateral F-T joint are also connected, but the medial and lateral F-T joints are not normally connected. As confusing as all this seems, the point is that the lateral F-T joint is separate from the other two joints in most horses. Even if the F-P joint connects with one or both of the F-T joints, the hole between the joint spaces is quite small. So, inflammation and effusion (accumulation of fluid) generally is confined to one joint, allowing the veterinarian to focus on that joint as the specific site of the problem.

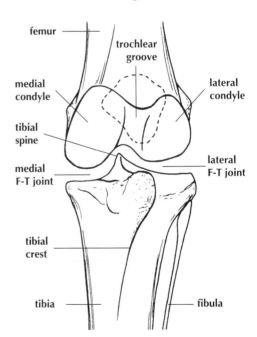

Fig. 21–11. Front view of the bones of the stifle, separated to show the joints. (The patella [dotted outline] has been removed to show the trochlear groove.)

It is also possible to block just one of the stifle joints (intra-articular anesthesia; *see Chapter 2*) and localize the site of the pain very precisely. To block the entire stifle the veterinarian must block all three joints. But most stifle problems occur in either the F-P or the medial F-T joint, so in most cases only one joint is blocked.

The F-P joint is the largest of the three. Effusion in this joint is obvious as a soft, fluidy swelling at the front of the stifle. Effusion in the F-T joints is far less obvious, and may not even be detectable because their joint capsules are much smaller and tighter than the "roomy" F-P joint capsule.

Menisci

A meniscus (plural: menisci) is a thick pad of fibrous cartilage. There are two crescent-shaped menisci in the stifle: one in each F-T joint, on either side of the tibial spine. They act as shock-absorbers and prevent friction between the joint surfaces of the tibia and femur. In people, the meniscus is the structure that is damaged when a person "tears a cartilage" in his or her knee.

Supporting Ligaments

There are three important sets of ligaments that support the stifle: the patellar, cruciate, and collateral ligaments.

Patellar Ligaments

The ligaments that connect the lower edge of the patella to the tibial crest are the medial, middle, and lateral patellar ligaments. On each side of the patella is a short ligament that anchors it to the femur. These are called the femoropatellar ligaments. The other supporting structures are the tendons of the quadriceps muscles. These muscles begin higher up on the femur

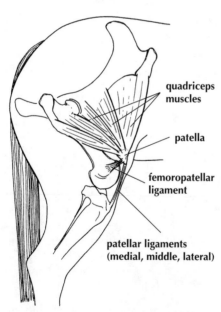

quadriceps muscles

patella

femoropatellar ligament

patellar ligaments (medial, middle, lateral)

Fig. 21–12. The structures that support the patella.

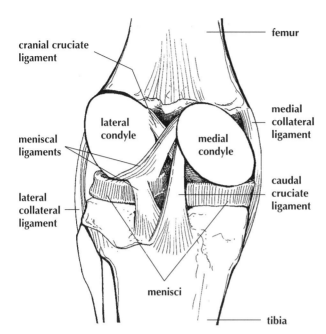

cranial cruciate ligament

femur

lateral condyle

medial condyle

medial collateral ligament

meniscal ligaments

lateral collateral ligament

caudal cruciate ligament

menisci

tibia

Fig. 21–13. The back of the stifle joint.

and pelvis, and they attach onto the top and front of the patella. When they contract they extend (straighten) the stifle.

Cruciate Ligaments

The cruciate ligaments are a pair of short, thick, rounded ligaments that connect the tibia and femur. They cross the F-T space from front to back, in between the two F-T joint capsules. The cranial cruciate begins on the tibial spine, toward the front of the joint, and attaches onto the femur at the back of the joint. The caudal cruciate does the opposite: it begins on the back of the tibia and attaches onto the femur toward the front of the joint. In the process, these ligaments cross over in the middle of the joint; the term, "cruciate" means cross-like. The cruciate ligaments prevent the tibia and femur from rotating in opposite directions and slipping too far forward or back.

Collateral Ligaments

The collateral ligaments are short, wide ligaments that span the femorotibial joints on each side of the leg: medial (inside) and lateral (outside). They prevent the tibia and femur from displacing to either side.

Gonitis

"Gonitis" means inflammation of the stifle. It is not a useful term because it does not distinguish between the many different causes of inflammation and swelling around the stifle. The swelling, which generally is easiest to see from the side, may involve soft tissue or bony structures within or around the joint. Thus, gonitis is a *symptom*, rather than a specific disease.

Osteochondrosis (Including OCD)

Osteochondrosis is a defect of developing bone that is often seen in young horses. The stifle is one of the more commonly affected joints. There are two types of osteochondrosis lesion that typically occur in the stifle: osteochondritis dissecans (OCD) and a bone cyst.

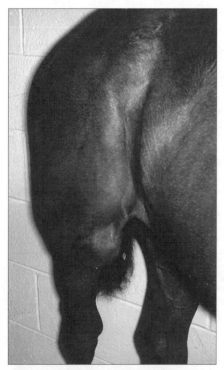

Fig. 21–14. OCD typically results in joint effusion, which causes a soft, fluidy swelling at the front of the stifle.

OCD

OCD is a fragment of bone and cartilage that breaks off the joint surface. In the stifle, these lesions are found in the femoropatellar joint, on the edges of the trochlear groove. Occasionally they also involve the patella. Consequently, most horses with stifle OCD have obvious effusion (accumulation of joint fluid) at the front of the stifle. Mild to moderate lameness (grade 2 – 3 of 5) is common with stifle OCD, although it may not show up until the young horse begins training or the workload is increased.

A femoropatellar joint block (discussed earlier) temporarily resolves the lameness in most cases. But radiographs are necessary to confirm the diagnosis. In most cases the OCD fragments are obvious.

Sometimes the only sign on radiographs is a flattened or irregular bone surface. When the joint is examined arthroscopically, it is not unusual to find cartilage fragments or erosions. These cartilage lesions are very common with osteochondrosis, but they cannot be seen on radiographs.

Osteochondrosis frequently is bilateral. So, most veterinarians radiograph both stifles, even though the signs may be obvious in only one leg.

> ## More Information
>
> Osteochondrosis, including possible causes, management, and prevention, is detailed in Chapter 14.

Treatment and Prognosis

These bone and cartilage fragments are often best removed using arthroscopy. Persistent effusion, lameness, and degenerative joint disease are likely if the fragments are left in the joint. The technique and post-operative care are discussed in Chapter 6. In most cases the surgeon recommends 1 – 4 weeks of stall rest after surgery, followed by 3 – 4 months of paddock or pasture rest. Joint medications *(see Chapter 5)* may also be recommended either immediately after surgery or when the horse resumes training.

The prognosis for athletic function is usually quite good once the fragments are removed. If the condition is managed with just rest and medication, the prognosis for athletic usefulness generally is not as good.

Bone Cysts

Bone cysts are cavities in the bone just beneath the joint cartilage. Most of these cysts have a small hole in the overlying cartilage that connects the cavity with the joint.

The most common location for a stifle bone cyst is on the bottom of the femur in the medial F-T joint. Joint effusion is difficult to detect in this joint, so the signs of a stifle bone cyst are nonspecific, merely consisting of moderate hindlimb lameness (grade 2 – 3 of 5).

Although blocking the medial F-T joint may temporarily improve the lameness, the diagnosis can only be made with radiographs. The view most likely to show the cyst is taken from back to front (a caudo-cranial view; *see Chapter 2*). The x-ray plate is held at the front of the stifle and the x-ray machine is positioned behind the horse. This view highlights the bottom of the femur, where a small, dark circle can be seen at the lower edge of the medial condyle. This lesion cannot be seen on the lateral (side) view of the stifle.

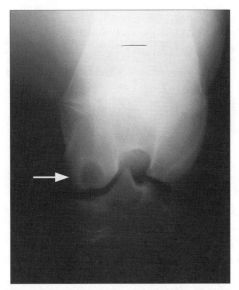

Fig. 21–15. Stifle bone cyst: a dark circle at the lower edge of the medial condyle.

Because of the size of the bones and the depth of muscle behind the stifle, a powerful x-ray machine is needed to get good quality caudo-cranial views of the stifle. The horse may need to be transported to a veterinary hospital to have these radiographs taken. Bone cysts often are bilateral, so most veterinarians routinely radiograph both stifles.

Treatment and Prognosis for Bone Cysts

In most horses surgery has a much better success rate than conservative management—rest and medication. One approach is to ream out the cyst with a surgical burr, then drill small holes in the bone around the cyst. This procedure is done with arthroscopy. Another approach is to drill through to the cyst from the side of the bone and fill the cavity with a bone graft. Some surgeons prefer this procedure because cleaning out the cyst and drilling into the surrounding bone from inside the joint sometimes causes the cyst to enlarge.

After surgery the usual recommendation is 2 – 4 weeks of stall rest, followed by 4 – 6 months of paddock or pasture rest. It takes several months for the cyst to fill in with bone and the cartilage defect at the joint surface to heal. Although some horses show obvious improvement well before the cyst has disappeared, it is usually not worth putting the horse back into work until these processes are completed. Repeat radiographs should be taken before the horse is returned to training.

The prognosis for a successful athletic career is fairly good with surgery. It is guarded at best with just conservative management.

Patella Problems

The patella is a small bone that is well protected behind the belly, so it is not often damaged. Most conditions involving the patella are due to developmental problems or poor conformation.

Upward Fixation (Locking) of the Patella
Definition and Causes

Upward fixation, or "locking" of the patella is a condition in which the horse's stifle is temporarily fixed in an extended (straightened) position. The quadriceps muscles *(see Figure 21–12)* extend the stifle when they pull up on the patella, and thus the tibia, via the patellar ligaments. This action causes the patella to slide up the trochlear groove in the end of the femur. When the patella slides up too far, its hook-shaped medial cartilage and the medial patellar ligament can be caught on the large medial condyle of the femur. As a result, the stifle is locked in that position and the horse cannot flex its stifle. When the stifle locks repeatedly, the medial patellar ligament may be stretched. This makes it even more likely that the patella will slide up and catch on the femur. Sometimes the middle patellar ligament is also stretched.

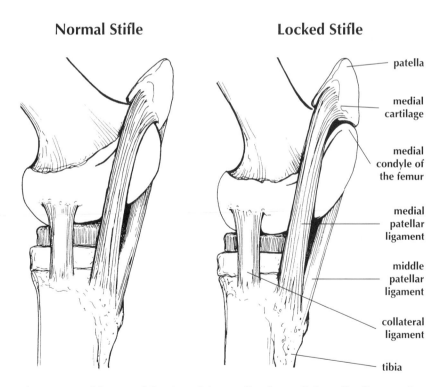

Normal Stifle   **Locked Stifle**

- patella
- medial cartilage
- medial condyle of the femur
- medial patellar ligament
- middle patellar ligament
- collateral ligament
- tibia

Fig. 21–16. With upward fixation of the patella, the medial patellar ligament is caught on the large medial condyle of the femur.

Contributing Factors

Upward fixation of the patella is seen in horses and ponies that have very upright, or straight hindlegs. In these animals the stifle is a little less angled than normal, so it is easier for the patella to slide up and catch on the femur. It has been suggested that this problem is hereditary. But it is probably only hereditary to the extent that conformation is dictated by genetics. That is, a straight-stifled horse is likely to produce straight-stifled offspring.

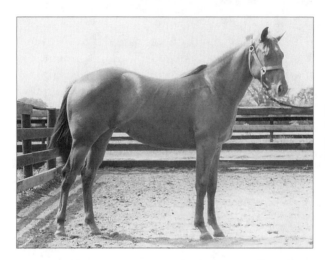

Fig. 21–17. Overly straight hindlegs predisposes to locking patellas.

Upward fixation is also seen in horses that are in poor body condition or have poor muscle tone. The quadriceps muscles put constant tension on the patellar ligaments while the horse is standing and moving. When the horse is malnourished or is not exercised regularly the quadriceps muscles lose tone and bulk, and become a little slack. As a result, the tension on the patellar ligaments is reduced, and they too may slacken a little. Loss of tone in the quadriceps muscles may also allow the patella a little extra mobility. This, and the slackened patellar ligaments make it more likely for the medial ligament to catch on the femur. With proper nutrition and regular exercise, the quadriceps muscles increase in tone and strength. Tension on the patellar ligaments increases, making it less likely that the patella will lock.

However, that does not explain why upward fixation is sometimes seen in very fit horses that, because of injury or another problem, are confined to a stall and not exercised at all. Within a week of confinement the horse's stifles may begin to lock. Why this occurs when the quadriceps muscles are obviously very well toned is poorly understood. Perhaps training increases quadriceps tone and strength so much that the muscles alter the stifle angle, keeping it slightly more extended than normal. This would make upward fixation more likely.

Another explanation involves insufficient blood flow to the quadriceps muscles. With training, the capillary (small blood vessel) network within these large muscles increases, as do the muscle cells' requirements for oxygen and nutrients. When the horse is just standing in a stall and not receiving any exercise, the blood supply to these muscles may be insufficient. As a result they may spasm and pull up on the patella. *(Muscle structure and function are discussed in Chapter 10.)*

These speculations on the role of the quadriceps muscles in upward fixation of the patella illustrate one important point: this condition has several possible causes and contributing factors, both structural and functional.

Signs and Diagnosis of Upward Fixation of the Patella

In severe cases of upward fixation, the horse's leg is extended behind it, and the horse cannot flex the leg and bring it back into the

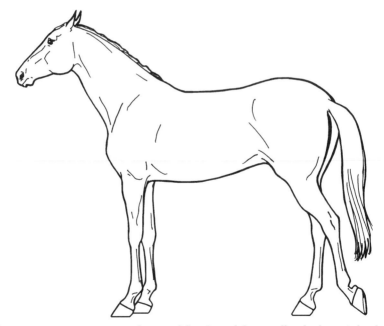

Fig. 21–18. In severe cases of upward fixation of the patella, the horse's leg is extended behind it, and the horse cannot bring it back into the normal position.

normal position. The horse may be stuck in that position for several hours and may need someone to manually release the patella. This can be done by pulling the patella over with the fingers, or by rotating the leg out and forward. In most cases, however, the horse can unlock the stifle without help.

More commonly, the fixation is intermittent; that is, the patella catches for only part of the stride, and not necessarily at every step. This gait is more pronounced when the horse walks slowly down a slope. Each time the patella is released, the stifle tends to collapse a little. When watching these horses from the side, their hindlegs buckle slightly at each step.

Although the problem may be seen in only one hindleg, it can often be produced in both because both stifles are structurally the same. Backing the horse or turning it in a tight circle can cause the stifle to lock in horses that are prone to upward fixation. To turn in a tight circle, the horse must pivot on the inside hindleg, which is only possible when the hock and stifle are fixed in a relatively extended position. This position makes it easier for the patella to catch on the femur. Pushing the patella up and over with the heel of the hand can also lock the stifle.

The diagnosis usually is clear from the signs, and the ease with which the stifles can be locked by backing or circling the horse, or manually. In some horses that repeatedly lock, there may also be effusion (excess joint fluid) in the femoropatellar joint. This indicates that the joint capsule lining is inflamed and/or the cartilage surface of the patella or femur is damaged. When effusion is present, the veterinarian may radiograph the stifles to check for other causes, such as OCD and bony problems with the patella (discussed later).

Treatment of Upward Fixation of the Patella

Veterinarians manage upward fixation of the patella either conservatively or surgically. Conservative management should always be tried first because surgery can have serious consequences.

Conservative Management

In many horses the problem can be resolved by improving their muscle tone with regular exercise. It is important to consider the possible cause of the condition and tailor the exercise program to suit the horse. An unfit or poorly-toned horse would benefit from a program of gradually increasing, daily exercise on a level, even surface. Tight circles, steep hills, and deep sand should be avoided until the horse's muscle tone and fitness improve. In a very fit horse that must be confined, daily hand-walking for at least 20 minutes twice per day may be all that is required, provided its primary injury allows.

Evaluating the horse's diet and modifying it as necessary also helps. A horse in poor body condition should be fed a balanced ration that supplies its energy and protein needs. A fit racehorse may benefit from having the energy and protein content of its ration reduced, particularly when training is suspended for any reason.

Some veterinarians and farriers have found that using wedges on the hindfeet to raise the horse's heels can reduce the incidence of upward fixation. The wedges make breakover easier, so the horse does not need to extend the leg as far to take a step. *(Breakover and shoeing options are discussed in Chapter 7.)*

When all of these measures prove unsuccessful after several weeks, some veterinarians inject an irritant substance around the medial and middle patellar ligaments. The irritant causes inflammation and fibrosis (production of fibrous, or scar tissue). This tightens the ligaments, preventing the medial ligament from catching on the medial condyle. This procedure is successful in some horses. However, it may not result in a permanent cure. Extreme care must be taken not to inject the irritant into the stifle joints; the inflammation and cartilage damage that results can be severe. For this reason, the procedure must only be performed by an experienced equine veterinarian.

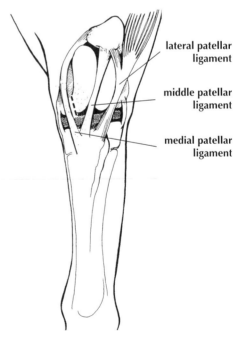

lateral patellar ligament

middle patellar ligament

medial patellar ligament

Surgery

In horses and ponies that repeatedly lock for hours at a time and must be manually released, surgery may be tried sooner rather than later. Sometimes regular exercise makes these episodes far less common. However, locking this severely can dam-

Fig. 21–19. The front of the stifle: the dotted line indicates the site of the skin incision for medial patellar desmotomy.

age the patella, and possibly even the cartilage on the femur. It can also stretch the patellar ligaments. Therefore, surgery may prevent more serious stifle problems in these animals.

Surgery involves cutting the medial patellar ligament; this procedure is called a medial patellar desmotomy. It is best done while the horse is standing (with sedation and local anesthetic) because weight on the leg puts tension on the patellar ligaments and makes them easier to feel. It is difficult to identify these ligaments when there is no tension on them, and it is very important that only the medial patellar ligament is cut. Severing the middle patellar ligament instead can result in instability of the stifle and degenerative joint disease.

The surgery is performed through a small skin incision, less than an inch (2.5 cm) long. The skin is then closed with one or two sutures. Most veterinarians prescribe a few days of antibiotics and NSAIDs following surgery. The horse's tetanus status should be reviewed before surgery *(see Chapter 5)*. Strenuous exercise should be restricted for about 4 weeks afterward. However, daily light exercise, such as hand-walking, during this time is beneficial. Because both hindlegs usually have the potential to lock, the veterinarian may recommend cutting the medial patellar ligament in both legs. The procedures can be done at the same time or a few weeks apart.

Potential Complications of Patellar Desmotomy. *This procedure can cause serious problems that are far more difficult to manage than upward fixation.* In a few horses and ponies in which upward fixation is the result of poor conformation, cutting the medial patellar ligament can allow the patella to dislocate (luxate) to the side of the stifle. Presumably, these animals have an abnormally shallow trochlear groove.

In all horses and ponies, cutting the medial patellar ligament alters the stability of the patella and concentrates the tension on the two remaining ligaments, instead of three. As a result some animals develop bone and cartilage abnormalities along the bottom of the patella weeks or months after patellar desmotomy. The bony changes can be seen on radiographs as irregular areas of new bone production (exostoses) and loss of bone density (lysis). In some cases small fractures may also be present. *(See Chapter 9 for more information on these bone problems.)*

Degenerative joint disease and chronic lameness commonly develop due to these changes. Sometimes it is possible to remove the bone fragments without damaging the remaining patellar ligaments or joint capsule. However, the problem of abnormal stresses on the patella remains, and more changes may develop over time. So, the decision to have this surgery performed should not be made without giving serious consideration to these potential problems.

Prognosis for Upward Fixation of the Patella

The prognosis for athletic function is very good in horses that respond just to regular exercise and dietary changes. (However, the problem may return if regular exercise ceases.) Persistent joint problems are very uncommon in these animals. The same cannot be said for horses that have had a patellar desmotomy.

Patellar Luxation

Luxation, or dislocation of the patella out of its groove at the lower end of the femur is rare in horses. Most reported cases have been in ponies and Miniature horses. In these animals it is usually caused by a congenital deformity of the patella or femur, and is first noticed soon after birth. If the deformity is present in both legs, the foal may be unable to get up or stand unassisted because it cannot fix its stifles in the standing position. If it is able to support itself, the foal stands with its hindquarters crouched.

When patellar luxation occurs in adult horses or ponies it is usually a consequence of either stifle trauma or patellar desmotomy (discussed in the previous section). When patellar luxation occurs due to trauma, it generally affects only one stifle. But as with young foals, the horse cannot bear weight on the leg because it cannot fix its stifle.

The medial (inside) condyle of the femur is larger than the lateral (outside) condyle, so it is more common for the patella to dislocate to the outside of the stifle. This condition can be diagnosed with palpation: the patella is out of place on one side of the stifle, or it can easily be slipped in and out of its groove. Radiographs are important because bone deformities or fractures can affect the choice of treatment and the outcome.

Treatment and Prognosis

Sometimes surgery to relocate the patella and tighten the femoro-patellar ligaments *(see Figure 21–12)* can prevent it from re-luxating. However, if radiographs show that the patella or femur is deformed, it may not be worth performing the surgery because, even after surgery, the foal may not be able to move normally. Euthanasia is usually recommended in these cases.

In all cases the prognosis is guarded. Patellar luxation due to trauma seldom occurs without other more serious problems, such as tearing of some of the patella's supporting ligaments or fracture of the patella. These problems often result in chronic lameness. This is also the case with luxation following patellar desmotomy.

The congenital condition may be hereditary, so even if the problem is corrected with surgery and the foal develops normally, it probably should not be bred as an adult.

Patellar Fractures

Fractures of the patella are uncommon but potentially serious injuries. They usually occur as a result of direct trauma to the front of the stifle. Examples include a kick, and hitting the stifles on a solid jump rail.

Signs and Diagnosis

Typical signs of a patellar fracture include moderate to severe lameness (grade 3 – 5 of 5), and painful swelling at the front of the stifle. Crepitus (crunching of bone-on-bone) may sometimes be heard or felt, although it is not common. A horse with a fractured patella tends to stand with the stifle (and therefore, the leg) flexed. If the patella is completely fractured across its center, the quadriceps muscles may pull the upper fragment away. As a result the horse cannot bear weight on the leg because it cannot fix its stifle in the standing position. With other types of patellar fracture, the horse can bear weight on the leg, although this can be very painful because it requires tension on the patella.

The swelling surrounding the stifle makes it difficult to palpate the patella, so radiographs usually are necessary to make the diagnosis. There are several possible fracture types. There may be a small fragment of bone off one edge, an incomplete crack, or a complete fracture through the front or center of the bone.

Treatment and Prognosis

If the fracture is not displaced (separated) the veterinarian usually recommends conservative management. Small fragments may be removed surgically, using arthroscopy *(see Chapter 6)* for fragments within the femoropatellar joint, and dissection for fragments outside the joint. Arthroscopy also allows the surgeon to examine the cartilage surfaces of the patella and femoral condyles for damage. This information is important in forming a long-term management plan, and making an accurate prognosis.

Following surgery, or with patellar fractures that are managed conservatively, the horse should be confined to a stall or small pen for at least 6 weeks. When repeat radiographs show that the fracture has healed well, the horse should be rested for at least another 3 months in a small paddock.

Note
Long-term NSAID use can have serious side effects. *See Chapter 9.*

There is constant tension on the patella, so patellar fractures heal slowly, often with just a fibrous union. Because the back of the patella forms the front of the femoropatellar joint, fractures that involve the joint surface can result in degenerative joint disease. This is a major limiting factor in the horse's return to full athletic function. Therefore, the prognosis for future athletic usefulness is guarded with fractures that involve the joint.

Cruciate Ligament Injuries

Definition and Causes

The cruciate ligaments help stabilize the stifle. They prevent the tibia and femur from rotating in opposite directions and slipping too far forward or back *(see Figure 21–13)*. The horse's cruciate ligaments can be strained or torn by sudden, forced rotation ("wrenching") of the joint. So, this injury is more likely in horses that must turn sharply on their hindquarters, particularly if the horse has hind shoes with traction devices. Heel caulks, toe grabs, etc. fix the foot and lower leg in place while the upper leg turns with the body. *(See Chapter 7 for more information.)*

Cruciate ligament injuries are relatively common in people

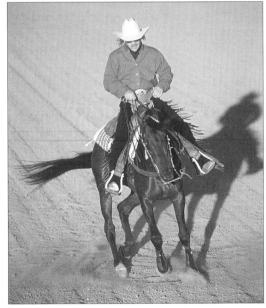

Fig. 21–20. Turning sharply on the hindquarters may injure a cruciate ligament.

and dogs, but they are not often diagnosed in horses. The condition is very difficult to confirm in horses, so its actual incidence is unknown. Strain of one or both of the cruciate ligaments may be more likely in some types of horses, although rupture of a ligament is probably very unusual in any horse.

Signs of Cruciate Ligament Injuries

When one or both of the cruciate ligaments is torn, the result is sudden, moderate to severe lameness (grade 3 – 4 of 5). The force required to tear these strong ligaments may also damage the collateral ligaments, which results in further joint instability and pain. The cranial cruciate ligament is attached to the tibial spine. When the ligament is strained or torn, the tension may be sufficient to also fracture the tibial spine. Furthermore, joint instability can result in damage to the menisci. So, there can be extensive damage within and between the femorotibial joints.

However, there may be no outward signs of this damage. Effusion (accumulation of fluid) in the femorotibial joints is not easy to detect. Unless the cruciates were damaged by a direct blow—which is very unlikely—there usually is no swelling around the stifle.

Diagnosis of Cruciate Ligament Injuries

The diagnosis is very difficult to make unless both ligaments are badly damaged. With a person or dog it is fairly easy to detect instability in this joint because there is an increased range of forward and backward movement of the top of the tibia. This test is very difficult to interpret in an adult horse, particularly while the horse is standing. The size of the bones and the strength of the thigh muscles make it difficult to detect stifle instability. To do this the veterinarian stands beside the horse and grasps the horse's tail for support. He or she then uses the heel of the other hand to push back on the front of the tibia, just below the stifle. Any pain, abnormal movement, or crepitus (crunching or grinding) as the pressure is applied means that one or both of the cruciate ligaments has been torn. If the horse is well behaved, the veterinarian may instead stand behind the horse, wrap his or her arms around the horse's thigh, and pull back on the tibia.

Sometimes the diagnosis is made with ultrasound. Radiographs are often unrewarding in an acute injury. However, they are worth taking in case there is a fracture of the tibial spine or changes in the width of the joint space. When a collateral ligament is stretched or torn, the joint space on the affected side may appear wider than normal. If the injury is chronic, there may also be bony changes around the joint, indicating osteoarthritis *(see Chapter 8)*.

Treatment and Prognosis for Cruciate Ligament Injuries

There is no specific treatment for cruciate ligament injuries in horses. Part of the cruciate ligaments can be seen with arthroscopy, but surgical repair is not possible. The only recommendation is stall rest for at least 6 weeks, followed by paddock rest for 4 – 6 months. Unfortunately, this approach is not often successful in allowing the horse to return to its former athletic activities, unless the ligaments were only strained.

Meniscus Injuries

The menisci are fairly well protected within the femorotibial joints *(see Figure 21–13)*. However, their supporting ligaments may be strained or torn when the cruciate ligaments are damaged. The menisci themselves can also be damaged when a cruciate or collateral ligament injury causes joint instability. Presumably, a meniscus could also become flattened and eroded if there is degenerative joint disease in one of the femorotibial joints.

The signs of meniscus injury are vague. Furthermore, they are likely to be masked by other more serious problems, such as cruciate or collateral ligament tears. Radiographs that show narrowing of the joint space may imply that a meniscus has been damaged. However, the only way to definitely diagnose this problem is with arthroscopy, which allows the surgeon to see the menisci. But unfortunately, there is little the surgeon can do to repair the damage. Removing the damaged meniscus is unlikely to improve the situation because meniscus injuries in horses typically are secondary to other more serious problems. Therefore, the prognosis for return to athletic function is poor.

Calcinosis Circumscripta

Calcinosis circumscripta is a small, hard mass that is occasionally found on the outside of the stifle in young horses, usually between 6 and 12 months old. The mass is calcified soft tissue that is firmly attached to the fascia (fibrous connective tissue) of the thigh muscles. The skin over the mass is usually not attached to it and can be freely moved. The cause of calcinosis circumscripta is not known, although some scientists speculate that it is an abnormal response to soft tissue trauma.

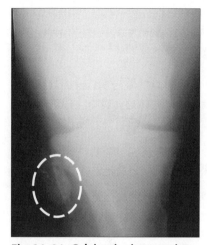

Fig. 21–21. Calcinosis circumscripta causes a small mass of calcified tissue on the side of the stifle.

The mass is not painful to touch and seldom causes lameness. In many cases it reduces in size or disappears after several months, so most veterinarians recommend surgical removal only for cosmetic reasons. Because the mass is firmly attached to the tissues surrounding the stifle, it can be difficult to remove without damaging the fascia and the underlying muscles and ligaments. Unless it is causing a problem for the horse, or the owner feels it is too unsightly, it is usually best to leave the mass alone.

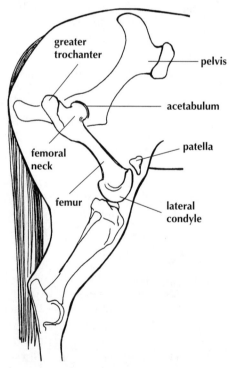

Fig. 21–22. The femur and pelvis.

FEMUR

The femur is a large bone that connects the stifle and the hip joint. It is well covered with muscle, so most of it cannot be directly palpated.

The lower end of the femur is discussed in the earlier section on the stifle. The top of the femur and the pelvis articulate to form the hip joint. It is a "ball and socket" joint, formed by the rounded head of the femur and the cup-shaped socket, called the acetabulum, on the lower side of the pelvis. Between the main part of the femur and the femoral head the bone narrows and bends toward the pelvis at a slight angle. This part of the femur is called the femoral neck. On the outside of the femur, at the same level as the neck, is a large knob of bone called the greater trochanter. The gluteal muscles attach onto the trochanter and extend the hip joint when they contract. These are the large muscles at the top of the rump.

The hip joint is located several inches behind, and a couple of inches lower than the point of the hip. Muscle overlies the hip joint, so it is not as prominent as the point of the hip. Nevertheless, in most horses the greater trochanter can easily be felt beneath the muscle. So, the trochanter is the landmark that indicates the approximate location of the hip joint.

Femoral Fractures

Femoral fractures can be devastating injuries in which the femur is shattered into several pieces. Incomplete fractures, in which the femur is just cracked, can also develop, although far less often. In most cases the fracture is the result of direct trauma to the side of the rump: for example, a fall or a trailer accident. Foals may sustain a femoral fracture when kicked by a mare or another adult horse. Fortunately, femoral fractures are uncommon in all age groups of horses.

Midshaft Femoral Fractures

The femur may be fractured anywhere along its length, although fractures are most common in the middle, or shaft, of the femur. These fractures usually have a very disappointing outcome. In most cases the force required to fracture a horse's femur shatters the bone. The large muscles that surround and attach onto the femur pull on the fracture pieces and cause them to displace and over-ride (overlap). It is very difficult for a fractured bone to heal when it has over-ridden. Even if the fracture is surgically repaired, tension from these muscles often results in repair failure.

Signs

Midshaft femoral fractures are classic longbone fractures *(see Chapter 9)*. The lameness that results is sudden and severe (grade 5 of 5). The horse cannot bear weight on the leg, and if the fracture has over-ridden, the leg appears shorter than the other. The point of the hock on the fractured leg is higher than that of the other leg. Swelling around the fracture is severe, but because of the muscle mass surrounding the femur, it may not seem very pronounced at first. However, by

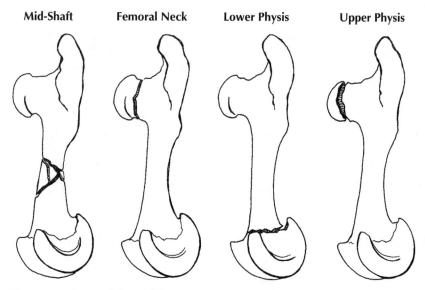

Mid-Shaft **Femoral Neck** **Lower Physis** **Upper Physis**

Fig. 21–23. Types of femoral fractures.

comparing both sides of the horse it usually becomes obvious.

Palpating the side of the thigh, between the stifle and the hip joint causes obvious pain, as does moving the leg. Crepitus (crunching of bone-on-bone) may also be heard or felt when the leg is moved. However, tension from the attached muscles and over-riding of the fracture pieces may restrict movement of the bone fragments and prevent crepitus.

A serious problem that sometimes occurs with midshaft femoral fractures is damage to the femoral artery. This artery runs along the femur, down the inside of the thigh. A sharp piece of bone may sever the artery and cause serious, sometimes fatal hemorrhage. Bleeding is not obvious unless the piece of bone also penetrated the skin. But hemorrhage should be suspected if the inside of the thigh swells dramatically and the horse shows signs of shock.

> **Note**
>
> **SIGNS OF SHOCK**
> - pale gums
> - high heart rate
> - cold extremities
> - weakness
> - collapse

Diagnosis of Midshaft Femoral Fractures

Diagnosing a midshaft femoral fracture usually is straightforward, based on the signs. However, if surgery is to be attempted, radiographs are necessary to determine the exact site and extent of the fracture. Sometimes it is possible to take radiographs of the lower half of the femur while the horse or foal is standing. However, in many cases it is necessary to anesthetize the animal to obtain good quality radiographs. But the problem with this approach is that the horse or foal must then get up after anesthesia on its fractured leg, unless it is taken straight to surgery or euthanized while under anesthesia.

Treatment and Prognosis for Midshaft Femoral Fractures

In young foals and small ponies it may be possible to repair some simple midshaft femoral fractures with bone plates or pins *(see Chapter 6)*. However, angular limb deformities often develop in foals when pain causes them to bear more weight on one leg *(see Chapter 14)*. So even with surgical repair of the femoral fracture, growth abnormalities may cause a problem in the opposite, weight-bearing leg. Surgical repair generally is impossible or unsuccessful in larger foals and adult horses because of their size and weight. *(See the discussions on radial and humeral fractures in Chapter 19.)*

The prognosis for successful fracture healing, normal growth, and future athletic usefulness with a midshaft femoral fracture in a foal is guarded. In adult horses the prognosis is grave, and for humane reasons euthanasia generally is recommended.

Fractures Across a Physis

The femur has two physes, or growth plates. One is at the bottom, just above the stifle; the other is at the top, just behind the head of the femur. Depending on the location and direction of the force, the femur may be fractured through one of these physes in foals less than about 12 months old.

Lower Physis

A direct blow to the side of the stifle may fracture the femur across the lower physis. This injury causes sudden, severe lameness (grade 5 of 5), and pain and swelling around the stifle. Because some problems involving the stifle cause similar signs, radiographs usually are necessary to confirm the diagnosis. For a satisfactory outcome—both in terms of fracture healing and future athletic function—these fractures must be repaired surgically. Treating the fracture with just stall rest generally is unsuccessful. These fractures are managed similar to physeal fractures in the tibia (discussed earlier), except that a cast or bandage cannot be used to support a physeal fracture in the femur.

Upper Physis and Neck

Fractures at the top of the femur in foals usually occur across the physis, although they may involve the femoral neck. With either of these fractures, the foal may still be able to put some weight on the leg, but the lameness is quite severe (grade 4 – 5 of 5). The large gluteal muscles that attach onto the trochanter of the femur help stabilize the fractured bone and so allow the foal to bear some weight on the leg. However, they also tend to pull the top of the femur up and forward, which shortens and rotates the entire leg. Because of the tension in these large muscles, crepitus (crunching of bone-on-bone) usually is not heard or felt with these fractures.

Based on the signs, it is impossible to tell the difference between a fracture through the upper physis or femoral neck and dislocation of the hip. Radiographs should be taken to differentiate between these conditions and determine exactly where the fracture is located. It is usually necessary for the veterinarian to anesthetize the foal to take these radiographs.

Surgical repair with bone pins or screws is needed if the foal is to have any chance of normal development and future athletic function. However, even with surgical repair, the prognosis is guarded to poor. Also, angular limb deformities are common in the opposite, weight-bearing leg *(see Chapter 14)*.

Dislocation of the Hip

Definition and Causes

The rounded head of the femur is held in the cup-shaped acetabulum by a tight, fibrous joint capsule, and a short, strong ligament called the round ligament. This ligament runs from the top of the "ball" to the center of the "socket." These two structures, together with the muscles that surround the hip joint, normally prevent dislocation (luxation) of the hip.

Luxation or subluxation (partial dislocation) of the hip is very uncommon in horses. In mature horses it takes extreme and unusual force, such as slipping and splaying the hind legs, to dislocate the hip. Even then, it is more likely for the femur to fracture than for the hip to luxate. Hip luxation is a little more common in young foals because they have less muscle mass to support the hip joint. Still, it is a very unusual injury. There have been cases in which the mare accidentally stepped on the foal while it was lying down, and dislocated the foal's hip by standing on the inside of its thigh. But again, a femoral fracture is more likely than hip luxation.

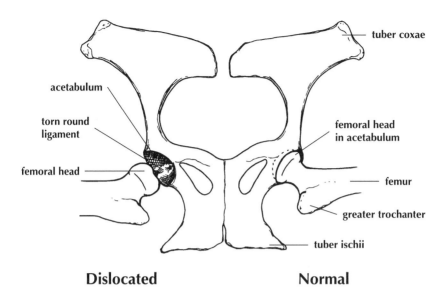

tuber coxae

acetabulum

torn round
ligament

femoral head
in acetabulum

femoral head

femur

greater trochanter

tuber ischii

Dislocated   **Normal**

Fig. 21–24. View of the pelvis from underneath (the horse is lying on its back
with its legs splayed).

Signs and Diagnosis

The signs of hip luxation include sudden, severe lameness (grade
4 – 5 of 5), and swelling over the affected hip joint. In most cases the
femur dislocates upward and forward because of the pull of the large
gluteal muscles that attach to the greater trochanter. Thus, the leg
appears shorter than the other, and the trochanter can be felt or seen
higher up and slightly further forward than normal. This is easiest to
detect by comparing the height of the trochanters when standing
behind the horse. Also, with a hand placed over the trochanter, it is
sometimes possible to feel a clunking or grinding sensation when the
leg is manipulated. However, this may be prevented by tension or
spasm in the surrounding muscles.

These signs are similar to those seen with a fracture through the
upper physis or neck of the femur, so radiographs are necessary to
confirm the diagnosis. To obtain good quality radiographs of the hip
joints, it is usually necessary to anesthetize the animal and lie it on
its back with its legs splayed. In some cases it may be possible to take
the radiographs while the foal is standing. But even with a powerful
x-ray machine, this technique usually is unsatisfactory in adult
horses.

Treatment and Prognosis for Hip Dislocation

Hip luxation is a serious condition. In adult horses tension in the muscle mass that supports the hip joint can make it nearly impossible to relocate the head of the femur into the acetabulum, even under general anesthesia. This is particularly true if the dislocation occurred more than a few hours ago. Furthermore, when the hip luxates, the round ligament and/or the joint capsule are stretched or torn. This makes it easy for the hip to luxate again.

Surgery to stabilize the hip joint may be attempted in young foals, although it is very difficult to prevent reluxation. Even if the surgery is successful, the unstable joint is prone to degenerative joint disease, which can cause chronic lameness. So, in all ages and sizes, dislocation of the hip carries a very poor prognosis for athletic function. A "pasture-sound" horse is generally the best that can be achieved. In many cases euthanasia is recommended for humane reasons.

Trochanteric Bursitis
Definition and Causes

The greater trochanter is the large, bony knob on the outside of the femur, just behind the hip joint. The gluteal muscles at the top of the rump attach onto the trochanter and extend the hip joint when they contract. Between the trochanter and the short tendons of the gluteal muscles lies a bursa (a fluid-filled sac). Its role is to protect the bone and tendons from excessive pressure and friction.

Trochanteric bursitis is inflammation of this bursa. It is an uncommon condition that is most often seen in Standardbred racehorses. Their

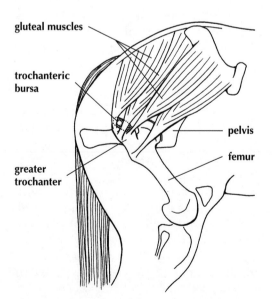

Fig. 21–25. Location of the trochanteric bursa.

gluteal muscles

trochanteric bursa

greater trochanter

pelvis

femur

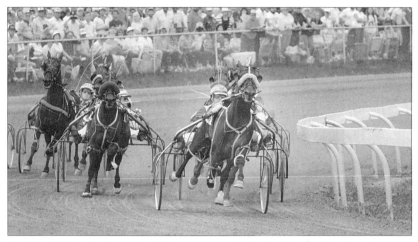

Fig. 21–26. Trochanteric bursitis is seen most often in Standardbred racehorses.

extreme stride length at race speeds may place excessive strain on the tendons of the gluteal muscles and therefore, on the trochanteric bursa. Pain in this area may also be caused by strain or tearing of the tendons, or damage to the top of the trochanter.

Many horses with trochanteric bursitis also have bone spavin *(see Chapter 20)*. It could be speculated that they alter their gait to reduce stress on the painful hock joints, but in the process they increase the load on the other structures in the upper hindlimb. Working on a track with tight turns may also contribute to strain of this bursa and its associated structures.

Signs and Diagnosis

The signs of trochanteric bursitis are vague. The lameness typically is moderate (grade 2 – 3 of 5) and difficult to localize. It may only be obvious when the horse is working at speed. In some cases there may be pain during palpation over the hip joint. But this can be difficult to assess because most horses are trained to move away when pressure is applied to the side of the rump. In chronic cases, there may be slight muscle atrophy (wasting) over the top of the rump on the affected side. However, several other conditions can cause muscle atrophy and chronic lameness, so it is not specific for trochanteric bursitis.

Diagnosing this condition can be difficult because the signs are so vague. It may be possible for the veterinarian to temporarily improve the lameness by injecting local anesthetic into the bursa or around the trochanter. Nuclear scintigraphy may also identify the trochanter as a source of pain. But the best way to confirm bursitis is by ultrasounding the area over the trochanter. When trochanteric bursitis is present, excess fluid is seen in the bursa. *(These diagnostic techniques are discussed in Chapter 2.)*

Treatment and Prognosis for Trochanteric Bursitis

Trochanteric bursitis can be very difficult to manage. In most cases the condition has been present for some time, and other damage may have occurred. Also, the hock problems that commonly plague these horses contribute to the chronic, intermittent or persistent lameness.

Inflammation in the bursa can usually be resolved with rest from regular training and a few days of anti-inflammatory therapy, such as cold therapy, NSAIDs, and DMSO *(see Chapter 5)*. However, the signs often return once training resumes. Corticosteroids injected into the bursa may improve or resolve the lameness for a few weeks, but this is only a short-term solution.

Successfully managing the lameness must involve identifying and treating any underlying or secondary hindlimb conditions. Because multiple problems may be present in these horses, the prognosis for return to the horse's former level of performance is guarded.

PELVIS

The pelvis is the connection between the hindlimb and the spinal column, and thus the rest of the horse. The pelvis also forms a solid base for the large rump muscles, which are the major locomotor muscles. The inner wall of the pelvis forms the roughly oval-shaped pelvic canal that protects the rectum, bladder, and some of the reproductive organs. In mares the pelvic, or "birth" canal forms the rigid passage through which the foal is delivered.

The upper part (wing) of the ilium is attached to the sacral portion of the spinal column by a pair of broad, dense ligaments, called the sacro-iliac ligaments *(see Chapter 22)*. Just above this point the top of each ilial wing forms a bony prominence called the tuber sacrale. These structures are the highest

More Information

The pelvis is a large, complex bone that is made up of three pairs of bones fused together: the ilium, ischium, and pubis.

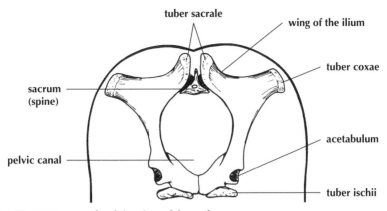

Fig. 21–27. A normal pelvis, viewed from the rear.

point on the rump. Below the wing of the ilium the point of the hip protrudes out the side. This bony prominence is called the tuber coxae. The portion of the pelvis that forms the point of the buttock is called the tuber ischii. The muscles at the back of the thigh attach onto this part of the pelvis.

In summary, there are three bony points on each side of the pelvis that act as "landmarks":

- the tuber sacrale at the top of the rump, just behind the loins
- the tuber coxae (point of the hip) at the side of the pelvis, just behind the flank
- the tuber ischii (point of the buttock) a few inches below the tail base

The greater trochanter of the femur is another landmark on

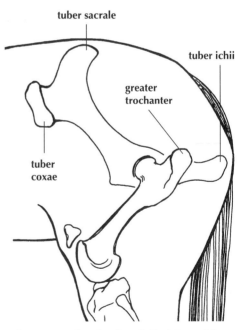

Fig. 21–28. The "landmarks" of the pelvis.

the side of the rump. It is not part of the pelvis, but it does indicate the position of the hip joint.

Pelvic Fractures

Fractures of the pelvis can occur as the result of a fall or other trauma to the side or top of the rump. But a recent study of Thoroughbred racehorses indicated that small, incomplete pelvic fractures may be fairly common in strenuously exercised horses. It is unlikely that trauma was the cause in every case. One explanation is chronic overloading of the bone by regular, intense exercise; that is, these fractures may be "stress" fractures. They are usually found near the sacro-iliac joint, where the ilium attaches to the sacrum. This joint supports the entire hindlimb, so the concussion from ground impact forces is concentrated in a very small area of the pelvis. This helps explain why fractures can occur in this part of the pelvis,

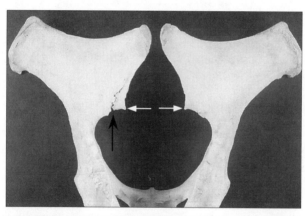

Fig. 21–29. An incomplete pelvic fracture in a racehorse [black arrow]. There are also bony changes on both sides [white arrows].

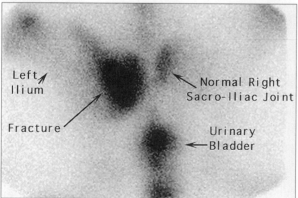

Fig. 21–30. Nuclear scintigraphy shows a "hot spot" that proved to be an incomplete pelvic fracture near the left sacro-iliac joint.

and also why nearby bony reaction was seen in many of the horses examined. *(Other findings of the study are given in Chapter 22.)*

Pelvic fractures may be incomplete or complete, simple or comminuted. Some pelvic fractures extend into the hip joint, causing an articular fracture. Others just involve the point of the hip (the tuber coxae).

Simple Pelvic Fractures
Signs and Diagnosis

Simple pelvic fractures can be very difficult to diagnose. They usually are not displaced and therefore do not result in asymmetry of the pelvis (discussed later). However, they can cause mild muscle atrophy after a few weeks. The muscle mass that covers the pelvis makes it difficult to detect swelling or pain. So, there may be no outward signs of a fracture, other than a mild to moderate lameness (grade 1 – 3 of 5) that is impossible to localize. A history of a fall or evidence of trauma, such as skin abrasions or bruising, adds weight to the possibility that the pelvis is fractured.

Rocking the horse from side to side is one way to check for pain and instability in the pelvis. The veterinarian gently pushes on the point of the hip with one hand then lightly pulls the horse back toward him or her with the tail. The push-and-pull can be repeated a few times in quick succession to make the pelvis rock back and forth. If the horse has a fractured pelvis, this procedure usually causes pain and an evasive move away from the veterinarian. However, most horses are trained to move away when pushed on the side of the rump, so the results of this test must be interpreted cautiously. Furthermore, pain associated with the hip joint, sacro-iliac area, and possibly the stifle may cause a response to this procedure. It is not specific for pelvic pain.

The veterinarian may perform a rectal examination and feel the inner surface of the pelvis while an assistant rocks the horse's pelvis from side to side. This technique may help identify subtle pelvic instability. If nothing else, it helps to rule out a comminuted, displaced fracture.

Definitions
Incomplete fracture: only one side of the bone is cracked. **Complete fracture:** the bone is broken completely. **Simple:** there is only one fracture line. **Comminuted fracture:** there are multiple fracture lines and several bone pieces. **Displaced:** the bone fragments are separated.
(See Chapter 9 for more information fractures.)

Nuclear scintigraphy is useful in these horses *(see Chapter 2)*. A "hot spot" over the pelvis identifies it as the location of the pain. However, the diagnosis cannot be confirmed without radiographs. In foals and small horses it is sometimes possible to take fairly good radiographs of part of the pelvis while the animal is standing and sedated. But in most cases good quality radiographs of the pelvis can only be obtained by anesthetizing the horse and lying it on its back with its legs splayed. However, the risk with this procedure is that the horse may extend fracture when it gets up after anesthesia.

Because of the difficulties in radiographing the pelvis, and the risks associated with anesthetizing the horse to confirm the diagnosis, the veterinarian may just assume that the pelvis is fractured from the history and the signs. However, it is important that other causes of obscure lameness, for example, an incomplete tibial fracture, are investigated and ruled out.

Treatment and Prognosis for Simple Pelvic Fractures

The usual recommendation for treating simple pelvic fractures is 3 – 4 months of rest in a small paddock. It is sometimes difficult to decide when the horse can begin regular exercise. The absence of lameness at the end of the rest period is usually the best way to tell that the horse is ready to resume training. If lameness persists or returns, the horse must be rested for longer.

The prognosis for return to full athletic function is usually very good, provided the fracture heals completely before exercise is resumed.

Comminuted Pelvic Fractures

Signs and Diagnosis

With complete, comminuted fractures, tension from the muscles that surround and attach to the pelvis often causes displacement of the fracture pieces. This can result in asymmetry of the pelvis: one or more of the bony landmarks are out of position. For example, the point of the hip on the fractured side may be higher or lower than normal.

To determine whether the pelvis is symmetrical, it helps to stand on a box behind the horse and look down onto the top of the rump. The horse must be standing as evenly as possible for this to be accurate. Standing on the ground behind the horse and comparing the height of the trochanter and the point of the hip on each side can also help to identify pelvic asymmetry. After a few weeks, muscle atrophy (wasting) often develops on the affected side. Loss of muscle mass on one side of the rump can make the pelvis look asymmetrical. So, it is important that the position of the bony points are compared, not just the overall shape of the hindquarters.

These fractures typically cause moderate to severe lameness (grade 3 – 4 of 5). In some cases the fracture can be felt when the veterinarian performs a rectal examination. Most of the inner surface of the pelvis can be palpated through the rectum, so it may be possible for the veterinarian to feel a displaced piece of bone. A less obvious fracture may be detected by having an assistant rock the horse from side to side while the veterinarian palpates the inside of the pelvis.

A definite diagnosis usually requires radiographs, although good quality radiographs of the pelvis are usually only possible after the horse is anes-

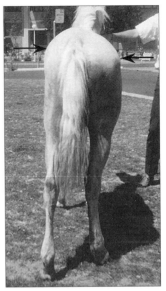

Fig. 21–31. Even though this horse is not standing squarely, pelvic asymmetry is obvious.

thetized. However, this procedure can create more problems if the horse further displaces the fracture as it gets up after anesthesia. For this reason, the veterinarian usually assumes that the pelvis is fractured based on the signs.

Other causes of muscle atrophy and gait abnormalities should also be considered if it is not clear that the pelvis has been fractured. Two possibilities are nerve damage and Equine Protozoal Myeloencephalitis, or EPM *(see Chapter 12).*

Treatment and Prognosis

Surgical repair of comminuted pelvic fractures is not practical. These fractures generally are managed with 2 – 3 months of stall rest, followed by at least another 3 months of paddock rest. Multiple, displaced fractures that involve the hip joint have a poor prognosis for athletic usefulness, or even for "pasture soundness." In these cases it is often more humane to euthanize the horse. Without radiographs it is impossible to be certain that the fracture involves the hip joint. However, the degree of lameness usually is a good guide: the more severe and persistent the lameness, the more likely that the hip joint is damaged.

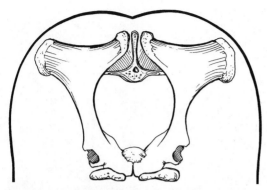

Fig. 21–32. The bony callus on the floor of the pelvis narrows the birth canal.

A potential complication of comminuted pelvic fractures in mares is narrowing of the pelvic ("birth") canal. Narrowing may be caused by either a displaced bone fragment or the bony callus that forms as the bone heals. Valuable broodmares can still be bred after the fracture has healed, but the foal may need to be delivered by cesarean section.

Fracture of the Tuber Coxae

Fracture of the tuber coxae, or the point of the hip, is a fairly common injury. It usually occurs when the horse knocks the side of its hip on a doorway or gate post.

Trauma to the point of the hip can have three possible results:

1. Bruising, with or without an incomplete fracture.
2. A displaced fracture.
3. Bone damage with an overlying wound.

In all cases it causes swelling over the point of the hip that is very painful during palpation. Stiffness, but not necessarily obvious lameness, is also common. This is because some of the large muscles at the front of the thigh attach onto the tuber coxae and put tension on it when they contract. With such similar signs it can be difficult to determine the extent of the damage at first, unless radiographs are taken.

Bruising and Incomplete Fractures

In many cases the injury just consists of bruising. If the bone is also fractured, it is an incomplete fracture. The pain is due to inflammation and bruising of the periosteum (the bone's fibrous, outer covering). This injury is painful, but not serious. With a few days of rest and anti-inflammatory therapy (cold therapy, NSAIDs, and DMSO; *see Chapter 5*), the swelling and pain subside and the point of the hip regains its normal appearance. If the bone has an incomplete fracture, the pain and stiffness may persist for a few weeks, but in time they disappear.

Displaced Fractures

Sometimes a piece of bone is fractured off the tuber coxae, causing a complete, displaced fracture. It may only be a

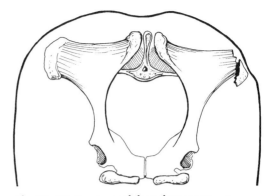

Fig. 21–33. Fracture of the tuber coxae—a "knocked down hip."

small chip of bone, but if the horse knocks its hip hard enough, the whole tuber coxae can be fractured off. When a large piece of bone or the whole tuber coxae is fractured, crepitus (crunching of bone-on-bone) may be felt when the point of the hip is palpated.

In most cases the horse catches its hip as it is going through a doorway or gateway. If the tuber coxae is completely fractured, the bone fragment is forced backward by the door jamb or gate post. At the same time, the muscles at the front of the thigh pull the bone fragment down. So, the point of the hip is usually displaced an inch or so down and back, hence the common name, "knocked down hip." This is easiest to detect when standing behind the horse and comparing the height of the tuber coxae on the left and right sides. The horse must be standing squarely, with equal weight on each hindleg for this observation to be accurate.

The amount of swelling that accompanies this injury can make it difficult to be certain how serious the fracture is. The veterinarian may recommend radiographs to confirm the diagnosis and determine the extent of the fracture. This part of the pelvis is easy to radiograph in the standing horse. The x-ray plate is placed in front of the tuber coxae and gently pressed into the flank to get more of the bone on the radiograph. The x-ray machine is positioned behind the horse, aiming forward. Alternatively, the x-ray plate can be placed over the top of the tuber coxae, and the x-ray beam directed upward and slightly inward from below the point of the hip.

When a large piece of bone is broken off the tuber coxae it may need to be reattached with a bone screw for best results. Smaller bone fragments can either be removed surgically, or left alone to heal back onto the bone. These fractures usually heal quickly and uneventfully, and often the horse can be returned to normal athletic activities within 2 – 3 months. But the "knocked down" appearance may remain if the fracture was not repaired surgically.

Wounds and Tuber Coxae Fractures

Sometimes the skin is also damaged when the tuber coxae is knocked. This wound may be a minor abrasion or a deep laceration. A common result of this injury is a sequestrum, which is an island of dead bone that the body treats as "foreign" material. Infection of the bone's outer surface often results (superficial osteomyelitis; *see Chapter 9*). The typical history in these horses is a small wound over the point of the hip that either fails to heal or begins to heal but then breaks open and oozes pus several days later. This history almost always means that a sequestrum, or other type of foreign material such as a piece of wood or metal, is present.

The wound will not heal until the bone fragment and any underlying damaged, infected bone is removed. Antibiotics are ineffective while the diseased bone is still in the wound. Usually, the veterinarian can surgically remove the fragment while the horse is standing. Sedation and local anesthetic are necessary if the veterinarian must explore the wound more thoroughly. Routine wound care is usually all that is required after this procedure. In most cases the horse can be returned to regular training within 2 – 3 weeks.

Two other minor points are worth making about injuries to the point of the hip. First, it is possible for the skin to be damaged without any bone damage if the horse just "grazes" its hip on a solid object. Although the point of the hip may be quite painful, the wound heals uneventfully, and no further problems develop. Second, the point of the hip is a very common site for pressure sores to develop *(see Chapter 13)*. If the horse is not observed every day, it can sometimes be difficult to tell the difference between a trauma-induced wound and a pressure sore. Both can be very painful and may be infected. The horse's history becomes important in such a case.

MISCELLANEOUS CONDITIONS
Exertional Rhabdomyolysis (Tying Up)

With exertional rhabdomyolysis (ER), or "tying up," the muscles of the thigh and rump are those most commonly, and usually most severely affected. The typical features of ER include muscle pain and cramps soon after the start of exercise. In some horses it takes very little exercise to bring on an episode. The affected muscles are swollen, firm, and painful, and the horse's gait is stiff and stilted. Most horses are reluctant to continue exercising, and some severely affected horses refuse to move at all. In these animals the urine may be dark, red-brown.

Fibrotic Myopathy

Fibrotic myopathy typically involves the muscles at the back of the thigh. Trauma to the semimembranosus, semitendinosus, or biceps femoris muscles can result in scarring and restriction of normal muscle activity. The resulting gait abnormality is quite distinctive: the horse abruptly places its foot too early when bringing the affected hindlimb forward.

More Information
ER is a complex problem with several possible contributing causes. See Chapter 10 for more information on diagnosis and management. More information about fibrotic myopathy, including its management, is also given in Chapter 10.

Aorto-iliac Thrombosis

Definition and Causes

A thrombus is a blood clot within an artery or vein. In aorto-iliac thrombosis, a thrombus develops or lodges in the last part of the aorta or the iliac arteries that supply the hindquarters. It is not known why these clots form, although it has been suggested that they are the result of damage to the vessel walls by migrating larvae of the redworm, or bloodworm *(Strongylus vulgaris)*. These larvae usually migrate up the wall of the blood vessels that supply the bowel. If they go too far and find their way into the aorta or iliac arteries they may damage these vessels and cause a blood clot to form.

Aorto-iliac thrombosis is very uncommon. It has probably been made even less common by the use of effective larvicidal anthelmintics (dewormers that kill the larval stages), such as Ivermectin.

Signs and Diagnosis

When a blood clot develops in the aorta or in one or both iliac arteries it reduces blood flow to the hindlegs. If the clot obstructs only one iliac artery, only that leg is affected. The signs are seen when the horse begins to exercise because at rest blood flow to the legs usually is adequate. The signs subside when the horse stops moving. Aorto-iliac thrombosis causes the following signs during exercise:

- painful muscle cramps which may be so severe that the horse crouches on its hindquarters
- sweating and anxiety, due to pain
- reluctance or inability to move
- cold skin on the affected leg

Some of these signs are similar to those that occur with exertional rhabdomyolysis (ER or "tying up"), so it is easy to confuse the two conditions. However, there are some differences:

1. The muscle cramps persist, and may even worsen after exercise in horses with ER. But the signs resolve within minutes once a horse with aorto-iliac thrombosis stops moving.
2. The skin temperature of the hindlegs is normal in horses with ER. In contrast, the skin on the affected leg is cooler than normal with aorto-iliac thrombosis.
3. The muscle enzymes, CPK and AST, are often greatly elevated in horses with ER. They may be only mildly elevated (if at all) after an episode of aorto-iliac thrombosis.
4. ER is very common; aorto-iliac thrombosis is very uncommon.

The diagnosis usually is based on the signs. Sometimes the veterinarian can feel the thrombus in the last part of the aorta or the first part of the iliac arteries during a rectal examination. However, if the clot is lodged further down the iliac arteries, it is not possible to palpate it. Ultrasonography via the rectum can sometimes be of use when the thrombus cannot be felt.

Treatment and Prognosis for Aorto-iliac Thrombosis

This condition is very difficult to manage. By the time the signs are obvious, the clot usually is large and well established. This makes it very difficult, if not impossible to break up the clot and restore normal blood flow. Nevertheless, anti-clotting drugs, such as aspirin, are important in preventing the clot from enlarging. Regular deworming with a larvicidal anthelmintic also helps prevent the clot from becoming larger.

Over time, the body creates new blood vessels to bypass and take over the role of the clotted artery. However, these vessels are much more narrow than the normal, healthy iliac artery, so they usually cannot accommodate the increased blood flow required by the working muscles during exercise. So, the prognosis for return to normal athletic activities is poor.

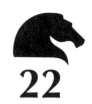

22

THE BACK

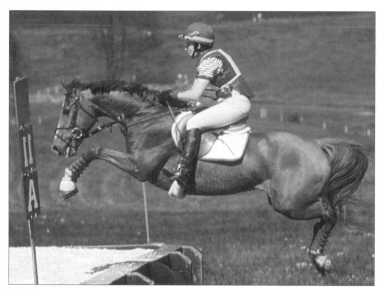

Fig. 22–1.

The spine is a bony column that surrounds and protects the spinal cord. It begins at the horse's poll and ends in the tail dock. By connecting the four limbs and head, the spinal column is the structural means of coordinated movement. In addition, the horse's back supports the ribcage and its contents, and the abdominal wall and organs. It also supports the rider.

The spine must be flexible enough to allow the horse to lower its head to graze, raise and turn its head to monitor its surroundings, and move freely and quickly when necessary. Yet it must be rigid enough to protect the spinal cord from damage and perform its other supporting functions.

The spinal column consists of a series of highly specialized bones called vertebrae. In between the vertebrae are the intervertebral joints. Like most other joints, the intervertebral joints have joint capsules and supporting ligaments, and muscles that overlie and/or activate them. Thus, the back can develop problems similar to those that occur in the limbs: bone, joint, ligament, and muscle problems. Nerve injuries can also be added to this list.

STRUCTURE & FUNCTION

The spinal column is so complex that an entire book could be devoted to this structure alone. For this reason, only the parts of interest in a discussion on lameness are mentioned here.

Vertebrae

The spinal column is divided into five sections:

- cervical—7 vertebrae in the neck
- thoracic—18 vertebrae (in a few horses, 19) to which the ribs attach
- lumbar—6 vertebrae (in a few horses, 5) in the loins
- sacrum—5 fused vertebrae that form the sacrum along the top of the rump
- coccygeal—15 – 25 vertebrae (average 18) in the tail dock

Most vertebrae consist of a solid, roughly cylindrical part called the body, and a thinner arch of bone above. The vertebral arch forms the top and sides of the spinal canal. Most have a ridge of bone along the upper (dorsal) surface, called the dorsal spinous process. All have bony projections, called transverse processes, at each side onto which muscles and ligaments attach. The size of these processes vary with the location. For example, the dorsal spinous processes of the first few thoracic vertebrae are very tall, and form the withers. The transverse processes of the lumbar vertebrae are quite long. Their tips can usually be palpated a few inches from the spine, just above the flank.

Intervertebral Joints

Each vertebra has three joint surfaces at either end: one major and two minor. The major joint surface is located on the vertebral body.

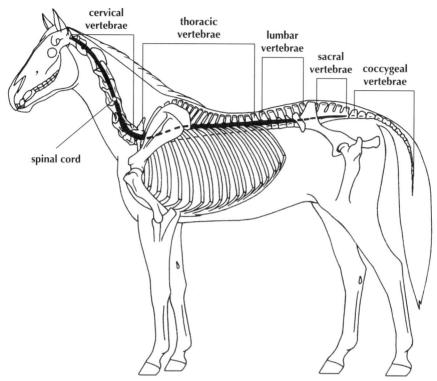

Fig. 22–2. The spinal column and cord.

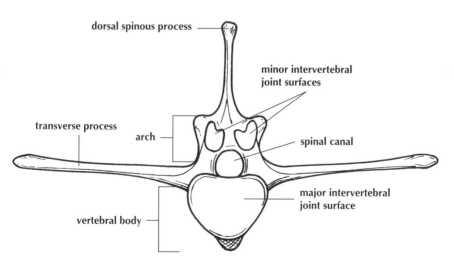

Fig. 22–3. A lumbar vertebra, viewed from behind.

In most vertebrae this cartilage surface is broad and rounded or oval-shaped. The minor intervertebral joint surfaces are on each side of the arch. These cartilage surfaces are small and irregular in shape.

The joints between the vertebral bodies (the major joints) are the main pivot-points for the spine. They are held together above and below by very strong ligaments that run along the floor of the spinal canal and the underside of the vertebral bodies. An intervertebral disc separates the vertebrae at each of these joints. This disc is composed of a ring of fibrous cartilage surrounding an elastic, "pulpy" center. The intervertebral discs act as shock absorbers. They also prevent excessive friction between the two joint surfaces.

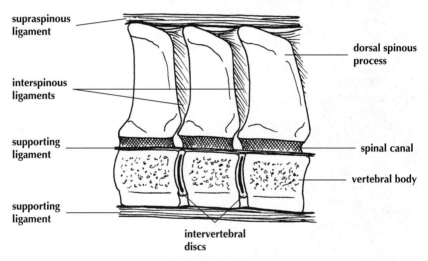

Fig. 22–4. Three thoracic vertebrae, cut in half lengthwise.

The location of the minor joints on each side of the vertebral arch allows a little independent movement of the vertebrae. Thus, the primary role of these smaller joints is that of a pad at the contact points between two vertebrae. These joints can become malaligned (out of position, or subluxated), and cause neck or back pain.

Supporting Structures

The minor joints are supported by thin joint capsules and small ligaments, and by the muscles that overlie the spinal column. Additional support is provided by the interspinous ligaments, which run between the spinous processes.

There is also a larger ligament that runs along the tops of the

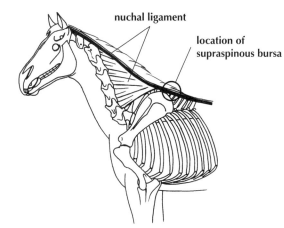

Fig. 22–5. Location of the nuchal ligament. The supraspinous bursa cannot be seen because the nuchal ligament covers it.

spinous processes, down the entire length of the spine; it is called the supraspinous ligament. Between the back of the skull and the withers this ligament is broader and thicker, and is called the nuchal ligament. It helps the horse support and raise its head. Beneath the nuchal ligament, both at the poll and at the withers, is a bursa. A bursa is a fluid-filled sac that protects the ligament and underlying bone from excessive friction and pressure. At the withers this sac is called the supraspinous bursa.

Muscles and Mobility

Except for the first couple of cervical vertebrae, the intervertebral joints have a very limited range of mobility. However, the small amount of movement in each of the many intervertebral joints means that, as a unit, the vertebral column is capable of a much larger range of mobility.

Movement is caused by the muscles that attach to the vertebrae; these muscles also assist in locomotion and spinal column support. There are many small muscles that connect only a couple of vertebrae. There are also some larger muscles that connect several vertebrae, and so move a large section of the spinal column. The longissimus dorsi—the pair of muscles that lie on each side of the spine along most of the back—is a good example of the latter.

The types of spinal column movement include:

- flexion and extension—rounding or hollowing the back
- lateral flexion—bending to the left or right

- rotation around the long axis of the spinal column—the individual vertebrae involved rotate clockwise or counterclockwise

These movements can occur together. In fact, because of the shape and location of the intervertebral joints, it is impossible for the spine to flex laterally without also rotating slightly.

Spinal Nerves and Reflexes

At each intervertebral joint, nerves exit/enter the spinal column through either a small hole in the vertebrae or a notch between the vertebrae. These spinal nerves can be irritated or compressed by inflammation or bony proliferation (osteoarthritis), or by malalignment of the vertebrae. Pain associated with this latter condition is often called a "pinched nerve."

As well as supplying the limbs and body, the spinal nerves supply the intervertebral joint capsules, supporting ligaments, and overlying muscles with sensation. (In the case of the muscles, they also stimulate motor function; *see Chapter 12.*) So, problems affecting these nerves can affect the supporting and mobilizing structures of the spinal column. The result is pain and/or loss of mobility in that part of the spine.

Sometimes the resulting muscle spasms occur several inches from the actual site of nerve compression; this is often called "referred pain." For example, pain over the rump may be due to compression of the spinal nerves in the loins. This is because some of the spinal nerves exit the spinal column and travel down the back to reach the tissues they supply. Thus, the nerve supply for a muscle may have its origin several inches forward of the muscle's location.

Spinal Reflexes

There are certain reflexes involving the spinal nerves that can be stimulated in every normal horse. There are two spinal reflexes that are of interest when evaluating back pain and lameness. The first occurs when the veterinarian runs a knuckle or a blunt object along the longissimus dorsi muscle, on either side of the back. This action causes the horse to hollow its back a little and bend away from the pressure. When both sides of the spine are tested at once, the horse simply hollows its back a little.

The second reflex occurs when the same procedure is applied alongside the spine over the rump and tail base (the sacral part of the spine). The horse hunches its back and tucks its rump under, away from the pressure.

These are normal responses; they do not mean the horse has a sore back. In fact, if the horse has back pain, it is more likely to brace itself by tensing the back muscles in an effort to suppress the reflex, protecting the painful area from movement. Therefore, the absence or suppression of a spinal reflex is sometimes more important than its presence.

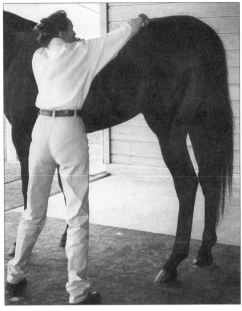

Fig. 22–6. Testing for normal spinal reflexes.

NECK & BACK PAIN

Although this chapter focuses on the back problems that can cause lameness, the neck is included for two reasons. First, the spinal column is a unit. While it consists of many individual structures, they are aligned such that the entire spinal column is continuous. So, the neck and back are inseparable parts of the same structure. Second, problems in the neck can sometimes cause lameness.

Pain associated with the neck or back is a significant cause of gait abnormalities or loss of performance in athletic horses. Neck or back pain may be the only cause, but sometimes the pain is secondary to a problem in the limbs. In these horses, resolving the lameness may be all that is required to resolve the back pain.

With over 30 bones, more than 100 joints, and many more associated soft tissue structures in the neck and back, pain can arise from many sources, including:

- vertebrae—e.g. fractures, over-riding spinous processes
- intervertebral joints and discs—e.g. malalignment, DJD, and osteoarthritis
- supporting ligaments—e.g. strain and tears, sacro-iliac instability
- muscles of the neck and back—e.g. muscle strain and spasms
- spinal nerves—e.g. compression ("pinched nerve")

In many cases neck or back pain is caused by a combination of these problems. For example, a sudden, evasive movement may cause strain and inflammation of an intervertebral joint capsule. This results in increased tension in the surrounding muscles, in an effort to prevent movement in the painful joint. The muscles may then spasm and become another source of pain. Or, the evasive move may have stretched or torn a supporting ligament, causing joint instability and malalignment of some of the small intervertebral joints. This, in turn, causes intervertebral joint pain, and inflammation or compression of the spinal nerves at that location. Muscle spasms often add to the pain.

Parts of the cervical vertebrae and their intervertebral joints can be palpated. However, in the back the overlying muscle (or shoulder blades and pelvis) prevent palpation of all but the tips of the dorsal spinous or transverse processes. So, it can be very difficult to determine which problems are present, and which is the primary injury. Muscle tension and spasm is a sign that there may be an underlying abnormality. However, it is difficult to know what problems (if any) lie beneath. A muscle spasm can develop in response to bone or soft tissue abnormalities, but it can also occur on its own.

Thus, specific diagnosis and treatment of back problems can be very difficult. Moreover, far less is known about the horse's back than the limbs, so some back conditions probably are under-diagnosed and inappropriately treated.

Identifying the Problem

Some general signs of neck or back pain include:

- change of posture or head carriage
- reduced ability or willingness to bend or flex the neck
- difficulty or resistance to turning in one direction
- difficulty or resistance to performing usual athletic activities, such as jumping, tight turns, and sliding stops
- shortened stride, reluctance to "stride out"
- vague gait abnormality (may or may not be obviously lame)
- apparent weakness or incoordination, such as "dropping" one leg out of cadence during the trot or canter
- pain during pressure over the neck, back, or rump

Before examining the neck and back, the veterinarian may request some information about the horse's use and work history. Traumatic incidents, such as a fall, collision with a solid object, or trailer accident, are important facts of which the veterinarian should be informed, regardless of how long ago they occurred. The veterinarian should also be informed of any current behavioral or performance problems.

Examining the Neck and Back

Problems in the limbs can cause back pain. So, a thorough physical examination and gait evaluation are important to rule out limb problems as either the primary cause of the gait abnormality or a contributing cause of the back pain.

More Information
Diagnostic tools and techniques, including physical examination and gait evaluation, are discussed in Chapter 2.

Observation can be useful in locating painful or otherwise abnormal areas of the horse's spine. For example, the horse's stance or head position may give a clue to the location of the problem. Asymmetry, such as that caused by muscle atrophy (wasting), swelling, or sacro-iliac subluxation (discussed later), is also an important finding.

Palpation

Detailed palpation is probably the most important skill needed for diagnosing problems of the neck and back. The veterinarian or chiropractor palpates the accessible parts of the vertebrae, such as the intervertebral joints in the neck and the dorsal spinous processes in the thoracic and lumbar spine. He or she also palpates the muscles that support and activate the spine. While palpating, the veterinarian or chiropractor is feeling for:

- pain
- muscle tension and spasms
- malposition of the bony prominences (dorsal spinous and transverse processes, and the top of the pelvis)
- unusual swellings or depressions
- asymmetry

Assessing Mobility

Finally, the range of spinal mobility can be assessed by evaluating the horse's willingness and ability to move its spine. This part of the examination focuses on the neck; the rest of the spinal column is far less mobile and much more difficult to assess. The mobility of the horse's neck can be evaluated manually, by physically moving the horse's head and neck through the normal range of motion. Alterna-

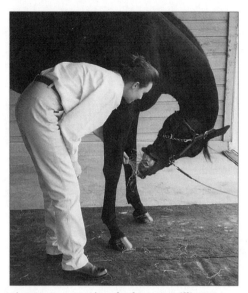

tively, it can be assessed by offering the horse a treat and observing its willingness to move its head and neck through a range of motions. For example, holding a handful of hay out in front of, or above the horse's head encourages it to extend, or stretch out its neck. Holding the hay between the horse's forelegs assesses its willingness and ability to flex its neck. Holding the hay at either flank requires the horse to bend its neck to the left and right. If the horse has difficulty with any of these

Fig. 22–7. Assessing the horse's willingness and ability to flex its neck.

maneuvers, it may have a neck problem.

The spinal reflexes can help assess the mobility of the thoracic and lumbar portions of the horse's spine. As mentioned earlier, suppression of these reflexes is often seen in horses with back pain.

Diagnostic Tools

Problems involving the vertebrae and intervertebral joints can sometimes be identified with radiography. But many parts of the horse's spine are very difficult to radiograph. For example, the first few thoracic vertebrae are hidden between the shoulder blades, and the first part of the sacrum is covered by the sides of the pelvis. Also, the size of the average adult horse makes it very difficult to take good quality radiographs of the bodies of the thoracic and lumbar vertebrae, even with a powerful x-ray machine. It is usually only possible to see the tops of the spinous processes clearly.

The size and shape of the adult horse also limits which views can be taken of the spinal column. Radiography can only provide a two-dimensional view of a three-dimensional structure. So at least two radiographic views, at right-angles to one another, should be taken of an area wherever possible. Two views can usually be taken of the cervical spine: one from the side (a lateral view) and one from underneath the neck (a ventro-dorsal view). However, only a lateral view can be taken of the thoracic portion of the spine. It is possible to take a ventro-dorsal view of the lumbo-sacral spine with a powerful x-ray machine. But the horse must be anesthetized and laid on its back for this procedure.

Nuclear scintigraphy is sometimes useful in identifying the site of the problem. Although a specific diagnosis is not possible with scintigraphy, it allows the veterinarian to confirm that there is a structural problem in the back. He or she can then investigate the specific area more thoroughly.

CT and MRI are useful for identifying bone and soft tissue problems in the spinal column in people and small animals. However, the size of the adult horse limits the use of these techniques (with respect to neck and back problems) to just the head and neck.

(See Chapter 2 for more information on these diagnostic tools.)

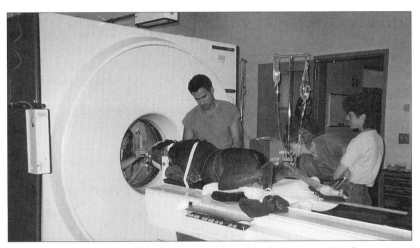

Fig. 22–8. An anesthetized foal being positioned in the computerized tomography (CT) machine.

Differences Between Horses and People

Many techniques that have been developed for diagnosing and managing neck and back problems in horses have been adapted from studies and experience with similar problems in people. However, all assumptions about the causes and management of spinal column problems in people may not be valid in horses, for at least three reasons.

First, the spinal column in people is aligned vertically, whereas it is horizontal in horses. Thus, the forces on the intervertebral joints and support structures are different. For example, human intervertebral joints and discs are subject to constant compression while the person is standing, moving about, and sitting. In horses, tension and shearing forces during flexion/extension, bending, and rotation of the spine are more important than compression.

Second, the load on the spine is less in people. Very few people carry heavy loads on their backs, and even when they do, most of the weight is borne on the shoulders and collar bones, rather than directly on the spinal column. The weight that is transmitted to the spinal column is distributed down the spine, which adds to the compressive load on the intervertebral joints. In contrast, horses that are ridden carry up to an additional 25% of their body weight (rider and saddle) across the middle of the spinal column. This adds to the tension and shearing forces on the intervertebral joints.

Third, most people are not athletes, so many of the neck and back problems human physicians and chiropractors address are chronic, degenerative conditions, such as arthritis and disc degeneration. Horses can also develop chronic neck or back problems. However, these problems usually result from some type of athletic activity or traumatic incident which caused an acute, potentially treatable injury that was left untreated.

Treatment Options

Several options are available for treating neck and back pain in horses. The choice of treatment depends on the primary problem.

Rest

The veterinarian or chiropractor usually recommends rest from strenuous exercise for most neck or back problems. In some cases as little as 1 – 2 days of rest may be all that is necessary. In other cases the horse may need to be rested for several weeks.

> **More Information**
>
> This discussion specifically relates to managing neck and back pain.
>
> For more general information on these treatment options, see Section II.

Exercise

Whether or not rest from regular training is recommended, some type of daily light exercise is beneficial in most horses with neck or back pain. Activity can relieve muscle spasms, and stimulates blood flow to the injured area. Hand-

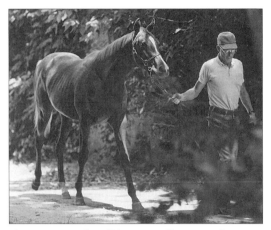

Fig. 22–9. Hand-walking can relieve muscle spasms and stimulate blood flow.

walking, longeing, "ponying," and pasture turnout are all preferable to ridden or driven exercise. This is because those activities do not place any extra strain on the horse's back.

"Mobilizing" the spine with gentle, specific exercises helps to restore and maintain flexibility with many neck and back problems in people. Inactivity can be detrimental to the recovery and long-term health of a damaged intervertebral joint. For this reason, some equine therapists recommend specific exercises that address the horse's particular problem. These "limbering" exercises can speed recovery and prevent reinjury in many cases.

Chiropractic Manipulation and Acupuncture

Sometimes neck or back pain is the result of malalignment of the vertebrae. In these horses, careful adjustment by an experienced equine chiropractor can restore the spine to normal mobility.

Acupuncture can provide temporary relief for neck or back pain. However, as with any therapy, a specific diagnosis should be made before treatment begins.

Physical Therapy

Several physical therapies can benefit horses with neck or back pain. Once a diagnosis is made, massage, heat therapy, magnetic field therapy, and therapeutic ultrasound can each help resolve the muscle spasms found with neck or back problems. These therapies can also increase blood flow to the injured area, which promotes healing.

Drugs

Veterinarians often prescribe pain-relieving medications, such as NSAIDs, DMSO, and corticosteroids, for neck or back pain. These

drugs relieve pain by relieving inflammation. If muscle spasms are
the result of soft tissue inflammation (such as an inflamed intervertebral joint capsule), relieving the inflammation can resolve the
painful muscle spasms. However, if a structural problem, such as a
fracture or malalignment, is present, these drugs may do little to resolve the pain.

Muscle relaxants are also occasionally used to relieve muscle spasms.

Surgery

Very few neck or back problems are treated surgically in horses.
Unlike in people, surgical fusion of an abnormal intervertebral joint,
removal of a damaged disc, or repair of a fractured vertebra is often
not an option in horses. There are two notable exceptions. One is
cervical vertebral malformation (CVM, or "wobbler" syndrome; *see
Chapter 12*). The other is over-riding spinous processes (discussed
later). Although conservative management is almost always the primary recommendation with these two conditions, surgery is occasionally done in unresponsive cases.

SPECIFIC CONDITIONS

It is not possible to discuss, or even list every problem that can
affect the spinal column. Only the more common conditions are included. A few unusual conditions are also briefly mentioned.

Neck Pain

More Information

Developmental abnor-
malities, vertebral frac-
tures, and infection
involving the vertebrae
or spinal cord are cov-
ered in Chapter 12.
These conditions prima-
rily cause neurologic
abnormalities, rather
than lameness.

Neck pain often develops during
breaking and training, particularly when
young horses are first taught to tie, and
when "tie-downs" or side reins are used
to teach the horse to accept the bit. In
many cases the neck pain is simply
caused by muscle strain and spasms, but
sometimes severe damage results from a
fall or violent resistance.

Neck problems are not restricted to
young horses. They are also found in
adult horses that perform demanding
activities, such as polo and Western
sports (reining, roping, cutting, etc.).

Even inactive horses can develop neck pain. For example, a pastured horse may get its head caught in a fence while trying to reach a patch of grass on the other side. Struggling to free itself can damage the supporting structures of the neck.

Sometimes neck pain is caused by structural abnormalities. These include cervical vertebral malformation ("wobbler" syndrome), osteoarthritis in the intervertebral joints, and malalignment of the vertebrae. Other abnormalities are functional, in that the vertebrae are structurally normal but the soft tissue components are functionally abnormal. Muscle spasms and inflammation of an intervertebral joint capsule are examples of functional problems that can cause neck pain.

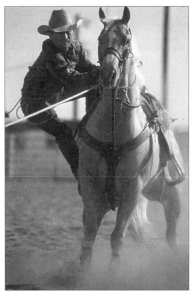

Fig. 22–10. Neck problems are often found in horses that perform demanding activities.

Malalignment of the cervical vertebrae can cause muscle spasms and pain in other areas (referred pain). A common site is in the muscles at the base of the neck. These muscles help bring the foreleg forward when the horse moves, so spasms in these muscles can cause a shortened stride on the affected side. Adjustment by a skilled equine chiropractor may be all that is necessary to resolve this problem.

Neck pain is not always directly related to the spinal column and its immediate structures. For example, an intramuscular injection reaction on the side of the neck can cause neck stiffness and pain for a few days after injection *(see Chapter 10)*. Other "non-spinal" problems that can cause neck pain include dermatitis, an allergic reaction to an insect bite, and tight braids in the mane.

Pain Over the Withers

The withers include the dorsal spinous processes of the first few thoracic vertebrae. Trauma to the withers can occur when the horse rolls against a solid object or hits the withers on a low-hanging tree branch. Flipping over backward can also damage the withers. Sometimes the force of impact fractures some of the spinous processes (see the later section on *Flip-Over Injuries*).

Malalignment of the first few thoracic vertebrae can cause pain over or behind the withers, particularly in the muscles on each side. Presumably, leverage from the forelegs causes this problem. Activities such as working cattle, turning quickly at speed (for example, polo and eventing), and working on slippery surfaces require the horse to set its forelegs wide apart. This action could rotate the thoracic vertebrae slightly because the shoulder blades lie against the ribs and spinous processes. The leverage on the vertebrae when the horse splays its forelegs and shifts its weight could be considerable. Adjustment by a skilled equine chiropractor may resolve this problem, provided the horse has sustained no other damage.

Another problem that may affect the withers is over-riding of the spinous processes. This condition is discussed in the later section on Midback Pain.

Pressure-Related Pain

Pressure from an ill-fitting blanket, saddle, or saddle pad can also cause pain over the withers. In some cases the pain is so severe that the horse cannot lower its head to eat or drink at ground level. These horses may strongly resent examination of the withers.

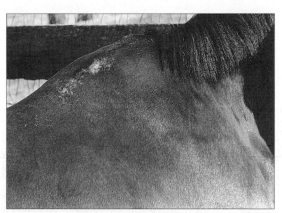

Repeated use of an ill-fitting saddle can cause chronic pressure on the top or sides of the withers. Over time, pressure-related damage to the hair follicles may cause permanent growth of white hairs. A common place for these patches to be found is in the slight depression at the base of the

Fig. 22–11. Saddle sores can leave areas of bare skin or white hair over the withers.

withers, just behind the shoulder blade. Any horse can develop this problem if the saddle does not fit correctly. Horses with high, prominent withers are probably more prone to it. But because the potential is obvious, most riders make sure that the saddle fits well, so this problem is less common than would be expected in these horses. It is seen more often in horses with flatter withers, such as Quarter Horses. This is because most riders do not anticipate a problem, so they may not take care to ensure that the saddle fits the horse properly.

In horses with low withers, the saddle may rotate slightly from one side to the other if the girth or cinch is not tight enough. This may cause an abrasion ("saddle sore") over or just behind the withers. If the girth or cinch is very tight, pressure-related problems are even more likely if the saddle does not fit the horse properly. In these horses, the saddle may cause pressure and muscle pain just behind the shoulder blades, rather than directly over the withers. As a result, the horse's stride may be shortened on one or both sides.

The supraspinous bursa lies between the tips of the spinous processes and the nuchal ligament *(see Figure 22–5)*. This bursa can be inflamed by chronic pressure if an ill-fitting saddle is repeatedly used. A common history is chronic pain over the withers, whether or not there is a "saddle sore." There may also be a small, soft swelling at the top of the withers, on either side of the nuchal ligament. The swelling may fluctuate in size, and may disappear when the horse is rested. This problem can persist for months or years, never getting much better or worse. However, in some horses it can progress to become fistulous withers.

Fistulous Withers

In this context, a fistula is an infected tract, or tunnel that begins or breaks out at the skin surface, and tracks infection through the tissues beneath the skin. In the case of fistulous withers, the infection involves the supraspinous bursa.

The bursa may become infected through a wound or deep abrasion over the withers, or through the bloodstream. In the past, when horses were used to pull carts and carriages, deep harness rubs over the withers were the most common cause. Fistulous withers is far less common now. (A similar condition, "poll evil," which involves the bursa at the back of the skull, is now rare.) Better management practices probably account for this progress.

For bacteria to invade the bursa from the bloodstream, the wall of the bursa must first be damaged. Chronic pressure from a poorly-fitted saddle is the most likely cause of this form of the disease.

Infection of the bursa results in further damage. Infected tracts form when the bursa ruptures and releases pus into the surrounding tissues. The infection travels between the muscles and ligaments, eventually breaking out through the skin as an oozing wound on the

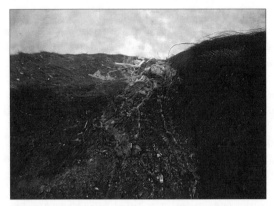

Fig. 22–12. The infection eventually breaks out on the side of the withers.

side of the withers. Mild lameness often is seen in these horses because movement places tension on the skin and underlying tissues in the infected area, and on the nuchal ligament and bursa.

Treatment and Prognosis for Fistulous Withers

This condition is very difficult to resolve. The infected tracts can be extensive, sometimes spreading down between the shoulder blade and the chest wall. The only way to resolve the infection is to anesthetize the horse and surgically open up all of the tracts. Antibiotics are important in controlling the infection, but on their own they are totally ineffective.

Even with aggressive surgery and several weeks of antibiotic therapy, the condition can persist, or return weeks or months later.

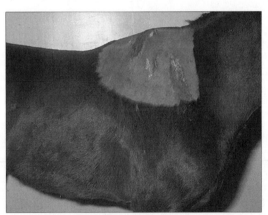

Fig. 22–13. Treating fistulous withers involves surgically opening all the infected tracts.

Therefore, the prognosis for complete resolution of the infection is guarded, as is the chance that the horse can return to training. This condition is far easier to prevent than treat.

Public Health Issues

In the past, it was common for the bacteria that cause brucellosis *(Brucella abortus)* to be found in these fistulous tracts. Brucellosis is a cattle disease that can be spread to people, causing fever, general illness, and joint pain. Thus, fistulous withers has long been a condition of public health importance. However, a recent survey of horses with fistulous withers found that only a few had been exposed to this organism. Although the veterinarian may take the precaution of testing for *Brucella,* it is generally safe to assume that the horse poses no great risk of transmitting the infection to people (or to other horses). Nevertheless, the precautions discussed in Chapter 4 for managing infected wounds should be followed in all horses with fistulous withers.

Midback Pain

The midback area primarily consists of the thoracic part of the spine, from the back of the withers to the loins. Spasms and pain in the longissimus dorsi muscles (which run down either side of the spine) are the hallmark of problems in this part of the back.

Malalignment of the vertebrae can occur along this part of the spine, although the ribs act as stabilizing struts to limit excessive rotation and bending. Nevertheless, activities or incidents that cause twisting of the spine can cause malalignment. Examples are kicking out to the side while bucking, or falling headlong over an obstacle.

Conformational faults can also lead to chronic back pain. They include:

- "wry back"—the spine is bent to the side
- "sway back"—the back is hollowed
- "roach back"—the back is hunched

These abnormalities alter the mechanics of the spine, making it less resistant to tension and shearing forces. Horses that have long backs are more prone to midback and lumbar pain for the same reason. Some horses hollow their backs when they jump, which adds to the load on these parts of the spine *(see Figure 22–1).*

Pressure-Related Pain

The saddle and rider can cause skin and muscle pain in this part of the back. Pain may be due to a poorly stuffed or badly positioned saddle, or an imbalanced rider. The rider does not need to be heavy to cause the horse back pain. He or she only needs to be off balance or "out of synch" with the horse's movements.

The pain associated with this problem usually is found in the muscles on either side of the spine. Very seldom is the pain directly over the vertebrae, unless the saddle is malpositioned and puts pressure on the spinous processes—which it should *never* do. Sometimes uneven or excessive saddle pressure causes an imprint of the pads and panels along the horse's back and sides. Swellings and depressions that match the saddle's shape can be seen immediately or within an hour after the saddle is removed. If the pressure is less severe, but the saddle moves about or the rider sits to one side, hair may be rubbed off in a patch on one or both sides of the horse's back. Repeated use of a badly-fitted or malpositioned saddle may cause white hairs to appear in this area, although a bare patch is just as common.

Recently, a conforming sensor pad has been developed to measure saddle pressure in horses. Sensors in a specially-designed saddle pad measure pressure at several points beneath the saddle, and transmit the information to a computer. This equipment allows the owner or trainer to identify areas of excessive pressure beneath the saddle, and select a saddle and pad that fit the horse properly. Having a saddler make or modify a saddle specifically for the horse is another way to ensure a proper fit.

Pommel

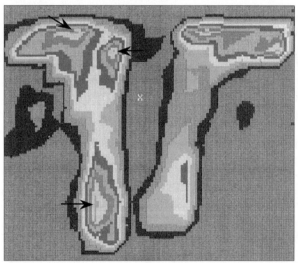

Fig. 22–14. A computer-generated image from the sensor pad. There is much more pressure on the left side of the horse's back, with islands of intense pressure [arrows].

Cantle

Cold Back

"Cold back" is a term used to describe a horse that sinks or hollows its back, or bucks when mounted. Other behaviors attributed to a cold back include flinching, bending away, or biting when groomed over the back, and having a short, stilted stride when the girth is tightened.

If palpation of the horse's back reveals tense, painful muscles on either side of the spine, then back pain most likely is the reason for these behavioral problems. However, in many of these horses the back feels normal when palpated, the saddle fits well, and the owner or trainer has investigated several other possibilities, without success. In these horses back pain probably is not the cause.

Possible Causes

On the surface, it makes sense to assume that if the horse has back pain, it would want to buck the rider off. However, bucking places a lot of strain on the back, and requires more flexibility than most horses with back pain have. So, bucking is one thing a horse with a sore back would probably not do. In fact, back pain is one of the main reasons why rodeo roughstock stop bucking well.

Flinching and biting when the back is brushed can have several possible explanations. First, the horse may have very sensitive skin, which is irritated by the brush. If the horse has very little fat cover over its ribs, too much pressure with the brush when grooming over the ribcage can also cause discomfort. Alternatively, brushing along the longissimus dorsi muscles may stimulate the normal spinal reflex that occurs in this part of the back (discussed earlier). Some horses resent repeated stimulation of this reflex. Another explanation may be found in the horse's attitude. Some horses express their dominant personality by trying to bite their grooms, particularly when they are feeling good. This behavior can quickly become a habit, especially as the horse's fitness improves.

Sinking when mounted can also be a persistent behavioral problem in some horses, as can bucking when mounted. Many of these horses settle down and behave themselves when they are longed for 15 – 20 minutes before the rider mounts. This would not be the case in horses with back pain.

Short-striding when the girth is first tightened may be due to irritation or pinching of the sensitive skin in the girth area. But it may also be due to pressure behind the withers. The girth exerts pressure around the horse's body, which may be greatest at the top of the spine. The girth can also put excessive pressure on the pectoral muscles that run up the sides of the chest wall, just behind the elbows. Stretching the horse's forelegs or walking the horse around before mounting moves the girth back slightly, into a more comfortable position.

Over-riding Spinous Processes

Definition and Causes

Most of the vertebrae have a ridge of bone along their upper (dorsal) surface, called the dorsal spinous process. These processes are tallest in the thoracic and lumbar vertebrae. They reach their great-

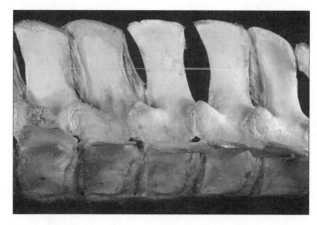

Fig. 22–15. Over-riding dorsal spinous processes in the thoracic spine. None of the processes should be touching.

est height at the withers, where the spinous processes of the fourth and fifth thoracic vertebrae may be over 7 inches (18 cm) high.

The spinous processes of the first 15 thoracic vertebrae lean backward. At the 16th, the process points straight up, and behind this, the processes of the remaining thoracic vertebrae and the lumbar vertebrae point slightly forward *(see Figure 22–2)*. Thus, there is opportunity at a few locations for the tips of the dorsal spinous processes to touch one another, or "over-ride." (This condition is also called impinging spinous processes.) The most common locations are:

- the last few thoracic vertebrae, which is about where the cantle of the saddle rests
- the first few lumbar vertebrae, over the loins
- the withers, where the spinous processes are very long

The spinous processes can over-ride if the small ligaments between them and the other ligaments that stabilize the spinal column are stretched or torn at that location. Trauma or excessive movement of the spinal column is a likely cause. In older horses, gradual stretching of these ligaments over several years may be the primary reason this problem develops. Poor conformation, such as a long back or a "sway" back, probably makes it more likely for the spinous processes to over-ride and interfere with one another.

Given that the most common location for this problem is beneath the saddle, it could be speculated that the weight of the rider also plays an important role by

> ## Of Interest
>
> Evidence of over-riding spinous processes has been found in the extinct equine species, *Equus occidentalis,* which existed long before horses were domesticated and ridden.

exerting downward pressure on the spine. This may cause hollowing of the spine at that location, which brings the spinous processes closer together. However, over-riding spinous processes are relatively common in Standardbred racehorses, so the weight of a rider must be only one of several possible factors.

When the stabilizing ligaments are stretched or torn, there is increased mobility of the affected intervertebral joints. Thus, pain can arise from at least four sources:

- inflammation of the periosteum (the bone's fibrous, but sensitive covering) on the tips of the over-riding processes
- strain on the joint capsules and supporting ligaments of the vertebrae
- malalignment of the vertebrae
- muscle spasms that develop in an effort to stabilize the intervertebral joints

The result of pressure from the neighboring spinous process is bone remodeling. This includes loss of bone density (lysis) at the contact point, and surrounding new bone production (exostoses; *see Chapter 9*). The tips of the processes are gradually eroded and reshaped. Over time, the body attempts to stabilize this painful area by bridging the affected spinous processes with fibrous (scar) tissue, and, in a few cases, a bony callus.

Signs and Diagnosis of Over-riding Spinous Processes

A firm or bony swelling may be felt or seen along the center of the back, directly over the affected spinous processes. The most common locations are the thoraco-lumbar area and the withers. In many horses this problem causes back pain. The muscles on either side of the spine are tense and painful when palpated, and the affected spinous processes may be painful when pressed with the fingers. The normal spinal reflex is often reduced or absent in these horses. They tend to brace their backs against this movement because it causes more pain. Although lame-

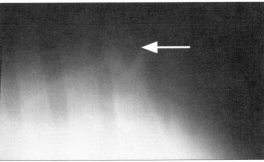

Fig. 22–16. Bone lysis in an over-riding spinous process at the withers.

ness is not common, a tense, sore back often alters the horse's stride, as well as its attitude and willingness to exercise. Poor performance, such as refusal to jump or loss of speed is common in these horses. Radiographs may show two or more spinous processes touching one another, and sometimes a loss of bone density or new bone production at the contact point(s).

However, *not all horses with over-riding spinous processes have back pain* or perform poorly. So, it is important to investigate other causes of performance problems and rule them out before this diagnosis is made. To confirm that the spinous processes are the problem, the veterinarian may inject local anesthetic around them. If over-riding spinous processes are a problem, the pain response should be reduced and the horse's gait should improve. Nuclear scintigraphy can also be used to determine whether inflammation and active bone remodeling are present.

Treatment and Prognosis for Over-riding Spinous Processes

Over-riding spinous processes is a permanent, degenerative condition. All treatment can do is relieve the horse's discomfort. Chiropractic manipulation and acupuncture can help many of these horses. Physical therapies, such as daily massage, heat therapy, and magnetic field therapy, may also help. They relieve pain by resolving the associated muscle spasms. Injecting long-acting corticosteroids into the area can also relieve the pain for a few weeks. However, because the problem is likely due to excessive mobility of the affected intervertebral joints, none of these therapies produce permanent results. *(See Chapter 4 for more information on these therapies.)*

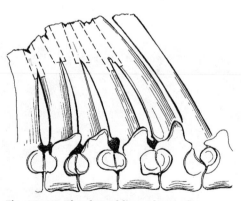

Fig. 22–17. The dotted lines show where bone would be removed.

Some veterinarians have tried surgically removing the parts of the spinous processes that touch. However, recovery to the stage where the horse can tolerate ridden exercise can sometimes take several months. Furthermore, this surgery does not address the cause: intervertebral joint instability. So, removing the over-riding parts of the processes may not completely resolve the back pain.

Reducing the intensity of the horse's exercise program may be necessary. In particular, demanding activities such as jumping, steep hill work, tight turns, and sliding stops should be restricted. Thus, the prognosis for continued athletic function at the previous level of performance is guarded if the back pain and gait abnormality persist or return despite treatment. In most cases the owner or trainer eventually has to find less strenuous activities for the horse.

"Non-Spinal" Causes of Midback Pain

Like neck pain, not all problems that cause back pain are directly related to the spinal column and its supporting structures. For example, bacterial dermatitis along the back can be very painful *(see Chapter 13)*. Topical DMSO can also cause painful skin irritation in some horses *(see Chapter 5)*. A far less common cause of back pain in horses is warble fly larvae ("cattle grubs"). These parasites migrate through the tissues and eventually break out through the skin along the back.

Fractured ribs and pleuritis can also cause midback pain and gait abnormalities. *(These conditions are mentioned in Chapter 1.)*

> ### Of Interest
>
> Nodular necrobiosis is a very common skin condition that causes multiple, firm skin lumps along this part of the back. These lumps are seldom painful and generally cause the horse no problems.

Pain Over the Loins and Rump

Pain during palpation over the lumbar area (the loins) or over the rump can be caused by many conditions. Only some of them are directly related to the spinal column and its support structures. The more common problems include:

- over-riding spinous processes
- malalignment of the lumbar vertebrae or the lumbo-sacral joint
- sacro-iliac pain
- exertional rhabdomyolysis (ER, or "tying up")
- muscle strain and tears
- intramuscular injection reaction
- pelvic fractures *(see Chapter 21)*

> ### More Information
>
> Muscle problems, including ER, muscle strain and tears, and IM injection reactions, are covered in Chapter 10.

Some mares and fillies appear lame or sensitive to palpation of the lumbar area and flank during various phases of the estrous cycle. This problem is mentioned in Chapter 1.

Some people believe that pain over the lumbar area means the horse has a kidney problem. However, the kidneys are further forward than most people think. They are well protected by the last few ribs and thoracic vertebrae, the transverse processes of the first two lumbar vertebrae, and several inches of muscle above and below the spine. It is impossible to "bruise the kidneys" by putting pressure on the horse's loins. Furthermore, painful kidney problems in horses are extremely uncommon.

Sacro-iliac Subluxation
Definition and Causes

In between the points of the hip, the sides of the pelvis slope upward and in toward the center of the back, like the sides of a steeply pitched roof (although they do not meet). The sides of the pelvis are called the ilial wings. At the top of each ilial wing is a bony prominence called the tuber sacrale. This is the highest point of the rump, whether looking at the horse from the side or the rear.

The sacrum runs between the ilial wings. This is the point where

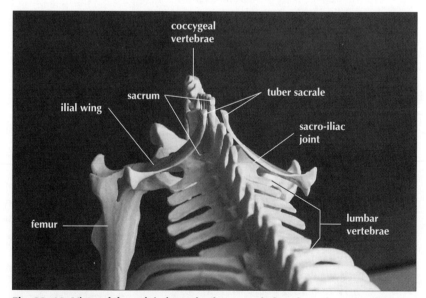

Fig. 22–18. View of the pelvis from the front, angled to show the sacro-iliac joints between the sacrum and ilial wing.

the pelvis attaches to the spinal column. In the forelimb the connection between the shoulder blade and the spinal column is composed entirely of muscles and ligaments. In the hindlimb this connection is bone-to-bone, at the sacro-iliac joints (one on each side of the sacrum). These joints are broad and flat. Although they have thin cartilage surfaces and a small joint capsule, their primary function is to support the pelvis, rather than allow a wide range of movement. To that end, these joints are supported and stabilized by broad, dense ligaments, called the sacro-iliac ligaments. The ligaments surround the sacro-iliac joints and connect the sacrum and the inside of the ilial wing. Movement in the sacro-iliac joints normally is negligible. In fact, there are even fibrous bands within the joint that help to hold it together and resist movement.

There is constant compression on the sacro-iliac joints and tension on the sacro-iliac ligaments while the horse is standing and moving. The more strenuous the activity, the more stress is placed on these structures. Speed combined with sharp turns or quick stops is most stressful. Such demanding activities can cause malalignment of a sacro-iliac joint, a condition called sacro-iliac subluxation (partial dislocation). In many cases chiropractic manipulation can restore the sacro-iliac joint to its normal position. However, if the sacro-iliac ligaments are stretched or torn, chronic joint instability can result.

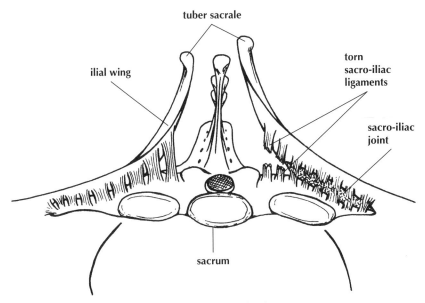

Fig. 22–19. The sacro-iliac area, viewed from the front.

Extra Information	
Abnormality	**Percentage of Horses Affected**
Over-riding spinous processes (lumbar)	92% (average of 4 vertebrae involved)
Degenerative joint disease in intervertebral joints	100%
Degenerative joint disease in sacro-iliac joints	100%
Asymmetric tuber sacrale	92% (1 – 10 mm difference) 8% (over 10 mm difference)
Stress fractures in spine or pelvis	50%

Fig. 22–20. A recent study of Thoroughbred racehorses found various abnormalities in the lower back or pelvis. Note: None of these horses showed obvious signs of back pain.

This condition can develop suddenly if the horse slips, falls, or flips over and lands on the top or side of its rump. In other cases it is the product of repeated strain on these ligaments.

Joint instability causes pain when the horse is moving, as does tension on a strained or torn sacro-iliac ligaments. The muscles in the lumbo-sacral area may spasm as a result of constantly trying to improve the stability and reduce the pain in the sacro-iliac area. This contributes to the horse's pain. Over time, degenerative joint disease can also develop in the damaged sacro-iliac joint. In racehorses, incomplete, or "stress" fractures are occasionally found in the ilium, over or next to the sacro-iliac joint *(see Chapter 21)*.

Signs and Diagnosis of Sacro-iliac Subluxation

Sacro-iliac joint or ligament damage causes chronic, low-grade pain, which may be seen as vague hindlimb lameness. Sometimes the horse merely shows a reluctance to perform its normal activities. For example, a dressage horse may be unwilling to perform an extended trot, or a show jumper may refuse jumps. A Standardbred racehorse may be reluctant to stride out, and so its race performance suffers.

The sacro-iliac joints are at least 5 inches (over 12 cm) below the tops of the tuber sacrale, in between the wings of the ilium. So, it is not possible to palpate this area or detect heat or swelling associated with it. Nevertheless, there are a few signs that the veterinarian uses to diagnose this condition.

Uneven Tuber Sacrale

When one of the sacro-iliac ligaments is overstretched or torn, the tuber sacrale become uneven in height: the damaged side is higher. This is easiest to see when standing behind the horse. To ensure that this observation is accurate, it is important to have the horse standing as square as possible on a level surface, with its weight evenly distributed on both hindlegs. Both hindfeet must be together, and the horse must not be resting a leg. It is easy to mistakenly conclude

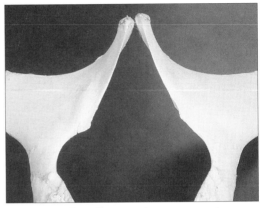

Fig. 22–21. The tuber sacrale are uneven in height. (The sacrum has been removed.)

that the tuber sacrale are uneven if the horse is not standing squarely.

Chronic sacro-iliac problems can also cause muscle atrophy (wasting) over the top of the rump, which makes the tuber sacrale stand out. This is called "hunter's bumps" or "jumper's bumps." These names illustrate the fact that sacro-iliac problems are more commonly seen in horses that perform strenuous or demanding activities. However, horses in poor body condition or with poor muscle tone from lack of regular exercise may also have prominent tuber sacrale. Thus, the asymmetry (difference in height) of these bony prominences is the most important piece of information.

Pain

If the sacro-iliac area is painful, pressure with the fingers or hand over the tuber sacrale may cause the horse to crouch away from the pressure. Sometimes it is easiest to place the thumb beside one tuber and the fingers beside the other and press down on both sides at the same time. This action puts pressure on the sacro-iliac joints, so if there is any pain or instability it causes an evasive response.

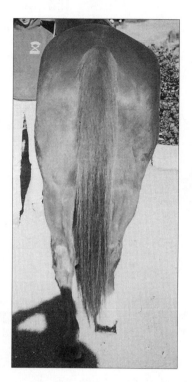

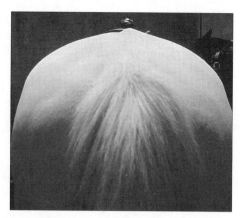

Fig. 22–22. Left: It is hard to tell if the tuber sacrale are even because the horse is not standing squarely. Above: The tuber sacrale of this roping horse are definitely uneven.

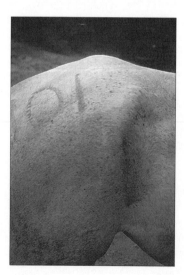

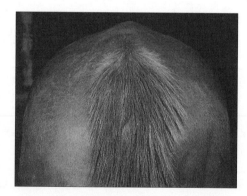

Fig. 22–23. Left: Chronic sacro-iliac problems can cause hunter's bumps. Above: Thin, poorly-muscled horses also have prominent tuber sacrale.

Other Tests

These signs usually are all that is necessary to make the diagnosis. However, if there is any doubt that the lameness is caused by the sacro-iliac problem, the veterinarian has a couple of other options. Lifting each hindleg in turn and raising it as high as possible often causes the horse pain, and it may also cause or worsen the lameness. Injecting local anesthetic directly into the sacro-iliac area may temporarily improve the lameness. But nuclear scintigraphy is likely to be more useful, and has less risk of infection.

Although lameness may result from sacro-iliac pain, horses with this condition often have other chronic hindlimb problems, such as bone spavin *(see Chapter 20)*. A thorough physical examination and gait evaluation are worthwhile in horses with sacro-iliac pain. Other causes of hindlimb lameness or back pain should be considered during this process.

Treatment of Sacro-iliac Subluxation

The pain and lameness may be due to ligament strain. But they could also be due to instability in the sacro-iliac joint, DJD, or a

stress fracture. Treatment should initially involve rest in a stall and/or small paddock for at least 6 weeks. The strained or torn ligaments, joint capsule, and bone must be given a chance to heal. Daily hand-walking is of benefit during this rest period in horses that are confined to a stall.

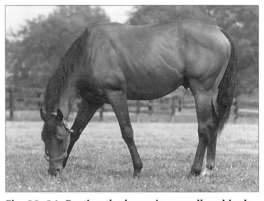

Fig. 22–24. Resting the horse in a small paddock gives the injured tissues time to heal.

Exercise

After this time, regular exercise is very important in restoring and maintaining the horse's usefulness. Extended rest periods do little to help this condition. Although the ligaments may eventually heal, they are not as strong as they were originally, so return to exercise after even months of rest may result in recurrence of the pain and lameness. This is because the sacro-iliac joints are also supported by the muscles in the lumbosacral area and over the top of the rump.

Long periods of inactivity (including pasture rest) result in loss of muscle tone and bulk, so the compromised joint loses yet another of its stabilizers.

Building up the muscles that support the sacro-iliac joints can restore some stability to the area. After the initial rest period, a program of gradually increasing, light exercise is usually more helpful than pasture turnout. Provided the horse is not lame, easy hill work or cavaletti work can help strengthen these muscles. Strenuous activities, such as jumping, working in deep sand, and steep hill work, should be avoided.

Medications

NSAIDs can make the horse more comfortable and willing to exercise. Some horses also improve when given intramuscular Adequan or oral GAGs *(see Chapter 5)*. Injecting corticosteroids into the sacro-iliac ligaments can help resolve the pain. However, it is counter-productive to continue working the horse without giving the ligaments time to heal. Further damage will likely result because this treatment does not improve the stability of the sacro-iliac joint. In fact, corticosteroids slow healing, so they can work against regaining joint stability.

Some veterinarians have attempted to strengthen these ligaments by injecting an irritant substance into them. The aim was to encourage fibrosis (thickening with fibrous tissue). However, more common results were increased pain and infection.

Other Options

Chiropractic manipulation and acupuncture can sometimes provide relief in these horses. But because the condition is caused by instability and excessive movement in a joint that should be essentially immobile, these therapies are unlikely to result in a permanent cure. In fact, improper chiropractic manipulation may cause further strain or damage to the ligaments.

Prognosis for Sacro-iliac Subluxation

Unless the sacro-iliac ligaments were only strained, the prognosis for high level athletic function without recurrent or persistent problems is guarded. The healed ligaments are not as strong or resilient as undamaged ligaments, so reinjury is fairly common in these horses. Also, because the early signs are vague, the problem may have been present for several months. Chronic problems are more difficult to resolve than acute injuries. Even with medications and the recommended exercise program, the horse may not be able to withstand training and competition at its former level.

FLIP-OVER INJURIES

"Flip-over" injuries occur when a horse flips over backward and injures its back, neck, or head. This is a fairly common injury in young horses, especially when they are first taught to tie. It also occurs during trailering, particularly when loading or unloading a nervous or unwilling horse. Occasionally, a horse may fall over backward when it rears or runs backward to avoid being caught. Sometimes a fall over a solid jump may cause a horse to flip forward and injure its spine.

The common denominators in most flip-over injuries are:

1. Force—the horse either pulls back hard against the object to which it is tied, or it runs backward quickly.
2. Insufficient traction—e.g. a slippery surface (such as concrete or wet rubber matting), and steel or aluminum shoes.

In general, the more force that is used to escape, the more damage the horse is likely to sustain. The type of surface the horse lands on can also be a factor in the degree of damage it sustains. More damage is likely when falling on a hard surface, such as concrete, than on a softer surface, such as sand or grass.

A horse may damage any part of its neck or back when it flips over. The likely location and severity of the damage are determined by the intensity of the force used to escape. This fact depends on:

- how securely the horse is tied
- how determined it is to break free
- how much force is required to break the equipment (halter, lead, buckles or clips) or hitching post
- how quickly the horse runs backward

Injury to the Tail Base

When only a little force is needed to escape, the horse may fall back onto its buttocks and the base of its tail, without flipping all the way over. For example, while being loaded into the trailer, the horse pulls back against the person holding the lead rope. If the person lets go or is pulled off balance, or if the halter breaks, the horse may fall back and land on its tail base.

This injury can result in fracture of the first few coccygeal vertebrae, or occasionally, the last part of the sacrum. The result is pain around the tail base and a reluctance or inability to move the tail. The nerves that supply the hindlimbs leave the spinal column further forward (in the lumbo-sacral area and the first part of the sacrum). So gait abnormalities are not often seen with this injury. The fractured vertebrae usually heal in 6 – 8 weeks, sometimes leaving a small depression (or a depression and a hard lump) at the tail base. The tail may also be crooked. Depending on the degree of damage to the nerves that control tail movement, the horse may lose the use of, and feeling in its tail. It may be left with a low tail carriage and a soiled tail. However, some tail base fractures heal without these harmless, but unsightly results.

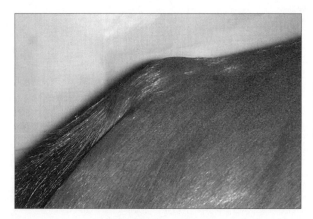

Fig. 22–25. Fracture of the tail base may leave a depression and a lump.

Injury to the Rump or Withers

If, in the previous example, the person had looped the lead rope once or twice around the breast bar of the trailer, the horse must use more force to break free. In this case the horse is more likely to flip over and land on its back if the person lets go or the equipment breaks. The first point of contact with the ground usually is the top of the rump (the sacrum or the bony prominences at the top of the pelvis). The second point is the withers.

Falling onto the top of the rump may damage the sacrum, pelvis *(see Chapter 21)*, or one of the sacro-iliac joints if the horse lands unevenly. But more commonly, it is the withers that are damaged.

Fractured Withers

A horse that flips over this way may fracture some of the dorsal spinous processes that form the withers. Fracture of these spinous processes results in swelling and severe pain during palpation. The

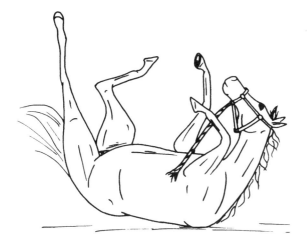

Fig. 22–26. If the lead breaks, the horse may land on its withers.

withers may appear misshapen or flattened, and when radiographs are taken, fractures may be seen in at least two spinous processes. The horse may not be obviously lame, although in most cases it is stiff and reluctant to move around for several days. Tension on the

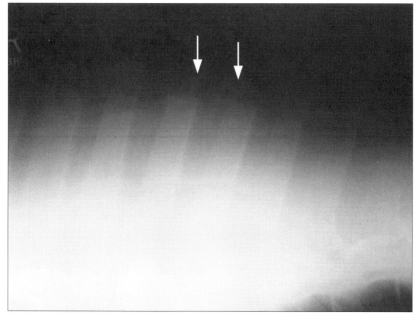

Fig. 22–27. Two spinous processes are fractured at the withers.

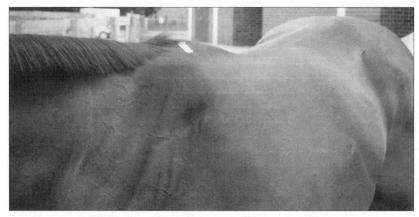

Fig. 22–28. Fractured spinous processes can leave the withers flattened.

fractured spinous processes from the nuchal ligament often makes the horse reluctant to lower its head to the ground to eat or drink.

Treatment and Prognosis for Fractured Withers

This injury usually heals with 2 – 3 months of paddock rest. It is important during the first few weeks to supply the horse with food and water at chest level if it will not lower its head all the way to the ground.

The prognosis for return to full athletic function usually is good. Once the fractures have healed, most horses do not resent the saddle because in most cases it sits behind the fractured spinous processes. Back pain usually does not persist, and the horse is able to return to its former level of performance. However, the distinctive flattened appearance of the withers may remain.

Injury to the Poll

A more serious injury can occur when the horse is securely tied to a solid object, such as a tree or fence post. It can also occur when the horse runs backward and slips. In these instances the horse generates explosive force, and in the process it may flip over and land on its poll. This can damage the first part of the neck or the skull. The first few cervical vertebrae may be fractured or dislocated. Or, the force of impact may stretch or tear the ligaments that support the intervertebral joints. This could allow subluxation (partial disloca-

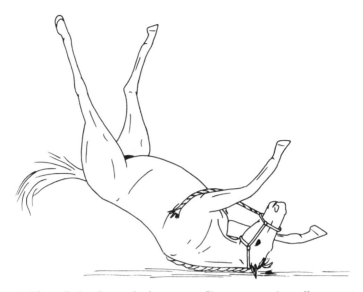

Fig. 22–29. With explosive force, the horse may flip over onto its poll.

tion) of the vertebrae. Each of these conditions can compress the spinal cord, causing various neurologic abnormalities, or even complete paralysis.

If the horse lands on its poll with sufficient force to fracture its skull, bone fragments may cause enough brain damage to kill the horse instantly. Bleeding from the ears or nostrils is sometimes seen with this type of injury. Clear cerebrospinal fluid may

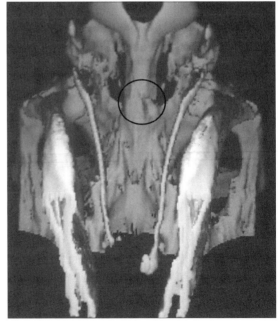

Fig. 22–30. A CT image of a fracture in the base of the skull, looking up toward the roof of the mouth.

More Information

Conditions of the brain, spinal cord, and peripheral nerves are discussed in Chapter 12.

instead be seen draining from the ears in some horses. In other cases the force may reverberate through the skull and fracture the bone along the floor of the cranium (the bony cavity that encloses the brain). This fracture can damage the brainstem, which is the area of the brain that controls consciousness. Damage to the brainstem can result in a coma. Damage to other parts of the brain and the cranial nerves may also occur. It is not uncommon for horses that recover from such an injury to be left with a temporary or permanent neurologic abnormality, such as a head tilt, blindness, or incoordination.

Whiplash Injury

There is another type of "pull-back" injury that may occur during transport. If the horse's head is securely tied with a fairly short lead or cross-ties, and the driver accelerates rapidly, the horse's hindfeet can slip forward underneath it. The horse may be thrown back onto its hocks or buttocks until it scrambles to its feet. This has a reverse "whiplash" effect on the vertebrae in the thoraco-lumbar area. The spine is suddenly wrenched into overextension, and the supporting intervertebral ligaments may be strained or torn. Presumably, sudden, forced extension of the intervertebral joints could also damage the intervertebral discs. However, this injury is very difficult to confirm in horses.

Muscle spasms and pain over the lumbar area are the usual findings during palpation. A vague hindlimb lameness may be seen, but more often the horse just resents the saddle and is reluctant to perform its normal activities. In severe cases the spinal cord may be bruised, which could result in some temporary neurologic abnormalities in the hindlimbs.

Treatment usually involves:

- a few weeks of rest from regular training
- anti-inflammatory therapy, e.g. NSAIDs, DMSO, or corticosteroids
- daily physical therapy, e.g. massage, heat therapy, magnetic field therapy, etc.

(These treatments are discussed in Section II: Principles of Therapy.)

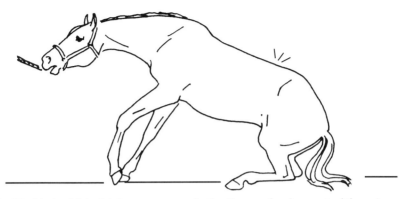

Fig. 22–31. A whiplash injury can occur in the thoraco-lumbar part of the spine.

Daily hand-walking or pasture turnout can help relieve the muscle spasms surrounding the damaged vertebrae, and ensure that the spinal column maintains its flexibility as the injury heals. Complete stall confinement can result in fibrosis (thickening with fibrous tissue) around the damaged intervertebral joints. This reduces the range of motion in that part of the spine. When regular exercise resumes, galloping, jumping, tight circles, steep hills, and sliding stops should be avoided for a few weeks to minimize strain on the previously injured area.

For the most part, each of these "flip-over" or "pull-back" injuries can be prevented by taking care when tying and transporting horses, especially if they are young, inexperienced, or nervous.

APPENDIX

Parts of the Horse

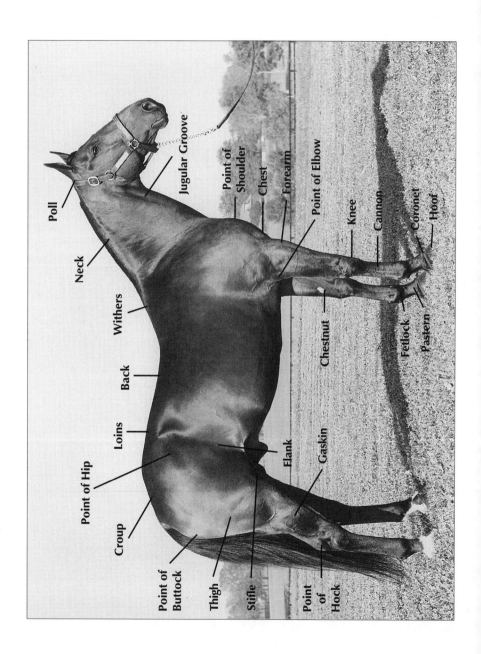

Skeleton of the Horse

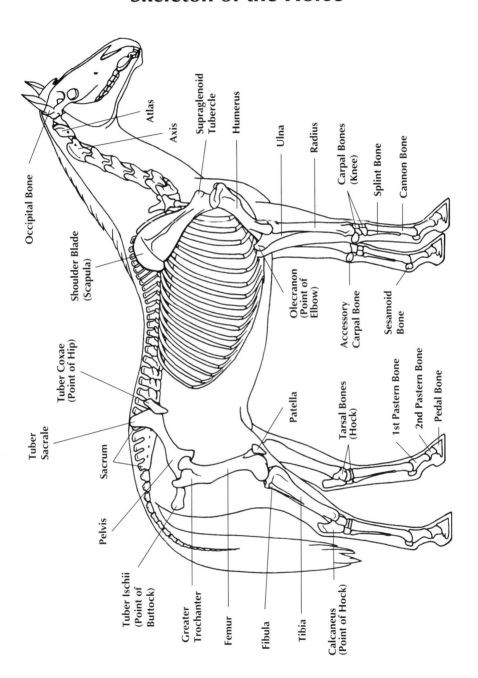

Occipital Bone
Atlas
Axis
Supraglenoid Tubercle
Humerus
Ulna
Radius
Carpal Bones (Knee)
Splint Bone
Cannon Bone
Shoulder Blade (Scapula)
Olecranon (Point of Elbow)
Accessory Carpal Bone
Sesamoid Bone
Tuber Coxae (Point of Hip)
Tuber Sacrale
Sacrum
Pelvis
Patella
Tarsal Bones (Hock)
1st Pastern Bone
2nd Pastern Bone
Pedal Bone
Tuber Ischii (Point of Buttock)
Greater Trochanter
Femur
Fibula
Tibia
Calcaneus (Point of Hock)

Directional Terms

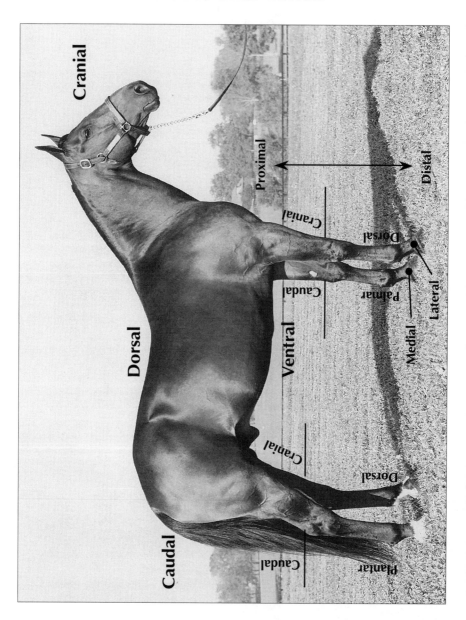

Weights and Measures Conversion Tables

Length

1 mm = 0.04 inch
1 cm = 0.4 inch
1 inch = 25.4 mm
1 inch = 2.54 cm
1 foot = 30.5 cm
1 foot = 0.305 meter
1 yard = 0.914 meter
1 meter = 3.3 feet
1 meter = 1.1 yards
1 mile = 1.609 km
1 mile = 8.0 furlongs
1 furlong = 0.13 mile
1 furlong = 220.0 yards
1 km = 0.6 mile

Volume

1 ounce = 0.13 cup
1 ounce = 29 ml
1 cup = 8.0 ounces
1 pint = 0.5 quarts
1 quart = 0.95 liter
1 quart = 0.25 gallon
1 ml = 1 cc
1 liter = 1.057 quarts
1 liter = 0.264 gallon
1 gallon = 3.79 liters

Weight

1 mg = 0.001 g
1 mg/kg = 0.4536 mg/lb
1 gram = 0.002 pounds
1 gram = 0.04 ounces
1 ounce = 28.35 grams
1 pound = 453.62 grams
1 pound = 0.4536 kilograms
1 kilogram = 2.20 pounds

Temperature

97.5°F =	36.4°C	101.9°F =	38.8°C
97.9°F =	36.6°C	102.3°F =	39°C
98.3°F =	36.8°C	102.7°F =	39.3°C
98.7°F =	37.0°C	103.1°F =	39.5°C
99.1°F =	37.3°C	103.5°F =	39.7°C
99.5°F =	37.5°C	103.9°F =	39.9°C
99.9°F =	37.7°C	104.3°F =	40.2°C
100.3°F =	37.9°C	104.7°F =	40.4°C
100.7°F =	38.2°C	105.1°F =	40.6°C
101.1°F =	38.4°C	105.5°F =	40.8°C
101.5°F =	38.6°C	105.9°F =	41.0°C

°F to °C: subtract 32 from °F and multiply by 0.556
°C to °F: multiply C° by 1.8 and add 32

Alternate Anatomic Terms

Structure	Alternate Terms
pedal bone	coffin bone, third phalanx, P3
navicular bone	distal sesamoid bone
coffin joint	distal interphalangeal joint
second pastern bone	short pastern bone, middle pastern bone, second phalanx, P2
pastern joint	proximal interphalangeal joint
first pastern bone	long pastern bone, first phalanx, P1
distal sesamoidean ligaments	XYZ ligaments
fetlock	ankle
fetlock joint	metacarpophalangeal joint (forelimb) metatarsophalangeal joint (hindlimb)
sesamoid bones	proximal sesamoid bones
palmar pouch (fetlock joint)	volar pouch
cannon bone	third metacarpal bone (forelimb), MCIII third metatarsal bone (hindlimb), MTIII
splint bones	second (medial) or fourth (lateral), metacarpal bones (forelimb), MCII or MCIV, second or fourth metatarsal bones (hindlimb), MTII or MTIV
suspensory ligament	interosseus muscle
inferior check ligament	carpal check ligament (forelimb), subtarsal check ligament (hindlimb)
intercarpal joint	midcarpal joint
radiocarpal joint	antebrachiocarpal joint
superior check ligament	radial check ligament
shoulder joint	scapulohumeral joint
tibiotarsal joint	tarsocrural joint
Achilles tendons	common calcanean tendon
hip joint	coxofemoral joint
tuber coxae	hook bone
tuber sacrale	sacral tubers
tuber ischii	ischiatic tuberosity, pin bone
coccygeal vertebrae	caudal vertebrae

List of Abbreviations

ALD Angular limb deformity
A-O Atlanto-occipital
AST Aspartate aminotransferase
°C Degrees Celcius, or Centigrade
C3 Third carpal bone
Ca:P Calcium-phosphorus ratio
cc Cubic centimeter
cm Centimeter
CNS Central nervous system
COPD Chronic obstructive pulmonary disease
CPK Creatine phosphokinase
CSF Cerebrospinal fluid
CT Computerized tomography
CVM Cervical Vertebral Malformation
DCP Dicalcium phosphate
DDFT Deep digital flexor tendon
DJD Degenerative joint disease
DMG Dimethyl glycine
DMSO Dimethyl sulfoxide
DNA Deoxyribonucleic acid
DOD Developmental orthopedic disorder
E. coli Escherichia coli
ECG Electrocardiogram
EDM Equine Degenerative Myelopathy
EEE Eastern Equine Encephalitis
EHV-1 Equine Herpesvirus type 1
EIA Equine Infectious Anemia
EMG Electromyography
EMND Equine Motor Neuron Disease
EPM Equine Protozoal Myeloencephalitis
ER Exertional rhabdomyolysis
EVA Equine Viral Arteritis
°F Defrees Fahrenheit
FE Urinary fractional excretion
F-P Femoropatellar
F-T Femorotibial
ft Feet
GAG Glycosaminoglycan
GTN Glyceryl trinitrate
HA Hyaluronic acid

HPP Hyperkalemic periodic paralysis
HO Hypertrophic osteopathy
IA Intra-articular, intra-articularly
ICL Inferior check ligament
IM Intramuscular, intramuscularly
IV Intravenous, intravenously
kg Kilogram
LEM Leukoencephalomalacia
L-S Lumbo-sacral
m Meter
mg Milligram
ml Milliliter
mm Millimeter
MRI Magnetic resonance imaging
MSM Methyl sulfonylmethane
NSAID Nonsteroidal anti-inflammatory drug
NSH Nutritional secondary hyperparathyroidism
OCD Osteochondritis dissecans
P1 1st phalanx, or pastern bone
P2 2nd phalanx, or pastern bone
P3 3rd phalanx; pedal bone
PBZ Phenylbutazone
PCR Polymerase chain reaction
PD Palmar Digital
PG Prostaglandin
PGE2 Prostaglandin E-2
PGI2 Prostaglandin I-2
PSGAG Polysulfated glycosaminoglycan
PTH Parathyroid hormone
SC Subcutaneous, subcutaneously
SDFT Superficial digital flexor tendon
SMZ Trimethoprim-sulfonamide
T3 Third tarsal bone or tri-iodothyronine (thyroid hormone)
T4 Thyroxin (thyroid hormone)
Tc Central tarsal bone
TENS Transcutaneous electrical nerve stimulation
TMPS Trimethoprim-sulfonamide
TSH Thyroid stimulating hormone
VEE Venezuelan Equine Encephalitis
VS Vesicular stomatitis
WEE Western Equine Encephalitis

Degrees of Lameness

Grade	Signs
Grade 1	Subtle lameness; may be inconsistent. Not apparent at the walk, and may not even be consistently seen at the trot.
Grade 2	Consistent, mild lameness at the trot.
Grade 3	Consistent, moderate lameness at the trot, with an obvious head nod (foreleg lameness) or hip hike (hindleg lameness).
Grade 4	Obvious lameness at the walk and trot, with a shortened stride and a pronounced head nod or hip hike. The horse is reluctant to trot.
Grade 5	Severe lameness; extremely reluctant or unable to bear weight on the affected leg during motion and at rest ("three-legged lame").

Lameness is described as the grade out of 5, for example, 3 of 5.

Understanding the Prognosis

The prognosis is the likelihood that the horse will recover satisfactorily. Sometimes it is possible for the veterinarian to be very precise; for example, the horse has a 75% chance of complete recovery. This figure usually is based on the veterinarian's experience with that condition, or on the results of scientific studies. However, many times it is not possible to be specific, and the prognosis is expressed in general terms.

The prognosis depends on the condition being treated. But it also varies with the horse and the circumstances. Thus, with very few exceptions, general terms are used throughout this book. These terms, and the approximate percentages they represent, are listed below.

Prognosis	Chance of Recovery
excellent	over 90% chance of full recovery
very good	over 80% chance of full recovery
good	over 70% chance of full recovery
fair	over 60% chance of full recovery
guarded	about a 50% chance of satisfactory recovery
poor	less than about 40% chance of satisfactory recovery
grave	little or no chance of recovery

Bibliography

Textbooks

Barragry, T.B. *Veterinary Drug Therapy.* Lea and Febiger, Philadelphia, PA, 1994.

Bramlage, L.R., Meagher, D.M., O'Brien, T.R., and Pool, R.R. "Athletic Injuries in the Performance Horse." *Proceedings of the 13th Bain-Fallon Memorial Lectures,* Australian Equine Veterinary Association, 1991.

Bromiley, M. *Equine Injury, Therapy and Rehabilitation.* Blackwell Science Ltd, Oxford, England, 1993.

Bromiley, M. *Natural Methods for Equine Health.* Blackwell Science Ltd, Oxford, England, 1994.

Butler, D. *The Principles of Horseshoeing II.* Butler Publishing, LaPorte, CO, 1985.

Clayton, H.M. *Conditioning Sport Horses.* Sport Horse Publications, Saskatoon, Saskatchewan, Canada, 1991.

Colahan, P.T., Mayhew, I.G., Merritt, A.M., and Moore, J.N., eds. *Equine Medicine and Surgery.* Fourth Edition. American Veterinary Publications, Inc., Goleta, CA, 1991.

Davies, H.M.S. *The Adaptive Response of the Equine Metacarpus to Locomotory Stress.* PhD Thesis, University of Melbourne, Australia, 1995.

Denoix, J.M. and Pailloux, J.P. *Physical Therapy and Massage for the Horse.* Trafalgar Square Publishing, North Pomfret, VT, 1996.

Getty, R., ed. *Sisson and Grossman's The Anatomy of the Domestic Animals.* Fifth Edition. W.B. Saunders Company, Philadelphia, PA, 1975.

Goodman Gilman, A., Rall, T.W., Nies, A.S., and Taylor, P., eds. *Goodman and Gilman's The Pharmacological Basis of Therapeutics.* Pergamon Press, New York, NY, 1991.

Harris, S.E. *Horse Gaits, Balance and Movement.* Howell Book House, New York, NY, 1993.

Hodgson, D.R. and Rose, R.J., eds. *The Athletic Horse: principles and practice of equine sports medicine.* W.B. Saunders Company, Philadelphia, PA, 1994.

Kobluk, C.N., Ames, T.R., and Geor, R.J., eds. *The Horse: diseases and clinical management.* W.B. Saunders Company, Philadelphia, PA, 1995.

Krook, L. and Maylin, G.A. *Race Horses at Risk* The Authors, Ithaca, NY, 1989.

Lameness in Equine Practice. Veterinary Learning Systems, Trenton, NJ, 1993.

Lane, J.G. and Dyson, S.J. "Equine Head and Hindlimb Medicine and Surgery." *Proceedings of the 15th Bain-Fallon Memorial Lectures,* Australian Equine Veterinary Association, 1993.

Mayhew, I.G. *Large Animal Neurology: a handbook for veterinary clinicians.* Lea and Febiger, Philadelphia, PA, 1989.

Mayhew, I.G. and Jackson, S.G. "Equine Neurology and Nutrition." *Proceedings of the 18th Bain-Fallon Memorial Lectures,* Australian Equine Veterinary Association, 1996.

Nichols, N., ed. *Detection of Therapeutic Substances in Racing Horses.* Australian Equine Veterinary Association, Sydney, Australia, 1992 (with updates to 1996).

Nutrient Requirements of Horses, 5th edition. National Research Council, Washington DC, 1989.

Pool, R.R. and Hurtig, M.B. "Pathogenesis of Equine Osteochondrosis." In *Joint Disease in the Horse,* McIlwraith, C.W. and Trotter, G.W. eds., W.B. Saunders Company, Philadelphia, PA, 1996.

Price, H. and Fisher, R. *Shoeing for Performance in the Sound and Lame Horse.* Trafalgar Square Publishing, North Pomfret, VT, 1989.

Proceedings of the American Association of Equine Practitioners, 1991– 1996.

Redden, R., ed. *Lecture Notes from the 10th Annual Bluegrass Laminitis Symposium,* International Equine Podiatary Center, Inc., Versailles, KY, 1996.

Robinson, N.E., ed. *Current Therapy in Equine Medicine 2.* W.B. Saunders Company, Philadelphia, PA, 1987.

Robinson, N.E., ed. *Current Therapy in Equine Medicine 3.* W.B. Saunders Company, Philadelphia, PA, 1992.

Rose, R.J. and Hodgson, D.R. *Manual of Equine Practice.* W.B. Saunders Company, Philadelphia, PA, 1993.

Smith, B.P., ed. *Large Animal Internal Medicine.* The C.V. Mosby Company, St Louis, MO, 1990.

Stashak, T.S. *Adams' Lameness in Horses.* Fourth Edition. Lea and Febiger, Philadelphia, PA, 1987.

Wagoner, D.M., ed. *Feeding to Win II.* Equine Research, Inc., 1992.

White, N.A. and Moore, J.N. *Current Practice of Equine Surgery.* J.B. Lippincott Company, Philadelphia, PA, 1990.

Veterinary Journals

American Journal of Veterinary Research, American Veterinary Medical Association, Schaumburg, IL.

Australian Equine Veterinarian, Australian Equine Veterinary Association, Sydney, Australia.

Australian Veterinary Journal, Australian Veterinary Association, Sydney, Australia.

Compendium on Continuing Education for the Practicing Veterinarian, Veterinary Learning Systems, Trenton, NJ.

Equine Practice, Veterinary Practice Publishing Company, Santa Barbara, CA.

Equine Veterinary Education, Equine Veterinary Journal Ltd, Newmarket, Suffolk, England.

Equine Veterinary Journal, Equine Veterinary Journal Ltd, Newmarket, Suffolk, England.

Journal of Equine Veterinary Science, William E. Jones, DVM, PhD, Wildomar, CA.

Journal of the American Veterinary Medical Association, American Veterinary Medical Association, Schaumburg, IL.

Figure Credits

Artwork by Dr. Robin Peterson, Dr. Marilyn Todd-Daniels, Tom Terrell, and Dawn Walker.

Thanks to Dr. Rick DeBowes, Kansas State University, for his photo contributions.

Figure 1–1. J. Noye.
Figure 1–2. Equine Sports Graphics, Inc.
Figure 1–5. Courtesy of the United States Trotting Association.
Figure 2–1. J. Noye.
Figure 2–9. Courtesy of Dr. Rebecca McConnico, Oklahoma State University.
Figure 2–17. Courtesy of Dr. Rebecca McConnico, Oklahoma State University.
Figure 2–18. Courtesy of Dr. Dan Steinheimer, Texas A&M University.
Figure 2–19. Courtesy of Dr. Rebecca McConnico, Oklahoma State University.
Figure 2–23. Courtesy of Dr. Karl Bowman, North Carolina State University.
Figure 2–24. Courtesy of Dr. Kathy Spalding, North Carolina State University.
Figure 2–25. Courtesy of Dr. Kathy Spalding, North Carolina State University.
Figure 2–26. Courtesy of Dr. Kathy Spalding, North Carolina State University.
Figure 2–28. Courtesy of Equine Only, Inc.
Figure 2–29. Courtesy of Dr. David Schmitz, Texas A&M University.
Figure 2–30. Courtesy of Dr. David Schmitz, Texas A&M University.
Figure 2–31. Courtesy of Dr. Dan Steinheimer, Texas A&M University.
Figure 2–32. Courtesy of Dr. Dan Steinheimer, Texas A&M University.
Figure 2–35. Courtesy of Veterinary Services, Inc.
Figure 2–36. Courtesy of Dr. Barrie Grant, San Luis Rey Equine Hospital.
Figure 2–37. Courtesy of Tom Ivers.
Figure 2–38. Courtesy of Laurie Fio, University of California, Davis.
Figure 3–1. J. Noye.
Figure 3–2. Cappy Jackson.
Figure 3–3. Courtesy of *Quarter Week.*
Figure 3–4. Katey Barrett.
Figure 3–6. Courtesy of the American Quarter Horse Association.
Figure 3–8. Barbara Ann Giove.
Figure 4–1. Barbara Ann Giove.
Figure 4–3. J. Noye.
Figure 4–4. Cappy Jackson.
Figure 4–5. Susan Lustig.
Figure 4–6. J. Noye.
Figure 4–7. Charlene Strickland.
Figure 4–10. Courtesy of Dr. Kathy Spalding, North Carolina State University.
Figure 4–19. J. Noye.
Figure 4–20. Kendra Bond.
Figure 4–21. Courtesy of Dr. Rebecca McConnico, Oklahoma State University.
Figure 4–24. Courtesy of Dr. Rebecca McConnico, Oklahoma State University.
Figure 4–26. Mimi Porter, Equine Therapy.
Figure 4–30. Mimi Porter, Equine Therapy.
Figure 4–31. Barbara Ann Giove.
Figure 4–32. Mimi Porter, Equine Therapy.
Figure 4–35. Courtesy of Dr. Rebecca McConnico, Oklahoma State University.
Figure 5–7. J. Noye.
Figure 5–9. Don Shugart.
Figure 5–14. Courtesy of Dr. Eleanor Green, University of Florida.

Figure 5–18. Cathy Nelson.
Figure 6–1. Courtesy of Dr. Barrie Grant, San Luis Rey Equine Hospital.
Figure 6–4. Barbara Ann Giove.
Figure 6–6. Courtesy of Dr. Kathy Spalding, North Carolina State University.
Figure 6–7. Courtesy of Dr. Rebecca McConnico, Oklahoma State University.
Figure 6–8. Courtesy of Dr. Rebecca McConnico, Oklahoma State University.
Figure 6–11. Courtesy of 3-M Animal Care Products.
Figure 7–1. Katey Barrett.
Figure 7–8. Courtesy of Dr. Ric Redden, International Equine Podiatry Center.
Figure 7–12. Cappy Jackson.
Figure 7–14. Courtesy of the United States Trotting Association.
Figure 7–15. Courtesy of the American Quarter Horse Association.
Figure 7–16. Kendra Bond.
Figure 7–19. Courtesy of W-Brand Products.
Figure 7–22. Courtesy of Dr. Karl Bowman, North Carolina State University.
Figure 7–23. Barbara Ann Giove.
Figure 7–25. Courtesy of Dr. Nancy Loving.
Figure 7–30. Courtesy of Dr. Ric Redden, International Equine Podiatry Center.
Figure 7–39. Courtesy of Dr. Karl Bowman, North Carolina State University.
Figure 7–53. Courtesy of Dr. Rebecca McConnico, Oklahoma State University.
Figure 7–55. Courtesy of Dr. Rebecca McConnico, Oklahoma State University.
Figure 7–60, top left. Courtesy of Dr. Rebecca McConnico, Oklahoma State University.
Figure 7–60, top right. Courtesy of Dr. Ric Redden, Int'l Equine Podiatry Center.
Figure 7–60, bottom left. Courtesy of Dr. Rebecca McConnico, Oklahoma State University.
Figure 7–63. Carol Kaelson.
Figure 8–1. Katey Barrett.
Figure 8–3. Courtesy of Dr. Kathy Spalding, North Carolina State University.
Figure 8–5. Equine Sports Graphics, Inc.
Figure 8–12, top left. Courtesy of Dr. Gary Nies, Oklahoma State University.
Figure 8–13. Courtesy of the American Quarter Horse Association.
Figure 8–16. Barbara Ann Giove.
Figure 8–18. Courtesy of the American Quarter Horse Association.
Figure 8–19. Charlene Strickland.
Figure 8–20. J. Noye.
Figure 8–21. Barbara Ann Giove.
Figure 8–23. Courtesy of Dr. Charles MacAllister, Oklahoma State University.
Figure 8–24. Courtesy of Dr. Rebecca McConnico, Oklahoma State University.
Figure 8–26. J. Noye.
Figure 8–28. Courtesy of Dr. Kathy Spalding, North Carolina State University.
Figure 9–1. Courtesy of *Quarter Week*.
Figure 9–6. Cathy Nelson.
Figure 9–12. Courtesy of Dr. Kathy Spalding, North Carolina State University.
Figure 9–14. Cappy Jackson.
Figure 9–16. Cappy Jackson.
Figure 9–18. Courtesy of Dr. Kathy Spalding, North Carolina State University.
Figure 9–19. Courtesy of Dr. Kathy Spalding, North Carolina State University.
Figure 9–21. Courtesy of Dr. Rebecca McConnico, Oklahoma State University.
Figure 9–23. Courtesy of Dr. Barrie Grant, San Luis Rey Equine Hospital.
Figure 9– 24. Courtesy of *Quarter Week*.
Figure 9–25. Courtesy of Dr. Rebecca McConnico, Oklahoma State University.
Figure 9–27. Courtesy of Dr. Kathy Spalding, North Carolina State University.
Figure 9–28. Barbara Ann Giove.

Figure 9–29, right. Courtesy of Dr. Kathy Spalding, North Carolina State University.
Figure 9–32. J. Noye.
Figure 10–1. J. Noye.
Figure 10–5. Cathy Nelson.
Figure 10–6. Courtesy of Cindy Dawkins.
Figure 10–9. Barbara Ann Giove.
Figure 10–12. Courtesy of the American Quarter Horse Association.
Figure 10–14. J. Noye.
Figure 10–18. Katey Barrett.
Figure 10–19. Barbara Ann Giove.
Figure 10–21. Courtesy of Darolyn Butler.
Figure 10–22. J. Noye.
Figure 10–29. Courtesy of the American Quarter Horse Association.
Figure 11–1. Barbara Ann Giove.
Figure 11–8. Cappy Jackson.
Figure 11–11. Courtesy of Dr. Nancy Loving.
Figure 11–12. Courtesy of Dr. David Schmitz, Texas A&M University.
Figure 11–13. Courtesy of Dr. David Schmitz, Texas A&M University.
Figure 11–16. J. Noye.
Figure 11–22. Courtesy of Dr. Rebecca McConnico, Oklahoma State University.
Figure 11–26. Courtesy of Dr. Kathy Spalding, North Carolina State University.
Figure 11–31. Courtesy of the United States Trotting Association.
Figure 12–1. Courtesy of Darolyn Butler.
Figure 12–8. Courtesy of Dr. Rebecca McConnico, Oklahoma State University.
Figure 12–9. Courtesy of Dr. Rebecca McConnico, Oklahoma State University.
Figure 12–13. J. Noye.
Figure 12–14. Barbara Ann Giove.
Figure 12–16. Courtesy of Dr. Rebecca McConnico, Oklahoma State University.
Figure 12–18. Courtesy of Dr. Rebecca McConnico, Oklahoma State University.
Figure 12–19. Courtesy of Dr. Rebecca McConnico, Oklahoma State University.
Figure 12–20. Courtesy of Dr. Rebecca McConnico, Oklahoma State University.
Figure 12–21. Barbara Ann Giove.
Figure 12–23. Courtesy of Dr. Rebecca McConnico, Oklahoma State University.
Figure 12–24. Barbara Ann Giove.
Figure 12–25. J. Noye.
Figure 12–26. J. Noye.
Figure 12–29. Cappy Jackson.
Figure 12–30. Courtesy of Dr. Charles MacAllister, Oklahoma State University.
Figure 12–31. Charlene Strickland.
Figure 12–33. Courtesy of Dr. Gary Nies, Oklahoma State University.
Figure 12–35. Courtesy of Dr. Rebecca McConnico, Oklahoma State University.
Figure 12–40. Courtesy of Dr. Rebecca McConnico, Oklahoma State University.
Figure 12–42. Courtesy of Dr. Gary Nies, Oklahoma State University.
Figure 12–43. J. Noye.
Figure 13–1. J. Noye.
Figure 13–2. Courtesy of Dr. Rebecca McConnico, Oklahoma State University.
Figure 13–3. Courtesy of Dr. Rebecca McConnico, Oklahoma State University.
Figure 13–4. Courtesy of the United States Trotting Association.
Figure 13–8. Courtesy of Dr. Kathy Spalding, North Carolina State University.
Figure 13–9. Courtesy of Dr. Rebecca McConnico, Oklahoma State University.
Figure 13–10. Courtesy of Dr. Rebecca McConnico, Oklahoma State University.
Figure 13–12. Don Shugart.

Figure 14–1. J. Noye.

Figure 14–4. J. Noye.

Figure 14–5. J. Noye.

Figure 14–6. J. Noye.

Figure 14–7, right. Courtesy of Dr. Charles MacAllister, Oklahoma State University.

Figure 14–12. J. Noye.

Figure 14–14, left. Courtesy of Dr. Rebecca McConnico, Oklahoma State University.

Figure 14–17. Courtesy of Dr. Ric Redden, International Equine Podiatry Center.

Figure 14–19. Courtesy of Dr. Charles MacAllister, Oklahoma State University.

Figure 14–20. Courtesy of Dr. Kathy Spalding, North Carolina State University.

Figure 14–22. Courtesy of Dr. Charles MacAllister, Oklahoma State University.

Figure 14–33. Courtesy of Dr. Ric Redden, International Equine Podiatry Center.

Figure 14–34. Courtesy of Dr. Kathy Spalding, North Carolina State University.

Figure 14–37. Courtesy of Dr. Rebecca McConnico, Oklahoma State University.

Figure 14–40. Cathy Nelson.

Figure 15–1. Equine Sports Graphics, Inc.

Figure 15–6. Courtesy of Dr. Kathy Spalding, North Carolina State University.

Figure 15–8. Katey Barrett.

Figure 15–11. Courtesy of Dr. Kathy Spalding, North Carolina State University.

Figure 15–17. Courtesy of Dr. Rebecca McConnico, Oklahoma State University.

Figure 15–20. Courtesy of Dr. Rebecca McConnico, Oklahoma State University.

Figure 15–22. Courtesy of Dr. Rebecca McConnico, Oklahoma State University.

Figure 15–26. Courtesy of Dr. Rebecca McConnico, Oklahoma State University.

Figure 15–29. Courtesy of Dr. Rebecca McConnico, Oklahoma State University.

Figure 15–30. Betty Jones.

Figure 15–31. Courtesy of Dr. Dan Steinheimer, Texas A&M University.

Figure 15–34. Courtesy of Laurie Fio, University of California, Davis.

Figure 15–36. Courtesy of Dr. Kathy Spalding, North Carolina State University.

Figure 15–37. Courtesy of Dr. Kathy Spalding, North Carolina State University.

Figure 15–41. Courtesy of Dr. Karl Bowman, North Carolina State University.

Figure 15–42. Courtesy of Dr. Rebecca McConnico, Oklahoma State University.

Figure 15–44. Courtesy of Dr. Rebecca McConnico, Oklahoma State University.

Figure 15–45. Courtesy of Dr. Rebecca McConnico, Oklahoma State University.

Figure 15–46. Courtesy of Dr. Rebecca McConnico, Oklahoma State University.

Figure 15–52. Courtesy of Dr. Rebecca McConnico, Oklahoma State University.

Figure 15–61. Courtesy of Dr. Rebecca McConnico, Oklahoma State University.

Figure 16–1. J. Noye.

Figure 16–8. Don Shugart.

Figure 16–11. Courtesy of Dr. Kathy Spalding, North Carolina State University.

Figure 16–15. Courtesy of Dr. Rebecca McConnico, Oklahoma State University.

Figure 16–22. Equine Sports Graphics, Inc.

Figure 16–24, top. Courtesy of Dr. Dan Steinheimer, Texas A&M University.

Figure 16–25. Courtesy of Dr. Dan Steinheimer, Texas A&M University.

Figure 16–27. Courtesy of Dr. Kathy Spalding, North Carolina State University.

Figure 17–1. Courtesy of the United States Trotting Association.

Figure 17–2. J. Noye.

Figure 17–5. Courtesy of Dr. Dan Steinheimer, Texas A&M University.

Figure 17–6. Courtesy of *Quarter Week*.

Figure 17–8. Courtesy of Dr. Kathy Spalding, North Carolina State University.

Figure 17–9. Courtesy of Dr. Dan Steinheimer, Texas A&M University.

Figure 17–10. Courtesy of Dr. Kathy Spalding, North Carolina State University.

Glossary

abrasion   Graze; superficial damage.

abscess   Pus-filled cavity beneath the skin or within a tissue, in many cases surrounded by fibrous tissue.

acepromazine   Tranquilizer that also lowers blood pressure; "ace."

acetabulum   Socket in the lower side of the pelvis; forms the hip joint with the head of the femur.

Achilles tendons   Superficial digital flexor and gastrocnemius tendons that run down the back of the gaskin and attach onto the point of the hock.

acquired   Not present at birth; developed afterward.

acrylic resin, acrylic repair   Synthetic material used to repair hoof wall defects; acrylic patch.

activated white blood cells   Immune system cells activated to kill bacteria and remove dead cells from a damaged area.

acupuncture   Chinese art of relieving pain and promoting healing by stimulating specific points on the body with needles or laser.

acute   Recent; injury that occurred only hours or a few days ago.

Adequan®   Commercial glycosaminoglycan used to treat joint disease; a joint medication.

adhesion   Band of fibrous tissue that fuses two structures.

adrenaline   "Stress" hormone produced by the adrenal glands.

aerobic   Using or requiring oxygen.

allergic reaction   Hypersensitivity, or over-reaction of the immune system to a substance.

anaerobic   Without, or lacking oxygen.

analgesia; analgesic   Pain relief; pain-killer.

anemia   Abnormally low red blood cell count.

anesthesia, anesthetic   Procedure or drug that removes feeling or awareness; anesthesia may be regional or general.

angular limb deformity   Deviation in the angle of the limb when viewed from the front or rear; "crooked legs," ALD.

ankylosis   Degenerative process resulting in bony fusion of a joint.

annular ligament   Ligament that wraps around a structure, e.g. the back of the fetlock and knee.

antibacterial   Able to inactivate or kill bacteria.

antibiotic   Drug that suppresses or kills micro-organisms.

antibiotic sensitivity testing   Laboratory test to determine which antibiotic(s) would be most effective in treating a specific infection.

antibodies   Specialized immune system proteins that help prevent or control infection.

antigen   Foreign substance to which the body mounts an immune response, such as viruses, bacteria, bacterial toxins, etc.

anti-inflammatory therapy   Treatment that prevents or relieves inflammation; includes cold therapy, NSAIDs, corticosteroids, DMSO, etc.

anti-oxidant   Substance that prevents or limits oxidant-related tissue damage.

antiseptic   Chemical that inactivates or kills micro-organisms.

apex   Tip; narrow end.

arteries   Blood vessels that carry oxygenated blood from the heart and lungs to the tissues.

arthritis   Inflammation of a joint; generally reserved for severe joint disease, such as septic arthritis and osteoarthritis.

arthrocentesis   Veterinary procedure in which a needle is inserted into a joint to sample the fluid or inject medication; joint tap.

arthrodesis   Surgical fusion of a joint.

arthroscopy, arthroscopic surgery   Surgical procedure using an endoscope to examine a joint and remove bone and cartilage fragments.

articular cartilage   *See joint cartilage.*

articular fracture   Fracture that involves a joint surface.

articulation   Joint; connection between two bones.

artifact   Man-made or artificial defect on an image.

aseptic   Free of micro-organisms; sterile.

AST   Aspartate aminotransferase; enzyme found in muscle, liver, and certain other cells.

astringent   Drying agent.

asymmetry   Unevenness in size or shape between the left and right sides.

ataxia   Incoordination; staggering or wobbly gait.

atrophy   Shrinking or wasting of a tissue.

auscultation   Listening to an internal organ with a stethoscope.

avulsion   Tearing away from a site of attachment.

avulsion fracture   Fracture in which a tendon or ligament pulls away a piece of bone.

axon   Long projection from a nerve cell.

"back at the knee"   Conformational defect in which the knee bends back slightly when seen from the side; "calf knee'd."

bacteria   Microscopic, single-cell organisms.

bacterial culture   Diagnostic procedure in which a fluid or tissue sample is incubated on a special culture plate to encourage any bacteria to grow.

bacterial dermatitis   Skin inflammation caused by bacterial infection.

bacterial toxins   Toxins produced by bacteria.

"bandage bow"   Swelling around a tendon caused by a bandage that is too tight.

bar   Part of the hoof wall that turns sharply at the back of the foot and runs forward along the side of the frog for a couple of inches.

bar shoe   Shoe in which the ends of the branches are connected by a metal bar.

baseline   Starting point; with radiographs, the appearance of a structure before it is altered by trauma or disease.

base-narrow   Conformational defect in which the feet are placed slightly to the inside of the points of the shoulders or buttocks.

base-wide   Conformational defect in which the feet are placed slightly to the outside of the points of the shoulders or buttocks.

"bench knees"   *See "offset knees."*

beveled   Angled or slanted.

bicarbonate   Substance that neutralizes excess acid.

bilateral   Occurring at the same place on both sides of the body.

biopsy   Minor surgical procedure in which a small sample of tissue is removed and examined microscopically.

"blister"   Compound that causes a chemical burn when applied to the skin; counter-irritant.

blood-brain barrier   Barrier that prevents cells and large molecules from leaving the bloodstream and entering the tissues of the brain and spinal cord.

blood culture   Bacterial culture of a blood sample.

blood pressure   Amount of pressure in the circulatory system; low blood pressure reduces blood flow to the tissues.

bog spavin   Nonpainful, soft, fluid-filled swelling of the hock. It is effusion in the tibiotarsal joint.

bone chip   Small piece of bone broken off the main part of the bone.

bone cyst   *See subchondral bone cyst.*

bone density   Amount of mineral deposited in the bone.

bone graft   Cancellous bone, harvested from another site and placed into a fracture to speed healing.

bone marrow   Jelly-like substance in the center of the longbones; produces red blood cells and some white blood cells.

bone pins, bone plates, bone screws   *See implants.*

bone quality   Combination of the thickness and density of the bone's cortex; determines the bone's strength and resilience.

"bone scan"   *See nuclear scintigraphy.*

bone spavin   Osteoarthritis in the lower hock joints; it causes bone spurs and narrowing of the affected joint space(s).

bone spur   Abnormal new bone growth at the edge of a joint.

botulism   Disease caused by bacterial toxins from *Clostridium botulinum*.

bowed tendon   Fiber damage and inflammation in one of the flexor tendons; the swelling gives it a bowed-out appearance.

"brace"   Mild counter-irritant used on the skin to stimulate blood flow to the tissues beneath; similar to a liniment.

brainstem   Base of the brain; responsible for awareness or consciousness.

"breakdown" injury   Severe damage to the fetlock's support structures; the fetlock drops and the horse cannot bear weight on the leg.

breakover   Phase of the stride in which the heel is lifted and the foot "rolls over" the toe.

breakover point   Part of the wall where the horse breaks over; ideally, the center of the toe.

bridle lameness   Gait abnormality seen only during ridden exercise; disappears when the horse is exercised without the rider.

broad-spectrum antibiotics   Antibiotics that are active against many different types of bacteria.

bruising   Leakage of blood from damaged vessels beneath intact skin or hoof.

bucked shins   Pain and new bone production at the front of the cannon bones on the forelegs of young racehorses; "shin soreness."

burns   Skin damage caused by heat, chemicals, or radiation; severity is graded from first-degree (mild, superficial damage) to third-degree (severe, full-thickness skin loss).

bursa   Small sac of fluid between a bone and a tendon; minimizes friction and pressure between the two structures. Plural: bursae.

bursitis   Inflammation and fluid accumulation within a bursa.

calcification; calcified   Replacement of cartilage or soft tissue with mineral deposits, which are mostly calcium.

calcium   Essential dietary mineral; needed for strong bones and normal muscle function.

calcium-phosphorus ratio   Number of calcium molecules for every molecule of phosphorus; Ca:P.

callus   Tissue thickening; a bony callus forms as a fracture heals.

cancellous bone   Lattice-like bone beneath the dense, outer cortex. Softer than cortical bone, it is sometimes called "spongy" bone.

capillaries   Microscopic blood vessels that supply the cells; blood flows from the arteries, through the capillaries, then into the veins.

capillary refill time   Time it takes for color to return to the gum after it has been briefly pressed with the thumb; should be less than 2 seconds.

capped elbow   Fluid-filled swelling over the point of the elbow; "shoe boil."

capped hock   Fluid-filled swelling over the point of the hock.

capsulitis   Inflammation of the joint capsule; usually includes synovitis.

carbohydrate   High-energy dietary component that consists of simple and complex sugars; grains are high-carbohydrate feeds.

cardiovascular fitness   Adaptation of the heart and circulation to regular exercise; increases the horse's exercise capacity.

cardiovascular system   Heart and blood vessels.

carpal valgus   Angular limb deformity causing "knock knees."

carpal varus   Angular limb deformity causing "bow legs."

carpometacarpal joint   Immobile lower knee joint, between the lower row of carpal bones and the top of the cannon and splint bones.

carpus   Knee.

cartilage   Special type of firm, non-bony tissue.

catecholamines   "Stress" hormones, such as adrenaline.

catheter   Hollow instrument for removing fluid from a body cavity or bloodstream, and administering fluid or medications.

cauda equina   Last part of the spinal cord.

cauda equina neuritis   Inflammation and degeneration of the nerves in the cauda equina area; polyneuritis equi.

caudal   Directional term meaning toward the horse's hind end.

cavaletti   Jump rails, raised a few inches off the ground; a training tool.

cell membrane   Outer covering of a cell.

cellulitis   Bacterial infection of the superficial tissues, causing a soft, warm, mildly painful swelling.

central nervous system   Control center of the nervous system, consisting of the brain and spinal cord; CNS.

cerebrospinal fluid   Special fluid that surrounds and protects the brain and spinal cord; CSF.

cervical muscles   Muscles on the side of the neck.

cervical vertebrae   Seven vertebrae in the neck.

Cervical Vertebral Malformation   Malformation of the cervical vertebrae, causing neurologic abnormalities; CVM, "wobbler" syndrome.

check ligament   Ligament that anchors the top of a flexor tendon to the bone, limiting overstretching of the tendon; accessory ligament.

chip fracture   Small piece of bone and cartilage, broken off within a joint; bone chip.

chiropractic manipulation   Manipulation of the spinal column to restore normal alignment of the small intervertebral joints.

chronic   Present for weeks, months, or even years.

chronic obstructive pulmonary disease   Allergic respiratory condition that results in constriction and plugging of the small airways in the lung; COPD.

chronic proliferative synovitis   Fibrous thickening (with or without calcification) of the pad of tissue in the front of the fetlock joint.

circulatory collapse   Large drop in blood pressure and blood flow to the tissues; shock.

clearance time   Time it takes for a drug to be eliminated from the body.

clefts of the frog   Grooves in the center and at each side of the frog.

cleft palate   Congenital abnormality in which the two sides of the hard palate (roof of the mouth) fail to fuse during development.

clench cutter   Chisel-like farriery tool for straightening or cutting off the clenches before removing the horse's shoe.

clenches   Turned-over ends of horseshoe nails, after the nails have been hammered through the hoof wall.

clips   Narrow flanges on the upper, outer edge of the shoe; they keep the shoe in place, and some restrict hoof wall expansion.

closed fracture   Fracture that does not involve a skin wound or a piece of bone penetrating the skin.

closed physis   Physis that is no longer producing bone.

clostridial myositis   Severe muscle damage and illness caused by the toxins of clostridial bacteria within a muscle.

"club foot"   Abnormal foot shape in which the heels grow very long, and the front of the hoof wall is close to vertical; the foot becomes box-shaped.

coccygeal vertebrae   Vertebrae that make up the tail dock.

coffin bone   *See pedal bone.*

coffin joint   Joint between the 2nd pastern bone and pedal bone.

Coggins test   Laboratory test for Equine Infectious Anemia (EIA).

colic   Sign of abdominal pain, usually due to a gastro-intestinal problem.

collagen   Microscopic fibers that give tissues, such as skin, tendons, ligaments, and joint cartilage their strength and resilience.

collateral ligament   Short, strong ligaments at the sides of a joint that help support it.

colostrum   Thick, sticky milk the mare produces just before foaling; contains very high levels of antibodies, which the newborn foal needs.

coma   Unconsciousness due to a brainstem abnormality.

comminuted fracture   Fracture with more than one fracture line and more than two pieces of bone.

common digital extensor tendon   Long tendon that runs down the front of the leg and attaches to the extensor process of the pedal bone; long digital extensor tendon, or extensor tendon.

complete fracture   Fracture that breaks the bone completely, into two or more pieces.

computerized tomography   Imaging technique giving a cross-sectional view of an area, or a three-dimensional view of a bone surface; CT.

concentration   Number of particles per unit of volume; e.g. grams per liter.

condylar fracture   Vertical fracture at the lower end of the cannon bone, which separates the condyle from the rest of the bone.

condyle   Rounded portion of bone at a joint surface.

congenital   Present at birth. Some congenital defects are hereditary, others are caused by conditions during pregnancy.

conservative management   Treatment that does not involve surgery.

contracted heels   Narrowing of one or both heels on the same foot.

"contracted tendons"   *See flexor contracture.*

contrast radiography   Radiographic technique in which contrast material is injected into a joint, tendon sheath, wound, etc. to outline or define the space.

core temperature   Temperature in the center of the body.

corium   *See coronary corium; laminar corium; solar corium.*

corn   1) Grain commonly included in horse rations. 2) Bruising of the sole at the heels, caused by an ill-fitting shoe.

cornified   Hardened, turned to horn.

coronary band   Rim of specialized skin around the top of the hoof wall; includes the coronary corium and blood vessels.

coronary corium   Cells that produce the horn tubules that make up the hoof wall.

cortex   Dense, outer layer of a bone.

corticosteroids   Potent anti-inflammatory drugs. They can also suppress the immune response; "cortisone."

counter-irritant   Compound that creates inflammation when applied to the skin.

"cow hocks"   Conformational defect in which the hocks angle in and the feet angle out when seen from the rear of the horse.

CPK   Creatine phosphokinase; enzyme found in muscle cells.

cranial   Directional term meaning toward the horse's head.

cranial nerves   Nerves that leave the base of the brain and supply the structures in the head.

cranio-caudal   Directional term meaning from front to back.

crepitus   Crackling, crunching, or grinding sensation that is heard and/or felt when a complete fracture or gas-filled wound is palpated or manipulated.

cruciate ligaments   Pair of short, thick ligaments in the stifle that attach the femur to the tibia, and cross over each other as they span the joint.

cuboidal bones   Block-shaped bones in the knee and hock.

"dead space"   Space within the tissues or beneath the skin, created by a wound.

debride   Trim away contaminated or devitalized tissue.

deep digital flexor tendon   Tendon that attaches to a muscle at the back of the forearm or thigh, runs down the back of the leg, and attaches onto the bottom of the pedal bone; DDFT.

degeneration   Breakdown of the normal structure of a tissue. In most cases the change is irreversible.

degenerative joint disease   Chronic joint disease involving cartilage damage and joint capsule thickening; DJD.

dehydration   Excessive loss of fluid from the body.

demineralization   Removal of mineral from the bones; loss of bone density.

density   How closely packed the molecules are in a structure.

dermatitis   Inflammation of the skin.

dermis   Deep layer of the skin; it contains dense collagen fibers that give skin its strength.

desensitize   Block sensation or feeling; numb.

desmitis   Inflammation of a ligament.

desmotomy   Surgical procedure that involves cutting a ligament.

developmental   Develops as the foal grows.

developmental orthopedic disorder(s)   Musculoskeletal abnormalities that develop as the foal grows; DODs.

deviation   Change in direction from the normal position or angle.

devitalized   Dead or dying.

diagonal bar shoe   Bar shoe in which one branch is shortened and a straight bar connects the ends of the branches; ¾ bar shoe.

diaphragm   Thin sheet of muscle that separates the chest and abdominal cavities; when it contracts air is drawn into the lungs.

dicalcium phosphate   Mineral supplement containing about twice as much calcium as phosphorus; DCP.

diffuse   Spread out; not very specific or localized.

digital arteries   Arteries that carry blood to the feet.

digital cushion   Dense, spongy tissue in the back half of the foot, between the frog and the deeper structures. It absorbs shock and helps move blood through the foot.

digital pulses   Pulses in the digital arteries.

dilation   To dilate or widen.

dimethyl glycine   Energy-based feed supplement; DMG.

dimethyl sulfoxide   Anti-inflammatory drug that is well absorbed through the skin; DMSO.

disinfectant   Chemical that inactivates or kills micro-organisms.

disinfection   Cleaning infected material from a surface then applying a disinfectant.

dislocation   *See luxation.*

displaced   Moved out of the normal position; separated.

distal   Directional term meaning away from the body; the part furthest from the body.

distal sesamoidean ligaments   Group of short ligaments that anchor the base of the sesamoid bones to the back of the pastern.

distention   To swell or expand from pressure within; mostly due to fluid accumulation.

distracting forces   Tension on a bone from the muscles, tendons, or ligaments that attach to it.

disuse atrophy   Wasting or shrinking of a muscle that is not used regularly.

DMSO   *See dimethyl glycine.*

DNA   Deoxyribonucleic acid; strands of complex molecules in the nucleus of every cell. They contain the genetic codes that direct all cell activities.

dorsal   Directional term meaning the upper surface; toward the top.

dorsal spinous processes   Ridges of bone along the tops of the vertebrae.

dorso-palmar   Radiographic view of the lower leg; the x-ray beam passes through the limb from front to back.

"dropped" elbow   Elbow joint that is lower than normal due to paralysis of the triceps muscles or complete olecranon fracture.

"dropped sole"   Sole that bulges toward the ground surface, instead of being slightly concave or level.

"dubbing"   Wearing down the hoof wall at the toe by either the horse dragging the toe or the farrier rasping the wall.

E. coli   *Escherichia coli.* Bacteria commonly found in the bowel, and one of the bacteria that cause endotoxemia.

edema   Accumulation of fluid within the tissues, resulting in soft swelling that stays dented (pitted) when briefly pressed.

effusion   Abnormal increase in fluid within a joint, tendon sheath, bursa, etc.; it expands the structure, causing a soft, fluidy swelling.

egg bar shoe   Bar shoe in which a curved piece of metal connects the shoe branches, making the shoe oval- or egg-shaped.

EHV-1 Myeloencephalitis   Inflammation and damage of the spinal cord and brain, caused by Equine Herpesvirus type one infection.

elasticity   Ability to stretch and return to the original shape without damage.

electrical muscle stimulation   Form of electrical tissue stimulation used to make a muscle contract.

electrical tissue stimulation   Use of a low voltage electrical current to stimulate cell activity, and hence healing.

electrocardiography   Diagnostic procedure that records the electrical activity of the heart; ECG (or EKG).

electrolyte   Any element with a positive or negative charge, e.g. sodium, potassium, and chloride.

electromyography   Recording of the electrical activity in a muscle; EMG.

electron   Negatively charged part of an atom; invisible particles that form an x-ray beam.

encephalitis   Inflammation of the brain, usually caused by infection.

endemic   Term used for a disease that is always present in an area.

endoscope   Instrument used to examine the interior of a body cavity.

endotoxemia   Build-up of endotoxin in the bloodstream, causing dehydration, shock, and possibly death.

endotoxin   Toxin consisting of the cell walls of dead Gram-negative bacteria.

enzymes   Complex molecules that aid cell reactions and digestion; can damage cell membranes when released from injured cells.

epidermis   Outer layer of the skin.

epiphysis   End of the bone, between the physis and the joint surface.

Equine Degenerative Myelopathy   Degenerative condition involving the spinal cord of young horses; EDM.

Equine Herpesvirus type one   Virus that can cause abortion in pregnant mares, mild respiratory disease (a "cold"), and neurologic disease; EHV-1.

Equine Infectious Anemia   Contagious viral infection that causes anemia. The blood test for EIA is a Coggins test.

Equine Motor Neuron Disease   Degenerative disease affecting the nerves that supply the muscles, causing weight loss, muscle tremors, pain, and weakness; EMND.

Equine Protozoal Myeloencephalitis   Inflammation and damage of the spinal cord and brain caused by the protozoa, *Sarcocystis neurona* or *falcatula*; EPM.

Equine Viral Arteritis   Contagious viral disease that causes fever, depression, nasal discharge, and limb edema; EVA.

ergot   Small, horn-like structure at the back of the fetlock.

estrous cycle   Female reproductive cycle; "heat" cycle.

euthanasia   Killing a hopelessly sick or injured horse for humane reasons.

excretion time   Time it takes for a drug to be eliminated from the body.

exercise capacity   Ability to continue to exercise; mostly relates to the horse's cardiovascular and muscular fitness.

exercise intolerance   Inability or unwillingness to exercise normally.

exertional rhabdomyolysis   Exercise-related muscle dysfunction and damage; ER, "tying up."

exostosis   New bone production on the surface of a bone. Plural: exostoses.

extension   Opening the angle of a joint by bringing the bones on either side toward or past the straight position.

extensor carpi radialis   Muscle and tendon at the front of the forearm that help to extend the knee.

extensor muscle   Muscle that causes joint extension.

extensor process   Small projection on the top of the pedal bone, at the front of the coffin joint.

extensor tendon   Tendon that is attached to an extensor muscle and causes joint extension when the muscle contracts.

"false bursa"   Swelling containing serum and surrounded by fibrous tissue; usually the result of chronic trauma.

fascia   Whitish, fibrous covering of a muscle.

fatty acids   Components of fat molecules, used by the muscles as a fuel.

femoral head   Rounded top of the femur, which fits into the acetabulum to form the hip joint.

femoropatellar joint   Joint between the femur and the patella, at the front of the stifle.

femorotibial joints   Two joints between the bottom of the femur and the top of the tibia, in the stifle.

fever rings   Horizontal rings in the hoof walls of all four feet, caused by severe stress or illness, especially when it includes a fever.

fibrin   Blood-clotting protein that can form adhesions between two structures or within a joint or tendon sheath.

fibroblasts   Cells that produce collagen, the fiber responsible for tissue repair.

fibrosis   Thickening or fusing with fibrous tissue.

fibrotic myopathy   Replacement of muscle tissue with fibrous tissue, which restricts normal muscle function.

fibrous tissue   Scar tissue; mostly consists of dense bundles of collagen fibers.

fibrous union   Fusion of a fracture with fibrous tissue instead of bone.

"firing"   Applying a hot iron to the skin to create a second- or third-degree burn.

fitness   Ability to exercise without tiring too soon.

flat-footed   Feet with soles that are flat or "dropped," instead of curving away from the ground surface.

flexion   Closing the angle of the joint by bringing the bones on either side toward each other.

flexor contracture   Failure of a flexor unit to lengthen at the same rate as the bones, resulting in persistent flexion of the affected joint(s); "contracted tendons."

flexor laxity   Slackness or looseness of the flexor unit, which allows the fetlock to drop and the toe to tip up.

flexor muscle   Muscle that causes joint flexion.

flexor tendon   Tendon that is attached to a flexor muscle and causes joint flexion when the muscle contracts.

flexor unit   Combination of a flexor muscle and its tendon.

flexural limb deformity   Abnormality of the limb angle when viewed from the side; may be flexor contracture or flexor laxity.

Foley catheter   Short plastic, rubber, or latex tube with a small, inflatable cuff just behind the tip.

folic acid   B vitamin that is essential for red blood cell production.

foot abscess   Infection and pus accumulation beneath the hoof wall or sole.

foot flight   Path the foot travels during a step.

formalin   Formaldehyde solution; used for drying and toughening the hooves.

"founder"   *See laminitis.*

"founder rings"   Horizontal ridges in the hoof wall due to laminitis.

"fracture-lame"   Severe lameness, like that seen with a complete fracture.

"free radicals"   Unstable oxygen molecules released by damaged cells; can damage other cells and continue or worsen inflammation.

free-school   Work a horse in an enclosed area without a rider, lead rope, or longe line.

frog   Rubbery, roughly triangular structure on the underside of the foot; the base of the frog lies between the heels.

frog support   Shoe or pad that uses the frog to support the foot.

full bar shoe   Bar shoe in which the branches are connected by a straight metal bar.

full sole pad   Synthetic, leather, or metal pad that covers the underside of the foot, between the hoof and the shoe.

full-limb cast   Cast that encases the limb to just below the elbow or stifle.

fullering   Groove in the ground surface of the shoe, in which the nails are set.

fungus   Large and diverse group of organisms. Those that cause infection in horses are microscopic. Plural: fungi.

furlong   Unit of distance; one furlong is 220 yards, or 200 meters.

gait abnormality, gait defect   Abnormal locomotory movement.

gait evaluation   Observing the horse as it moves to determine whether the gait is normal, and if not, where the problem lies.

gastric ulcers   Ulceration or erosions in the stomach lining.

gastrocnemius tendon   Tendon that runs down the back of the gaskin and attaches to the point of the hock. It is one of the Achilles tendons; "gastroc" tendon.

gastro-intestinal problems   Abnormalities involving the stomach and/or intestines; often caused or worsened by the diet.

general anesthesia   Using drugs to temporarily make the horse unconscious, and unable to feel or respond.

generalized   Covering a large area, or in some cases the entire body.

generalized allergic reaction   Severe, possibly fatal hypersensitivity reaction, usually caused by a drug, insect bite, etc.

generalized infection   Infection that affects the entire body; systemic infection. Signs include fever, depression, and loss of appetite.

genetic   Inherited; a trait that is passed down from parent to offspring.

germinal   Area from which cells develop, or germinate.

glucose   Simple sugar; it is used by cells as fuel.

gluteal muscles   Large muscles at the top of the rump.

glycogen   Glucose-based molecule that muscle cells use for energy.

glycosaminoglycans   Complex molecules that aid cartilage repair; GAGs.

graded exercise   Increasing the amount and intensity of exercise in a stepwise manner, over a period of days or weeks.

grade of lameness   Relative severity of the lameness; usually graded on a scale of 1 to 5, with 5 being the most severe.

gram-negative bacteria   Bacteria that do not absorb Gram stain in the laboratory. These bacteria, which include *E. coli* and *Salmonella* species, cause endotoxemia.

granulation tissue   Pink, irregular tissue that fills in an open wound. It is composed of collagen fibers, fibroblasts, and new blood vessels.

"gravel"   Hoof wall abscess.

ground impact forces   Force of impact when the foot lands, which increase with the horse's speed.

growth plate   *See physis.*

gum color   Color of the horse's gums; used to evaluate health. In a healthy horse, the gums are light pink.

half-round shoe   Shoe made out of half-round metal, instead of a flat strip of metal.

head nod   Increase in head movement during motion; usually indicates lameness in the forelimb that is bearing weight when the head goes up.

head tilt   Abnormal angle of the head caused by a neurologic abnormality in the brain or a cranial nerve.

heart bar shoe   Shoe with a V-shaped piece of metal connecting the ends of the branches; the V-bar sits over the frog.

heavy metals   Metals with a high molecular weight, such as lead, mercury, iron, etc.

heel caulks   Patches of metal welded onto, or worked into the heels of the shoe to increase traction.

heel extension   Lengthening the branches of the shoe or welding a metal bar to the back of the shoe to add length; trailers.

hematoma   Pool of blood within a tissue or beneath the skin/hoof, generally the result of direct trauma.

hemorrhage   Excessive or uncontrolled bleeding.

high-motion joint   Joint that normally has a wide range of motion, e.g. fetlock, knee, and hock.

hip hike, hip lift   Increased movement of the pelvis during motion; usually indicates hindlimb lameness on the side with greatest movement.

hip joint   "Ball and socket" joint between the femur and the pelvis.

hobbles   Harness used in pacers to connect the forelimb and hindlimb on the same side; hopples.

hoof knife   Tool used to trim the wall, sole, and frog.

hoof-pastern angle   Relationship between the angles at the front of the hoof wall and the pastern; they should be the same.

hoof tester Wide, pincer-like tool used to examine the hoof for painful areas.

hoof wall angle Angle of the front of the hoof wall in relation to the ground, often measured with a protractor.

hoof wall crack Narrow, vertical or horizontal defect in the hoof wall; it may be superficial or full-thickness.

hoof wall–pedal bone bond Tight connection between the sensitive and insensitive laminae, which holds the hoof wall and the pedal bone together.

hoof wall resection Removal of an abnormal area of hoof wall.

horizontal rings Horizontal ridges in the hoof wall, beginning at the coronary band and growing down the hoof.

horn Hard substance of which the hoof wall and sole are made; it mostly consists of hair-like tubules of keratin.

hospital plate Metal plate attached with bolts to the bottom of an egg bar shoe. It protects the sole, yet allows the foot to be treated.

"hot spot" Area of increased tissue uptake of the radioactive particles during nuclear scintigraphy; indicates inflammation or increased cell activity.

"hot walker" Machine that allows several horses to be walked at the same time. Overhead arms slowly move the horses in a circle.

hyaluronic acid Substance that gives joint fluid its lubricating properties. Commercial HA (or "acid") preparations are used to treat joint disease and tendon sheath inflammation.

hygroma Fluid-filled swelling over a bony surface, caused by trauma.

hyperflexion Exaggerated joint flexion; overflexion.

hyperkalemic periodic paralysis Inherited muscle disorder of Quarter Horses. It causes episodes of muscle tremors and weakness; HPP (or HYPP).

hypermetria Exaggerated flexor muscle activity and increased joint flexion, causing a poorly-coordinated, high-stepping gait.

hypertrophy Normal increase in size of a tissue.

hypocalcemia Low blood calcium concentration.

hypometria Exaggerated extensor muscle activity and reduced joint flexion, causing a stiff-legged, "toy soldier" gait.

ilium Top part of the pelvis.

immune complex Combination of an antigen and an antibody; e.g. virus-and-antibody.

immune system Body system that defends against invading micro-organisms; the major components are white blood cells and antibodies.

immunosuppression Suppression of the immune response.

implants Stainless steel (or other alloy) bone pins, plates, screws, etc. specifically designed for surgical fracture repair.

incision Wound made by cutting the skin with a sharp instrument, such as a scalpel blade.

incomplete fracture Fracture that involves only one side of the bone, so the bone remains intact.

incubation period Time between invasion of a micro-organism and the first signs of infection.

infectious, infective Able to cause or spread infection; contagious, or transmissible.

inferior check ligament Ligament that begins at the back of the knee (or hock) and fuses with the deep digital flexor tendon about halfway down the cannon.

inflammation Body's response to cell or tissue damage. The five signs are pain, heat, swelling, redness, and loss of function.

inflammatory substances Compounds released by cells in inflamed tissue, causing the outward signs of inflammation; include prostaglandins, leukotrienes, and "free radicals."

insensitive laminae Tiny corrugations on the inside of the hoof wall. They are not supplied with blood vessels or nerves.

intercarpal joint Middle knee joint, between the two rows of carpal bones.

intercarpal ligaments Pair of supporting ligaments in the back of the intercarpal joint.

intervertebral joints Joints between the vertebrae.

intra-articular Into a joint; IA.

intra-articular anesthesia Injecting sterile local anesthetic into a joint to temporarily block feeling in that joint; joint block.

intramuscular Into a muscle; IM.

intramuscular injection reaction Muscle inflammation caused by an intramuscular injection.

intravenous Into a vein; IV.

intravenous fluid therapy Giving large volumes of fluids intravenously to treat dehydration or shock.

iodine solution Dilute solution of iodine, usually containing between 1% and 7% iodine.

joint block *See intra-articular anesthesia.*

joint capsule Fibrous, outer covering of a joint. It helps stabilize the joint, and supports and protects the synovium.

joint cartilage Thin layer of cartilage on the bone surfaces within a joint; articular cartilage.

joint fluid Fluid that fills the joint space; synovial fluid.

joint medications Drugs used to treat inflammatory or degenerative joint conditions; corticosteroids, hyaluronic acid, Adequan®.

joint mobility Range of joint motion; e.g. flexion and extension, bending from side to side (lateral flexion), and rotation.

"joint mouse" Fragment of cartilage, floating free within a joint.

joint space Area enclosed by the joint capsule.

joint tap *See arthrocentesis.*

keg shoes Mass-produced steel shoes.

keratin   Dense protein that makes up the horn of the hoof wall, the outer layer of the skin, and hair.

laceration   Traumatic wound that cuts or tears the skin, and sometimes the tissues beneath.

lactate   1) Substance produced by cells that must function anaerobically. 2) To produce milk.

lactic acid   Molecule containing lactate and hydrogen ions.

"lag screw" fixation   Method of fracture repair using bone screws.

laminae   Layers or folds of tissue; e.g. the tiny corrugations on the inside of the hoof wall.

laminar corium   Layer of tissue between the surface of the pedal bone and the hoof wall.

laminitis   Painful foot condition in which the blood supply to the hoof wall is interrupted, and the hoof wall–pedal bone bond breaks down; "founder."

laser therapy   Use of a low-level ("cold") laser to promote healing.

lateral   Directional term meaning the outer side of a limb.

lateral cartilages   Firm pieces of cartilage, protruding up from the sides of the pedal bone.

lateral digital extensor tendon   Tendon that runs down the outside of the leg and joins the common digital extensor tendon at the front of the leg.

lateral radiograph   Radiograph taken from the side; a latero-medial view.

latero-medial   Radiographic view in which the x-ray beam passes through the limb from outside to inside.

latero-medial balance   Aspect of foot conformation; the left and right sides of the hoof wall are identical in shape, height, and angle.

lavage   Liberally flush with water or saline solution.

laxity   Looseness; slackness.

"leg paint"   Mild counter-irritant, similar to a "blister."

legume hay   Hay produced from a legume crop, such as alfalfa and clover.

lesion   Physical defect or structural abnormality.

leukotrienes   Inflammatory substances released by damaged cells; they attract and activate white blood cells.

lifecycle   Stages of growth and reproduction of an organism.

ligament   Dense, fibrous structure that connects two bones.

Lily Pad™   Vinyl frog-shaped pad taped to the bottom of the foot to put pressure on the frog and support the underlying structures.

liniment   Mild counter-irritant that is rubbed into the skin to improve blood flow to the skin and the tissues beneath.

loading capacity   Amount of weight or force a structure can withstand without being damaged; strength.

local anesthetic   Drug that, when injected, temporarily blocks sensation in the area.

localize   Pinpoint; narrow down to a specific area.

longbones   Long, thick bones that are shaped roughly like a cylinder, with a medullary cavity in the center. They include the cannon bone, radius, humerus, tibia, and femur.

long toe–low heel   Abnormal foot shape in which the heels are low and the hoof wall grows longer at the toe. The hoof wall angle is lower than normal.

"low bow"   Tendonitis in a flexor tendon, just above the fetlock.

lower hock joints   Horizontal, immobile joints in the lower part of the hock: the tarsometatarsal, distal intertarsal, and proximal intertarsal joints.

lower motor neuron   Motor nerve that leaves the spinal cord to supply the tissues, especially muscles.

low-motion joint   Joint that normally has a limited amount of motion; e.g. the pastern joint.

lumbar vertebrae   Five or six vertebrae in the the loins, or lumbar area of the back, between the ribcage and the rump.

lumbo-sacral   Junction between the last lumbar vertebra and the sacrum.

luxation   Dislocation of a bone or tendon out of its normal position.

lymph   Tissue fluid, collected by the lymphatic system.

lymphatic system   Network of tiny vessels that collect excess fluid from the tissues and return it to the bloodstream.

lysine   Amino acid that can aid hoof wall growth when added to a lysine-deficient diet.

lysis   Degenerative process of breaking down or dissolving a tissue.

magnetic field therapy   Use of a magnetic field (either solid magnets or electromagnetic energy) to promote healing.

magnetic resonance imaging   Diagnostic imaging procedure that provides excellent soft tissue detail; MRI.

maleolus   Small projection of bone on the lower end of the tibia. Plural: maleoli.

mammary glands   Udder.

manipulate   Moving a body part through its normal range of motion.

maternal antibodies   Protective antibodies the foal received from its mother's colostrum.

medial   Directional term meaning the inner side of the limb.

medullary cavity   Relatively hollow center of the longbones; called the "bone marrow" cavity sbone marrow.

meninges   Membranes that surround the brain and spinal cord.

meningitis   Inflammation of the meninges, usually due to infection.

meniscus   Thick pad of fibrous cartilage in the stifle; one in each femorotibial joint. Plural: menisci.

metabolic bone disease   Condition affecting bone metabolism, in particular calcium and phosphorus storage.

metabolic disorder   Abnormality of function, rather than structure.

metabolic rate   Rate of cell activity.

metabolism   Physical and chemical processes involved in cell function.

methionine   Essential amino acid that can aid hoof wall growth when added to a methionine-deficient diet.

methyl sulfonylmethane Anti-inflammatory substance derived from DMSO; MSM.

microfracture Small, incomplete fracture that only involves the outer surface of the bone; may not be visible on radiographs.

micro-organisms Microscopic organisms, such as bacteria, fungi, viruses, protozoa, etc.

mineral Elements that are required by the body; e.g. calcium, phosphorus, magnesium, and copper.

mismatching, mismatched feet Difference in size, shape, and angle between the left and right feet.

moist dermatitis Inflammation of the skin caused by constant moisture.

molecular weight Weight of a molecule; the larger the molecule, the higher the molecular weight.

motor nerve Nerve that transmits signals from the brain and spinal cord to the tissues; motor neuron.

mucous membranes Pink membrane that lines the mouth, nasal passages, eyelids, vulva, etc. Its color is used to gauge the horse's health and circulatory system function.

muscle enzymes Enzymes that are found in muscle cells; include CPK and AST.

muscle fatigue Inability of a muscle to continue to contract with normal speed and strength.

muscle spasm Sustained contraction of part or all of a muscle; the muscle remains contracted, rather than relaxing.

muscle strain Damage caused by overstretching of a muscle.

musculoskeletal Relating to the bones, joints, muscles, tendons, and ligaments of the limbs and spine.

mushroom shoe Bar shoe consisting of a half circle at the toe, with a flat plate that sits over the frog.

myelitis Inflammation of the spinal cord.

myeloencephalitis Inflammation of the spinal cord and brain; usually caused by bacterial, viral, or protozoal infection.

myelogram, myelography Injecting sterile contrast material into the spinal canal, then taking radiographs of the neck to check for narrowing of the spinal canal.

myelopathy Degenerative condition of the spinal cord.

myofilament Contracting units within muscle cells.

myopathy Degenerative muscle disorder.

myositis Inflammation of a muscle.

nail puller Farriery tool for removing horseshoe nails one at a time.

nasogastric tube Long plastic, rubber, or latex tube that is passed through the nostril, down the esophagus, and into the stomach; "stomach tube."

navicular bone Small bone at the back of the coffin joint.

navicular bursa Small, fluid-filled sac between the back of the navicular bone and the deep digital flexor tendon.

navicular bursitis   Inflammation of the navicular bursa.

navicular syndrome   Degenerative condition of the navicular bone and supporting structures.

neck cradle   Wooden or metal restraint device that prevents the horse from flexing its neck; used to stop bandage chewing.

nerve   Collection of microscopic axons (nerve fibers), traveling together in a protective, outer sheath.

nerve block   Injecting local anesthetic around a nerve to temporarily block sensation in the skin and other tissues supplied by that nerve; used to localize lameness to a specific area.

nerve ending   Junction between a nerve and the cell it supplies.

nerve root   Nerve bundle that emerges from the spinal canal; consists of several nerves that then branch off to specific tissues.

"nerving"   *See Palmar Digital neurectomy.*

nervous system   Brain, spinal cord, and nerves.

neurectomy   Surgically cutting a nerve for long-term pain relief.

neuritis   Inflammation of a nerve or group of nerves.

neurogenic atrophy   Muscle wasting due to loss of nerve supply.

neurologic   Relating to the nervous system.

neuromuscular junction   Connection between a nerve ending and a muscle cell.

neuron   Nerve cell; the basic unit of the nervous system. It consists of a cell body and an axon.

neuropathy   Degenerative condition involving a nerve or group of nerves.

non-articular fracture   Fracture that does not involve a joint surface.

non-displaced fracture   Fracture in which the bone pieces are in their normal position, and are not separated.

nonsteroidal anti-inflammatory drug   Drug other than a corticosteroid that relieves or prevents inflammation; NSAID. Examples include phenylbutazone, aspirin, ibuprofen, and flunixin.

nonsupporting bone   Bone that does not directly support the body or bear weight; e.g. splint bones and accessory carpal bone.

non-union   Failure of a fracture to repair completely, usually caused by instability or infection.

nonweight-bearing lameness   Lameness so severe that the horse will not or cannot bear weight on the limb; grade 5 of 5 lameness.

nuchal ligament   Broad, thick ligament that runs from the poll to the withers, beneath the mane.

nuclear scintigraphy   Injecting a harmless radioactive substance into the horse and measuring its uptake into the tissues; "bone scan."

oblique   At an angle; with radiographs, when the x-ray beam is aimed midway between the front (or back) and side of the leg.

"offset knees"   Conformational defect in which the forearm and cannon bone are not aligned when seen from the front—the cannon is slightly offset to the outside of the knee; "bench knees."

open fracture   Fracture that involves a skin wound or a piece of bone penetrating the skin; "compound" fracture.

open physis   Physis that is still "active" and producing bone.

open wound   Unsutured wound; a wound that is left open.

oral   Relating to the mouth; a drug administered orally is given into the horse's mouth.

organic material   Material originally from a live organism, either plant or animal; e.g. manure, pus, blood, bedding, and feed.

orthopedic   Relating to the musculoskeletal system.

orthopedic wire   Sterile stainless steel wire used for orthopedic surgery, such as fracture repair.

"osselet"   Literally, a small piece of bone; general term for various bony changes at the front of the fetlock.

ossify   Turn into bone or become bone-like.

osteoarthritis   Severe degenerative joint disease with bony abnormalities within and around the joint.

osteoblasts   Bone-forming cells.

osteochondral   Bone-and-cartilage; an osteochondral fragment is a piece of bone with cartilage attached.

osteochondritis dissecans   Osteochondrosis lesion in which a fragment of bone and cartilage is broken off the joint surface; OCD.

osteochondroma   Bone spur with a cartilage cap, found near a physis.

osteochondrosis   Abnormality of developing bone; results in bone and/or cartilage defects at the joint surface.

osteomyelitis   Bone infection and destruction, usually caused by bacterial invasion of a damaged bone.

osteoporosis   Abnormal loss of mineral (calcium and phosphorus) from a bone; it weakens the bone.

"over at the knee"   Conformational defect in which the horse or foal stands with the knee slightly flexed (bent); "tied in at the knee."

overextension   Excessive extension of a joint.

overflexion   Excessive flexion of a joint.

"over-reaching"   Interference in which a hindfoot catches the heels of a forefoot during exercise.

over-ride   Overlap.

oxidant   Cell by-product or chemical that causes oxidation—a reaction that can cause cell damage.

oxytetracycline   Broad-spectrum antibiotic that is also used to treat flexor contracture in young foals.

paddock   Fenced area less than ⅛ acre (48 square feet).

pain threshold   Point at which the horse shows awareness of pain.

palmar   Directional term meaning the area at the back of the foreleg, below the knee.

Palmar Digital nerves   Nerves that run down the back of the pastern and supply the back half of the foot; PD nerves.

Palmar Digital neurectomy   Surgical procedure to cut the Palmar Digital nerves and provide long-term pain relief; "nerving."

palpate   Feeling an area with the fingers or hands, checking for pain, swelling, heat, etc.

paralysis   Complete loss of muscle function, usually caused by loss of nerve supply.

parasite   Plant or animal that lives upon or within another living organism at that organism's expense.

paring   Trimming away a little at a time.

"parrot mouth"   Conformational defect in which the upper jaw is longer than the lower jaw; "overshot jaw."

passive motion   Physical therapy in which part of the horse's body is moved by the therapist.

pastern joint   Joint between the first and second pastern bones.

"pasture sound"   The horse is chronically lame but comfortable enough for pasture turnout.

patellar ligaments   Three ligaments (medial, middle, and lateral) that anchor the bottom of the patella to the top of the tibia.

pathogenic   Disease-causing; usually applied to harmful bacteria, such as *Salmonella* and *E. coli*.

pectoral muscles   Muscles at the front of the chest and under the girth area.

pedal bone   Bone within the hoof; coffin bone.

pedal bone rotation   Downward displacement of the tip of the pedal bone during acute laminitis.

periople   Thin, cuticle-like layer that covers the top part of the hoof wall, just below the coronary band.

periosteum   Membrane that covers the bones; it consists of fibrous tissue, blood vessels, nerves, and osteoblasts.

peripheral   Directional term meaning at or near the outer edge.

peripheral nerves   Nerves that supply the tissues; that is, the nerves outside the central nervous system.

permeability   Leakiness.

peroneus tertius   Tendon that runs from the lower end of the femur to the front of the hock. It ties the stifle and hock together, such that flexing the stifle also flexes the hock.

phenylbutazone   NSAID that is commonly used in horses; PBZ or "bute." (The old name is butazolidin, or BTZ.)

phosphorus   Essential mineral; combined with calcium, it produces mineral deposits that give bones their strength and resilience.

physeal cartilage   Specialized growth cartilage in the physes of young horses. Bones grow in length as this cartilage produces new cells that mature into bone.

physeal fracture   Fracture that begins in, or extends into a physis.

physical examination   Examination of the body by physical means: observation, palpation, manipulation, auscultation, and measurement of the rectal temperature.

physical therapy   Therapy that uses physical tools (cold, warmth, the hands, magnetic fields, etc.) on the body surface.

physis Area of specialized cartilage near the ends of the bones in young horses; commonly called the growth plate because it is responsible for bone growth. Plural: physes.

physitis Inflammation or abnormal cell activity in a physis, causing painful swelling.

pigeon-toed *See toe-in.*

pigmented skin Dark-colored skin; contains many pigment cells.

pincers Farriery tool for clipping off excess hoof wall at the ground surface.

"pinched nerve" Compression of a spinal nerve as it leaves the spinal canal.

plantar Directional term meaning the area at the back of the hindleg, below the hock.

plasma Liquid portion of the blood.

plastic shoes Horse shoes that are made of plastic or some other synthetic material; they are usually glued onto the foot.

plateau When discussing recovery from illness, it means that no further improvement is seen.

platelets Microscopic particles in the bloodstream that assist blood clotting.

pleuritis Inflammation of the membrane (the pleura) that lines the chest cavity and covers the lungs, caused by bacterial infection.

pneumonia Infection of the lungs.

polymerase chain reaction Diagnostic test that detects the presence of an invading micro-organism's DNA; PCR.

"ponying" Leading one horse while riding another; sometimes the safest way to hand-walk high-spirited racehorses.

post-operative care Management of the horse following surgery.

potassium Essential electrolyte, required for normal function of all cells, especially muscle.

Potomac Horse Fever Disease caused by the micro-organism, *Ehrlichia risticii;* causes diarrhea, which can lead to laminitis.

predispose, predisposition Inclined to; more likely to.

pressure sore Wound caused by excessive pressure, which obstructs blood flow to the skin.

procaine penicillin Type of penicillin specifically formulated for intramuscular injection.

progesterone Female hormone that maintains pregnancy.

prognosis Prediction of the outcome; the chances that the horse will recover. *See **Understanding the Prognosis.***

proliferation Outgrowth, extra growth.

prophylactic Treatment or management decision undertaken to prevent a particular problem.

proprioception Awareness of where the limbs are placed in relation to each other and to the ground surface.

proprioceptive deficits Mistakes made in limb movement and placement due to a neurologic abnormality.

prostaglandins   Inflammatory substances; certain prostaglandins also help protect the stomach lining and kidneys.

prosthesis   Artificial body part, fitted after amputation.

proteoglycans   Large, complex molecules that trap water within the cartilage, making it a more effective shock absorber.

protozoa   Primitive, bacteria-like micro-organisms that have only a single cell.

"proud flesh"   Excessive granulation tissue in a wound.

proximal   Directional term meaning toward the body; the part closest to the body.

pulse pressure   Strength of the pulse; may be strong ("bounding"), normal, or weak (faint).

puncture wound   Deep, narrow wound caused by a penetrating object.

pus   Collection of tissue fluid, white blood cells, bacteria, fibrin, and cell debris; forms as a result of bacterial infection.

quadriceps muscles   Large group of muscles at the front of the thigh; they begin on the pelvis or top of the femur, and attach onto the patella at the front of the stifle.

quarter   Part of the hoof from the widest point back to the heels.

quarter clips   Narrow flanges raised on the upper, outer edge of the shoe at the quarters; prevent the hoof wall from expanding.

quarter crack   Vertical hoof wall crack at the quarters or heel; often complete, full thickness cracks.

quilted leg wrap   Rectangles of quilted cotton or synthetic fabric.

rabies   Deadly viral disease of all warm-blooded animals; it affects the brain, although early signs can be highly variable in horses.

rabies suspect   Animal that potentially has been exposed to rabies, or is showing signs similar to those seen with rabies.

racing plates   Lightweight shoes used on racehorses; usually made of aluminum or other lightweight alloy.

radial nerve   Nerve that supplies the skin and extensor muscles at the front of the forearm, and the triceps muscles on the side of the shoulder.

"radiating" wound   Minor skin wound that conceals more extensive soft tissue, and possibly bone damage beneath.

radiography, radiographs   Images produced by x-rays striking special film; the images are commonly called "x-rays."

raised heel shoe   Shoe or shoe-and-pad combination that raises the horse's heels.

raised rim shoe   Shoe with a low metal rim around the upper, outer edge. It prevents the hoof wall from expanding.

rectal examination   Veterinary examination of the organs in the pelvic canal and abdomen by inserting a hand into the horse's rectum.

recumbent   Lying down and unable to get up.

referred pain   Pain in one area caused by a problem in another.

regional anesthesia   Temporarily desensitizing a specific area with local anesthetic; includes joint blocks, nerve blocks, and tissue blocks.

remodeling   Changes in a tissue's size, shape, or structure in response to the load on it.

"repair" cartilage   Cartilage that fills in an erosion or other defect in joint cartilage; it is not as strong or as resilient as healthy cartilage.

"repair" tissue   Tissue that fills in a defect or heals a damaged area; it mostly consists of fibrous tissue.

resection   Surgical removal of a portion of tissue.

respiratory infection   Infection of the respiratory system; e.g. a "cold."

respiratory muscles   Muscles needed for breathing, including the diaphragm and the muscles between the ribs (intercostal muscles).

retina   Network of specialized cells and nerve endings that lines the back of the eyeball; responsible for vision.

reverse shoe   Regular shoe that is nailed on backward, so the toe of the shoe is at the horse's heels; open-toe egg bar.

rim pad   Pad that is the size and shape of a shoe, and is nailed on between the shoe and the hoof.

rim shoe   *See raised rim shoe or traction rim shoe.*

ringbone   Bony proliferation around the pastern; often osteoarthritis of the pastern and/or coffin joint.

"roach back"   Conformational defect in which the back is hunched, or bowed up slightly.

rocker shoe   Shoe that is tipped up slightly at the toe, to make breakover easier.

roll cotton   Cotton padding that comes in a roll.

rolled toe shoe   Shoe in which the ground surface at the toe is curved to make breakover easier.

rotational forces   Twisting or wringing forces on a structure; torque.

rubbing alcohol   Isopropyl alcohol; used as a liniment or "brace."

sacral vertebrae   *See sacrum.*

sacro-iliac joints   Pair of joints between the sacrum and the ilium; they are located several inches below the tuber sacrale.

sacro-iliac ligaments   Ligaments that connect the sacrum to the ilium, and stabilize the sacro-iliac joints.

sacro-iliac subluxation   Displacement or malalignment of the sacro-iliac joint(s).

sacrum   Portion of the spinal column along the top of the rump, consisting of five fused sacral vertebrae.

sagittal fracture   Fracture that runs vertically into, or through the center of a bone.

saline solution   Salt dissolved in water; to make the concentration like that of tissue fluid, add 1 heaped teaspoon salt to 1 quart water.

salvage procedure   Treatment of a serious condition simply to save the horse's life or make it useful in some limited capacity, such as breeding.

"sawhorse" stance   Standing with the forelegs stretched out in front, and the hindlegs out behind, like a sawhorse.

scapula   Shoulder blade.

scapular spine   Narrow ridge of bone that runs down the center of the shoulder blade.

scar tissue   *See fibrous tissue.*

schoolmaster   Experienced horse used to teach a less experienced rider.

sclerosis   Abnormal hardening of a tissue, such as an increase in bone density beneath the cortex.

secondary   As a result of another problem.

secondary ossification center   Separate area of growth cartilage, other than the physis, that matures into bone as the foal grows.

sedation   Giving a drug that makes the horse more relaxed and less responsive; tranquilization.

"seedy toe"   *See white line disease.*

selenium   Essential trace mineral; deficiency can cause muscle degeneration.

sensation   Feeling; awareness of pain, temperature, pressure, tension, etc.

sensitive laminae   Tiny corrugations in the laminar corium of the hoof wall; they are supplied with blood vessels and nerves, so they register pain.

sensory nerve   Nerve that transmits signals, such as pain, temperature, pressure, and tension, from the tissues to the brain; sensory neuron.

septic arthritis   Severe joint infection, usually caused by bacterial invasion.

septicemia   Generalized bacterial infection, causing severe, life-threatening illness.

septic tenosynovitis   Severe bacterial infection of a tendon sheath.

sequestrum   Piece of bone that has become separated from the main part of the bone, loses its blood supply and dies. Plural: sequestra.

serology   Diagnostic test for an infectious disease; involves measuring antibodies in a blood or fluid sample.

seroma   Collection of serum beneath the skin or within the tissues.

serum   Clear, yellow, liquid portion of the blood once it has clotted.

sheared heels   Inflammation and tearing of the sensitive hoof wall tissues when the heels on a foot are different in height.

sheath   1) *See tendon sheath.* 2) Fold of skin surrounding the penis.

sheet cotton   Thin sheets of cotton fiber.

shock   Circulatory collapse.

shoe puller   Farriery tool used for removing horseshoes; it looks like pincers.

shoulder joint   Shallow "ball and socket" joint between the top of the humerus and the bottom of the shoulder blade.

"sickle hocks"   Conformational defect in which the cannons in the hindlimbs angle forward slightly when seen from the side.

side clips   Narrow flanges raised on the upper, outer edge of the shoe between the toe and quarter; they help keep the shoe in position and prevent hoof wall expansion.

side extension   Piece of metal, plastic, or acrylic resin attached to the side of the shoe to correct angular limb deformities; "wing."

signs   Symptoms that can be seen, heard, or felt without special equipment.

simple fracture   Fracture that has only one fracture line.

sinuses   Air-filled cavities beneath the facial bones; they open into the nasal passages.

skyline   Radiographic view in which the x-ray beam is directed down along the outer edge of a structure.

slab fracture   Fracture in which a piece is broken off the front of the bone, like a slab of rock from a cliff face; usually restricted to the cuboidal bones.

slough   Lifting away of dead tissue.

"slow, distance work"   Preliminary fitness work, performed at low speed (trot and canter).

sodium   Essential electrolyte, necessary for the normal function of all cells, and for normal fluid balance.

soft tissue   Any tissue other than bone, teeth, hooves, and abnormal mineral deposits; e.g. skin, subcutaneous tissue, tendons, ligaments, and muscles.

solar corium   Tissue that produces the horn which forms the insensitive layer of the sole.

solar margin   Lower edge of the pedal bone, facing the sole.

sole   Horn and sensitive tissue on the underside of the foot, between the hoof wall and the frog.

sole bruise   Bruising or hematoma in the sensitive tissues of the sole; "stone bruise."

sonogram   Image produced by diagnostic ultrasound.

spinal canal   Tunnel in the vertebrae through that the spinal cord runs; vertebral canal.

spinal column   Bones that surround the spinal cord; spine, vertebral column.

spinal nerves   Nerves that leave the spinal canal to supply the tissues.

splay-footed   *See toe-out.*

splint   1) Bony swelling on the side of the cannon bone or splint bone, caused by trauma or concussion. 2) Device or action aimed at immobilizing an area with external support, such as PVC pipe or pieces of wood.

sporadic   Describes disease that is only occasionally seen, and affects only one or two horses at a time.

spores   Dormant, resilient stage of a micro-organism's lifecycle.

stance   Way the horse chooses to stand.

Staphylococcal bacteria   Bacteria commonly found on the skin; "staphs."

stay apparatus   Tendons and ligaments that support the limbs, allowing the horse to stand with little or no muscular effort.

sterile technique   Methods used to minimize the amount of bacteria that are introduced into the tissues during a procedure.

"stocking up"   Harmless fluid buildup in the lower legs, usually caused by inactivity.

stocks   Structure designed for restraining horses, consisting of a frame of boards or bars that is a little longer and wider than the average adult horse.

"stomach tube"   *See nasogastric tube.*

"stone bruise"   *See sole bruise.*

strain   Abnormally large amount of tension on a structure, which could lead to tissue damage.

strangles   Infectious respiratory disease caused by the bacteria, *Streptococcus equi.* It causes abscesses in the glands under the jaw and in the back of the throat.

Streptococcal bacteria   Bacteria commonly found on the skin; "streps."

stress   1) Abnormally large amount of force on a structure, whether tension, compression, or rotation. 2) Physical or psychological influences that affect the entire body.

"stress" fracture   Incomplete fracture that involves only the cortex on one side of the bone; generally caused by strenuous exercise.

stride length   Distance that a foot travels with each step.

stringhalt   Gait abnormality in which the horse's hocks are overflexed when it walks or trots.

Strongylus vulgaris   Scientific name for redworms, or bloodworms; large strongyles.

subchondral bone cyst   Rounded cavity within a bone near the joint surface (subchondral = below the cartilage).

subcutaneous   Beneath the skin; SC.

subluxation   Partial dislocation.

sulcus   Groove or crevice; usually refers to the grooves either side, and down the center of the frog. Plural: sulci.

superficial   On or near the surface.

superficial digital flexor tendon   Tendon that attaches to a muscle at the back of the forearm or thigh, runs down the back of the leg, then splits and attaches onto the sides of the pastern; SDFT.

superficial osteomyelitis   Bone infection on the surface of an otherwise healthy bone.

superior check ligament   Ligament that anchors the top of the superficial digital flexor tendon to the back of the radius, just above the knee.

support bandage   Bandage that supports an injured leg, or supports the opposite, weight-bearing leg if the horse is very lame.

supporting bones   Bones that support the body, or bear weight.

suspensory apparatus   Structures that support the fetlock:
  • superficial and deep digital flexor tendons (SDFT and DDFT)
  • superior and inferior check ligaments
  • suspensory ligament
  • sesamoid bones
  • distal sesamoidean ligaments

suspensory ligament   Ligament that originates at the back of the knee/

hock and cannon bone, runs down the back of the cannon, and divides into two branches that attach onto the top and outside of the sesamoid bones.

"sway back"   Conformational defect in which the back is hollowed.

"sweat"   Medication applied to the skin and covered with plastic wrap and a bandage.

sweeney   Damage to the suprascapular nerve at the front of the shoulder blade, causing atrophy of the shoulder muscles and instability of the shoulder joint.

symmetry   Evenness or balance of proportions; the left and right sides are identical in shape and size.

symptom   Sign of an abnormality or disease.

syndrome   Combination of symptoms that are consistently seen together, regardless of the cause.

synovial fluid   Fluid that fills a joint space, tendon sheath, or bursa; it nourishes, lubricates, and protects the structures within or around it.

synoviocentesis   Sampling the fluid from a joint or tendon sheath.

synovitis   Inflammation of the synovium, causing effusion.

synovium   Membrane that lines the joint capsule, tendon sheath, or bursa, and produces synovial fluid; synovial membrane.

systemic   Affecting or involving the entire system, or body.

systemic antibiotics   Antibiotics given by a route that results in distribution to the entire body; e.g. oral, intramuscular, and intravenous.

tail base   Where the tail joins the rump.

tail carriage   Height at which the horse carries its tail; may be low, normal, or high.

tail dock   Top part of the tail, which contains the coccygeal vertebrae.

talus   Large hock bone that articulates with the lower end of the tibia to form the tibiotarsal joint.

tendon   Fibrous structure that connects a muscle to a bone.

tendonitis   Inflammation and swelling of a tendon, usually with tendon fiber damage; bowed tendon.

tendon sheath   Thin sheath that surrounds and lubricates a tendon as it runs over a joint or irregular bony surface; it has a synovial lining that produces fluid.

tendon splitting   Surgical procedure in which small incisions are made into the tendon to release blood and fluid in its core, and improve blood supply to the damaged tendon.

tenosynovitis   Inflammation of the synovial lining of a tendon sheath, causing effusion.

tension   Force that pulls on a structure.

tetanus   Disease in which toxins from bacteria, *Clostridium tetani*, cause generalized muscle spasms, respiratory paralysis, and death; "lockjaw."

tetanus status   Whether the horse is currently vaccinated against tetanus.

therapeutic ultrasound   Ultrasound used to promote healing (in contrast to diagnostic ultrasound).

third carpal bone   Large, flat cuboidal bone in the center of the lower row of carpal bones; C3.

thoracic vertebrae   Vertebrae along the back; the ribs attach to these bones.

thoroughpin   Non-painful, fluidy swelling at the back of the hindleg, just above the point of the hock.

three-quarter bar shoe   *See diagonal bar shoe.*

thrush   Foul-smelling, superficial infection of the frog; when severe it can cause frog deterioration and mild lameness.

tibia   Major bone in the gaskin, between the hock and the stifle.

tibial crest   Ridge of bone along the front of the tibia, just below the stifle.

tibial spine   Narrow peak of bone on the top of the tibia, between the tibia and the femur.

tibiotarsal joint   Large, hinge-type joint between the bottom of the tibia and the talus; the major hock joint.

"tied in at the knee"   *See "over at the knee."*

tissue block   Injecting local anesthetic into an area to temporarily block sensation in those tissues.

titer   Level of antibodies in a blood or fluid sample; it is the result of serology.

toe clip   Small, raised flange on the outer, upper edge of the shoe at the toe. It helps keep the shoe from slipping back.

toe extension   Piece of metal, plastic, or acrylic resin attached to the front of the shoe. It is used to treat foals with a "club foot" and horses with a severed extensor tendon.

toe grab   Narrow metal bar that protrudes from the bottom of the shoe at the toe; used to increase traction.

toe-in   Conformational defect in which the foot is skewed so that the toe points slightly inward; pigeon-toed.

toe-out   Conformational defect in which the foot is skewed so that the toe points slightly outward; splay-footed.

topical   Applied to the skin surface.

toxemia   Accumulation of bacterial toxins in the bloodstream.

toxin   Poisons produced by living things, such as bacteria, fungi, and plants.

trace mineral   Essential mineral that is needed in only very small amounts; e.g. selenium.

tracking up   The hindfoot print lands on, or in front of the forefoot print.

traction devices   Modifications to the horse's shoes to improve traction on loose or slippery surfaces; e.g. toe grabs or heel caulks.

traction rim shoe   Shoe in which one edge of the fullering (or the outer edge of the shoe) is raised all the way around the ground surface to provide extra traction.

trailers   *See heel extension.*

tranquilizer   Drug that tranquilizes, or sedates the horse.

transducer   Ultrasound probe; the part of the machine that sends out ultrasound signals.

trauma   Physical damage, often caused by a fall, a kick, running through a fence, etc.

triceps muscles   Large, flat group of muscles on the side of the shoulder, between the back of the shoulder blade and the point of the elbow.

trimethoprim-sulfonamide   Commonly-prescribed broad-spectrum antibiotic; TMPS, SMZ.

trochlear groove   Shallow channel at the lower end of the femur; the patella slides up and down this groove at the front of the stifle.

tuber coxae   Bony point at the side of the pelvis, just behind the flank; point of the hip.

tuber ischii   Bony point at the back of the pelvis, a few inches below the tail base; point of the buttock.

tuber sacrale   Bony point at the top of the pelvis; the highest point on the rump.

"twisted bowel"   Twisting or knotting of the intestines, causing severe colic, shock, and death if it is not corrected.

"tying up"   *See exertional rhabdomyolysis.*

ultrasonography   Diagnostic technique using ultra-high frequency sound waves to image soft tissues and bone surfaces; often just called ultrasound.

under-run heels   Abnormal foot shape in which the heels are lower than normal and are at a lower angle than the front of the hoof wall.

unpigmented skin   Pink skin, with few or no pigment cells.

upper motor neuron   Motor nerve within the brain or spinal cord. It connects with other upper motor neurons, and with lower motor and sensory neurons.

urinary fractional excretion   Measurement of electrolytes or minerals excreted in the urine; fractional excretion, FE.

vaccination   Using a vaccine to provide immunity against an infectious disease by stimulating the body to produce specific antibodies.

vaccine   Purified preparation containing a specific micro-organism (or cell fragment) or the toxin it produces.

valgus   Angular limb deformity in which the limb below the affected joint deviates to the outside; e.g. carpal valgus causes "knock knees."

varus   Angular limb deformity in which the limb below the affected joint deviates to the inside; e.g. carpal varus causes "bow legs."

vasculitis   Inflammation of blood vessel walls, allowing leakage of plasma or blood into the tissues.

vasoconstriction   Constriction, or narrowing of a blood vessel.

vasodilation   Dilation, or widening of a blood vessel.

vasodilator   Drug or other substance that causes vasodilation.

veins   Blood vessels that carry de-oxygenated blood from the tissues back to the heart and lungs.

ventral   Directional term meaning the underside; away from the top.

ventro-dorsal   Radiographic view in which the x-ray beam is directed upward from underneath.

vertebra   Bone of the spine, or vertebral column. Plural: vertebrae.

vertebral body   Solid portion of the vertebra; the top of the vertebral body forms the floor of the spinal canal.

vertical load   Downward force, such as weight-bearing.

virus   Micro-organism that is little more than DNA; it must invade cells to survive and multiply.

virus isolation   Diagnostic test to identify a virus in a blood, fluid, or tissue sample.

viscosity; viscous   Slippery quality, like clean motor oil.

vitamin D   Vitamin that is involved in calcium and phosphorus balance.

web   Width of the shoe branch.

wedge pad   Wedge-shaped plastic or rubber pad, fitted between the shoe and the hoof to raise the heels a few degrees.

weight-bearing forces   Load on the limbs from the horse's body weight; it increases with the horse's speed, and with a rider.

white blood cell count   Concentration of white blood cells in a blood or fluid sample.

white blood cells   Immune system cells that respond to tissue damage and infection.

white line   Pale inner layer of the hoof wall, visible at the ground surface of the hoof, between the main part of the wall and the sole.

white line disease   Crevice between the hoof wall and sole that begins at ground surface and may spread up or around the hoof wall; "seedy toe."

"wind puffs," "wind galls"   Small fluid-filled swellings around the fetlocks; may be effusion in the fetlock joint or the flexor tendon sheath.

wing   1) *See side extension.* 2) Side of the pedal bone.

wing fracture   Fracture in the wing of the pedal bone.

wing of the ilium   Part of the pelvis that curves up from the point of the hip to the tuber sacrale.

withdrawal time   Length of time a drug should be withheld before competition; it is based on the clearance time.

"wobbler" syndrome   *See Cervical Vertebral Malformation.*

wound breakdown   Loosening, tearing, or breaking of the sutures, allowing a sutured wound to gape open.

"wry back"   Conformational defect in which the spine is bend to the side.

xeroradiography   Special radiographic procedure that gives excellent bone detail.

"x-rays"   *See radiography.*

Index

Symbols

A

C